AIDS

SEXUAL BEHAVIOR AND INTRAVENOUS DRUG USE

Charles F. Turner, Heather G. Miller, and
Lincoln E. Moses, *Editors*

Committee on AIDS Research and the
Behavioral, Social, and Statistical Sciences

Commission on Behavioral and Social Sciences
and Education

National Research Council

NATIONAL ACADEMY PRESS
Washington, D.C. 1989

National Academy Press • 2101 Constitution Avenue, N.W. • Washington, D. C. 20418

NOTICE: The project that is the subject of this report was approved by the Governing Board of the National Research Council, whose members are drawn from the councils of the National Academy of Sciences, the National Academy of Engineering, and the Institute of Medicine. The members of the committee responsible for the report were chosen for their special competences and with regard for appropriate balance.

This report has been reviewed by a group other than the authors according to procedures approved by a Report Review Committee consisting of members of the National Academy of Sciences, the National Academy of Engineering, and the Institute of Medicine.

The National Academy of Sciences is a private, nonprofit, self-perpetuating society of distinguished scholars engaged in scientific and engineering research, dedicated to the furtherance of science and technology and to their use for the general welfare. Upon the authority of the charter granted to it by the Congress in 1863, the Academy has a mandate that requires it to advise the federal government on scientific and technical matters. Dr. Frank Press is president of the National Academy of Sciences.

The National Academy of Engineering was established in 1964, under the charter of the National Academy of Sciences, as a parallel organization of outstanding engineers. It is autonomous in its administration and in the selection of its members, sharing with the National Academy of Sciences the responsibility for advising the federal government. The National Academy of Engineering also sponsors engineering programs aimed at meeting national needs, encourages education and research, and recognizes the superior achievements of engineers. Dr. Robert M. White is president of the National Academy of Engineering.

The Institute of Medicine was established in 1970 by the National Academy of Sciences to secure the services of eminent members of appropriate professions in the examination of policy matters pertaining to the health of the public. The Institute acts under the responsibility given to the National Academy of Sciences by its congressional charter to be an adviser to the federal government and upon its own initiative, to identify issues of medical care, research, and education. Dr. Samuel O. Thier is president of the Institute of Medicine.

The National Research Council was established by the National Academy of Sciences in 1916 to associate the broad community of science and technology with the Academy's purposes of furthering knowledge and of advising the federal government. Functioning in accordance with general policies determined by the Academy, the Council has become the principal operating agency of both the National Academy of Sciences and the National Academy of Engineering in providing services to the government, the public, and the scientific and engineering communities. The Council is administered jointly by both Academies and the Institute of Medicine. Dr. Frank Press and Dr. Robert M. White are chairman and vice-chairman, respectively, of the National Research Council.

The work that provided the basis for this volume was supported by grants from the Rockefeller Foundation, the Russell Sage Foundation and by a contract with the U.S. Public Health Service.

Library of Congress Catalog Card Number 88-43331

ISBN 0-309-03948-7 (paperbound); 0-309-03976-2 (hardbound)

Printed in the United States of America

Committee on AIDS Research and the Behavioral, Social, and Statistical Sciences

LEWELLYS F. BARKER *(NRC Fellow)*, National Research Council and American Red Cross, Washington, D.C.

MARSHALL H. BECKER, School of Public Health, University of Michigan

ROBERT BORUCH, Departments of Psychology and Statistics, Northwestern University

TRACY L. BRANDT *(Administrative Secretary)*, National Research Council

LESTER BRESLOW, Division of Cancer Control, School of Public Health, University of California at Los Angeles

J. BROOKS-GUNN, Education Policy and Research Division, Educational Testing Service, Princeton, New Jersey

THOMAS J. COATES, Division of General Internal Medicine, Center for AIDS Prevention Services, University of California at San Francisco

ROBYN M. DAWES, Department of Social and Decision Sciences, Carnegie Mellon University

DON C. DES JARLAIS, New York State Division of Substance Abuse Services, New York City, and Rockefeller University

JOHN H. GAGNON, Department of Sociology, State University of New York at Stonybrook

ALBERT R. JONSEN, Department of Medical History and Ethics, University of Washington at Seattle

SHIRLEY LINDENBAUM, Department of Anthropology, Graduate Faculty, New School for Social Research

GARDNER LINDZEY, Center for Advanced Study in the Behavioral Sciences, Stanford, California

ROBERT M. MAY, Department of Zoology, University of Oxford

JANE MENKEN, Department of Sociology, University of Pennsylvania

HEATHER G. MILLER *(Senior Research Associate)*, National Research Council

LINCOLN E. MOSES *(Chair)*, Department of Statistics, Stanford University

CHARLES F. TURNER *(Study Director)*, National Research Council

BAILUS WALKER, School of Public Health, State University of New York at Albany

LAURIE SCHWAB ZABIN, Department of Population Dynamics, Johns Hopkins University School of Hygiene and Public Health

Panel on Statistical Issues in AIDS Research

JOAN L. ARON, Department of Population Dynamics, Johns Hopkins University School of Hygiene and Public Health

LYNNE BILLARD, Department of Statistics, University of Georgia

RON S. BROOKMEYER, Department of Biostatistics, Johns Hopkins University School of Hygiene and Public Health

JANE MENKEN *(Chair)*, Department of Sociology, University of Pennsylvania

LINCOLN E. MOSES, Department of Statistics, Stanford University

BRUCE D. SPENCER, Department of Statistics, Northwestern University

MICHAEL A. STOTO, Division of Health Promotion and Disease Prevention, Institute of Medicine

CHARLES F. TURNER *(Study Director)*, National Research Council

Panel on AIDS and IV Drug Use

LEWELLYS F. BARKER *(NRC Fellow)*, National Research Council and American Red Cross, Washington, D.C.
LAWRENCE S. BROWN, JR. Addiction Research and Treatment Corporation, and Department of Medicine, Harlem Hospital, New York City
DON C. DES JARLAIS *(Chair)*, New York State Division of Substance Abuse Services, New York City, and Rockefeller University
SAMUEL R. FRIEDMAN, Narcotics and Drug Research, Inc., New York City
ROBERT L. HUBBARD, Center for Social Research and Policy Analysis, Research Triangle Park, North Carolina
SHIRLEY LINDENBAUM, Department of Anthropology, Graduate Faculty, New School for Social Research
HEATHER G. MILLER *(Senior Research Associate)*, National Research Council
JOHN A. NEWMEYER, Haight-Ashbury Free Medical Clinic, San Francisco

Liaison Representatives, U.S. Public Health Service

WENDY BALDWIN, National Institute of Child Health and Human Development
WILLIAM W. DARROW, Centers for Disease Control
LLOYD KOLBE *(Chair)*, Centers for Disease Control
KEVIN O'REILLY, Centers for Disease Control
MARK ROSENBERG, Centers for Disease Control
STANLEY F. SCHNEIDER, National Institute of Mental Health
ERNESTINE VANDERVEEN, National Institute on Drug Abuse
RONALD W. WILSON, National Center for Health Statistics, Centers for Disease Control

Consultants

MARION EATON, Program in Mathematical Methods in Educational Research, Stanford University
ROBERT E. FAY, National Research Council
SUSHAMA GUNJAL, National Research Council
SAHR JOHN KPUNDEH, Department of Political Science, Howard University
BARBARA BRYAN LOGAN, College of Nursing, University of Illinois at Chicago
DEBORAH MALOFF, Hinsdale, Illinois
JOHN L. MARTIN, School of Public Health, Columbia University
LEAH MAZADE, National Academy Press
LAURA RUDKIN-MINIOT, Department of Sociology, Princeton University
STEPHEN SAUNDERS, Department of Psychology, Northwestern University
JEFF STRYKER, School of Public Health, University of Michigan

Preface

Statistics on the spread of the human immunodeficiency virus (HIV) and, consequently, of acquired immune deficiency syndrome (AIDS) tell a grim tale. As of November 14, 1988, 78,312 cases of AIDS had been reported in the United States, and 44,071 people had died as a result of the disease. Moreover, there is no end in sight: projections of the number of AIDS cases and deaths show large increases in the years to come, and it is estimated that as many as 54,000 Americans may die from AIDS during 1991 alone.

Yet HIV infection/AIDS is more than a biomedical phenomenon. It is also a social phenomenon—an epidemic rooted firmly, some fear intractably, in human behavior. The vital need for data to help in designing, implementing, and evaluating programs to curb the epidemic's spread transcends numerical tallies of people infected and lives lost. Understanding the human behaviors that transmit HIV infection (and thereby AIDS), as well as the social contexts in which those behaviors occur, calls for action by the disciplines that constitute the behavioral, social, and statistical sciences.

The creation of this committee highlights the central importance of behavior in the HIV/AIDS epidemic. Because HIV/AIDS is a sexually transmitted disease, it must be opposed with behavioral weapons—education, counseling, and persuasion, among others—a fact that will not change even when effective therapies or vaccines are discovered. In this respect, the HIV/AIDS epidemic is similar to outbreaks of other, nonfatal sexually transmitted diseases. For example, gonorrhea and syphilis persist in the United States, despite the availability for the past 40 years of drugs that are effective against them. The challenges facing us are great, especially given the severity of the AIDS epidemic.

In its charge, the Committee on AIDS Research and the Behavioral, Social, and Statistical Sciences was asked to

- describe what is known about the spread of HIV and AIDS in the United States, with special attention to the quality of the information at hand and to the kind of additional information that is needed;
- identify critical populations and indicate objectives and tasks related to them;
- describe existing research findings in the behavioral and social sciences that should be useful in planning and choosing among interventions designed to control the spread of HIV infection;
- describe existing research on (a) interventions intended to facilitate behavior changes and (b) ways to evaluate their effectiveness; and
- identify new research that should be undertaken to design, implement, and evaluate better interventions in the future to control the spread of HIV.

This three-part report is the committee's answer to that charge. Because it is important to know the prevalence and incidence of HIV infection in planning strategies to control its spread, the first part, "Understanding the Spread of HIV Infection," begins with a review of the extent of HIV infection within the U.S. population today. The two subsequent chapters discuss the sexual and IV drug-use behaviors that contribute to transmission of the virus and thus alter the prevalence and incidence of HIV in the United States. The second part of the report, "Intervening to Limit the Spread of HIV Infection," details principles of behavioral change that might prove useful in designing and implementing intervention strategies to slow disease transmission. A separate chapter discusses methods for measuring the effectiveness of such interventions. The third part, "Impediments to Research and Intervention," reviews the barriers that may compromise the nation's ability to control the spread of the disease. One chapter considers barriers to research efforts; another chapter discusses obstacles that threaten to hinder effective AIDS prevention.

As biomedical scientists continue to search for effective therapies and vaccines to combat HIV/AIDS, behavioral, social, and statistical scientists must invest their energies in understanding and affecting the behaviors that transmit the virus. It is well to remember that, as we write, HIV continues to spread. As part of the nation's response to this complex disease and its devastating consequences for individuals and for society as a whole, we confront the urgent task of turning ignorance into understanding and understanding into action.

—Charles Turner, Heather Miller, and Lincoln Moses
Editors

Acknowledgments

During the course of this study, our committee has been assisted by many scientists who took time to share their insights and expertise. Without this generous assistance, the committee would not have been able to complete its task.

The birth of this study benefited from the support and goodwill of many people. At critical moments in the study's gestation, Samuel Thier of the Institute of Medicine and our former colleagues David Goslin and Roy Widdus interceded to ensure that the project was not stillborn. Kenneth Prewitt of the Rockefeller Foundation and Eric Wanner and Peter de Janosi of the Russell Sage Foundation generously and quickly provided funds for the committee's start-up costs. The Public Health Service provided subsequent financial support for the undertaking, and their liaison representatives made important contributions to the committee's work. To all those who have assisted us in our work, the committee extends its sincere thanks and appreciation.

Note on Authorship

The list below identifies the persons who shared the responsibility for preparing the first draft of each chapter in this volume. The committee reviewed all contributions, and they have been revised and edited in light of committee reactions and the comments of outside reviewers. The purpose of the following alphabetical list, therefore, is to give credit to individuals but not to assign final responsibility for the published text. It should also be noted that, although the list covers major sections of this volume, these sections frequently contain additional paragraphs or pages from other hands.

SUMMARY: This is the collective product of the deliberations of the entire committee, and it presents our recommendations.

CHAPTER 1: Aron, Billard, Brookmeyer, Menken, Moses, Spencer, Stoto, Turner

CHAPTER 2: Gagnon, Lindenbaum, Martin, May, Menken, Turner, Zabin

CHAPTER 3: Barker, Brown, Des Jarlais, Friedman, Hubbard, Lindenbaum, Miller, Newmeyer, Stryker

CHAPTER 4: Becker, Brooks-Gunn, Coates, Dawes, Lindenbaum, Miller, Zabin

CHAPTER 5: Boruch, Dawes, Miller, Moses

CHAPTER 6: Miller, Turner

CHAPTER 7: Coates, Dawes, Jonsen, Miller, Turner, Walker, Zabin

Primary responsibility for the revision and editing of this volume was shared by Charles Turner, Heather Miller, and Lincoln Moses.

Contents

APPENDIXES

BACKGROUND PAPERS

AIDS

SEXUAL BEHAVIOR AND INTRAVENOUS DRUG USE

Summary

The human immunodeficiency virus (HIV), now known to be the cause of acquired immune deficiency syndrome, or AIDS, is only one element of the complex problem that is commonly called the AIDS epidemic. The spread of HIV infection and, consequently, AIDS is the product of human behaviors enacted in social contexts. Both the behaviors and the circumstances in which they occur are conditioned and shaped by culture and larger social structures. The epidemic is thus as much a social and behavioral phenomenon as it is a biological one.

Understanding how HIV infection is spread, encouraging behavioral change so as to retard this spread, and coping with the social consequences of the epidemic raise questions that lie within the domain of the social, behavioral, and statistical sciences. Following publication of the 1986 report on AIDS of the Institute of Medicine/National Academy of Sciences,[1] the present committee was established in the fall of 1987 to provide a focus for AIDS activities within these disciplines at the National Research Council. At the request of the Public Health Service (PHS) and with additional support from the Rockefeller and Russell Sage Foundations, the committee

[1]This committee's review of the behavioral, social, and statistical issues related to HIV/AIDS builds on the work of the Institute of Medicine/National Academy of Sciences, which has produced two reports that focused on public health, biological research, and medical care issues: *Confronting AIDS: Directions for Public Health, Health Care, and Research* (1986) and *Confronting AIDS: Update 1988* (both published by the National Academy Press, Washington, D.C.).

The committee also wishes to acknowledge the related activities being carried out or planned by the Academy complex. Some of the efforts under consideration—including the future activities of our own committee and of the Institute of Medicine—address topics that will be of concern to readers of this report, including drug and vaccine development, AIDS research policy, and the social impact of the AIDS epidemic.

has begun its work by reviewing the contributions that can be made by the paradigms, data, and methods of the social, behavioral, and statistical sciences[2] in mounting an effective national response to the HIV/AIDS epidemic.[3]

The committee's report is divided into three parts. The first part presents evidence on the current extent of HIV infection in the U.S. population (Chapter 1) and on the patterns of sexual behavior and drug use (Chapters 2 and 3) that spread HIV infection. The second part describes intervention strategies and principles that hold promise for producing behavioral change to slow the spread of HIV infection (Chapter 4) and methods for evaluating the effectiveness of such interventions (Chapter 5). The third part (Chapters 6 and 7) discusses some of the barriers that impede effective research and intervention programs. The organization of this summary follows that of the report, and it includes some of the report's key recommendations. (All of the committee's recommendations are listed in Appendix A.)

At the outset of its report, the committee believes it is important to comment on the term *epidemic*, which is sometimes misunderstood in connection with HIV/AIDS. During an epidemic, the occurrence[4] of *new cases* of a disease in a community follows a well-known pattern: it may increase dramatically in a short period of time, peak, and then decline. During the course of an epidemic, there may be cycles of rise and decline in the number of new cases.

In 1989 the United States stands at the base of a rapidly rising curve of AIDS cases and deaths. Barring a dramatic breakthrough in treatment, it is projected that more than 50,000 Americans will die of AIDS during 1991. The number of deaths during this 12-month

---

[2]Including anthropology, economics, political science, psychology, sociology, and statistics, and their subdisciplines (e.g., demography, social psychology, biostatistics, etc.).

[3]Specifically, the committee was charged to (1) describe what is known about the spread of HIV infection and AIDS in the United States; (2) identify critical groups at risk of infection and how to reach them; (3) describe research findings from the social and behavioral sciences that should be helpful in planning and choosing among ways to intervene successfully to control the spread of HIV infection; (4) describe ways to evaluate the effectiveness of such interventions; and (5) recommend new research that can expand our understanding of the spread of HIV infection and improve the nation's ability to control this spread in the future.

[4]Two technical terms are frequently used in discussions of epidemic diseases: incidence and prevalence. *Incidence* denotes the rate of occurrence of new infections per unit of time (e.g., per year). Thus, an incidence of .03 per year in some group means that new infections occurred in 3 percent of the group during the year in question. *Prevalence* denotes that proportion of a group that is currently infected. A prevalence of .10 means that 10 percent of the group is currently infected.

period alone will exceed the total number of deaths in this country from the beginning of the epidemic through 1988.

Such rapid growth in the occurrence of a disease is the defining characteristic of an epidemic, but it is important to recognize two further points about the HIV/AIDS epidemic.

First, the occurrence of AIDS cases lags behind the spread of HIV infection. Several years typically elapse between the time an adult is infected with HIV and the appearance of clinical signs sufficient to warrant the diagnosis of AIDS. The contemporary spread of HIV cannot therefore be discerned from the current counts of new AIDS cases. So, for example, in the absence of therapies that retard the progression from HIV to AIDS, the epidemic of AIDS cases will continue to rise for several years after the spread of HIV infection begins to decline in a population. Similarly, a sharp decline in the occurrence of new AIDS cases in a given year would not preclude the possibility that the occurrence of new HIV infections had increased during that same year. Unfortunately, the barriers that impede tracking of the spread of HIV infection exceed those that impede tracking of the spread of AIDS cases. Hence, currently available information about the spread of HIV infection is considerably less reliable than information about the occurrence of AIDS cases.

Second, the committee would emphasize that a decline in either the spread of HIV infection or the occurrence of new AIDS cases (or both) would not signal that the danger has passed. HIV is already substantially seeded in the U.S. population—the number of people who are now infected may surpass 1 million—and the virus is likely to continue to spread, if not in epidemic form, then in a persistent, more stable "endemic" form (literally, "dwelling with the people"). The threat of epidemic and endemic disease will be most serious for those groups that are most heavily seeded with HIV infection, including IV drug users and men who have sex with men, as well as for their sexual partners and offspring. Currently available data also indicate that the black and Hispanic populations of the United States are experiencing a disproportionate burden of AIDS cases (in particular, cases associated with IV drug-use, heterosexual, and mother–infant transmission). The AIDS case data suggest that these populations may be more heavily seeded with HIV infection than are other ethnic groups and may be disproportionately threatened with further spread of the virus.

Our committee is concerned with understanding and reducing the spread of HIV infection, whether this spread be epidemic or endemic in character.

MONITORING THE SPREAD OF HIV AND AIDS

The overall dimensions of the current HIV/AIDS epidemic in the United States (or anywhere) are hard to determine because the most observable component—people who have AIDS—is only a small part of the total epidemic. The largest component by far is composed of all those who have been infected by HIV, but the magnitude of this component is difficult to estimate because most infected persons are asymptomatic for several years after their infection.

A key first step in controlling the spread of HIV infection and AIDS is the collection of reliable data on the prevalence and incidence of HIV infection and AIDS in the population. A further step requires an understanding of the sexual and IV drug-use behaviors that spread HIV from one person to another and thereby produce changes in HIV prevalence and incidence. The committee believes that more reliable systems must be developed for tracking the course of the epidemic. It also wishes to emphasize—in the strongest possible terms—that the development of such systems is a prerequisite for mounting a fully effective and efficient national response to AIDS.

Statistics on AIDS

Weekly data from the Centers for Disease Control (CDC) report past and current cases of AIDS. As of November 14, 1988, 78,312 cases of AIDS had been reported to CDC, and 44,071 people had died as a result. Such statistics are important, and the panel recommends that the system for collecting them be maintained and strengthened. Yet the committee concludes that a fully adequate system for monitoring the course of the epidemic must go beyond the current system for reporting AIDS cases and deaths: it must also provide reliable monitoring of the prevalence and incidence of HIV infection in the U.S. population. Developing accurate statistical systems to monitor HIV infection is critical for several reasons.

- Counts of AIDS cases are out-of-date indicators of the present state of the epidemic because there is a long, asymptomatic latency period between HIV infection and the development of AIDS. For example, most adults who will be counted as new AIDS cases in 1989 were probably infected with HIV prior to 1986.
- The lives of a substantial proportion of persons infected with HIV will be substantially shortened as a result

of that infection. However, these people do not always manifest sufficient symptoms to be captured by the AIDS reporting system.

- All HIV-infected individuals have the potential to transmit the infection and thereby spread the epidemic.

Statistics on HIV Infection

At present, there are no reliable data on the current prevalence of HIV in the United States, although rough estimates have been constructed using two quite different methods. One method aggregates estimates of the size of each major risk group (e.g., the number of persons who regularly inject IV drugs) multiplied by estimates of the HIV prevalence rate for that group. The second method exploits the necessary mathematical links among three time series: (1) the cumulative cases of AIDS to a given time; (2) the cumulative number of cases of HIV infection to that time; and (3) the distribution of the lengths of time that may elapse between infection with HIV and the appearance of AIDS (the latency, or incubation, period).

These two methods agree that the most plausible estimates of prevalence lie in the vicinity of 1 million infected persons (with a range of 0.5–2 million). Admittedly, both of these estimation methods are vulnerable to many sources of uncertainty. These uncertainties are of very different kinds, however. The first method is subject to uncertainties about, for example, the number of persons who regularly use IV drugs. The second method is subject to uncertainties about the probabilities that an HIV-infected person will develop AIDS (i.e., 1, 2, 3, $\cdots n$ years after infection). Confidence in the rough estimate produced by the two methods is strengthened by the fact that the uncertainties affecting each method are quite different. The committee concludes, nonetheless, that more reliable data on HIV prevalence are needed.

In recommending that reliable systems be developed for tracking the course of the HIV/AIDS epidemic, the committee wishes to reiterate its firm belief that such systems are prerequisites for mounting an effective and efficient national response to AIDS. Without better information on the incidence of new HIV infections in the population, the United States will lack adequate means for determining whether current strategies for controlling the spread of the virus are working. Without better information on the prevalence of HIV infection, the nation will be unable to prepare adequately for future demands for hospital beds and other health care services. Without better data, scientists and the American public can anticipate endless debates about whether the disease is spreading "rapidly" or "slowly." To the extent that opposing sides in these debates produce "evidence" from convenience samples,[5] inconsistency in conclusions is to be expected, and there is no basis for an informative scientific debate. Reliable assessment of the prevalence of HIV infection in a population requires drawing a sample from that population, obtaining a blood specimen from each person in the sample, and accurately testing the specimens for the presence of HIV.

The validity and hence the usefulness of such HIV prevalence data depend critically on how the sample is chosen from the population. Fifty years of theory and practice have provided a valuable statistical tool for this purpose: probability sampling. Drawing probability samples of U.S. households is a well-developed art; drawing probability samples of populations of special interest (for example, clients of sexually transmitted disease clinics and drug treatment centers) is also within the reach of current statistical technology.[6] The use of such methods will allow the monitoring of prevalence over time and the estimation of the incidence of infection, not only for the national population but for specific geographic areas and for groups defined by demographic characteristics and behavior.

CDC's Family of HIV Seroprevalence Surveys

CDC has launched a program to survey HIV prevalence among several population groups, including clients of drug treatment centers, clinics for sexually transmitted diseases (STDs), tuberculosis clinics, and clinics serving women of reproductive age; patients at general hospitals; and newborn infants. With the exception of the newborn survey, the clinics, centers, and hospitals that will furnish data in this survey program have been purposively selected to facilitate public health management of the epidemic, and many survey sites have been chosen because they serve populations that are presumed to be especially vulnerable to infection. Such purposive selection, however, compromises the usefulness of the data for estimating prevalence and

---

[5]In a "convenience" sample, respondents are selected in a manner that precludes generalization of the statistical findings (e.g., prevalence of infection) with known margins of sampling error to any population beyond the particular individuals included in that sample.

[6]As discussed in the following section, "National Seroprevalence Survey," the execution of such surveys requires that survey designers grapple with the potential problem of sample bias owing to selective nonresponse in the survey.

incidence in any well-defined population of interest. With the exception of the survey of newborns, the committee finds that none of these surveys (as currently designed) will provide estimates of HIV prevalence that can be generalized with known margins of error to the population groups of interest (e.g., all clients of STD clinics or patients at general hospitals).[7] It is likely, however, that some or all of these surveys can be augmented so as to become probability samples. In such augmented surveys, the present sample elements (the clinics or hospitals included in the present surveys) would constitute one stratum in a stratified probability sample of the populations of general hospitals, STD clinics, and so on.

The committee recommends that efforts be made to reformulate the CDC family of seroprevalence surveys as probability samples. The committee recognizes that these surveys may serve other purposes, and it acknowledges the difficulties and effort involved in such a reformulation and the operational constraints that undeniably weigh heavily on CDC. Nevertheless, the committee believes that wider, if not total, use of probability samples is feasible. Greater involvement of the National Center for Health Statistics (which has recently been made a part of CDC) in the design and execution of these surveys may be helpful in achieving this objective.

One component of the family of seroprevalence surveys tests blood specimens from newborn babies, and the committee considers this effort to be a very promising enterprise. Because data are obtained from *all* newborns, the survey is free of many kinds of bias. In addition, this survey provides a basis for monitoring the seroprevalence of childbearing women, a substantial and important component of the sexually active adult population.[8] **The committee recommends that the newborn infant seroprevalence survey be extended to include all children born in the United States.**

Supplementing the newborn survey with surveys of probability samples of women who have abortions would provide a more complete picture of HIV prevalence among sexually active women of reproductive age. **The committee recommends instituting a continuing anonymous probability survey of the HIV serostatus of**

[7] Chapter 1 of the main report discusses problems that affect the use of data from special populations (e.g., military recruits, blood donors, etc.) to infer HIV prevalence or changes in prevalence in the population at large.

[8] Newborns of HIV-seropositive women carry the maternal antibody to HIV, even though the infants themselves may not be infected. After some time, the maternal antibodies disappear from the infant's blood if the baby is not infected. The Institute of Medicine/National Academy of Sciences 1988 report estimated that there is a 30–50 percent risk of perinatal HIV transmission from an infected mother to her child (p. 35).

women who are clients of clinics that provide abortion services. This survey will be most valuable if the universe surveyed includes *all* women who have abortions.

National Seroprevalence Survey

A seroprevalence survey based on a national probability sample of households is currently undergoing feasibility testing at CDC's National Center for Health Statistics. The idea of such a survey has much appeal, but there are formidable barriers that will have to be overcome before implementation could proceed. A pilot test in Washington, D.C., was recently canceled after protests from the community and the city health department. This experience suggests the extreme sensitivity of all such data collection programs; it also underscores the need to fully inform and involve local communities, public health departments, and all groups that might be at risk if the confidentiality of the data collections were to be compromised.

The greatest technical barrier to obtaining an accurate estimate of HIV prevalence is the possibility of bias from selective nonresponse. This kind of bias can plausibly occur if, for example, individuals who belong to groups with elevated HIV prevalence rates (e.g., gay men, IV drug users) are more likely than people in other segments of the population to refuse to supply a blood specimen.

Although the obstacles to conducting a national seroprevalence survey are substantial, they are not necessarily impossible to overcome, and success, if obtained, would be rewarding indeed. Thus, the committee commends the exploratory spirit in which CDC has begun the development of this survey, and it applauds the strategy of using pilot experiments to test the survey's capacity to provide useful direct estimates of prevalence—and, ultimately, of trends in prevalence. The outcome of these experiments should play a decisive role in the final decision of whether to go forward with the national survey.

Assuring Confidentiality

Much of the information needed to understand and cope with the spread of HIV infection is obtainable only with the consent of a person who may be harmed if confidentiality is breached. Thus, guaranteeing confidentiality helps protect individual respondents, and it also serves society's interest in obtaining statistical information to help combat the disease.

To maintain confidentiality, safeguards to prevent both deliberate disclosure and inadvertent "deductive" disclosure must be put into place. Deductive disclosure can be precluded by coarsely grouping, modifying, or withholding part of the information before releasing or publishing the data. The committee believes that policies for sharing statistical data on HIV and AIDS must provide absolute protection of confidentiality and should seek to provide this protection at the least practical cost in information.

Three additional strategies can help in this regard. First, confidentiality can be buttressed with legal penalties in the event of a breach. Second, legal protection against discrimination based on HIV status can be established. Third, anonymous testing can be conducted so that the identity of the donor is neither known nor traceable to the blood specimen.[9] The committee believes that each of these strategies should be vigorously pursued.

Sexual Behavior and AIDS

The need to control the spread of HIV infection has forced a recognition of the underdeveloped state of sex research in the United States. Information about sexual conduct is necessary to understand both the epidemiology of the spread of the disease and the social processes that are involved in behavioral change. Yet current understanding is fragmentary, and the underlying research data are often unreliable.

Alfred Kinsey and his colleagues pioneered the use of social science techniques to document the sexual behavior of Americans in the 1940s. The defects of this work are widely known: for example, respondents were disproportionately drawn from the Midwest and from college campuses, and the research did not use probability sampling. Still, there can be no denying the crucial historical importance of that work in ushering in a new era in which social science has played a larger role in understanding human sexuality.

Since the original Kinsey studies were published in 1948 and 1953, there has been an uneven effort in sex research, in terms of volume and quality, and especially in research relevant to the behaviors that are known to spread HIV. The paucity of solid research contributes to the dilemma now faced by scientists and policy makers

[9]Blind testing has been widely employed in studies using blood specimens that have been collected for *other* purposes. It is, however, feasible to use analogous methods in studies that collect blood specimens for the *specific purpose* of testing for HIV. In this case, all identifying information would have to be destroyed prior to the HIV test to ensure anonymity.

who are trying to develop intervention strategies to retard the spread of the virus. Studies are especially lacking on at least five topics:

1. sexuality outside of marriage;
2. sexuality with persons of the same gender;
3. sexuality with persons of both genders;
4. sexual contacts for pay; and
5. variations in sexual techniques among the various types of sexual partnerings.

In the past, federal agencies have supported some behavioral research on sexual practices, but much of it has been focused on the sexual behavior of female adolescents, with the goal of preventing teenage pregnancies. The committee believes such research is a valuable and necessary part of the federal research portfolio, but basic knowledge of human sexual behavior is needed in many other areas as well. **The committee recommends that the Public Health Service support vigorous programs of basic social and behavioral research on human sexual behavior, particularly through such agencies as the National Institutes of Health; the Alcohol, Drug Abuse, and Mental Health Administration; and the Centers for Disease Control.**

Same-Gender Sex Among Men

Because the initial spread of the HIV epidemic was first identified among men who have sex with other men, there has been an upsurge of interest in the number of such men, their sexual practices, and the organization of their social life. The relationship of persons with same-gender sexual orientation to the larger U.S. society has been undergoing substantial change during this century, and that change in itself has affected the sexual and social lives of these men.

Estimates of the number of men who engage in same-gender sexual behavior figure prominently in the attempts (mentioned earlier) to calculate HIV prevalence. The estimates used in those attempts were derived from Kinsey's studies on male sexual behavior in the period 1938–1948. In addition to the defects in that work that were noted above, the committee finds that the Kinsey studies are not an adequate base on which to formulate estimates of the number of persons in the contemporary population who have sexual relations with persons of the same gender.

New data, however, are available from two national surveys conducted in 1970 and 1988. These studies have their own methodological difficulties, but data from both of them suggest that a minimum of 2–3 percent of American men have sex with other men with some frequency during adulthood. Data from the 1970 survey also suggest that a minimum of 20 percent of adult American males had at least one sexual experience to orgasm with another male during their lives, and 7 percent of men have such an experience in adulthood (age 20 or older).

The long history of social intolerance toward same-gender sexuality introduces considerable uncertainty about the accuracy of these estimates, which are derived from self-reports obtained in two national surveys. The committee believes that the foregoing estimates are best treated as setting "lower bounds" on the actual number of men who have such experiences. This conclusion follows from the assumption that the number of men in a survey who will conceal the homosexual experiences they have had is greater than the number of men who will report homosexual experiences that never actually occurred.

Although our understanding of AIDS in the male homosexual population is far from complete, longitudinal studies initiated during the early years of the epidemic have provided a rich and expanding data base on patterns of HIV transmission and sexual behavior. Early studies among gay men, including the Multicenter AIDS Cohort Studies (MACS), established AIDS as a sexually transmitted disease and identified important risk factors for its spread, including multiple sexual partners and unprotected anal intercourse.

In addition to the longitudinal studies that have delineated the risk factors and natural history of AIDS, other studies have been following cohorts of gay men to compile detailed behavioral data over time. These studies offer some indication that behavioral changes to reduce the risk of HIV infection have been occurring in many groups of gay men. Significant decreases in the prevalence of unprotected anal intercourse have been reported in studies undertaken in such urban areas as San Francisco, New York City, Chicago, and Boston. In addition, significant declines in numbers of sexual partners have been reported in numerous studies of gay male sexual behavior as it relates to AIDS. Unfortunately, changes in risk-associated behavior have not been universal: high rates of unprotected anal intercourse have been reported in areas that are not foci of the epidemic (e.g., upstate New York and New Mexico).

Identifying the factors responsible for behavioral change among gay men is methodologically and conceptually complex. The factors responsible for initial reductions in risk-associated behavior may not be the same factors that are involved in maintaining those behaviors.

Studies have suggested that initial behavioral change is facilitated by knowledge about AIDS and HIV transmission, a supportive social environment, and personal experience with someone who has developed AIDS.

The data gathered during the early days of the epidemic indicate that gay men are making changes in specific sexual practices instead of adopting monogamy or eliminating sexual contact altogether. Geographic variation in infection rates and in the acceptance of safer sex behaviors, however, point to the need for continued behavioral studies in diverse regions of the country.

Teenage and Adult Heterosexuals

Understanding the sexual conduct of young people is also important for an understanding of HIV transmission. Evidence from national studies of contraception and teenage pregnancy suggests that young people are not particularly skilled in managing their sexual lives. Other evidence from those studies indicates two additional patterns: (1) a steadily increasing proportion of young people begin heterosexual intercourse in their mid-teens and (2) an increasing proportion begins intercourse very early in their teenage years. In addition, there is evidence that this earlier onset of heterosexual intercourse has been accompanied by an increase in the number of heterosexual partners people have before marriage. (No reliable data are available on trends in homosexual experience among adolescents, but the evidence cited earlier in the discussion on same-gender sex suggests that such experiences are not uncommon.)

Changes in the sexual behavior of young persons have two implications for the transmission of HIV. First, there is a large group of heterosexually active and relatively inexperienced young people with some tendency toward risky conduct. Second, there is little understanding of how to encourage change in the risky sexual behaviors many of them practice. Sexual intercourse now seems to be a recognized fact in the lives of the majority of young people. Intercourse is no longer linked to marriage or to forming a permanent couple, and such intercourse is often undertaken with inadequate precautions to forestall unwanted pregnancies or to prevent sexually transmitted diseases.

Increases in sexual activity and in the number of heterosexual partners among teenagers have been paralleled by similar changes in sexual activity among older individuals. The rise in the age of

Americans at first marriage and the increase in cohabitation among persons in their early to mid-20s have resulted in a greater rate of turnover in coupled relationships during what was, for many individuals in the past, a period of marriage and family formation. Another change is the increase in divorces (the rate of which now approaches 50 percent of all first marriages). There is little evidence on the acquisition of new sexual partners during the period after a divorce, but what little there is suggests that some individuals are relatively sexually active "in between" more permanent relationships.

Finally, the committee finds very little information about sexual relationships maintained concurrently with an apparently monogamous coupled relationship. That such relationships occur is apparent, but there are few reliable data from representative samples on their rate of occurrence or other relevant aspects of these relationships.

The impact of programs promoting "safer sex" for sexually active segments of the population—both teenagers and adults—is currently unknown. Given present levels of sexual activity, such programs—in particular, promotion of the use of condoms and spermicides—appear to be important areas on which to focus educational efforts and resources. **The committee recommends that local public health authorities ensure that condoms are readily available to all sexually active persons.** Promotion of condom use might be facilitated if condoms were sold in a wider variety of retail outlets, including supermarkets, convenience stores, and vending machines placed in diverse locales. Furthermore, because there is evidence suggesting that STDs may play a role as cofactors in the transmission of HIV, it is important to offer STD treatment as part of HIV/AIDS prevention efforts and to make that treatment as attractive as possible to those who need it. **The committee recommends that local public health authorities ensure that treatment for all sexually transmitted diseases is readily available to all persons who may seek such treatment.**

The committee recognizes that programs to promote safer sex practices are still hampered by a lack of knowledge about the actual effectiveness of those practices. Condom failure rates for contraception are known to vary, with some groups of users experiencing high failure rates. The committee believes more research is needed to understand the reasons people do or do not use condoms and spermicides and to determine the factors associated with their improper use. **The committee recommends that the Public Health Service immediately begin a research program to determine**

the extent to which the use of condoms and spermicides reduces the risk of HIV transmission. This program should include investigations of the current use of these products, how that use might be modified, and—equally important—how these products themselves may be modified to encourage uses compatible with human skills and dispositions.

Female Prostitution

Many female prostitutes are at high risk of HIV infection because of their use of IV drugs, their associations with IV drug users, their large number of sexual partners, and their increased likelihood of contracting other sexually transmitted diseases. Yet despite a general consensus about their high level of risk, little research has focused on prostitution: there are few data on female prostitutes and virtually no scientifically adequate data on male prostitutes. Even the size of these groups is unknown. Although estimates have occasionally been made of the number of female prostitutes in the United States, the committee finds that the lack of careful research to support these estimates makes them unreliable guides to the actual number of women in this group.

Despite the lack of data on the number of female prostitutes, however, available data suggest that the majority of prostitutes who have become infected with HIV in the United States have not become infected through sexual behavior. Most AIDS cases among women in the United States have occurred in women who use IV drugs. Although it is seldom possible to disentangle completely the effects of sexual transmission from drug-related transmission, the fact that there are relatively few women with HIV infection who are not IV drug users suggests that shared injection equipment—rather than sexual activity—has been the most significant transmission factor among female prostitutes.

Research and Data Needs

The committee finds that the long history of unfunded and underfunded research on human sexual behavior in this country has resulted in deficiencies in substantive knowledge, in the appropriate tools for scientific investigation of this topic, and in researchers who are expert in this area. Yet now, the nation is confronted with an epidemic that requires such knowledge, such tools, and such people. In its report, the committee details a number of specific research needs.

The committee recommends that the Public Health Service support research in those subsets of the population that are at increased risk of HIV infection. Research should include prostitutes and their clients, minorities, young gay men, gay men living outside the current epicenters of the epidemic, socially vulnerable adolescents, the different groups that make up the heterogeneous IV drug-using population, and the sexual partners of IV drug users. It is particularly important to obtain information from the people in these groups because of their potential role as conduits for the spread of HIV—through sexual activity—from groups with higher rates of prevalence to groups with lower rates.

It can be expected that some of the groups will be difficult to reach and count. It is also likely that it will be difficult to elicit the cooperation of these groups in data collection efforts and to obtain valid information concerning sensitive (and sometimes illicit) behaviors. **The committee recommends that resources be invested in methodological research to develop better procedures to obtain information from hard-to-reach groups.**

There is also a pressing need for greater sharing of the sexual behavior research data that do exist. The value of any data set can be effectively multiplied by making it available to other researchers for secondary analysis; consequently, the sharing of research data has become a standard practice in many disciplines. **The committee recommends that funding agencies, both public and private, encourage the sharing of data relevant to HIV infection and AIDS that have been gathered by federal and extramural researchers, within the limits set by scientific priority and confidentiality. To facilitate such sharing, the committee recommends that a data archive be established to support secondary analyses of these data.** The resources of this archive and the documentation accompanying the archived data sets should be sufficient to allow future researchers to understand the limitations of the archived data.

Data on Sexually Transmitted Diseases

The behaviors that favor or inhibit the transmission of HIV also favor or inhibit the transmission of other STDs. As a result, other things being equal, the transmission rates for STDs other than HIV should respond to the same behavioral interventions that are being designed to reduce HIV transmission.

Reliable data on the incidence of other STDs might also be useful for validating time-series measurements derived from surveys of individual sexual behavior. Unfortunately, statistics on STDs have been a subject of concern for many years. Underreporting is known to be quite common (particularly for cases diagnosed by private physicians), and this situation may have been exacerbated in recent years by the diversion of public health resources from tracking syphilis and gonorrhea to AIDS (thereby reducing the numbers of new cases of gonorrhea and syphilis that are counted). Improving these statistics would be a sound investment, given the potential usefulness of STD statistics as a surrogate measure of the behavioral changes that will ultimately reduce the number of AIDS cases. **The committee recommends that an independent review of STD data collection systems be undertaken and sufficient resources provided to undertake any improvements that may be required.**

IV Drug Use and AIDS

Since AIDS was first recognized, there has been growing appreciation of the critical role played by IV drug use in the spread of HIV infection. As of November 14, 1988, 20,752 cases of AIDS—approximately one quarter of all cases—had been diagnosed in individuals who reported using IV drugs.

The main factor in the spread of infection by this group is the practice of sharing injection equipment, which acts as a vector for HIV-contaminated blood. Sharing occurs for a variety of economic, cultural, and practical reasons, but whatever the individual causes of the behavior, almost all IV drug users report "needle-sharing"[10] at some time during their drug-use "careers."

HIV infection among IV drug users also poses a threat to their sexual partners and offspring, as well as to persons with whom they share injection equipment. Nearly 70 percent of the reported cases of heterosexually acquired AIDS in the United States have been associated with IV drug use, and almost 75 percent of pediatric AIDS cases have been diagnosed in cities with high seroprevalence rates among IV drug users. These data, combined with the potential (through needle-sharing) for the rapid spread of HIV infection among IV drug users, define a problem whose solution requires both immediate action and long-term research. The current state of knowledge suggests that there will be no immediate resolution to the problem of IV drug

[10]This practice includes the sharing of needles, syringes, and various other paraphernalia used for dissolving drugs and straining impurities.

use itself; nevertheless, existing research provides a basis for establishing programs to slow the spread of HIV infection among those who inject drugs.

Obviously, primary prevention of drug use could be an extremely effective prevention strategy for drug-associated HIV transmission. Relying on primary prevention *alone* is not realistic, however, given the uneven record of past efforts to control drug use and the threat of a continued epidemic of HIV transmission in the United States among persons who inject drugs, their sexual partners, and their children. The committee recommends that the nation adopt a three-pronged strategy to control the spread of AIDS through IV drug use.

First, drug treatment programs should be available to all who desire treatment. Several studies conducted prior to the advent of AIDS show that treatment can reduce IV drug use. Moreover, studies conducted during the AIDS era have shown that entering and remaining in drug treatment programs are factors associated with significant reductions in the rates of HIV infection among IV drug users.

Second, the committee concludes that, regardless of the availability of treatment opportunities, a substantial number of people in the United States will continue to inject drugs, at least in the short run. Consequently, the committee also recommends expanding programs for "safer injection" (including sterile needle and syringe exchanges and the promotion of injection equipment sterilization using bleach). None of the current studies on safer injection programs has shown increased IV drug use. Indeed, it appears that safer injection programs may indirectly encourage IV drug users to seek treatment. Furthermore, although results are still preliminary, many studies indicate that such programs do reduce the risk of HIV transmission among IV drug users. Finally, action should also be taken to provide a better understanding of the effects of these programs. **The committee recommends that well-designed, staged trials of sterile needle programs, such as those requested in the 1986 Institute of Medicine/National Academy of Sciences report *Confronting AIDS*, be implemented.**

Thus, the committee believes it is necessary to establish better data collection systems to monitor current AIDS prevention efforts for IV drug users. The quality of existing data on IV drug use is not adequate to answer the difficult questions AIDS poses. Assessing the scope of the problems associated with HIV transmission among IV drug users is difficult when neither the number of IV drug users nor the seroprevalence rate is known with any certainty. Current estimates rely on data that were collected for other purposes and that were acquired through efforts intended to measure only crude trends.

In sum, the committee recommends that the appropriate government authorities take immediate action to

1. **provide drug treatment upon request for IV drug users throughout the country;**
2. **sustain and expand current programs that provide for "safer injection" to reach all current IV drug users in the nation on a continuing basis and with appropriate research evaluation; and**
3. **establish data collection systems for monitoring present AIDS prevention efforts for IV drug users.**

The IV drug-using population is also at risk of acquiring and spreading HIV infection through unprotected sexual behaviors. Little is known about the sexual, contraceptive, and childbearing practices of IV drug users, although early studies indicate that more risk-reducing change has occurred in injection practices than in sexual behaviors. **The committee recommends that high priority be given to studies of the sexual and procreative behavior of IV drug users, including methods to reduce sexual and perinatal (mother–infant) transmission of HIV.**

Although the committee urges that more basic behavioral research be undertaken to improve understanding of risk-associated behaviors and how to change them, it also finds that the implementation of intervention programs cannot wait upon the findings of such research. The severity of the AIDS epidemic demands innovative approaches to prevent the spread of infection among IV drug users, with special attention to collecting good evaluation data. Reaching and serving IV drug users will require innovative methods and additional resources.[11] Slowing the spread of HIV infection in this country depends on the ability to find new ways to reach and influence this population. Planned variations of intervention strategies, accompanied by sound evaluation measures, will enable a determination of which kinds of programs are most successful in facilitating change in risky behaviors in this population.

---

[11] For example, some AIDS intervention programs use mobile vans and cadres of "outreach workers"—who can go into "shooting galleries" and other places in which drug use occurs—which have proven helpful in serving people who have not been reached by other services or agencies.

LIMITING THE SPREAD OF HIV INFECTION

Facilitating Change in Health Behaviors

Preventing the spread of HIV infection will require changing those behaviors that are known to transmit the virus and then maintaining those changes over time. Whether these goals can, in fact, be accomplished will depend in large part on the effectiveness of the intervention strategies that are brought to bear on the problem.

Providing accurate, appropriate information is a logical starting point for any intervention program, although information by itself is unlikely to be sufficient to alter risk-associated behavior. Yet even the accomplishment of this prologue to more complex efforts requires an understanding of the target audience in order to formulate and deliver persuasive messages. To produce action (in this case, behavioral change), a message must reach the appropriate audience and be understood. **The committee recommends making information available in clear, explicit language in the idiom of the target audience. Furthermore, the committee recommends that sex education be available to both male and female students and that such education include explicit information relevant to the prevention of HIV infection.**

Health education campaigns of the past, notably those to prevent STDs and drug use, have tended to rely on fear to motivate those at risk. Research has shown, however, that fear alone is unlikely to succeed. Fear-arousing health promotion messages must also provide specific information on the steps that can be taken to protect an individual from the threat to his or her well-being. The excessive fear generated by heightened perceptions of seriousness and susceptibility can be offset by providing assurances that there is, indeed, something that can be done to prevent infection. Therefore, AIDS prevention messages should strike a balance in the level of threat that is conveyed: the level should be sufficiently high to motivate individuals to take action but not so high that it paralyzes them with fear or causes them to deny their susceptibility.

The mass media can play an important role in providing information about risk, as well as in molding both the skills and behavior of individuals and the norms of the community to support that behavior. **The committee recommends that television networks present more public service messages on those behaviors associated with HIV transmission and practical measures for interrupting the spread of infection. The committee further**

recommends that television networks accept condom advertisements. Efforts should be made to link media representatives with local public health agencies to ensure that the messages are appropriate for the local audiences and that well-designed evaluations of media efforts are conducted.

Although public information campaigns are a sound first step for prevention programs, they are generally insufficient on their own to induce widespread behavioral change. For people to initiate changes in their behavior, they must be motivated, they must believe that the changes being proposed will do some good, and they must believe they have a reasonable chance of successfully accomplishing those changes. Past research on behavioral change indicates the following:

- Changes that are consistent with an individual's existing beliefs and values are more likely to be adopted.
- For some people, modifying behavior through incremental changes is easier to achieve than a global change in life-style.
- Offering alternative courses of behavior from which an individual can choose is preferable to dictating one "appropriate" behavior.
- For those who believe in the efficacy of a particular behavior but do not believe they can successfully execute it, skills training can be helpful.
- Most people need assistance and support to change unhealthy behaviors, and most will not be completely successful in adhering to new patterns.

AIDS prevention programs should also incorporate what is already known about the adoption and diffusion of new ideas. For example, opinion leaders of target populations should be identified and used to maximize a program's credibility and persuasiveness with the target audience and to shape more effective messages and programs. Also to be considered is the community context in which a prevention program is implemented. If they are to be successful, new programs should be carefully reviewed before being implemented for characteristics that might impede their acceptance in the community.

Targeting programs to the community rather than to individuals may bring additional benefits. Community-level programs have two important points of impact: (1) they can reach a critical mass of individuals to provide information, motivation, and skills training; and (2) by working through a variety of community agencies, they can foster changes in the norms that stipulate appropriate behavior for community members.

One further approach to facilitating behavioral change is the use of HIV antibody testing, an approach that has been found to be helpful in changing behaviors in some groups. **The committee recommends that anonymous HIV antibody testing with appropriate pre- and posttest counseling be made available on a voluntary basis for anyone desiring it.** However, to maximize the usefulness of antibody testing in facilitating behavioral change, more knowledge is needed about why individuals seek testing, how testing affects behavioral change in different populations, and how it affects psychiatric morbidity. The committee also emphasizes that HIV testing is not a substitute for broader efforts in education and intervention.

Evaluating Interventions

The role of evaluation is to allow a determination of which strategies actually change people's behavior and which do not. Making these determinations requires a systematic process that produces a reliable account of a program's effectiveness. Indeed, preparing for an evaluation can often increase program specificity and quality at the outset. Program innovations that are informed by feedback from careful (and prompt) evaluations can lead to the more rapid discarding of poor ideas and the adoption of good ones. The eventual result is a more effective intervention program.

The committee recommends that the Office of the Assistant Secretary for Health take responsibility for an evaluation strategy that will provide timely information on the relative effectiveness of different AIDS intervention programs. Such a strategy should consider both short- and long-term benefits and should be applied to a variety of programs.

When possible, for at least each major type of intervention and each major target population, a minimum of two intervention programs should be subjected to rigorous evaluations that are designed to produce research evidence of the highest possible quality. Variants of intervention programs should be developed for and tested in different populations and in different geographic areas using random assignment strategy accompanied by careful evaluation. When ethically possible, one of the variants should be a nontreatment control.

Randomized Field Experiments

One of the most crucial aspects of evaluation involves inferring whether an intervention has had an effect on the target population. To determine such effects, one must compare what did happen with what would have happened if the intervention had not taken place. Because it is not possible to make this comparison directly, inference strategies turn to various proxies—for instance, extrapolating a trend from past history (before treatment) or using comparison groups. Frequently, however, no similar comparison group can be defined or recruited. Moreover, although adjustments can be made for known differences between two groups, such adjustments may be difficult to make, and there is no way to account for unrecognized differences in two differently constituted groups.

The remedy for this problem is to establish a singly constituted group in which to assess treatment effects. To be included in the group, a person must satisfy the criteria for inclusion in the program. Then, a subset of that one group is randomly chosen to receive the intervention, thus producing two comparable subgroups that are not identical but are as alike as two random samples drawn from the same population.

To maintain the comparability of the two groups, outcome measurements must be performed symmetrically for all program participants (treated and untreated). This idea underlies randomized clinical trials and randomized field experiments. The design is a powerful tool, although there will be some cases in which it cannot be applied. **The committee recommends the expanded use of randomized field experiments for evaluating new intervention programs on both individual and community levels.**

Resources for Evaluation

Carrying out evaluations that produce reliable data about the effectiveness of interventions to stop the spread of HIV infection requires creative leadership on the part of the management of an organization and an attitude among its staff that evaluation is positive and constructive. In addition, priorities must be set, and adequate resources must be made available for evaluation activities. Unfortunately, there are seldom enough dollars, expert people, or time to evaluate everything in detail. The selection of a particular intervention for in-depth evaluation should depend on several criteria: the importance of the intervention, the extent of the knowledge already in hand, the perceived value of additional information, and the estimated feasibility of the assessment. To use available program evaluation resources most efficiently, **the committee recommends that only the best-designed and best-implemented intervention programs be selected to receive those special resources that will be needed to conduct scientific evaluations.**

There is also a need to upgrade the capacity for evaluation at the local level. Producing quality data that will allow program planners to learn from ongoing intervention efforts will require additional resources, including appropriately trained personnel. Individuals with expertise in program evaluation need to be identified and brought into the AIDS prevention arena. Unfortunately, many state and local agencies have few connections with individuals in this field and will need assistance to identify appropriate people and recruit them. The committee believes it is critical that technical assistance for evaluation activities be made available. **The committee recommends that CDC substantially increase efforts, with links to extramural scientific resources, to assist health departments and others in mounting evaluations.** CDC (and any other agency that undertakes AIDS prevention programs) should assign to some administrative unit the responsibility for ensuring the use of planned variants of intervention programs and for overseeing a system of evaluation.

OVERCOMING BARRIERS TO RESEARCH AND INTERVENTION

Much needs to be done to improve available knowledge about the behaviors that transmit HIV and to control further spread of the infection. The committee finds, however, that some of the needed actions have encountered and will continue to encounter resistance. Some obstacles arise from the structure of the scientific disciplines involved and the historical lack of support for the kinds of research that are now urgently needed. Other barriers come from within our culture, and they find practical expression in political decisions that restrict the types of AIDS education and intervention activities that governments are willing to fund or permit.

Barriers to Research

Although there is growing appreciation of the need for behavioral and social research related to HIV transmission, the personnel to conduct such efforts are currently in short supply at agencies involved in AIDS activities. CDC, for example, is managing more than

$150 million of AIDS behavioral research and intervention programs with a small and severely overextended cadre of people trained in relevant disciplines. Of approximately 4,500 total employees at CDC's Atlanta facility, fewer than 40 are Ph.D.-level behavioral and social scientists, and only a few of those individuals are working on AIDS-related projects. **The committee recommends that the number of trained behavioral and social scientists employed in AIDS-related activities at federal agencies responsible for preventing the spread of HIV infection be substantially increased.**

Since the early years of the epidemic, CDC has had primary responsibility for AIDS data collection. Some surveys have involved only the collection of physical specimens (e.g., blood) along with a very restricted set of demographic characteristics (e.g., age, sex, residence). At present, CDC's Atlanta staff does not include a sampling statistician. The agency's recent acquisition of the National Center for Health Statistics (NCHS) can provide some of the needed statistical expertise, but the role of NCHS in CDC's data collection programs is still being defined. **The committee recommends that the CDC AIDS program increase its staff of persons knowledgeable about survey sampling and survey design, and that it exploit the methodological expertise of the National Center for Health Statistics.** Finally, in addition to experienced survey scientists, CDC needs technical assistance to evaluate currently funded intervention programs.

The committee recognizes that it may be difficult to attract a sufficient number of senior scientists to Atlanta on a permanent basis. One- or, preferably, two-year visiting scientist appointments might provide quick access to needed personnel and allow CDC management greater flexibility in meeting changing staff needs. **The committee recommends the use of PHS fellowship programs and Intergovernmental Personnel Appointments (IPAs) as an interim means for rapidly enlarging the cadre of senior behavioral and social scientists working on AIDS programs at CDC and other PHS agencies.**

Collaborative Research

Much of the best behavioral and statistical research on AIDS has occurred through collaborations among scientists from universities, the staffs of government agencies (at all levels), and organizations rooted in the communities that have borne the brunt of the AIDS epidemic. Collaborations of this kind are seldom without conflict; differences of social origin, ethnicity, economic status, or sexual orientation may sometimes lead to misunderstandings. Yet such misunderstandings should not deter collaboration; they should be seen as part of an indispensable process of accommodation of varying viewpoints. Efforts to design and implement effective AIDS education without taking into account the idioms and milieu of the target population are doomed to failure. The active and equitable collaboration of persons in the target populations with "outside" scientists and researchers can provide an important safeguard against such failures.

Talented, well-trained, and dedicated workers will be needed for research and intervention efforts at all levels of involvement, from the coordination and funding centers of the federal government to local outreach and education programs. To have credibility in the communities suffering the highest rates of HIV infection and to maximize the likelihood of successfully preventing the further spread of infection, intervention programs at all levels must increase the involvement of minority researchers and minority health care workers in the black, Hispanic, and gay communities. In addition, the committee recommends that special support be provided to foster what are often weak linkages among practitioners (those best positioned to deliver services) and researchers and to remove or reduce organizational impediments to the establishment of those relationships.

One creative mechanism that has been developed to foster collaboration is the multidisciplinary AIDS research center. Much of the needed behavioral and social research on AIDS prevention requires large, multidisciplinary teams of scientists with close working relationships with many of the different communities in which interventions must be conducted. Recent initiatives, particularly those of the National Institute of Mental Health (NIMH), have been designed to stimulate the formation of multidisciplinary AIDS research centers in those cities that are the current foci of the AIDS epidemic. The committee believes that these initiatives are an appropriate component of rational strategies for the support of behavioral research on AIDS. The NIMH centers have shown evidence of involving scientists who have valuable links to the communities in which prevention research is needed. **The committee recommends that support of multidisciplinary centers for research on AIDS prevention be viewed as a long-term commitment to allow sustained collaborative efforts, including valuable prospective studies.**

Social Barriers to Intervention

Because AIDS and HIV infection are mainly transmitted by sexual activity and IV drug use, controlling the epidemic requires both a scientific understanding of these behaviors and a social commitment to behavioral interventions that are sufficient to reduce the transmission of HIV infection to a level that cannot sustain epidemic growth. As noted at the beginning of this summary, epidemic disease refers not so much to the number of people who are affected but rather to the sudden appearance and rapid spread of a disease in a community, a phenomenon that usually evokes strong political and social responses.

AIDS education efforts provide a number of examples in which potentially effective prevention activities have become entangled in social conflicts that caused delays in their implementation or a weakening of their message. Specific controversies have involved restrictions on the use of explicit language in educational materials, conflict between providing scientific information or promoting particular moral values in AIDS prevention messages, and prohibitions against condom advertising on network television.

Conflicts of this sort are not unique to this epidemic. Indeed, there are a number of similarities between the AIDS epidemic and epidemics of the past. For example, history suggests that cultural, political, and economic institutions faced with the need to respond quickly to catastrophe often cling to familiar practices, even in the face of an unusual threat. Certainly, instances of such institutional "behavior" can be noted in efforts to mobilize society's forces against AIDS and HIV infection.

A further similarity between this epidemic and most others is the disproportionate effect on the poor. Because education is critical to controlling the spread of HIV/AIDS, the ability to reach across class boundaries is vital. Yet those who must design and provide this education sometimes have little knowledge of the culture or conditions of poorer people. Differences of language, values, and lifestyle can make effective collaboration and communication difficult.

Complicating these factors is the additional element of stigmatization—the phenomenon of marking individuals or groups as warranting exclusion from human society. In its sociological meaning, stigma is the set of ideas, beliefs, and judgments the dominant group in a society holds about another group that it has selected as deserving of scorn or blame (in this case, those who are infected or who have the disease). These beliefs are not merely negative; often, members of the stigmatized group are characterized as dangerous or as deserving of punishment for some vague offense or moral improbity, a pattern of thought that has led throughout human history to the blaming and persecuting of minorities as the cause of plagues or scourges.

The HIV epidemic has led to stigmatization since its beginning. The fact that the disease has been largely confined to male homosexuals and IV drug users has made stigmatization almost inevitable, for these groups were already the objects to some degree of the deprecating judgments that constitute this phenomenon. Fortunately, even though stigmatization has occurred, the public thus far has repudiated the worst forms of stigmatizing punishment. Calls for quarantining those infected with HIV have been rejected, and some protections for ensuring confidentiality have been erected in the areas of antibody testing and serostatus disclosure. Nevertheless, more remains to be done. Health professionals have a particular responsibility to counter stigmatization, especially in light of their past success in destigmatizing other conditions: leprosy, epilepsy, and, to some extent, mental retardation. The media also bear a particular responsibility in what they present and how they present it. Similarly, churches and educators have important roles to play.

Finally, politicians and the American legal system can affect the extent to which any group in society is subject to stigmatization. A politician who becomes an advocate for the stigmatized obviously takes on an unpopular task. Laws, however, can retard the social process of stigmatization by prohibiting some of the behaviors that are inspired by it. Research has shown, for example, that the possibility of legal prosecution can alter discriminatory behaviors in various settings even in the presence of discriminatory attitudes. The law can also protect those who are infected with HIV from discrimination, and the educational message conveyed by such protection can help to reduce the underlying current of stigmatization that pushes those infected with HIV and AIDS to the outskirts of society.

* * *

In closing, we return to the theme with which we began: the HIV/AIDS epidemic is partly a social phenomenon, and the major weapons that are currently available to contain it seek to change the behaviors that spread the disease. Even if fully effective therapies or vaccines were to be found, it is likely that there will be a continuing role for behavioral intervention. It is more than 40 years since effective drugs against syphilis and gonorrhea became widely available, but those diseases have not yet been eradicated in the United States. Similarly, the struggle to retard the spread of HIV is likely to persist well into the next century. Improved understanding and prevention of the behaviors that spread HIV/AIDS will be needed—not only in the short run, however many years that may be, but in the decades that follow any medical breakthrough as well.

NOTE: Reference documentation for the material in this Summary is presented in the respective chapters of the full report.

Part I

Understanding the Spread of HIV Infection

In Part I, we discuss key aspects of the scientific knowledge required to understand the spread of the human immunodeficiency virus (HIV) and the epidemic of acquired immune deficiency syndrome (AIDS). Chapter 1 reviews estimates of the current size of the epidemic and evaluates the statistical data systems that have been established to monitor the spread of HIV in the United States. Chapters 2 and 3 discuss the two major classes of behavior that have spread HIV infection and thereby sustained the epidemic: sexual behavior and intravenous (IV) drug use.

1

Monitoring the Epidemic's Course

This chapter reviews the statistics and statistical systems that provide the nation with information about the current state and future course of the AIDS epidemic.[1] To conduct this review, the committee appointed a special panel on statistical issues in AIDS research. The material in this chapter constitutes the parent committee's findings after consideration of the technical panel's work.

The panel was asked to evaluate the adequacy of current statistics (and those likely to be available in the near future) for assessing the present state and monitoring the future course of the AIDS epidemic. Early on, the panel concluded that a fully adequate monitoring system must go beyond the current system for reporting AIDS cases and AIDS deaths. Rather, an adequate system of information on the current state of the epidemic must provide reliable monitoring of the prevalence and incidence of HIV infection in the population.

Developing accurate statistical systems for monitoring HIV infection is important for a number of reasons:

- Counts of AIDS cases are out-of-date indicators of the present state of the epidemic. There is a long, asymptomatic latency period between HIV infection and the development of AIDS (in most persons). Consequently, the statistics on *new* AIDS cases reflect *old* cases of HIV infection. For example, most of the adults who will be

[1]In this chapter, we focus on HIV and AIDS statistics. In Chapter 2, we discuss the potential value of reliable statistics on other sexually transmitted diseases that should (other things being equal) respond to the same behavioral changes that would reduce the transmission of HIV.

counted as new AIDS cases in 1989 are likely to have been infected with HIV prior to 1986.

- Persons whose life spans are significantly shortened by HIV infection do not always manifest sufficient symptoms to be captured by the AIDS reporting system. Thus, some persons dying of HIV-related illnesses do not qualify for inclusion in the statistics on AIDS deaths.[2]
- HIV-infected persons without overt AIDS symptoms can transmit the virus to others.
- The future magnitude of the AIDS epidemic will be determined primarily by the current extent and future spread of HIV infection in the population.

These considerations, and the fact that the AIDS reporting system is functioning reasonably well (although not perfectly, as noted in the following paragraphs), led the panel to concentrate its attention on what is currently known about the prevalence and incidence of HIV infection in the United States.

Notwithstanding this focus, the committee notes the need for constant vigilance to ensure the efficient functioning of the AIDS case reporting system. The time lag between the diagnosis of a case and the reporting of it to the Centers for Disease Control (CDC) appears to be increasing. At present, CDC estimates that only 85 to 90 percent of AIDS cases are reported within one year of diagnosis, and

---

[2]A review of death certificates in Boston, Chicago, New York, and Washington, D.C., during 1985 found that the reporting of AIDS cases (those meeting the 1985 surveillance definition) was 89 percent complete; that is, in 89 percent of all AIDS deaths, the decedent had already been included in the AIDS case registry. However, an additional 13 percent of deaths thought to be HIV related did not meet the CDC criteria for AIDS diagnosis (Hardy et al., 1987); that is, 13 percent of all deaths originally attributed to AIDS, *Pneumocystis carinii,* or Kaposi's sarcoma on the death certificate did not meet the surveillance definition for AIDS but were judged "clinically suspicious" (p. 388) because they had an opportunistic infection included in the surveillance definition but the infection had not been confirmed by the required methods. It is also suspected that such HIV-related deaths are responsible for an epidemic of non-AIDS deaths among IV drug users in New York City. The eightfold increase in non-AIDS deaths (from 257 in 1978 to 1,607 in 1985) is presumed to be due to the fatal consequences of HIV infection in cases that did not meet the surveillance definition for AIDS. Increases in non-AIDS deaths among New York City IV drug users between 1981 and 1985 occurred in the following HIV-related categories: pneumonia (not *Pneumocystis carinii*), from 15 to 193; tuberculosis, from 3 to 35; and endocarditis, from 4 to 64 (Des Jarlais et al., 1988:155).

Ultimately, some of these HIV-related deaths might be captured by the reporting system through the use of the new HIV codes for classifying causes of death from death certificates. This assumes, of course, that the physician completing the certificate is aware of the decedent's HIV status. In any event, even if this system were entirely reliable, it would count people only at the point of death.

it is thought that this percentage is declining.[3] Such a decline would be a reasonable consequence of the growing demands the epidemic is making on the state and local public health departments that handle AIDS surveillance and reporting. Indeed, the increasing delays noted in the reporting of AIDS cases might be taken as direct evidence of the stresses being placed on the personnel and institutions who must cope with the epidemic. Additional resources appear to be needed now (and more will probably need to be added incrementally in the future) so that case reporting delays do not continue to increase.

The panel also identified a need for special methodological studies to assess the reliability and validity of the categorization of AIDS cases by mode of transmission. Accurate data on transmission modes are crucial because they identify the behaviors and populations that must be targeted to control the spread of infection. Although some careful work has been done to explore the accuracy with which such determinations are made, further research could provide much valuable information. Given the difficulties in obtaining accurate information on sexual behavior (particularly in some subpopulations), there is good reason to believe that some error and bias contaminate the tabulation of AIDS cases by transmission mode. Methodological studies to assess the magnitude and direction of such inaccuracies could provide useful information that would aid in the interpretation of the AIDS case data.[4]

PREVALENCE AND INCIDENCE OF HIV INFECTION

Prevalence denotes that proportion of a population that is currently infected; it is usually expressed as cases per 1,000 or per 10,000, or it may be written as a percentage (e.g., 0.4 percent, or 4 cases per 1,000). Incidence denotes the rate of occurrence of new cases of infection per unit of time (e.g., per year). Thus, an incidence of .03 per year in some population group means that new cases of infection occurred in 3 percent of the initially uninfected members of the group during the year in question. Incidence may be estimated

[3]The median reporting delay (i.e., the time from diagnosis to report) has, for example, increased from 2 to 3 months in the past year (M. Morgan, Statistics and Data Management Branch, AIDS Program, CDC, personal communication, September 26, 1988).

[4]These studies would be important to conduct even if they were to conclude that the inaccuracies themselves were, in fact, inconsequential.

directly by tracking new cases (as can be done with AIDS) or indirectly by observing changes in prevalence and adjusting for deaths (as might be done with HIV).

In November 1987, CDC transmitted a report to the President and his Domestic Policy Council that summarized in a clear, comprehensive fashion the state of present knowledge of HIV incidence and prevalence (CDC, 1987b).[5] The report performed a great service in pulling together and organizing a massive amount of disparate information, much of which was unpublished. In summarizing current knowledge, the report highlighted the substantial gaps in our understanding of the HIV epidemic and made it quite clear that almost all that is known about HIV incidence and prevalence comes from research samples that have been recruited in a manner that precludes generalizations to well-defined segments of the population. (Such non-population-based samples are sometimes called "purposive" or "convenience" samples.)

Uses of HIV Prevalence and Incidence Data

There are three important uses for reliable HIV prevalence and incidence data. First, such data can be used to compare population groups in terms of current HIV prevalence and, subsequently, to target prevention services to those groups that are most in need. Second, reliable HIV prevalence and incidence data can be helpful in assessing the effects of prevention services and other interventions. A third, less direct use of such data is in calibrating forecasting models. These models in turn may allow us to better anticipate the future course of the epidemic and the demands it will make on health care and other social systems.

Prevalence Data

At present, data on the prevalence of HIV infection come principally from two sources: (1) blood samples derived from programs testing special populations (e.g., military applicants and blood donors) and (2) testing of anonymous blood specimens from smaller studies of convenience samples. Table 1-1 summarizes the seroprevalence data from four testing programs, two large and two small. As the table shows, there is some consistency across the estimates generated from

---

[5] The "Review of Current Knowledge" section of this report has been issued as a supplement to the *Morbidity and Mortality Weekly Report* of December 18, 1987 (CDC, 1987a).

TABLE 1-1 HIV Seroprevalence Rates Among all Blood Donors, Military Recruits, and Samples of Hospital Patients and Job Corps Applicants

Sample	Number Tested	Year	Percentage Seropositive
Blood donors	12.6 million	1985–1987	0.02
		1985	0.035
		1987	0.012
Military recruits	1.25 million	1985–1987	0.15
Hospital patients[a]	8,668	1986–1987	0.32
Job corps applicants	25,000	1987	0.33

[a]Non-self-selected samples from the general population at four hospitals in the Midwest. The actual prevalances ranged from 0.09 percent to 0.89 percent across hospitals. The prevalance among military recruits in the same four cities (adjusted for age and sex) is 0.11 percent.

SOURCE: CDC (1987a).

three of these programs. In particular, testing of applicants for military service, of patients in four Midwestern hospitals, and of participants in the Job Corps program all produced HIV prevalence estimates in the range of about 10 to 30 per 10,000. Estimates of HIV prevalence among blood donors, however, were an order of magnitude lower—1 to 3 per 10,000.

Despite the large number of persons screened in the four testing programs shown in Table 1-1, the results are not representative of the population. Military recruits, for example, come from particular age and educational strata, and persons reporting homosexual behavior or drug use are barred from enlistment. Such selection factors introduce large and numerically unknown biases; consequently, data from the military screening program cannot be used to make inferences about HIV infection in the national population.

Similarly, residential Job Corps entrants are drawn from the disadvantaged 16- to 21-year-old population, and they overrepresent racial and ethnic minorities. Hospital samples in turn have more old and sick people than the general population, and this group may be socioeconomically biased because the patterns of health care utilization are correlated with socioeconomic status (Andersen et al., 1987; Secretary's Task Force on Black and Minority Health, 1985:194).

The operation of biasing factors in these samples may be strongest in the blood donor group because people who believe they are at high risk for HIV infection have been asked not to donate blood.

Potential blood donors at Red Cross sites are interviewed for risk factors, and they are given several opportunities to elect not to donate their blood for use in transfusions. Thus, it is not surprising that HIV prevalence among blood donors is much lower than that in other samples. The 10-fold lower prevalence rate for blood donors illustrates the problems that can arise when volunteer samples are used to make inferences about the general population.

An example of the misunderstandings that may result from the use of such samples is the reports in the popular media[6] that the prevalence of infection detected among military recruits in the United States did not increase during the first 15 months of the military's testing program. Although this result appears encouraging, it is actually quite difficult to interpret because it is not known whether the population of military recruits was stable over time. It is possible that potential military recruits who had engaged in high-risk behaviors were discouraged from volunteering by publicity about the mandatory HIV testing of recruits. A more subtle source of possible bias may be the changes that often occur in the pool of military applicants with respect to the mix of population subgroups in the pool. These changes may be the result of a number of outside influences. For example, when the recruitment needs of the armed forces are great, the minimum educational standards for enlistment are relaxed. Similarly, when the economy fluctuates, the pool of those seeking entry to the military services may enlarge or shrink. Such changes have unknown effects on the HIV infection rates among applicants in different years.

Monitoring Trends

It is sometimes asserted that, although available HIV prevalence data are biased, they may be sufficient for following trends. Yet there are good reasons to be skeptical of this assertion. First, there is usually no assurance that the characteristics of the measurement techniques used to determine HIV prevalence have been stable over time. Given the great advances in basic knowledge and practical expertise in AIDS research since 1981, it is likely that measurement techniques have changed, although the magnitude of the differences generated by such changes is not known. Unfortunately, when comparisons are

[6]See, for example, "AIDS Rate Remains Stable Among U.S. Military Recruits Since Testing Started in 1985; Statistics Puzzle Experts," *Washington Post*, May 15, 1987:A1.

made across studies that lack well-defined protocols,[7] differences in measurement procedures are often impossible to recognize or control.[8] Second, the populations being tested may not be stable over time. The CDC report notes, for example, that HIV prevalence in blood donors has decreased over time because people who tested positive dropped out of the donor pool.

Incidence Data

Measures of HIV incidence are not generally available, but they would be particularly valuable for tracking the epidemic's course, making long-term projections about its future spread, and evaluating the overall effectiveness of efforts to control AIDS. For example, reliable data on the incidence of HIV infection would make it possible to test the hypothesis that the incidence of new cases has peaked (or is now peaking) in certain population groups. In this regard, the committee notes that data included in the CDC report suggest that incidence rates may be declining among gay men (see, in particular, CDC [1987a:Table 12 and Figure 13]). It is unclear, however, how much of this peaking results from the saturation with HIV infection of small cohorts of gay men, particularly in instances in which the cohorts were selected because of their high levels of sexual activity.

Variation in Estimated HIV Prevalence for Selected Groups

The CDC report noted substantial differences in the estimated prevalence of HIV infection on the basis of the following:

- "risk factors"—homosexual sex among men, IV drug use, hemophilia, or heterosexual sex with persons at risk;
- source of the sample—blood donors, applicants for military service, patients at clinics for sexually transmitted diseases (STDs), newborns, and so forth;
- geographic location; and

[7]This problem frequently arises when comparisons are made across different research studies. However, data from screening programs that use highly standardized measurement procedures and careful quality control of laboratory testing (e.g., in the armed forces) are less vulnerable to this problem.

[8]The inability to recognize or control these differences also makes it impossible to recalibrate the prevalence estimates (i.e., by replicating the two measurement procedures and observing the resulting variation in prevalence estimates).

- demographic factors—in particular, sex, age, and race.

The differences in reported prevalence estimates ranged over two orders of magnitude. It is unlikely that biases in the data could account for *all* of the observed differences. Furthermore, the reported variations in HIV prevalence often mirrored differences in the number of reported AIDS cases, suggesting that the estimates may be sufficiently accurate to provide a crude ranking of various groups in terms of HIV prevalence.

Major groups for whom HIV prevalence and incidence data are presented in the CDC report include homosexual and bisexual men, IV drug users, hemophiliacs, heterosexual partners of HIV-infected persons (or persons in recognized risk groups), patients at general care hospitals, tuberculosis patients, prostitutes, heterosexuals without identifiable risk factors, and newborn infants and their mothers. In addition, by reporting the data according to locale, CDC provides implicit information about variations in HIV prevalence across the country. The rest of this section summarizes the data presented on each of these groupings in the CDC report. The next section considers uncertainties that limit the usefulness of these data for making inferences about the prevalence and incidence of HIV infection in the overall population.

Homosexual and Bisexual Men. In 50 surveys and studies conducted in 23 cities in 16 states, HIV prevalence rates ranged from under 10 to 70 percent, with most of the estimates falling between 20 and 50 percent. Prevalence estimates were highest in San Francisco, but the CDC report found that HIV was not concentrated in any one region of the country. It should be noted that most of the samples were drawn from patients at STD clinics, so the observed rates probably overstate prevailing rates in the population of men who have same-gender sexual contacts.

IV Drug Users. The prevalence of HIV infection among IV drug users showed marked geographic variation ranging from 50 to 60 percent in New York City, northern New Jersey, and Puerto Rico to less than 5 percent in areas distant from the East Coast. These estimates were derived primarily from samples obtained at facilities treating heroin addicts. (Some evidence suggests that IV drug users who are not in treatment may be at greater risk of infection; see Chapter 3.)

Hemophiliacs. Prevalence rates among hemophiliacs appear to be uniformly distributed across the United States. There are indications, however, that the likelihood of infection in a given sample will be correlated with the type and severity of coagulation disorder: reported HIV prevalence rates were 70 percent for hemophilia A and 35 percent for hemophilia B.

Heterosexual Partners of Persons with HIV Infection or at Recognized Risk. The prevalence rates for this group varied from under 10 to 60 percent in a limited number of studies. The reasons for these large differences are unclear.[9] Recent evidence suggests that infectiousness increases with the deterioration of the immune system. The relative efficiency of male-to-female and female-to-male transmission may also be important, but there are insufficient data to assess this possibility. For heterosexual partners of high-risk persons of unknown HIV status, HIV prevalence ranged from 0 to 11 percent.

Patients at General Care Hospitals. Non-self-selected samples of 8,668 blood specimens from the general population at four hospitals in the Midwest gave an age- and sex-adjusted prevalence of 0.32 percent. The actual prevalences ranged from 0.09 to 0.89 percent. (HIV prevalence among military applicants in the same four cities, adjusted for age[10] and sex, was 0.11 percent.)

Newborn Infants and Women of Reproductive Age. In a Massachusetts study, methods were developed to detect HIV infection in women who have borne live infants.[11] On the basis of 30,708 tests in 1986–1987, the weighted average prevalence was 0.21 percent (unadjusted for the mother's age and race), varying from 0.80 percent at inner-city hospitals to 0.09 percent at suburban and rural hospitals. Female military applicants from Massachusetts had a crude prevalence of 0.13 percent (adjusted for age and race). As discussed later

[9]Subsequent to the publication of the CDC report, Peterman and coworkers (1988) reported a study of 55 wives of HIV-infected men. Ten of these women seroconverted during the course of the study. The women who seroconverted reported fewer instances of unprotected intercourse than those who did not seroconvert, suggesting that other factors in addition to exposure affect the probability of HIV transmission.

[10]It should be noted that adjustment of the military sample for age introduces considerable uncertainty because the age distribution of military recruits and military personnel includes only a very small percentage of persons in older age groups.

[11]The risk of HIV transmission from an infected mother to her infant is estimated to range from 30 to 50 percent. However, all infants of infected mothers carry maternal antibodies to HIV—whether or not they are actually infected with the virus.

in this chapter, these prevalence estimates represent the population of childbearing women and are unbiased in terms of self-selection or exclusion related to HIV risk factors.

Prostitutes. HIV prevalence among female prostitutes ranged from 0 to 45 percent, with the highest rates in large inner-city areas in which drug use is common, such as New York City, Miami, and Detroit. The prevalence of HIV infection was three to four times higher in female prostitutes who were also drug users, and it was twice as high in black and Hispanic prostitutes as in white and other prostitutes. The geographic pattern of HIV infection in prostitutes appeared to parallel the geographic distribution of AIDS among women in general.

Tuberculosis Patients. HIV infection is thought to have caused an increase in the number of persons with clinical tuberculosis (TB). In one study that was not limited to self-selected groups, 19 percent of 276 TB patients in Dade County, Florida (which includes Miami) tested positive for HIV. In four studies of TB patients at high risk, the prevalence ranged from 0 to 50 percent.

Heterosexuals Without Known Risk Factors.[12] The prevalence of HIV infection among heterosexually active persons in the absence of known risk factors in either partner appears to be low. Two small studies of seropositive military applicants found that 20 of 24 applicants in New York City who sought counseling actually had recognized risk factors, and 11 of 12 applicants in Colorado had risk factors (e.g., male homosexual contacts). In addition, 30 of 33 seropositive male active-duty military personnel revealed recognized risk factors when interviewed. Among seropositive blood donors interviewed in Los Angeles, Baltimore, and Atlanta, 153 of 186 donors (82 percent) had risk factors; of those interviewed in New York City, 97 of 109 (89 percent) had risk factors. These data suggest that as few as 15 percent of infected military applicants and blood donors acquired their infection heterosexually. This would imply that the prevalence rate for *heterosexually acquired* HIV infection was 0.021 percent for military applicants (adjusted for age, sex, and race) and 0.006 percent for blood donors.

[12] "Without known risk factors" means without histories of IV drug use, male homosexual contacts, sexual contact with persons known to be infected, or hemophilia or transfusions prior to the adoption of universal blood donation screening.

Variation by Age. There were marked differences in the cumulative AIDS incidence and available measurements of HIV prevalence by age, sex, race, and ethnicity. For age, the available cross-sectional data indicated a differential prevalence of HIV infection that rose from the mid-teens to a peak in the early 30s, and then declined in the 40s and 50s. In theory, such a pattern might arise from two opposing age trends:

- The young have been exposed to the risk of infection for less cumulative time, which might tend to produce lower prevalence at younger ages.
- With increasing age, there may be decreased frequency of behaviors that risk infection. For example, a 20-year-old is apt to be more sexually active, to have more partners per year, and, perhaps, to be more likely to use IV drugs than a 50-year-old. Some of these patterns may be hard to verify. Nonetheless, to the degree that they apply, they suggest that, during the years since AIDS appeared, the sexual activities of older persons may have been, on average, less risky than those of their younger contemporaries.

One implication that follows from these opposing trends is that the age distribution of persons infected with HIV might be quite different in a region to which HIV came late (versus a region that was affected earlier) because the tendency on the part of the young to accumulate risky experience would exert less influence.

Variation by Gender. The cumulative prevalence of AIDS cases (i.e., the total number of cases for each gender divided by the number of cases) was 13 times higher among men than among women. However, the cited HIV prevalence rates varied widely; the male-to-female ratio of prevalence was 5.5:1 among military applicants (adjusted by age and race), 4.6:1 among blood donors, 2.3:1 among sentinel hospital patients, and the ratio apparently approaches 1:1 among IV drug users. In theory, the variation in these ratios should reflect (1) the sex composition of the underlying risk groups plus (2) the extent to which these risk groups may be included in the population being considered. Considering the entire population, the 13:1 preponderance of men among AIDS cases reflects the fact that most AIDS cases in the United States have occurred among men who have sex with men and among IV drug users. If, however, only women and men who already belonged to one of the risk groups (e.g., IV drug users) were considered, a different result would be expected (e.g., the approximately 1:1 ratio reported for this group).[13]

Variation Among Blacks, Whites, and Hispanics. Although blacks constitute only 11.6 percent of the national population, approximately one quarter of reported AIDS cases in adults and one half of cases in children have been among blacks. Similarly, more than one tenth of adult cases and two tenths of pediatric cases have been diagnosed among Hispanics, who account for 6.5 percent of the national population. Estimates of HIV prevalence rates have been more variable, but the disproportion is consistent (see CDC [1988a:Table 10]). In the four hospitals studied in the Midwest, the seroprevalence rate for blacks was 3.2 times higher than that for whites. Among IV drug users, the reported seroprevalence rates for blacks were 1.7 to 5.1 times higher than those for whites; for Hispanics, the rates were 1.7 to 3.3 times higher. Similarly, seroprevalence rates among black and Hispanic military recruits were 6.9 and 3.0 times higher, respectively, than the seroprevalence rate for white recruits.

Geographic Spread of the Epidemic. Although there is a geographic correlation between AIDS prevalence and HIV prevalence, there are also important discrepancies that suggest that the AIDS case data will have only limited usefulness as a proxy measure of HIV infection. (Indeed, it may be possible to obtain important insights about the epidemic's spread by studying the divergences between the picture of the epidemic provided by the AIDS case reports and that provided by programs monitoring HIV infection.) The AIDS statistics for a particular locale are the manifest expression of the unseen history of HIV infection in the population of that locale. The cumulative count of AIDS cases increases with the number of infections and their duration. Other things being equal, a large disparity in the ratio of AIDS cases to cases of HIV infection in two areas (given accurate data) may suggest that the time course of infection was different in the two locales.[14]

---

[13]The roughly 1:1 ratio cited for IV drug users is inferred from the statement (CDC, 1987a:10) that "[b]y contrast, in the one principal risk group that includes women—IV drug users—the prevalence does not differ appreciably by sex." The 1:1 ratio cited for IV drug users could be produced in a number of ways, among them equivalence in needle-sharing behaviors and random mixing (by gender and HIV status) of sharing groups.

[14]The disparity is not, however, definitive evidence. That conclusion would require several strong assumptions—for example, that there were no differences across the populations in the two locales in the distribution of probabilities of progressing from HIV infection to AIDS in year 1, 2, 3, 4, . . ., and so on. Yet it has been suggested that the

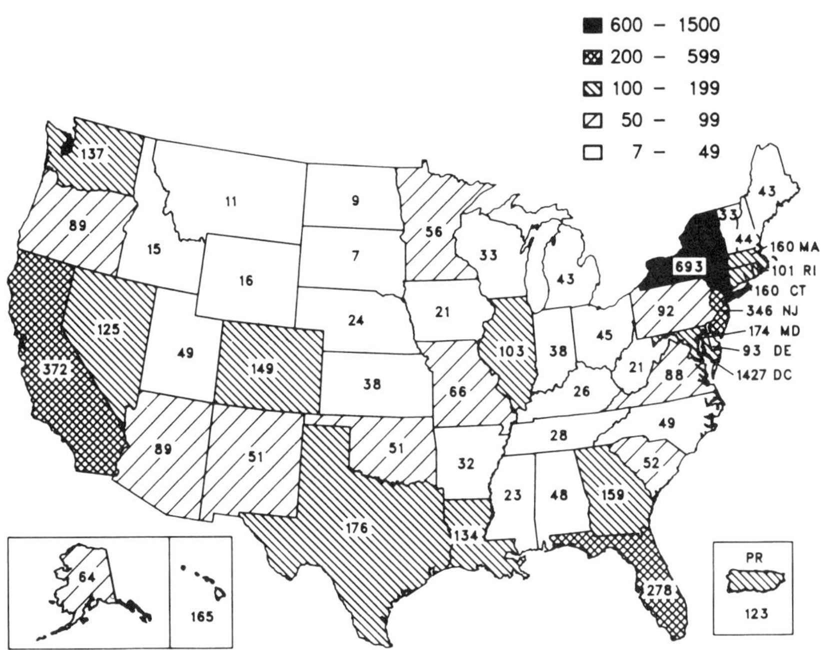

FIGURE 1-1 Incidence of AIDS cases ($N = 44{,}745$), by state, per million population, November 2, 1987. SOURCE: CDC (1987a).

Recognizing that there are competing hypotheses and that the available data on HIV prevalence are imperfect, it may nonetheless be instructive to consider the state-level data presented by CDC (Figures 1-1 and 1-2). As shown in Figure 1-1, the locales with the highest cumulative incidence of AIDS for the population were

1. District of Columbia — 1.43 per 1,000
2. New York — 0.69 per 1,000
3. California — 0.37 per 1,000
4. New Jersey — 0.35 per 1,000
5. Florida — 0.28 per 1,000

The five locales with the highest HIV prevalence rates among military recruits (Figure 1-2) were

distribution may be different for adults and children; thus, a crude comparison of rates in two populations could be misleading if there were differences in the relative numbers of infected children. There are many other possible confounding factors for which there are no data.

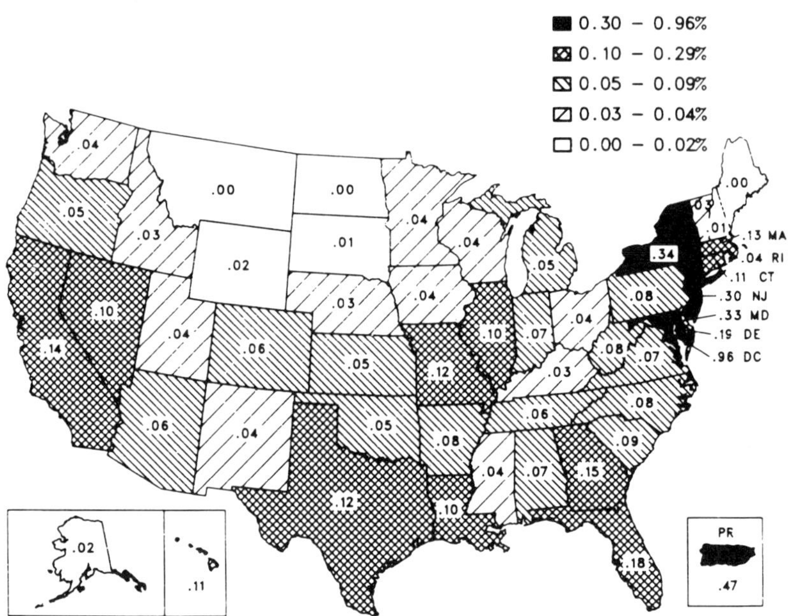

FIGURE 1-2 Sex-adjusted HIV antibody prevalence (percent positive) among applicants for military service (N = 1,253,768) by state for the period from October 1985 to September 1987. SOURCE: CDC (1987a).

1. District of Columbia	9.6 per 1,000
2. Puerto Rico	4.7 per 1,000
3. New York	3.4 per 1,000
4. Maryland	3.3 per 1,000
5. New Jersey	3.0 per 1,000

Two jurisdictions that were included among the top five in the HIV rankings—Puerto Rico (no. 2) and Maryland (no. 4)—were not ranked in the top five in cumulative AIDS incidence. (Puerto Rico had a cumulative AIDS incidence rate of .12 per 1,000; the Maryland rate was .17 per 1,000.)

These data begin to suggest hypotheses about the timing of the geographic spread of the epidemic between adjacent jurisdictions (e.g., D.C. and Maryland) and jurisdictions that comingle segments of their population through migration and tourism (e.g., New York and Puerto Rico). Although these data can suggest hypotheses, they cannot provide a fully reliable indicator of the timing of the geographic spread of HIV. Military recruits do not fairly represent the population; thus, data about their rates of HIV prevalence may not provide accurate rankings of jurisdictions in terms of the prevalence of infection.[15]

These data demonstrate the inconsistencies that can arise in using prevalence and incidence rates obtained from the testing of special populations. If another source of state-level HIV prevalence data had been used, the picture might have been different. For example, Mississippi, which has one of the lowest HIV prevalence rates among military recruits (0.4 per 1,000) would be near the top of a ranking of HIV prevalence on the basis of tests of blood donors.[16]

Uncertainties About HIV Prevalence

Although the above "patterns" can provide some crude guidance as to the relative prevalence of HIV infection in different groups, there are substantial difficulties in the interpretation of these data. It is clear, for example, that the various studies of HIV prevalence included in the CDC report sometimes used different exclusion criteria. Some studies compared rates based on all individuals, while other studies specifically excluded patients diagnosed with AIDS, AIDS-related condition (ARC),[17] or "recognized" HIV infection. For instance, the Multicenter AIDS Cohort Study (MACS) specifically excluded AIDS patients. HIV seroprevalence rates from the MACS are based on 5,000 homosexuals who were free of AIDS at their initial visit. Other studies, such as seroprevalence studies of emergency room patients, may have included some AIDS patients in the calculation of prevalence rates. This lack of consistent criteria introduces

---

[15] For example, to the extent that states vary in the distribution of infected individuals across risk groups (e.g., homosexual men and IV drug users) and members of these groups vary in their likelihood of volunteering for military service, the recruit data will provide a different ranking of HIV prevalence.

[16] Mississippi's rate for blood donors is .25 per 1,000, which is the fifth highest rate shown in the CDC figure. Some of the states were combined, however, so the comparison is not precise. Nonetheless, Mississippi's rate of .25 exceeds that of New Jersey (.20 for blood donors), which ranked among the top five on both cumulative AIDS incidence and HIV prevalence among military recruits.

[17] A term formerly used to describe a variety of symptoms and physical findings that may occur subsequent to HIV infection but that do not satisfy CDC's surveillance definition of AIDS (Institute of Medicine/National Academy of Sciences [IOM/NAS], 1986:353). Today, with a better understanding of the natural history of HIV infection, the term *ARC* is falling into disuse. Another IOM/NAS committee has recently recommended that use of the term ARC be discontinued and that HIV infection itself be considered a disease (IOM/NAS, 1988:37).

considerable uncertainty in the comparison and synthesis of findings from the studies in the CDC report.

The prevalence data also indicate, as would be expected, that there can be large differences in the results obtained from convenience samplings of what might appear to be the same population. So, for example, estimates of the prevalence of HIV infection among female prostitutes in New York City are reported as 14.3 percent on the basis of an "outreach" study conducted during 1985–1987 and 1.5 percent on the basis of a different outreach study conducted during 1986–1987.

There are also problems in using such data to target interventions to specific groups. First, there are the obvious selection biases. Prevalence estimates based on samples of gay men recruited at STD clinics will probably be higher than those that would apply to gay men in general because men recruited at an STD clinic are being treated for a disease whose mode of transmission parallels that of HIV infection. Similarly, as noted earlier, most potential blood donors in high-risk groups will presumably avoid donating blood, thereby reducing the prevalence of HIV among blood donors to a rate below that of the population in general. These biases subvert the usefulness of such data for decision making.

The committee also notes that discussions of the source, direction, and magnitude of biases in these samples are largely conjectural. Very little empirical research has been done to characterize these biases. Because HIV prevalence data will continue to be available from military recruits and blood donors, it would be valuable to explore these biases empirically. Careful studies documenting the nature of the interrelationships between trends across time in HIV prevalence in well-defined populations (estimated from probability samples) and trends in HIV prevalence found in these special groups would be especially valuable. Over time, such studies might provide an empirical basis for broadening the interpretation of trend data derived from these screening programs.[18]

In addition to the problems introduced by bias in the composition of the groups studied, the committee notes that other uncertainties about the data arise in the laboratory. The procedures used to determine HIV seroprevalence in the various studies cited in the CDC

[18]Attempts to develop seroprevalence maps for local areas and to model HIV prevalence for regions by combining estimates from a multiplicity of screening programs and convenience samples might also be pursued. A key challenge in such efforts, however, will be providing clear and convincing rationales for the estimates of self-selection probabilities (i.e., the probability that a given member of the target population will appear in a particular convenience sample; see Manton and Singer [1988]).

report were not standardized across studies. Furthermore, HIV antibody tests may be sensitive to non-HIV infections and other biological factors that may introduce further inaccuracies into comparisons across studies. These inaccuracies are especially problematic in the study of low-prevalence populations. Finally, clerical errors (even if rare) can seriously distort already low prevalence estimates.

When the Department of Defense instituted HIV testing of applicants for enlistment in the armed forces, it established a system to standardize the HIV testing used in the program and to monitor the quality of testing done at laboratories. Similarly, CDC has established a system for testing the proficiency of laboratories conducting HIV tests as part of CDC's surveillance program. Such quality assurance programs were these agencies' responses to the widely documented experience of noncomparability of laboratory measurements performed in different places with different personnel and equipment, even on much less exacting tests than those used to detect HIV infection. Because all prevalence statistics (and clinical diagnoses) rely on test results, the level of accuracy of such results should be as high as is technically possible. What is needed is a system for monitoring the quality of HIV testing, *wherever it is performed.* **The committee recommends that an appropriate federal agency mount a continuing program to monitor HIV testing at all laboratories doing such testing.** In making this recommendation, the committee records its support for the recent recommendation on this same topic by the Presidential Commission on the Human Immunodeficiency Virus Epidemic (1988:Recommendation no. 6-33).

Principles and Methods of Estimating Prevalence

This section begins by describing an "ideal" survey for measuring HIV prevalence in a defined group. It then identifies some of the obstacles that inevitably arise in conducting surveys and the ways in which such obstacles can be overcome. The section also offers recommendations for a realistic program to measure HIV prevalence.

An ideal survey of HIV prevalence would include four steps: (1) select a probability sample from the group of interest; (2) obtain a blood specimen from each person in the sample; (3) accurately assess the HIV serostatus of each blood specimen; and (4) combine the individual results using the statistical formulas applicable to the kind of probability sample that produced the data.

Probability Samples

The theory and practice of probability sampling—"coin of the realm" in efforts to describe a population—are well developed. The Consumer Price Index (CPI), the National Health and Nutrition Examination Survey (NHANES), and the statistics on unemployment all use this method, primarily because it yields unbiased estimates (when execution is flawless) and valid indications of the uncertainty of those estimates. When the cooperation of institutions—such as hospitals—is needed to reach the sample, however, there may be complications. Some institutions may be more cooperative than others, some may keep better records, and some may be more desirable targets because, for example, past data may exist that can provide a historical context for the new measurements. Such considerations may demand recognition and accommodation. Fortunately, the accommodation need not be to abandon probability sampling; it may instead call for giving preferred institutions large probabilities of selection (even certainty can be provided), with less preferred institutions receiving smaller selection probabilities (although the selection probability may not be zero for any institution). Much expertise regarding issues of this kind resides in the National Center for Health Statistics, which is now a component of CDC.

Full Coverage of the Sample

Obtaining blood from each person in the sample may not be easy. Indeed, some people in a sample will not let their blood be drawn, and such refusals (nonresponse) can seriously distort prevalence estimates. Hull and colleagues (1988) report a survey in which 18 percent of a group declined to provide a blood specimen; among those 18 percent, there were more HIV positive results than among the 82 percent who did provide specimens.[19] Thus, even modest nonresponse can gravely compromise the accuracy of results.

One device for coping with possible nonresponse is to assure respondents of the confidentiality (or even anonymity) of the information they are to provide—and then to ensure that such assurances

---

[19]Every person in the group had previously given a blood specimen, and the specimens had been anonymously tested (i.e., the specimens had no personal identifiers); consequently, the total number of HIV positives was known. The number of positive results among the 18 percent who declined to give a blood specimen ($n = 9$) was more than that found among the identified specimens of the 82 percent who did not refuse the second time ($n = 8$).

are realized. Such methods as replacing names with in-house identification numbers and restricting access to files help ensure confidentiality. Provisions must also be made to forestall the possibility of "deductive disclosure." For example, a report that two 35-year-old women at hospital B gave birth to seropositive male infants on January 4 might allow the identification of the mothers from public birth records if the hospital is small (because there might have been only two male births to 35-year-old mothers in that hospital that day).

There are many ways to "coarsen" data to prevent deductive disclosure, and some methods are more effective than others. Replacing the date of birth with the month of birth introduces a 30-fold reduction in specificity and seems to lose very little useful information; removing the mother's race, however, would yield less reduction in specificity at a cost of more valuable information. Data release and reporting standards for the protection of confidentiality deserve thorough deliberation and careful policy making. Such procedures can easily develop through an ad hoc process and be suboptimal. Finding ways to safeguard confidentiality while permitting scientists to use these important data to the maximum extent feasible requires detailed study. **The committee recommends that CDC and other agencies with HIV/AIDS data gathering and reporting functions review their data disclosure practices, searching for rules and setting policies that continue to safeguard confidentiality but do so at the least practical cost in information.** It should be recognized, however, that no matter how strong the assurance of confidentiality and the measures to ensure it, some people will continue to refuse to furnish blood specimens (or other information).

A second approach to the goal of obtaining a blood specimen from each person in the sample is to use blood specimens that have no patient identifiers—that is, "blind" blood specimens that have already been obtained for some other purpose. This approach guarantees that the identity of the donor will neither be known nor be traceable to the blood specimen. Carefully considered minimal personal information such as the donor's gender, race, and age (but not date of birth) may accompany the sample. No ethical problem of violating an individual's privacy arises with this approach because no one's HIV status becomes known to anyone (including the donor, who will need another test if that knowledge is desired). The disadvantages to this approach are that individuals cannot be followed over time, and only meager information about the donor can be related to his or her HIV status. Still, a blind survey may deal with the nonresponse bias problem quite effectively. (It is feasible to use analogous methods in studies that collect blood specimens for the specific purpose of testing for HIV. In that case, all identifying information would have to be destroyed prior to the testing of the blood specimens. For further discussion, see Turner and Fay, in this volume.)

Accurate Testing

Good laboratory tests for HIV serostatus exist, but long experience shows that it is difficult to maintain high levels of accuracy. The committee reaffirms its recommendation that an appropriate federal agency establish an effective surveillance and quality-monitoring program that includes every laboratory permitted to do HIV testing.

Combining Results

A rather subtle difficulty attends the step of combining results in a survey. Some few individuals who are not infected will nevertheless test seropositive—because of laboratory error, clerical error, or perhaps some phenomenon known only to virologists (or future virologists). In short, some false positives are inevitable, a factor that is particularly significant in the case of a low-prevalence condition such as HIV infection, for which even a small false-positive rate can be important. Thus, if 1 truly uninfected person in 500 gave a false-positive test result and the actual prevalence of HIV infection in the group being tested were 1 in 1,000, the list of seropositives would include three times as many individuals as it should, two thirds of whom are actually infection free. It will be impossible to tell which individuals are true positives and which are false positives. Furthermore, any change in testing error rates will appear to be a change in prevalence. This contingency can be dealt with in two steps: (1) by systematically monitoring HIV testing labs to obtain information about the magnitude of the HIV false-positive rate at each facility and (2) by using that information to adjust the observed prevalence rates.

THE 1989 HIV SURVEILLANCE SYSTEM

The present HIV surveillance system consists of six components that constitute what CDC calls its "comprehensive family of surveys." The data produced by this survey program are intended to accomplish the following objectives:

- "to obtain information on the incidence [of new cases of infection] and prevalence of HIV infection in risk groups and other defined populations" (CDC, 1987b:Appendix p. 2);[20]
- to provide early warning of the possible emergence of HIV infection in new populations;
- to assist in targeting prevention activities and planning for future health care and other service needs; and
- to evaluate the effectiveness of AIDS prevention activities.

This surveillance program was put in place in 1987–1988;[21] it will survey HIV prevalence (and, where possible, related behavioral risk factors) for six groups: IV drug users, patients at general hospitals, patients treated at STD clinics, patients at TB clinics, patients at clinics serving women of reproductive age, and newborn babies. These surveys are being conducted in the 20 metropolitan areas of the United States that report 75 percent of the current AIDS cases and in 10 other metropolitan areas with moderate to low AIDS prevalence. The survey program will be the nation's major source of HIV surveillance statistics for the next several years.[22]

Because of the importance of this program, the committee's Panel on Statistical Issues in AIDS Research undertook a review of the six protocols that describe the individual surveys and how they will be conducted. As a result of this review, the committee has concluded that—with the exception of the screening of newborns—none of the surveys will remedy the major deficit that exists in our current knowledge: *these surveys cannot characterize (with knowable margins of error) the prevalence or incidence of HIV infection in any well-defined population.* As was true of all of the studies reported in CDC's 1987 review of HIV prevalence, five of the six components of the family of surveys program gather data from non-population-based samples that cannot be generalized to any larger population of interest.

---

[20]From the appendix entitled "Summary of HHS Plan to Determine the Incidence, Prevalence and Risk Factors for HIV Infection in the United States"; see p. 2, Point IV.

[21]Elements of the "sentinel hospital" surveillance component (CDC, 1988c) were begun during 1986.

[22]Developmental programs to test the feasibility of other strategies (e.g., HIV testing of stratified probability samples of the population) are just now beginning. However, even if preliminary testing demonstrated that these strategies were feasible, data gathering could not begin until late 1989, and the first results would probably not be available until 1990 at the earliest.

This conclusion, although strong and adverse, describes the results of a natural flow of events. Let us consider the four listed objectives of the "comprehensive family of surveys"; they serve two purposes—and those purposes are in tension. One is to help *manage* the public health problem of HIV spread at the local level. This purpose is well served by choosing study sites that have a high prevalence of infection or that are judged to be especially liable to large increases in prevalence; this purpose is also well served by selecting from among many clinics in a metropolitan area the one or two that offer the most cooperation, have the best records, and so on. Yet the second purpose (actually listed first), "to obtain information on the incidence and prevalence of HIV infection in risk groups and other defined populations," is severely compromised by the same purposive selections. Fortunately, the tension between the two purposes might be eased by suitably enlarging the surveys to become *probability samples* (i.e., involving the already chosen study sites as certainty strata). The opportunity to improve the family of surveys in this way is too important to bypass without serious investigation. To forego this opportunity would threaten the scientists and policy makers of 1995 with the same data problems that bedeviled the 1987 report on HIV prevalence: imponderable uncertainty about the prevalence and incidence of HIV infection in nearly every group of interest.

The committee recommends that efforts be made to reformulate the CDC family of seroprevalence surveys as probability samples. We believe this reformulation should be done as expeditiously as is compatible with good work.

To familiarize readers with the current family of surveys program, we describe in some detail the design and problems of two of the surveys and briefly note our concerns about three of the others. This section concludes with a description of the neonatal screening survey, the one component that is not subject to the criticisms of the other five parts of the family of surveys program. Indeed, the committee recommends that the neonatal program be expanded nationwide as soon as is practical (see the discussion later in this section).

Surveillance of IV Drug Users

Two kinds of cross-sectional surveys[23] will be conducted to monitor HIV prevalence among users of IV drugs: surveys of IV drug

[23]These surveys will supplement other studies by the National Institute on Drug Abuse (NIDA), which is currently supporting seroprevalence surveys in six cities of those IV

users who are currently in treatment and surveys of those who enter treatment in the future. These surveys will include clients at approximately 50 drug treatment centers in 30 metropolitan areas.

The in-treatment and entrant samples have the same stated objectives:

1. to estimate seroprevalence and correlate it with the demographic characteristics of individuals;
2. to obtain risk factor data from individuals where feasible and correlate risky behavior with seroprevalence; and
3. to establish benchmark estimates of behavior so that changes in behavior over time can be noted (see CDC/National Institute on Drug Abuse [NIDA], 1988:11).[24]

The reason for conducting the in-treatment surveys in addition to entrant surveys is to "rapidly ascertain HIV seroprevalence by sampling IVDUs [IV drug users] currently enrolled in drug treatment—populations that are relatively large and accessible" (CDC/NIDA, 1988:13). The in-treatment surveys are to be conducted only in situations in which seroprevalence among IV drug users is unknown and in which "relatively few IVDUs enter treatment, thus making rapid seroprevalence ascertainment from the 'entrant' survey difficult" (p. 14).

The entrant surveys will be conducted in two versions: blinded and nonblinded. In the blinded surveys, the IV drug users entering treatment will neither be informed of the survey nor of the results of their blood test. The nonblinded study will obtain informed consent prior to testing from the persons entering treatment. The nonblinded studies should be able to obtain more detailed information about "risky" behavior; in addition, trained personnel will be able to inform participants of their test results and provide counseling. The blinded studies will have higher (within-center) participation rates, however, because persons entering the center will not have the opportunity to refuse to participate. The CDC/NIDA protocol for this survey expresses the hope that "[i]deally, both blinded and non-blinded surveys should be conducted simultaneously in a treatment center. In this way, a non-biased estimate of HIV seroprevalence will be obtained . . ." (1988:16).

---

drug users who are either in treatment or who are reached by AIDS community outreach demonstration projects. The NIDA surveys are based on a nonrandom selection of sites.

[24]It should be noted that objective (3) might be accomplished without coupling the measurement of "risky" behavior to blood testing.

The estimate of seroprevalence from the blinded survey should yield an unbiased estimate of seroprevalence for that particular center. Yet unbiased estimates of seroprevalence among all IV drug users in treatment cannot be obtained under the proposed design. The major problem with the survey design is what appears to be a vaguely specified but unquestionably nonrandom selection method for choosing the drug treatment centers that will be included in the sample.[25] The lack of randomization is disturbing for two reasons. First, estimates of seroprevalence will be subject to biases, the magnitudes of which are unknown and most likely cannot even be estimated. Second, estimates of sampling error will miss what could be the major source of sampling variability—variability in seroprevalence across treatment centers within a metropolitan area.

A further problem with the survey design is the small number of drug treatment centers in the sample. A 50-center sample (the size proposed by CDC/NIDA) allows the surveying, on average, of only one or two centers from each of the 30 metropolitan areas. Using so few centers could make comparisons among metropolitan areas quite imprecise if there were substantial variability in seroprevalence among treatment centers in a given area. Indeed, this potentially important source of variability will not be assessed in the study. The documents that describe how local contractors should conduct the survey ignore entirely the component of sampling variability that arises in the selection of treatment centers. Thus, the protocol's specification of required sample sizes (CDC/NIDA, 1988:21ff) presumes that individual drug users are the sampling unit in a single-stage random selection. The protocol provides tables that purport to show the sample sizes necessary to detect differences with prespecified levels of statistical power. Yet the calculations that were used to produce these tables employ a statistical model appropriate for simple random sampling of individual IV drug users, which is not the type of sampling that is being used in the survey design.

If treatment centers were sampled (rather than selected), the design would be a multistage (cluster) sample of IV drug users with treatment centers defining the clusters. The (probably positive) intraclass correlation within treatment centers would imply that sample sizes larger than those envisioned in the proposal would be needed to attain the power indicated. Unequal selection probabilities for IV drug users in different centers would compound this problem.

[25]Some kind of stratified allocation of treatment centers is envisioned but only vaguely described in the proposal (CDC/NIDA, 1988:12).

Sentinel Hospital Surveillance

The Sentinel Hospital Surveillance program (CDC, 1988c) is intended to obtain estimates of HIV prevalence using a general hospital population sample that is not self-selected. Eight medical facilities were included in the program in 1986–1988; the survey design calls for the extension of this network to include 40 hospitals nationally, with at least 30 located in the metropolitan areas targeted by the other HIV surveys. Participating institutions must be either a short-term general hospital, a health maintenance organization, or a consortium of hospitals in the same area. They must have adult, pediatric, and emergency services, and they must receive a minimum of 17,500 annual admissions (including emergency room visits).

The general survey procedure includes a number of essentials. Infection is indicated by serologic positivity, which is established by a positive ELISA[26] confirmed by a Western blot test.[27] Only blood specimens that have already been collected for other purposes are eligible for testing. These specimens must be drawn from patients on hospital clinical services with little recognized association with AIDS.[28] An aliquot (0.5 milliliter minimum) will be drawn off from the blood specimen and labeled with the patient's sex, race or ethnic group,[29] age in years, and the month and year of collection. The clinical service will be indicated on a separate label.

Each month a random subsample of 300 specimens will be selected independent of clinical service according to a specified age/sex stratification. The stratification ensures that equal numbers of men and women are selected within each age group, and it counteracts

---

[26] Enzyme-linked immunosorbent assay, a test used to detect antibodies against HIV in blood specimens (see the 1986 and 1988 IOM/NAS reports).

[27] The Western blot technique involves the identification of antibodies against specific protein molecules. It is believed to be more specific than the ELISA in detecting antibodies to HIV; it is also more difficult to perform and considerably more expensive. (For further information, see IOM/NAS [1986, 1988].)

[28] Eligible services include cardiovascular, endocrinology, obstetrics, ophthalmology, orthopedics, pediatric ear–nose–throat (excluding middle-ear infection), adult ear–nose–throat (except patients hospitalized for cancer or biopsy), emergency (except patients hospitalized for infectious diseases), gynecology (except patients hospitalized for infections, STDs, cancer, or biopsy), general surgery (except patients hospitalized for cancer or biopsy), and pediatric surgery (except patients hospitalized for cancer or biopsy). Also eligible are patients hospitalized for accidents, poisoning, burns, trauma (excluding gunshot and stab wounds), drowning, asthma, cerebrovascular accidents, and hernias.

[29] The coded race and ethnic groups are "white (not Hispanic)," "black (not Hispanic)," "Hispanic," "other," and "not specified." If at least 10 percent of the blood specimens are from an identifiable racial or ethnic group (other than black, white, or Hispanic), that group is to be coded.

the overrepresentation of the aged in hospital populations. In addition, the design requires that hospitals with fewer than 50 percent nonwhite patients oversample blood specimens from these patients.

Seroprevalence rates will be calculated by age group, sex, and race. Composite rates adjusted by age and sex for each hospital, for the region, and for the nation will also be calculated. Data for individual hospitals and cities will not be published; instead, ranges of values for institutions and regions will be offered. State and local authorities and participating hospitals will receive summaries of data for their own specimens, as well as regional and national results.

Because the surveillance uses blind testing of blood specimens with no personal identifiers retained, self-selection biases will be avoided. However, once again, the hospitals themselves will be selected rather than sampled. In selecting the participating hospitals, CDC (1988c:45) states that "weight will be given to the offeror's breadth of representativeness and the probable consistency of representativeness." To this end, potential sites are asked to provide information on the geographic and socioeconomic characteristics of the population they serve and the "approximate proportion" of nonwhites among their patient populations. Although such data may guide the survey designers to choose hospitals with particular types of population diversity, it does not overcome the major inadequacy of the design.

Like the survey of IV drug users, the sentinel hospital surveillance system eschews the sampling of hospitals within the 30 metropolitan areas. Because only 40 hospitals will be chosen to participate, in most cities this surveillance system will be monitoring prevalence in one hospital, HMO, or consortium. If there is considerable variation in seroprevalence rates for hospitals within the same metropolitan area, there must be doubts about the ability of this system to meet its explicitly stated objective "to obtain information to indicate current prevalence of HIV infection in the United States, and more importantly, changes in prevalence over time" (CDC, 1988c:1). This does not imply, of course, that the resultant data would not be suggestive or that this type of surveillance system would not provide information that could be obtained rapidly and economically. Yet the value of this information would be immeasurably enhanced if the study design were altered so that prevalence data could be projected to the entire hospital population and not merely to the 40 hospitals included in this sample.

Surveys of STD and TB Clinics and Clinics Serving Women of Reproductive Age

In its review of the other components of the CDC family of surveys program (CDC, 1988a,b,d), the committee's statistical panel determined that these components (with the exception of neonatal screening) shared the deficiency in sampling that characterizes the surveys of IV drug users and sentinel hospitals. Consequently, we do not describe these components of the survey in detail but instead raise certain other issues that pertain particularly to them.

For the surveys targeted at clinics serving women of reproductive age, the committee is concerned about the substantive justification for including all of the different types of clinics: family planning, prenatal, abortion, and the Special Supplemental Food Program for Women, Infants, and Children (WIC). We find little reason to conduct blinded surveys in prenatal clinics. The screening of newborns (discussed later in this chapter) will provide better information on the HIV status of women giving birth, and such a screening captures the entire population of these women. However, representative data on the serostatus of women who have abortions would be extremely valuable. Unfortunately, as with the other components of the survey program, the study of women attending abortion clinics will not be generalizable to the population of women using such clinics.

The panel was surprised to find that the survey designers did not stratify their selection of clinics by type (e.g., prenatal, abortion, etc.). Without controlling the mix of clinics in different geographic areas, it becomes difficult to make comparisons across areas.

In reviewing the protocol for the blinded HIV prevalence surveys of patients at TB clinics, the committee felt that further consideration might be given to the use of *confidential* rather than *anonymous* testing. Current standards of medical practice dictate HIV testing for all TB patients because preliminary evidence suggests that TB patients with HIV infection require a modification of the standard antituberculosis therapy. Thus, both CDC and the American Thoracic Society have recommended a more aggressive approach to the treatment of TB in HIV-infected patients. It might reasonably be argued that if it is good medical practice to test for HIV infection in all TB patients, then clinics should perform such tests and patient permission should be sought to use these data for statistical purposes. If so, confidentiality, rather than anonymity, would be important.

One cannot rule out the possibility, of course, that such testing would lead to substantial rates of nonresponse, but it is also possible that people who come to a clinic for treatment of a major disease will be less likely to refuse to participate. They may be even less likely to refuse when they learn that HIV testing is necessary for the effective treatment of their condition. In any event, a small amount of anonymous testing could be used as a check on selection bias.

While we do not wish to recommend unequivocally a confidential (nonblinded) survey of TB patients, we do believe that CDC should reconsider this option if the major purpose of this survey is to assess the prevalence of HIV in patients of public TB clinics. In this reconsideration, it would be desirable for CDC to pilot-test a nonblinded screening procedure to determine whether it produces high levels of nonresponse. The committee recognizes, however, that the data gathered from TB clinics may have other uses (see the discussion later in this chapter) and these uses may legitimately influence the data collection strategy.

Data Management

A final area of concern to the committee regarding the family of surveys program involves the program's proposed data management plan. This plan seems to ensure that some data will be discarded to ensure confidentiality.[30] This outcome would result from the requirement that there be a minimum number of persons per stratum (e.g., black men aged 20–24), which is applied to the smallest possible group by month and by site. Considering that yearly (or half-yearly) trends are likely to be the data of interest, it should be possible to wait until a year's worth of data has accumulated before transmitting it to the central data collection site. Alternatively, some central facility within each metropolitan area could aggregate data for that area, and restrictions could be placed on the availability of results for specific clinics.

Neonatal Screening

The neonatal screening (CDC/NIH, 1988) is unique among the surveys planned for the 30 target cities included in the family of surveys

[30]Discussions with CDC staff indicate that this aspect of the plan probably resulted from attempts to guarantee anonymity *at the clinic level* in the blended surveys. Because HIV test results will be identifiable by clinic, the data disclosure possibilities are great (particularly since some of the clinic samples will be small). Although the committee has no solution to propose, it does believe further study of this issue is warranted. Among the alternative strategies that might be considered are relaxation of the requirement that *all* HIV test results be identifiable by clinic.

program. It is the only survey to provide seroprevalence data that, by design, can be generalized to an identifiable population.

The CDC/National Institutes of Health (NIH) neonatal survey will perform HIV tests using the dried blood specimens that are routinely collected from all (hospital-born) newborns (to test for metabolic disorders). Because children born to HIV-infected mothers carry the mother's antibodies (without necessarily being infected themselves),[31] the HIV seroprevalence rates derived from this screening can be projected both to the population of newborns and to the population of childbearing women. (Estimates of the number of newborns who are actually infected, as opposed to the number who are passively carrying the mother's antibodies without infection, will require ancillary studies; these studies might be performed on small subsamples, however.) The statistics derived from this survey will provide a basis both for projecting future AIDS cases among infants and, perhaps most importantly, for monitoring the prevalence of infection among an important part of the population of heterosexually active women.

Although the neonatal survey is unique in its ability to provide seroprevalence estimates that reflect rates of infection in an important, identifiable population, it is not perfect. The group of women represented by these statistics will not include all women who may be at risk of infection. For example, the group does not include women who choose not to bear children, women who abort or miscarry prior to delivery,[32] or women who have ceased childbearing. Because serostatus may influence a woman's decision to avoid pregnancy or to abort after conception, biases of uncertain magnitude may occur when these data are generalized beyond the operational definition of the population studied (i.e., all women who delivered a live child in a hospital during a particular time period). The magnitude and direction of one of these biases may be estimated, however, by conducting ancillary studies of the serostatus of probability samples of, in particular, women who abort. Consequently, **the committee recommends instituting a continuing anonymous probability survey of the HIV serostatus of women who are clients of clinics that provide abortion services.**

---

[31] All newborns of HIV-seropositive women carry the maternal antibody to HIV, even though the infants themselves may not be infected. It is estimated that there is a 30–50 percent risk of perinatal HIV transmission from an infected mother to her child and subsequent diagnosis of AIDS in the infant (IOM/NAS, 1988:35).

[32] The draft protocol (CDC/NIH, 1988:20) notes that attempts will be made in another program to monitor seroprevalence in aborted fetuses; no details are given of this effort.

Other aspects of the neonatal survey also require attention. Interpretation of the seroprevalence statistics derived in this survey will require that analysts grapple with the systematic differences between women who bear children (particularly those who bear many children) and those who do not. For example, the seroprevalence rates that are obtained in the newborn screening survey will be affected by childbearing women in proportion to the number of children they bear. Obtaining and recording information on the birth order of the infant may permit estimation of the size of this bias so that the HIV seroprevalence estimates for childbearing women can be adjusted to correct for it. Interpreting the results of the neonatal screening will be greatly assisted by the various reliable sources of statistical data on the characteristics of childbearing women already in existence (e.g., the National Survey of Family Growth and the registry of births).

The newborn survey will be conducted statewide in all of the states that encompass the 30 cities included in the family of surveys program. These blinded surveys will be conducted by the states' public health departments; CDC/NIH is also urging state health departments in the rest of the nation to participate in this survey. The survey protocol calls for a quarter-inch "punch" to be removed at the processing laboratory from the filter paper containing blood obtained from a newborn heel stick. This small sample will be tested for HIV; the remainder of the filter paper will continue to be used in tests for neonatal metabolic disorders. The protocol asserts that "virtually 100 percent of babies born in the United States are screened [in this manner] for phenylketonuria and congenital hypothyroidism" (CDC/NIH, 1988:6).

The protocol also describes various alternatives for sampling the blood specimens. We believe it would be best to include all infants in the sample. First, it is not an impracticably large task because every baby is already tested (from the same specimen) for other purposes. Second, a large sample is helpful because of the low prevalence of HIV infection. Seroprevalence in women is in the .001 to .01 range; let us use .003 for the purposes of this example. In a county with a population of 1 million, about 16,000 births can be expected annually. Of those, approximately 48 will be seropositive. Even with 100 percent HIV testing, as soon as subgroups are considered (e.g., "older white mothers" or "younger Hispanic mothers"), there will be only a dozen or so cases annually that will provide evidence about HIV prevalence in such subgroups. Moreover, comparisons of year-to-year changes in the number of cases will be less precise than the rates themselves. In this instance, the opportunities for economy through the use of samples are not large; furthermore, administrative simplicity, lower costs, and greater effectiveness can probably be attained by routinely treating all births in exactly the same fashion.

Basic demographic information to be collected in the newborn survey includes the month and year of the infant's birth, the county (or parish) of the mother's residence, and the county (or parish) in which the hospital is located. The protocol notes that, for counties with few births or for those with only a single hospital, data should be aggregated to ensure that there will be no inadvertent disclosure of the mother's or infant's identity. In addition to the basic demographic information, the protocol specifies that "when available and provided that inadvertent disclosure [of identity] cannot occur, the zip code of mother's residence and hospital locations, and/or mother's race and age should be included" (CDC/NIH, 1988:11). The committee believes these provisions provide good illustrations of the need for a carefully considered policy on the collection of identifying data (which is already the subject of a recommendation appearing earlier in this chapter).

Because CDC's proposed neonatal screening will provide unbiased estimates of HIV prevalence for a population of great interest, **the committee recommends that the newborn infant seroprevalence survey be extended to include all children born in the United States.**

It should be recognized, however, that the interpretation of trends in the prevalence rates obtained through this survey will lead immediately to questions about transmission. High (or rising) rates of infection will prompt the question of whether such increases are due to infection through IV drug use and needle-sharing among women of childbearing age, whether they are a consequence of heterosexual transmission of HIV infection, whether they are the result of increased childbearing among female IV drug users, or whether they arise from still other factors. As it is presently constructed, the neonatal survey can pose such questions effectively, but it will not provide answers regarding the causes of any trends that are observed. To provide such answers will require a different sort of data gathering (which might build on the neonatal survey). These data gathering efforts might target areas with high prevalence rates (or with rapid changes in prevalence rates); targeted follow-up surveys would then be needed to establish the causes of transmission in these areas. One strategy might regard the neonatal survey as a "screener" to identify areas in which more specialized studies should be conducted to answer questions of causality. This type of strategy would not be overly difficult to implement after some experience is gained with the basic neonatal survey.

ESTIMATES OF NATIONAL HIV PREVALENCE AND INCIDENCE

There are three methods of estimating the current extent of HIV infection in the United States.

1. Divide the population into groups or strata, and for each stratum estimate both the size of the group and its rate of seroprevalence. Combine these estimates for an estimated number of infected persons in the stratum; obtain a national total estimate by adding the estimates for all strata.
2. Exploit the necessary mathematical connections among three time series: $A(t)$, the number of AIDS cases seen by time t; $H(t)$, the number of HIV infections that have occurred (mostly unseen) by time t; and $l(x)$, the probability distribution for the "latency," the length of the interval between acquiring HIV infection and being diagnosed with AIDS.
3. Conduct a sample survey of the population of the United States, collecting and testing blood specimens.

This section considers each of these methods in turn, calling them (1) the components model, (2) the epidemiological model, and (3) the sample survey method.

The Components Model

The components model was used to derive the most widely quoted estimate of HIV prevalence in the United States (see Table 1-2), which was presented in the Public Health Service's 1986 "Coolfont Report" (Public Health Service, 1986). That report concluded: "[B]y extrapolating all available data, we estimate that there are between 1 and 1.5 million infected persons in those groups [IV drug users and homosexual men] at present" (p. 343). Although explicit calculations were not shown in the original document, the Coolfont report indicated that its authors estimated that 2.5 million American men between the ages of 16 and 55 are "exclusively homosexual" throughout their lives and that 5–10 million more have some homosexual

TABLE 1-2 Estimates of the Number of Persons Infected with HIV in the United States

Source	Population	Date	Estimate
PHS Coolfont report[a]	IV drug users and homosexual men	June 1986	1.25 million[b]
CDC Domestic Policy Council report[c]	IV drug users and homosexual men	Nov. 1987	1.17 million[d]

[a]Public Health Service (1986:341–348).
[b]Estimated as the interval 1.0 million to 1.5 million; the midpoint of the interval is shown in the table.
[c]CDC (1987b).
[d]Estimated as the interval 945,000 to 1.41 million; the midpoint of the interval is shown in the table.

contact.[33] Similarly, they estimated (without explicit reference to a source) that 750,000 Americans inject heroin or other drugs at least once a week and that similar numbers inject drugs less frequently. These estimates of population size were then multiplied by estimates of the prevalence of HIV infection among these groups[34] to generate the widely quoted estimate that there are from 1–1.5 million infected persons in these two groups. Changes in estimates of population size and HIV prevalence led CDC (1987a) to revise its estimate for 1987 (see Table 1-2) to 945,000–1.41 million infected individuals.

Estimates derived using the components model are vulnerable to errors of unknown magnitude in both multiplicands. For example, the 1986 Coolfont estimate used data collected by Kinsey and colleagues (1948) in the 1940s to estimate the *current* number of male homosexuals in the United States. Even 30 years ago, the Kinsey data were widely regarded as unreliable for making such estimates because the research that produced them did not use probability sampling and because the respondents in the Kinsey studies were disproportionately drawn from the Midwest and from the college-educated segment of the population (e.g., Terman, 1948; Wallis, 1948; Cochran et al., 1953). Today, a further leap of faith is required

[33]The subsequent CDC report (1987a) provides the explicit breakdown used in the 1986 calculations.

[34]The prevalence rates used in these calculations were not published in the original report (Public Health Service, 1986), but the report states that HIV prevalence estimates range from 20–50 percent for homosexual men and from 10–50 percent for users of IV drugs.

to assume that the relative size of the (self-reported) homosexual population has not changed since the 1940s (see Chapter 2 and Fay and colleagues [in press]). Furthermore, the committee notes that estimates of the prevalence of HIV infection among homosexual men were not derived from probability samples. Identical problems afflict the estimates of HIV infection among IV drug users (see Spencer [in this volume]).

The Epidemiological Model

The epidemiological model depends on a necessary mathematical relationship among these three time series:

- $A(t)$, the (cumulative) number of AIDS cases that have appeared by time t;
- $H(t)$, the (cumulative) number of cases of HIV infection that have occurred (mostly unseen) by time t; and
- $l(x)$, the probability[35] that a person will be diagnosed with AIDS after the passage of x years from time of infection with HIV.[36]

Before discussing the mathematical relation, let us note what is known about these series. First, from CDC statistics, $A(t)$ is known for the period since 1981. The data are not quite exact because revisions must and do occur. (For example, a major revision of the AIDS case definition was adopted in 1987 [CDC, 1987c]). Because of reporting delays, the most recent portion is most susceptible to revision. Second, almost nothing is known about $H(t)$ because there are such meager data about HIV prevalence. Third, $l(x)$ can be known only for x from 0 up to about 10 years, for there has been no opportunity to see the relative frequency of latencies longer than 10 years. What is known about this latency distribution comes largely from studies of hemophiliacs, transfusion recipients, and a few other

[35] The function $l(x)$ is a probability density function that ordinarily sums to 1.0 if integrated from 0 to infinity. However, because not all of those infected with HIV may eventually be diagnosed with AIDS, the integral of $l(x)$ from 0 to infinity may be less than 1.0.

[36] Implicit in this definition of $l(x)$ is the assumption that latencies (intervals between time of infection and time of AIDS diagnosis) have had the same probability distribution over time; thus, the definition tacitly assumes that changes in the ratio of men to women among infected individuals or in the relative proportions of IV drug users, homosexuals, and blood product recipients are all immaterial with respect to the distribution of latencies. (With the exception of latencies for newborns, we are not aware of convincing information that contradicts—or supports—these assumptions.) Also involved is the assumption that diagnostic practices have not altered in a way that shortens or lengthens latencies.

special groups. By assuming that $l(x)$ has a specific functional form, such as that of the Weibull distribution, it is possible to extend our estimate of $l(x)$ beyond $x = 10$ years.

The epidemiological model sets out to estimate the curve $H(t)$ by using $A(t)$, which is approximately known, and $l(x)$, which is somewhat known. The relation among these three series is

$$A(t) = \int_0^t H(t-x)l(x)dx. \tag{1}$$

Thus, if any two of $A(t)$, $H(t)$, and $l(x)$ are known exactly, the other can be calculated exactly. We do know $A(t)$ more or less exactly and $l(x)$ can be estimated; thus, it is possible to produce an *estimate* of $H(t)$, the cumulative incidence of HIV infection up to time t. An estimated solution of equation (1), then, consists of two estimated series, $H(t)$ and $l(x)$; the adequacy of this solution can be judged by how closely the resulting $A(t)$ (from the solution) corresponds with the observed $A(t)$. Unfortunately, quite different pairs of estimates of $H(t)$ and $l(x)$ provide equally good fits to $A(t)$ but carry very different values for the cumulative incidence $H(t)$ and for the latency distribution $l(x)$.

In practice, using equation (1) to estimate $H(t)$ is fraught with difficulties. In particular, $l(x)$ is very small for the first two or three years. Thus, as equation (1) shows, AIDS cases that have been diagnosed by, for example, 1988, are primarily a function of the number of HIV infections through 1985. Therefore, even a perfectly accurate count of the AIDS cases diagnosed through the previous year provides little reliable information on new HIV infections during the past three or four years. Because HIV incidence may be growing rapidly and because it is not possible to estimate precisely the number of new cases of HIV in the past few years, estimates of the cumulative incidence $H(t)$ could be far off the mark. This imprecision does not matter very much for predicting the number of new AIDS cases in the short-run because such predictions do not depend heavily on the incidence of HIV infection in the past few years (Brookmeyer and Gail, 1986). In terms of predicting current HIV prevalence, however, and for estimating trends in prevalence over time, this imprecision can be costly.

Clearly, the epidemiological and the components models approach the estimation of HIV prevalence quite differently. Each has its problems, but they are of quite different kinds. Both produce estimates of HIV prevalence of "about 1,000,000"—meaning, within the range of 0.5–2 million infected persons. Confidence in this rough estimate is strengthened by the fact that the uncertainties affecting the two methods of estimation are quite different.

Sample Survey Method

The Public Health Service recently embarked on a developmental program to test the feasibility of obtaining direct estimates of HIV infection by means of a survey that would seek blood specimens (and associated questionnaire data on risk) from a probability sample of the national population. This undertaking is necessarily complex and difficult, and it cannot be foreseen whether such a survey will produce the desired estimates.

Among the most important of the attendant difficulties will be ensuring a sufficiently high rate of response to the survey. Because less than 1 percent of the population is thought to be infected with HIV, nonresponse could have a debilitating impact if it were to come disproportionately from population subgroups with elevated prevalence rates. In that case, the estimates produced by such a survey program could be seriously biased, even if the initial sample of designated respondents were unbiased. (Turner and Fay [in this volume] explore in greater detail the complexities involved in such a survey.)

The committee commends the exploratory spirit in which the Public Health Service has begun the development of this survey, and it applauds its strategy of using experiments to test whether or not such a survey might provide useful direct estimates of prevalence (and, ultimately, trends in prevalence). The outcome of these experiments should play a decisive role in the ultimate decision of whether to go forward with such a survey.

CONCLUSION

The committee believes that there is a pressing national need for better statistical systems to monitor the spread of the AIDS epidemic and, more particularly, the spread of its precursor, HIV infection. The development of such systems will require time and adequate resources—both in dollars and in appropriately trained scientific staffs. If the nation is to have a better understanding of the HIV/AIDS epidemic in 1999 than it has in 1989, the investment *must* be made. Delays in committing resources to the development of these systems would be false economy. Such a policy would only postpone unavoidable expenditures while forcing scientists and policy makers to continue to "make do" and work without accurate information on the current magnitude and future course of the epidemic.

The development of a more reliable system for tracking the spread of HIV infection is a prerequisite for mounting a fully effective and efficient national response to AIDS. Without better information on the incidence of new HIV infections in the population, the nation will lack adequate means to determine whether current strategies for controlling the spread of HIV are working. Without better information on the prevalence and spread of infection in the population, it is difficult to prepare adequately for future demands for hospital beds and other health care services. Without better data, it is easy to anticipate endless debates about whether the disease is spreading "rapidly" or "slowly." To the extent that opposing sides in these debates produce "evidence" from convenience samples, inconsistency in conclusions is to be expected, and there is thus no basis for an informative scientific debate.

What we require for more informative debates, for better planning for future health care needs, and for improved evaluation of the effects of national AIDS-control strategies are *data derived from research designs that can provide reasonably unbiased estimates of the prevalence and incidence rates for HIV infection in well-defined populations of substantive interest.*

Attributes of an HIV Monitoring System

Such designs for monitoring HIV would have two characteristics that set them apart from the procedures ordinarily used for tracking epidemics. These attributes follow directly from the nature of the disease under consideration. A *passive* reporting system is not adequate to monitor the spread of a fatal infection that is asymptomatic (for almost all infected individuals) for a long period of time. This fact requires a conceptual departure from the way in which epidemic diseases have traditionally been monitored. Traditionally, such diseases have been classified as "reportable" by public health officials. After such a determination, health care workers (physicans, testing laboratories, etc.) were legally required to report all new cases of the disease to the local department of public health. These reports, when aggregated by federal disease control officials, provided crucial information for monitoring the course of many past epidemics. Part of the reason for the success of this type of system followed from the fact that many of these infections quickly caused symptoms that required medical attention. The outcome (in a substantial fraction of cases) was swift, and the size of the public health problem posed by the spread of the infection could be monitored by counting the number of new cases reported to health authorities.

Unfortunately, a passive reporting system does not work as well for diseases that in most infected individuals are slow to require medical attention. These diseases do not provide sufficient motivation to the infected person to seek medical care quickly and thereby be captured by the statistical reporting system; consequently, the statistical system must actively "ferret out" information on new cases. This more active method of case gathering and reporting is the first way in which an HIV monitoring system would differ from more traditional case-reporting systems.

A second difference is that an adequate measurement system for HIV cannot rely exclusively on the routine functioning of the medical infrastructure to count infected persons. This requirement has important institutional consequences because it mandates the organization of surveillance outside of traditional medical settings.

Other Uses of Data on HIV

This committee has listened with interest to arguments that population-based estimates of HIV incidence and prevalence are unnecessary from a public health perspective. Rather, it has been suggested that targeted samples of convenience could suffice to provide "sentinels" that could be used to guide the nation's response to the AIDS epidemic.

The committee recognizes that there may be public health uses of prevalence data whose purposes can be served by other methodologies. In reviewing the protocol for HIV testing of patients at TB clinics, for example, the committee was initially perplexed by the choice of blind testing; reasonable standards of medical treatment would dictate routine HIV testing of all TB patients because preliminary evidence suggests that standard antituberculosis therapy should be modified for persons infected with HIV. After discussions with CDC staff, the committee came to understand that a major purpose of the blind testing was to convince reluctant clinics to begin routine HIV screening of TB patients. The evidence from the blind screening was intended to stimulate local clinic staff to recognize the extent of HIV prevalence in their clinic and to adopt the Public Health Service's recommendation for routine HIV screening of all TB patients.

In this case, there was a clear public health use for numerical information on prevalence in particular clinics. That purpose could be well served without attempting to estimate accurately the true prevalence of HIV among all patients at TB clinics. While recognizing this important public health use of such data, the committee would observe that the *stated objectives* of this survey, as with other components of the family of surveys program, were to determine HIV prevalence and monitor trends in prevalence.[37] These more demanding objectives require a survey design appropriate to these tasks.

It is the opinion of this committee that the public health mandate to monitor the spread of HIV *requires* that reliable statistical data be gathered on HIV infection. Gathering such data necessitates the use of methods that ensure (to the extent technically possible) that the resultant estimates will reflect, with known margins of error, the actual incidence and prevalence of infection in specific populations. *The committee concludes that it would be a serious mistake for the Public Health Service to continue to "make do" with estimates derived from convenience samples.*

The committee would also emphasize that much of the information needed to understand and cope with the spread of HIV is obtainable only with the consent of a person who may be harmed if test result confidentiality is not maintained. Thus, maintaining confidentiality serves not only fairness but also society's interest in access to information to help combat the disease. Two steps can help: (1) confidentiality can be buttressed with legal penalties in the event of its breach, and (2) legal protection against discrimination can be established for persons infected with HIV. In this regard, the committee wishes to note that it endorses the approaches to protecting confidentiality and opposing discrimination proposed by the Presidential Commission on the Human Immunodeficiency Virus Epidemic (1988).[38]

The Presidential Commission has provided the President and the American people with 35 specific recommendations on the steps that should be taken to halt discrimination against persons with HIV infection and AIDS and to guarantee the confidentiality of

---

[37] The protocol (CDC, 1988a:4) states: "The objectives of this survey are the following: (1) to determine the prevalence of HIV antibodies among persons with confirmed or suspected tuberculosis by age, sex, race, ethnicity, metropolitan area, TB clinic site, country of origin, clinical status (confirmed or suspected TB), anatomic site of infection (pulmonary, extrapulmonary, or both) and (in the non-blinded surveys) AIDS risk factor; and (2) to monitor trends in infection levels over time. Implementation of a standard protocol will facilitate comparison of data from different clinics."

[38] See Chapter 9, Sections I and II.

information about individuals' HIV status. The committee believes that the approaches recommended by the commission could serve the nation well by improving the climate in which future research and interventions will be conducted.

Finally, the committee and its Panel on Statistical Issues in AIDS Research wish to end this chapter by offering two observations: one about the past and one about the future.

The Public Health Service has met an unexpected, challenging, and complicated epidemic with vigor and ingenuity and has much to be proud of. Moreover, its achievements have been accomplished in the face of considerable adversity on a number of fronts—physical, diplomatic, political, and administrative. As always, however, the past must give way to the future. The HIV/AIDS problem is not going to disappear soon, if ever. Its most visible component, AIDS, will surely increase for years to come. Now is the time to prepare for the future, and good data will be indispensable in future efforts to control this epidemic. No postponement should be accepted in implementing the clearly necessary steps to markedly improve the data on this disease. CDC should be given the resources needed to promptly initiate the appropriate steps to improve the nation's HIV/AIDS information base.

REFERENCES

Andersen, R. A., Chen, M., Aday, L., and Cornelius, L. (1987) Health status and medical care utilization. *Health Affairs* 6:136–156.

Brookmeyer, R., and Gail, M. H.. (1986) Minimum size of the acquired immunodeficiency syndrome (AIDS) epidemic in the United States. *Lancet* 2:1320–1322.

Castro, K., Lieb, S., Jaffe, H., Narkunas, J., Calisher, C., Bush, T., Witte, J., and the Belle Glade Field-Study Group. (1988) Transmission of HIV in Belle Glade, Florida. *Science* 239:193–197.

Centers for Disease Control (CDC). (1987a) Human immunodeficiency virus infection in the United States: A review of current knowledge. *Morbidity and Mortality Weekly Report* 36(Suppl. S-6):1–48.

Centers for Disease Control (CDC). (1987b) Human Immunodeficiency Virus Infections in the United States: Review of Current Knowledge and Plans for Expansion of HIV Surveillance Activities. Report to the Domestic Policy Council. Centers for Disease Control, Atlanta, Ga. November 30.

Centers for Disease Control (CDC). (1987c) Revision of CDC surveillance case definition for AIDS. *Morbidity and Mortality Weekly Report* 36 (Suppl. 1S):3S–15S.

Centers for Disease Control (CDC). (1988a) Protocol for Estimating HIV Seroprevalence in Patients with Confirmed or Suspected Tuberculosis Attending Tuberculosis Clinics. CDC Protocol No. 839. Centers for Disease Control, Atlanta, Ga.

Centers for Disease Control (CDC). (1988b) Protocol for Estimating HIV Seroprevalence from Surveys in Clinics Which Serve Women of Reproductive Age. CDC Protocol No. 842. Centers for Disease Control, Atlanta, Ga.

Centers for Disease Control (CDC). (1988c) Protocol: Sentinel Hospital Surveillance System for HIV Infection. RFP 200-88-0623(P). Centers for Disease Control, Atlanta, Ga.

Centers for Disease Control (CDC). (1988d) Survey of HIV Seroprevalence and Assessment of Associated Risk Behaviors in Patients Attending Sexually Transmitted Disease Clinics. CDC Protocol No. 843. Centers for Disease Control, Atlanta, Ga.

Centers for Disease Control/National Institute on Drug Abuse (CDC/NIDA). (1988) Proposal for Monitoring HIV Seroprevalence in Intravenous Drug Users in Treatment. CDC Protocol No. 840. Centers for Disease Control, Atlanta, Ga.

Centers for Disease Control/National Institutes of Health (CDC/NIH). (1988) HIV Seroprevalence Survey in Childbearing Women Utilizing Dried Blood Specimens Routinely Collected on Filter Paper for Neonatal Screening Programs (draft protocol). Centers for Disease Control, Atlanta, Ga.

Cochran, W. G., Mosteller, F., and Tukey, J. W. (1953) Statistical problems of the Kinsey Report. *Journal of the American Statistical Association* 48:673–716.

Des Jarlais, D. C., Friedman, S. R., and Stoneburner, R. L. (1988) HIV infection and intravenous drug use: Critical issues in transmission dynamics, infection outcomes, and prevention. *Reviews of Infectious Diseases* 10:155.

Dondero, T. J., Pappaioanou, M., and Curran, J. W. (1988) Monitoring the levels and trends of HIV infection: The Public Health Service's HIV surveillance program. *Public Health Reports* 103:213–220.

Fay, R. E., Turner, C. F., Klassen, A. D., and Gagnon, J. H. (In press) Prevalence and patterns of same-gender sexual contact among men. *Science.*

Hardy, A. M., Starcher, E. T., II, Morgan, W. M., Druker, J., Kristal, A., Day, J. M., Kelly, C., Ewing, E., and Curran, J. W. (1987) Review of death certificates to assess completeness of AIDS case reporting. *Public Health Reports* 102:386–390.

Hull, H. F., Bettinger, C. J., Gallaher, M. M., Keller, N. M., Wilson, J., and Mertz, G. J. (1988) Comparison of HIV-antibody prevalence in patients consenting to and declining HIV-antibody testing in an STD clinic. *Journal of the American Medical Association* 260:935–938.

Institute of Medicine/National Academy of Sciences (IOM/NAS). (1986) *Confronting AIDS: Directions for Public Health, Health Care, and Research.* Washington, D.C.: National Academy Press.

Institute of Medicine/National Academy of Sciences (IOM/NAS). (1988) *Confronting AIDS: Update 1988.* Washington, D.C.: National Academy Press.

Kinsey, A. C., Pomeroy, W. B., and Martin, C. E. (1948) *Sexual Behavior in the Human Male.* Philadelphia: W. B. Saunders.

Manton, K. G., and Singer, B. M. (1988) Forecasting the Impact of the AIDS Epidemic on Elderly Populations. Department of Epidemiology and Public Health, School of Medicine, Yale University.

Peterman, T. A., Stoneburner, R. L., Allen, J. R., Jaffe, H. W., and Curran, J. W. (1988) Risk of human immunodeficiency virus transmission from heterosexual adults with transfusion-associated infections. *Journal of the American Medical Association* 259:55–58.

Presidential Commission on the Human Immunodeficiency Virus Epidemic. (1988) *Final Report of the Presidential Commission on the Human Immunodeficiency Virus Epidemic.* Washington, D.C.: Government Printing Office.

Public Health Service. (1986) Coolfont report: Public Health Service plan for combating AIDS. *Public Health Reports* 101:341–349.

Secretary's Task Force on Black and Minority Health. (1985) *Report of the Secretary's Task Force on Black and Minority Health,* Vol. 1, U.S. Department of Health and Human Services. Washington, D.C.: Government Printing Office.

Terman, L. M. (1948) Kinsey's "Sexual Behavior in the Human Male": Some comments and criticisms. *Psychological Bulletin* 45:443–459.

Wallis, W. A. (1948) Statistics of the Kinsey report. *Journal of the American Statistical Association* 44:463–484.

2

Sexual Behavior and AIDS

It is now widely recognized that controlling the spread of the AIDS epidemic will require a national effort to persuade a sizable fraction of the population to modify their sexual behavior. The effort will be most crucial for those individuals who are now sexually active with multiple partners (concurrently or serially) and for young persons who will become sexually active in future years. This urgent need, in turn, has generated a renewed awareness of the lack of an adequate scientific understanding of human sexual behavior (including its emergence and development) and the necessity for rigorous programs of basic research in this field. In this chapter, we describe what is currently known about (past and present) human sexual behavior and the types of data collection efforts needed to provide basic information from which to fashion the kind of understanding that is now required.

STATUS OF THE RESEARCH FIELD

In the United States, research on human sexual behavior has always been a high-risk undertaking in which there has been little public investment. Earlier in this century, the paucity of scientific research on human sexual behavior led to an effort at the National Research Council (NRC) to organize and promote such research. In 1922, with the support of the Rockefeller Foundation, the NRC established the Committee for Research in Problems of Sex, which played a major role in identifying and supporting fundamental research on sexual behavior. Until it was disbanded in 1963, the committee provided research grants and in some cases made arrangements for direct funding by the Rockefeller Foundation for efforts ranging from studies of hormones and the biology of sex to the pioneering social research of Albert Kinsey and his collaborators (Aberle and Corner, 1953).

Despite the committee's efforts, however, the AIDS epidemic has highlighted the gaps in scientific knowledge about the sexual behavior of contemporary Americans. These gaps compromise practical attempts to cope with the AIDS epidemic and handicap efforts by health scientists to predict its future course. For example, as noted in Chapter 1, estimates of the number of persons infected with HIV (Public Health Service, 1986; CDC, 1987) have used Kinsey and colleagues' (1948) data to estimate the number of men in the United States who have sex with men. As Chapter 1 also noted, however, Kinsey's data have been widely regarded as unreliable for use in making such estimates because they were not collected by probability sampling and because they pertain to the population of 1938–1948.

Similarly, promising mathematical models of the dynamics of the spread of HIV infection require data on a wide range of sexual behaviors; these data currently are not available. For example, the distribution of the number of sexual contacts (both current and new partners) among individuals in a population has been shown to be important to the spread of the virus (May and Anderson, 1987). The number of contacts is a key determinant of the "reproductive rate" (R_0) of the epidemic, which is defined as the average number of new cases of infection generated by a single infected individual. There are currently no reliable data on sexual contacts for the national population; there are also no such data for groups with elevated risks of transmitting or contracting HIV infection (e.g., men who have sex with men, IV drug users, heterosexuals with many sexual partners). Indeed, there is no reliable information on the size of the nonmonogamous heterosexual population. The lack of such data makes predictions about the future spread of AIDS extremely uncertain.

These examples illustrate but two of a large number of crucial needs for reliable data on human sexual behavior. AIDS and HIV-related concerns present the most pressing needs for better data; yet over the longer term, we anticipate that the outcomes of such research will find application in many areas besides AIDS—for instance, in population studies and in the treatment of sexual dysfunction.

In this chapter, we review the types of data on human sexual behavior that will be needed to understand and predict the course of the epidemic and to design effective interventions to bring about the behavioral changes required to control the epidemic. We also describe the available data on sexual behavior in the United States, including trends in adolescent and adult sexual behavior, same-gender sex, and prostitution; the methodological and other problems that need to be overcome to obtain more reliable and valid data about relevant aspects of sexual behavior in the United States; and the role of anthropological techniques in this effort. Finally, we present a series of recommendations intended to improve understanding of the sexual behaviors that spread HIV infection.

NEEDED DATA

Two classes of data are urgently needed in the confrontation with AIDS/HIV. One class of data is required to understand the dynamics of HIV transmission that sustain the epidemic so as to predict the epidemic's future course. This class includes a mix of biological and social data. Although there may be differences of opinion on detail, there is widespread agreement on the common core of basic information needed for these purposes.

Another class of data is needed to control the epidemic's spread by reducing the frequency of behaviors that are likely to transmit the virus. This class is not as well defined as the first class of data because the task calls for a fundamental understanding of the factors that explain the development and expression of human sexuality (including its variety, social malleability, and other aspects).

Data Needed to Understand the Epidemic's Future Course

Understanding the future course of the HIV/AIDS epidemic requires —both at present and at regular intervals in future years—a variety of data on sexual behavior. Purely statistical extrapolations of current trends, such as those used by CDC (Public Health Service, 1986), can provide useful short-term predictions of the number of AIDS cases in the future, and they do not require a model of the underlying dynamics of disease transmission. For long-term predictions, however, it is necessary to understand the underlying dynamics of transmission within particular risk groups (see, e.g., May and Anderson, 1987). Such understanding in turn requires more extensive knowledge of three key elements of HIV transmission.

First, it is necessary to know the probability that an infected individual will transmit the infection to a partner (including male-to-male, male-to-female, female-to-male, or female-to-female transmission through sexual acts or by needle-sharing). The transmission probabilities in these instances depend on the kind of contact in question and the duration of the partnership, as well as on a variety of other factors. Transmission probabilities are not well understood at present; they are probably most uncertain for heterosexual transmission.

Second, data are needed on the rates of acquiring new sexual partners (or needle-sharing partners) among specific groups. Such data include not only the average number of new sexual partners acquired each year but the variation in this number as well. Persons who acquire new partners at a high rate play a disproportionate role in the transmission of infection, as they are both more likely to acquire and more likely to transmit infection. Thus, in both an epidemiological and a mathematical sense, sexual contacts (or needle-sharing contacts) in a group cannot accurately be characterized by "average" individuals or "average" behavior. Data are also needed on the relative frequency of behaviors that have markedly different likelihoods of transmitting infection (e.g., anal, vaginal, or oral sex). Similarly, information is needed about the extent to which awareness of HIV/AIDS transmission has altered behavior (particularly with respect to the use of condoms and spermicides) in ways that may reduce transmission.

Third, it is essential to know some key facts about the natural history of HIV infection, an area of knowledge in which, currently, uncertainties abound. There is considerable variation in the time that elapses between a person's acquiring HIV infection and the appearance of full-blown AIDS. The current best estimate is that the mean incubation period is 8 years, but as data spanning more time become available, it seems likely that this estimate will increase.[1] There is also uncertainty about the time-course of infectiousness. Evidence is now accumulating that suggests that infectiousness varies over the course of the disease. It appears that it may be elevated in the early phase of HIV infection and again at the onset of AIDS itself (as the immune system collapses) but that it may remain relatively

[1] The current estimate is that the majority of HIV-seropositive individuals will go on to develop AIDS, and it is not impossible that 100 percent of seropositive individuals may eventually develop full-blown AIDS (IOM/NAS, 1988:35–36). See also the projections of Lui and colleagues (1988).

low at other times (e.g., IOM/NAS, 1988:38; Anderson and May, 1988:Figure 1).

The basic reproductive rate (R_0) of an infection within a particular population determines whether the infection has the potential to generate an epidemic in that population. The reproductive rate is essentially the number of new cases of infection produced, on average, by each infected individual in the early stages of the epidemic, when essentially all contacts are themselves not infected. So, for example, if R_0 is less than 1.0 for heterosexual transmission of HIV in the United States, on average, each case of HIV infection will produce fewer than one subsequent case, and the process will not be self-sustaining. There will be some chains of HIV transmission in which men will infect women who will then infect men and so on, but they will be few and short. If R_0 is larger than 1.0, however, such chains will be more numerous and longer, and a "chain reaction," or epidemic, will be generated. The larger the value of R_0, the shorter the time it takes for the number of cases of infection to double.

It is clear that R_0 exceeded 1.0 among gay men in large U.S. cities in the late 1970s and early 1980s and that it exceeds 1.0 today among IV drug users who share needles. It is also clear that R_0 exceeds 1.0 among the heterosexual populations of many parts of Africa. At present, it is unknown whether R_0 is large enough (greater than 1.0) to engender a self-sustaining epidemic with purely heterosexual chains of transmission in the United States.

The basic reproductive rate for a defined risk group depends on the three factors discussed earlier: the transmission probability, contact rates, and duration of infectiousness in that group. In the early stages of an epidemic, R_0 can be estimated by multiplying the values of these three factors: the probability that infection will be transmitted to any one new contact (sexual or needle-sharing partner), the average number of new contacts each year, and the number of years over which the infected individual remains infectious. It should be noted that the reproductive rate for HIV infection combines the fundamental biology of the virus (which determines the incubation interval, for example) with behavioral factors (e.g., rates of acquiring new sexual partners, whether condoms are used, and so forth). Thus, R_0 can differ from one risk group to another and can change over time in response to behavioral changes.

If R_0 for heterosexually transmitted HIV in the United States is less than 1.0, no "second-wave" epidemic, spread purely by heterosexual contact, is possible. Moreover, even if R_0 does exceed 1.0 in the heterosexual population, the doubling time for the second-wave epidemic may bear little relation to that of the "first wave," which spread mainly among gay men and IV drug users. Furthermore, if the doubling time of this second, heterosexual wave is much longer than that of the first wave—for example, 5–10 years or more—the resulting patterns of spread among heterosexuals may go unnoticed against the much larger background of cases among homosexuals and IV drug users.

Data Needed to Understand the Epidemic's Dynamics

Estimating future demands on hospitals and other public health services requires reliable models of HIV transmission dynamics. Such epidemiological models, in conjunction with knowledge of the underlying biological and behavioral variables, can also help in assessing the relative effectiveness of different kinds of behavioral change and guiding the development of effective public health education.[2]

Data needs are driven by immediately relevant questions of disease transmission, progress, and control. The resulting intellectual strategy is to design new research looking for the "facts about sex" in order to answer those questions. Such facts, particularly when reliably collected and combined with a sensitive understanding of the cultural boundaries between social groups, may be of considerable use in the medical and social management of the HIV/AIDS epidemic. Yet the committee would point out that there are risks in a strategy of proceeding from an interest in disease to research on the "facts" of sexual conduct. These risks involve the possibility that concerns about disease will reinforce the tradition of treating some aspects of sexual conduct as social or medical "problems."

To understand the motives, development, and varieties of human sexual behavior, it is crucial to understand the systems of meaning and action—the cultural context—in which the "facts of sex" are embedded. The facts remain the same, but understanding may differ. Different understandings in turn may have important consequences for designing effective educational efforts to encourage self-protective behaviors.

---

[2]Efforts to reduce risky behavior in individuals often do not require detailed knowledge of the transmission dynamics of the epidemic. Nevertheless, efforts directed toward accessible individuals can go hand in hand with broader, population-level studies of the relative effectiveness of different broad categories of public education. Individual counseling and activities to reduce risky behavior in particular groups that are accessible to AIDS prevention efforts are not alternatives to mathematical modeling, given that such modeling may lead to the development of intervention strategies that make maximal use of scarce resources.

In the following sections of this chapter, we review available data (largely collected prior to the onset of the AIDS epidemic) on sexual behavior in the United States. The history of research on human sexuality, at least in the United States, can be divided somewhat crudely into the pre-Kinsey and post-Kinsey eras. Despite the fact that Kinsey himself cited a number of questionnaire and interview surveys of sexual behavior conducted in a variety of countries as early as the first decade of the twentieth century (Kinsey et al., 1948, 1953), it was the publication of the two "Kinsey reports"—*Sexual Behavior in the Human Male* (1948) and *Sexual Behavior in the Human Female* (1953)—that dramatically shifted the study of human sexuality away from its predominantly clinical and psychopathological concerns. In doing so, Kinsey and his coworkers responded to the call of Havelock Ellis in the 1920s, who proposed that sex researchers expand their interests beyond the asylum, the prison, and the clinic to study "fairly normal people" (Gagnon, 1975). In the attempt to accomplish this task, no matter how provisionally, the Kinsey studies helped to change the way in which sexuality was approached in American society: first, by establishing sexuality as a legitimate object of scientific inquiry; second, by offering a blurred but still discernible "snapshot" of what some people were doing sexually; and third, by offering a different definition of what was thought to be *normal* sexuality.

THE KINSEY STUDIES

It is not easy for those who have grown up in the 1960s and later to understand the extraordinary impact of the Kinsey studies in a society in which ignorance about sexuality was pervasive. Even those who were already adults when Kinsey's work first came to the nation's attention probably find that their memories of that world have been corroded by time and the deluge of sexual materials and references that have characterized the past three decades. The Kinsey studies engendered extensive, if not always thoughtful, discussions of sexuality in a society in which public talk about sex had been restricted to the vulgar, the moralistic, or the psychoanalytic. After their publication, words such as masturbation, homosexuality, orgasm, vagina, extramarital sex, clitoris, and penis could be spoken of in more or less polite company (although not in the *New York Times* of the period). People knew (or thought they knew) that one man in three had had sex at least once with another man; one married woman in four had sex outside of marriage; and the average rate of intercourse in marriage was between three and four times a week for couples in their 20s. The "facts" were out of the closet and seemed unlikely to be put back in. The vast outpouring of public discussion was based on what were two long and seemingly indigestible books, the first reporting approximately 3,000–5,000[3] face-to-face interviews with men, the second reporting 5,940 similar interviews with women.

Quality of the Kinsey Data

Because the Kinsey studies[4] are cited even today as a primary source of information on sexual behavior, it is valuable to review their design. To assess the quality of these data and their appropriateness for estimations of contemporary sexual behavior, it is important to examine two methodological aspects of the Kinsey studies: (1) the interview schedule, including its topical coverage, the interviewing procedures, and the interviewers; and (2) sampling—the method of gathering cases. These two aspects are discussed below; a third major aspect, the impact of the Kinsey studies on conceptions of sexual normality, is discussed later in the chapter.

The Interviews

The greatest strengths of the Kinsey studies were probably their coverage of a wide variety of sexual topics and the quality of the interviewing. The theories that informed the interview were quite general; they primarily reflected Kinsey's prior training as a taxonomist who had made his reputation in the ecological and evolutionary study of the gall wasp. Kinsey was fundamentally interested in the behavioral events (as opposed to the attitudes, motives, or emotions) that composed an individual's sexual history, and he saw those events as expressions of the interaction between the universals

---

[3]This range reflects the fact that different analyses reported in the first volume were done at different times and that during the intervals, additional cases accumulated. Gebhard and Johnson (1979:9) note: ". . . in those days we lacked computers and our card sorters were slow. A relatively simple table could easily take a full day or two of sorting—assuming the machine was available. Consequently, some tabulations were made a year or more before others and since our interviewing continued, our Ns varied. Thus, Table 62 in the *Male* volume [*Sexual Behavior in the Human Male*] shows 3,012 white males in our earliest age category (which should include all post-pubescents), yet in Table 63, the number is 3,925. Still later in Table 92 the N has risen to 4,625. This particular table was made in May 1947—one of the latest prepared."

[4]Additionally, the volumes *Pregnancy, Birth and Abortion* (Gebhard et al., 1958), *Sex Offenders: An Analysis of Types* (Gebhard et al., 1965), and *The Kinsey Data: Marginal Tabulations of 1938–1963 Interviews Conducted by the Institute for Sex Research* (Gebhard and Johnson, 1979) contain important information about these studies.

of the mammalian heritage and the specifics of social learning in a cultural context. The interview thus embodied a general scientific perspective rather than a specific set of hypotheses to be tested.

The interview schedule consisted of a dozen topical areas that could be covered in approximately 300 questions (Gebhard and Johnson, 1979:13–14). Interviewers were not restricted to the specific framework of the schedule, however, as the goal was to obtain information in an area rather than to ask precisely worded questions. The interviewers memorized the schedule, changed wording to conform with usage by the interviewee, and recorded only coded responses (to maintain confidentiality). The schedule was designed by Kinsey in the late 1930s and was consolidated by the early 1940s. Its continuing use had the benefit of maintaining comparability in data that were collected over nearly 25 years, although at some cost to the ability to learn from mistakes or adapt to new knowledge.

Kinsey wanted the social interaction involved in the interview process to be businesslike and nonjudgmental. Nothing was to be disapproved of or found shocking by the interviewers. Interviews were most often conducted outside the home, in institutional or commercial settings in which appointments could be made and anonymity preserved.

Almost every possible sexual topic was included: people were routinely asked about masturbation, nocturnal orgasm, intercourse (in all its variations), homosexual contacts, animal contacts, and sexual fantasies. Respondents were asked in considerable detail about the ages at which they engaged in these behaviors, frequencies, techniques, partners (when appropriate), and rates of orgasm. Those individuals with extensive histories of homosexuality, prostitution, sex offenses, sadomasochism, and the like were queried still further. Few studies conducted since that time have been as sharply focused on sexual behavior or so exclusively interested in sexual conduct for its own sake. More recent studies of sexual behavior have often asked only a few questions about sexuality, usually in the context of another inquiry that was defined by some social problem (e.g., adolescent pregnancy).

There are significant differences between the Kinsey interview and the interviews that characterize most modern surveys. Current surveys that use face-to-face data gathering usually have fixed interview schedules; interviewers are required to conform to the precise wording and order of questions printed on the survey questionnaire. In addition, a changing technology of data gathering has produced other variations:

- survey interviewers are most often women, many interviewers are involved in each survey, and interviews are often done in the subject's home;
- most surveys—even studies that have some relation to sexuality (e.g, studies of reproduction and fertility)—do not focus entirely on sexual matters but instead ask such questions infrequently and usually as modest additions; and
- in many cases, interviews are conducted by telephone.

Sampling

It has long been recognized that one of the greatest faults of the Kinsey research was the way in which the cases were selected: the sample is not representative of the entire U.S. population or of any definable group in the population. This fault limits the comparability and appropriateness of the Kinsey data as a basis for calculating the prevalence of any form of sexual conduct.

The population segment best represented by the Kinsey interviews can be described as a "chunk" of the white, youthful, college-educated U.S. population whose adolescence and young adulthood were lived during the late 1920s, the Great Depression, and World War II. Of those interviewed, 96 percent were white, and their median age was 24;[5] moreover, 68 percent of those interviewed were 30 years of age and younger—and were thus able to offer evidence on only the first quarter of adult sexual life. Some respondents were specifically chosen because they were delinquents, criminals, or sex offenders;

[5]This and subsequent characterizations of the Kinsey cases are taken from Gebhard and Johnson (1979:47–51, Tables 1–3). This particular description refers to Kinsey cases interviewed at any time from 1938 to 1963. (Table 2-1 shows the number of cases collected during different periods.) Gebhard and Johnson's (1979) tabulations are restricted to what they call Kinsey's "basic sample," which they define as including "postpubertal individuals who were never convicted of any offense other than traffic violations and who did not come from any sources which we knew to be biased in terms of sexual behavior" (p. 41). This basic sample included 177 black men, 223 black women, 4,694 white men, and 4,358 white women, all of whom had attended college for at least one year. The basic sample also included 766 white men and 1,028 white women who had not attended college.

Kinsey's basic sample does not include cases identified by Gebhard and Johnson as (1) homosexual (defined as "postpubertal individuals who had at least 50 homosexual contacts or who had at least 20 sexual partners of the same gender as the individual" [p. 43]); (2) delinquents (defined as "postpubertal individuals who have been convicted of a felony or misdemeanor other than a traffic violation" [p. 45]); and (3) "special groups," which are described as "simply residual categories of individuals who cannot be assigned elsewhere because of some sample bias or because of some other special characteristic" (p. 45). This last "residual" group included 380 prepubertal and 999 postpubertal males, and 156 prepubertal and 717 postpubertal females.

TABLE 2-1 Year of Interview by Gender for Persons Interviewed Using the Original Kinsey Interview Schedule

	Males		Females	
Year	Number	Percentage	Number	Percentage
Prewar, 1938–1941	1,910	19.5	436	5.6
Wartime, 1942–1945	3,353	34.3	3,740	48.4
Postwar, 1946–1952	2,907	29.7	3,413	44.2
Early 1950s 1953–1956	1,461	14.9	58	0.8
Post-Kinsey, 1957–1963	146	1.5	78	1.0
Total	9,777		7,725	

SOURCE: Gebhard and Johnson (1979).

most of the remainder were, in the tradition of most sex research, college educated. About 84 percent of the men and women interviewed had some college education, and 45 percent were in college at the time of the interview. Perhaps most striking is that 25 percent of the college-educated women had been to graduate or professional school, as had 47 percent of the college-educated men. About one half of the female sample was interviewed during World War II, and many others were interviewed shortly afterward (see Table 2-1).

Perhaps more important than the composition of the sample were the methods by which the cases were collected. Both the difficulties of sampling on a sensitive topic and Kinsey's confidence that the sheer force of accumulated cases[6] would eventually translate into representativeness severely compromised the usefulness of the data for making estimates of prevalence that could be generalized to any larger group or to the overall population.

Kinsey gathered cases in a variety of ways. Many respondents were interviewed as the result of gaining access to a group through a contact person: for example, a faculty member sympathetic to Kinsey's goals might allow him to speak to a class to recruit students, or a prison administrator would offer access to an inmate population.

[6]Kinsey hoped to gather 100,000 interviews to complete his research (see the dedication to the 1948 volume); some 17,000 had been completed by the time of his death.

In other cases, lectures to less organized groups such as PTAs were used as occasions to ask for volunteers. These two types of groups became what Kinsey later described as "100 percent groups"—that is, groups in which he estimated that he interviewed all (or almost all) of those exposed to his request for cooperation. In these "sample" groups, Kinsey believed that he was solving some of the problems of sampling, particularly those of volunteer bias. Yet neither the contact persons nor the groups to which they offered access were sampled from some larger list; consequently, the final sample could never, in principle, have been a probability sample. In addition, many of the cases were friends of friends who were recruited through networks of referrals.

It is difficult even to begin to consider how these cases could be added together or "corrected" to make what at best could only be marginally satisfactory population estimates. This point is made most trenchantly in the major statistical review of the Kinsey research (Cochran et al., 1953).

Utility of the Kinsey Data

Despite their limitations, the Kinsey data published in 1948 and 1953 (based largely on those individuals in the sample who grew up in the 1920s and 1930s)[7] remain the most widely known and referenced data on American sexual behavior. Portions of the studies have been used as historical benchmarks for the estimation of sexual change over the last half century (e.g., the rates of premarital and marital sexual conduct). Other results, particularly those relating to the prevalence of extramarital intercourse, masturbation, intercourse with female prostitutes, and homosexual conduct by men and women, are sometimes cited as if they applied to the contemporary U.S. population. *Given the inadequate samples on which the estimates are based, the committee believes these uses are inappropriate even for the periods in which the data were gathered.*

It is also likely that the quality of the data varies across various sexual topics and measures. One might expect common forms of conduct (e.g., masturbation and heterosexuality before and within marriage) to be reasonably well reported. However, information on conduct that is relatively rare (e.g., homosexuality, intercourse

[7]The apparent discrepancy in the times of "growing up" cited here (1920–1930) and those cited earlier (1920–World War II) reflects the different periods during which data were gathered. The earlier characterization referred to the entire body of Kinsey data, which was gathered between 1938 and 1963.

outside of marriage, contact with prostitutes, and bisexuality) is quite sensitive and more likely to be misreported. Yet these are the very forms of sexual conduct that are pertinent to an understanding of the spread of HIV/AIDS. There is a tendency to use Kinsey (and other) inadequate numbers in the absence of good data, but in so doing, there is a serious risk of making wrong predictions and creating the illusion that more is known about sexual behavior than is in fact the case.

Another problem with the Kinsey data is a result of focus rather than method. Kinsey was most interested in the frequency of various sexual activities, expressed primarily in terms of orgasm. His work was based on a concept of differential "energy" (including sexual energy) of the individual organism, which led to a concern with these measures. A more social model of sexuality would focus on sexual partners and networks of sexual partnering, as it is likely that types and numbers of partners actually shape frequencies of conduct and the specific sexual practices performed. A partner-driven model of sexuality might also satisfy more adequately the needs of epidemiology in relation to the transmission of HIV.

Kinsey and the Issue of Sexual Normality

The public uproar that greeted the publication of the Kinsey reports was a signal that something more than a scientific event had occurred. Kinsey was violently assailed by representatives of religious groups, conservative congressmen, and some social research methodologists. He and his work were caricatured in the press. Some people have claimed that the ferocity of this attack may well have shortened Kinsey's life (W. B. Pomeroy, 1972:381). Given Kinsey's dual claims—that sexuality could and should be the object of detached scientific inquiry and that sexual normality rested ultimately on the mandates of the mammalian origins of the human species—this attack might have been expected.

Indeed, there is evidence that some conflict was foreseen. In setting forth arguments for the legitimacy of sex research, Alan Gregg of the Rockefeller Foundation argued in the preface to *Sexual Behavior in the Human Male* (Kinsey et al., 1948) that

> [c]ertainly no aspect of human biology in our current civilization stands in more need of scientific knowledge and courageous humility than that of sex. As long as sex is dealt with in the current confusion of ignorance and sophistication, denial and indulgence, suppression and stimulation, punishment and exploitation, secrecy and display, it will be associated with a duplicity and

> indecency that lead neither to intellectual honesty nor human dignity.

This was no neutral claim but an assertion of the legitimacy of objective, detached, dispassionate inquiry as against the indecent and dishonest social arrangements that were then current. Moreover, these were and are "fighting words" because they stake out a large area of human conduct for scientific inquiry and judgment. The very claim for the legitimacy of science in the area of sexuality was an attempt to change the "rules of the game" that defined what conduct was normal and what was abnormal.

Kinsey went even further, however. He attempted to counter the traditional religious view that sexual virtue was entirely composed of heterosexual activity in the pursuit of reproduction inside the bonds of marriage, as well as the orthodox psychoanalytic revision of this traditional view, which admitted the existence of other forms of sexual expression but treated them as either perversions from or preludes to the sexual "normality" found in mature heterosexual committed relationships. Kinsey's counter to these views was to take a strong biological line that emphasized the evolutionary history of the species rather than the defective status of the individual. He argued that homosexuality, masturbation, and oral sex (to take the triad he most often discussed when dealing with these issues) were common activities in "the mammalian heritage" as well as among human groups in which sexual behavior was not culturally repressed. Hence, such activities represented the diversity of nature rather than perversions and deviations from biological or cultural standards for the sexually correct individual (Kinsey et al., 1948).

This extraordinarily original argument allowed Kinsey to bring what was thought to be unnatural behaviors under the umbrella of a broad, evolutionary perspective. Sexuality could thus be treated as part of a natural world that should not be limited by the artifices of culture.

The Kinsey research reflected an important moment in the history of science and society in the United States. It opened the door to further work and changed the way in which sexuality was talked about in this country. Yet for reasons of method and history, it cannot provide answers to the questions that have been raised by the AIDS crisis: it cannot replace carefully conducted, contemporary research.

After the Kinsey Studies

The various social and cultural forces of the 1930s and 1940s that prompted the original Kinsey studies, and the example of those studies, did not produce a continuing tradition of sex research. Particularly lacking are contemporary studies of

- sexuality outside marriage,
- sexuality with persons of the same gender (homosexuality),
- sexuality with persons of both genders (bisexuality),
- sexual contacts for pay (female and male prostitution), and
- variations in sexual techniques across various types of sexual partnerings.

There is somewhat better information on heterosexuality among adolescents and young people (although these data are usually restricted to young women and to such topics as ages of initiation and rates of intercourse rather than partners and techniques) and coital rates in marriage. Both of these topics have been included in national surveys as well as in studies of more limited populations that cover a more extensive range of questions. In addition, since the publication of works by Masters and Johnson (1966), sexual dysfunction among married couples has received a great deal of attention, largely in clinical or experimental studies.[8]

The lack of a robust scientific tradition of research on sexuality has not, however, reduced the demand for and the supply of "facts" about sexuality. Research quackery abounds. "Surveys" have been conducted by journalists, women's and men's magazines, and enterprising professionals using invalid and unreliable questionnaires and collections of respondents whose population characteristics and response rates are unspecified. (Smith [in this volume] provides a review of one well-publicized report on sex in contemporary America [Hite, 1987].) Individually, such "reports" are transient sources of

[8]Other research programs in sexuality of less immediate relevance to the committee's concerns have included studies of sexual offenders, sexual contacts between adults and children, sexually explicit materials (studies of both their availability and their effects), and sexual violence against women. Such studies are important in a number of ways, and they may merit careful review in future work. Studies of sexually explicit materials, for example, are important for measuring change in the sociosexual climate in the society. Studies of sexual abuse and violence will be critical elements in understanding some of the sources of sexual difficulties experienced by both children and adults. In addition, there has been a steady growth of research on sexual psychophysiology, particularly as it relates to sexual dysfunction.

fun, fantasy, and profit—a short flash in the media pan. Collectively, they may have a more negative character. They become part of the penumbra of nonfacts and fake knowledge that informs the media and the public. Indeed, in the absence of scientific data, numbers from some of these surveys have been cited in research, textbooks, or serious science journalism. To the degree that science has abandoned the task of sexual enlightenment, others have filled the gap.

TRENDS IN HETEROSEXUAL BEHAVIOR IN ADOLESCENCE AND YOUNG ADULTHOOD

The extensive transformation of the role of sexuality in the lives of young people since the turn of the century has generated widespread social concern, especially since World War II. Kinsey found changes among young people during 1920–1945. His studies were followed by a surge of sociological interest in the premarital sexual conduct of young people as an element in changing courtship patterns (see reviews by Cannon and Long [1971] covering the 1960s and Clayton and Bokemeier [1980] covering the 1970s). Since the 1970s, research has been undertaken by both sociologists and demographers, motivated primarily by a concern for the rising rate of births among young unmarried women (e.g., Zelnik and Kantner, 1980; Hofferth et al., 1987). Although the data used in the various studies are not always strictly comparable, taken as a whole, they document impressively the increase in premarital sexual activity in the United States.

Kinsey's Findings

Figure 2-1 shows the cumulative percentage of women reporting premarital sexual intercourse by their decade of birth. Among ever-married women[9] who were still not married by age 20, only 8 percent of those born before 1900 reported premarital intercourse; however, for women born during the first three decades of the twentieth century, 18, 23, and 21 percent reported premarital intercourse. Commenting on these results, Kinsey and his collaborators (1953:298) observed: "This increase in the incidence of pre-marital coitus, and the similar increase in the incidence of pre-marital petting, constitute the greatest changes which we have found between the patterns of sexual behavior in the older and younger generations of American

[9]Ever-married women include those currently married and those who have been married at some point in their lives (e.g., widows, divorcées).

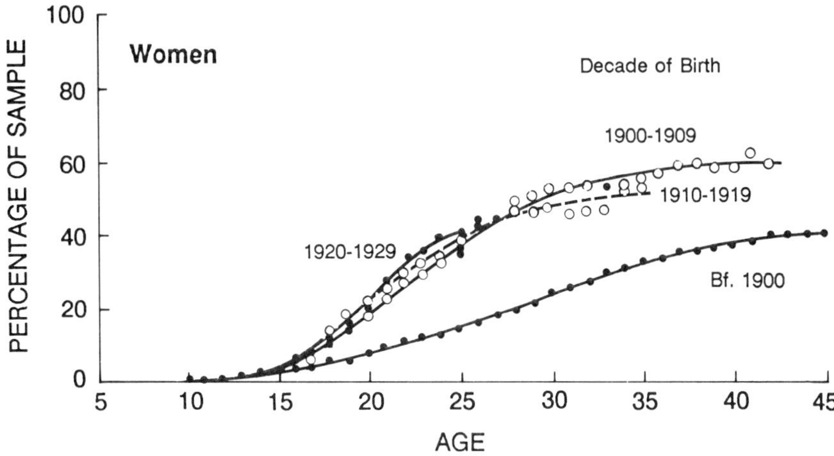

FIGURE 2-1 Cumulative percentage of women reporting premarital sexual intercourse by their decade of birth. Samples were restricted to ever-married women who had not married by the age shown in the figure. SOURCE: Kinsey and colleagues (1953:Figure 50 and Table 83).

females." In contrast, they found much smaller changes in the reported prevalence of premarital intercourse among young men in this same period. Figures 2-2a and 2-2b show the cumulative percentages of men, by education, reporting premarital sexual intercourse.[10]

Kinsey reports more substantial changes in male frequency of sex with "companions" than in frequency of sex with prostitutes. The difference consisted mainly of a change in the frequency with which men reported having sex with prostitutes—not a change in the percentage of men who had at least one such experience. Complementing the finding that women born after 1900 were more likely than those born before 1900 to report premarital sex, men in the younger cohort reported greater frequencies of sex with companions and reduced frequencies of sex with prostitutes. These differences

[10]The figures for men and women are not strictly comparable because the men were split into two groups by age at the time of the interview and the women were grouped by year of birth. The older generation of men are those "who were 33 years of age or older at the time they contributed their histories" (Kinsey et al., 1948:395). The point of division of the men by birth year can very roughly be estimated as a birth year in the range 1906–1912.

Because the interviewing stretched over several years, the two groups overlapped in birth dates. Gebhard and Johnson's (1979:32–35) history of the interviewing suggests that most of the interviews reported in Kinsey's 1948 volume were conducted from 1939 to 1945 or 1946. In the sample interviewed in 1939, those older than 33 were born in 1906 or before; men interviewed in 1945 were over 33 if they had been born in 1912 or earlier.

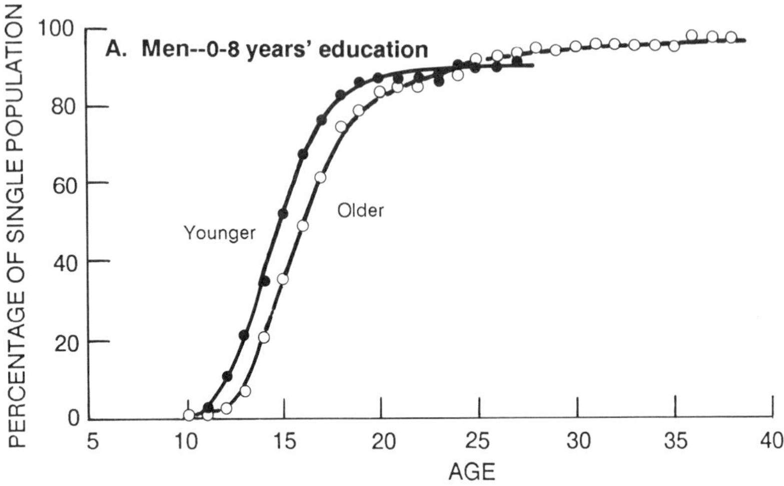

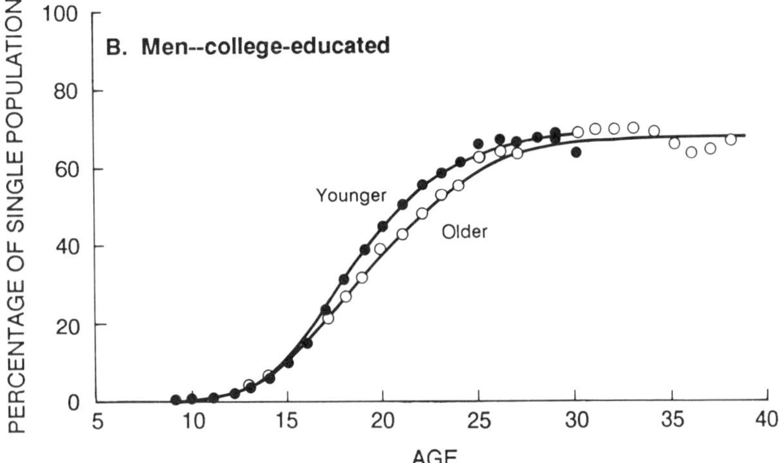

FIGURES 2-2a and 2-2b Cumulative percentages of men reporting premarital sexual intercourse by educational level. NOTE: In their text, Kinsey and colleagues imply that Figures 2-2a and 2-2b are based on a sample of men who were single at the time of the interview. This sample would be somewhat different from that used to construct the graph for women shown in Figure 2-1. SOURCE: Kinsey and colleagues (1948:Figures 111 and 116).

led Kinsey to the curious speculation that the "sexual outlet" formerly spent on prostitutes was now to be spent on companions: "The drives against prostitution have succeeded in diverting a third to a half of the intercourse that males used to have with prostitutes to pre-marital activities with other girls" (Kinsey et al., 1948:413). This image of male sexual energy waiting to be expended in one place or another is an important example of the asocial character of Kinsey's basic sexual theory.

Studies After Kinsey

The Kinsey studies were followed and extended by a number of social and behavioral researchers who investigated patterns of association, emotional intimacy, attitudes toward premarital sex, and premarital intercourse (e.g., I. Reiss, 1960, 1967; see also the reviews by Cannon and Long [1971], and Chilman [1978]). These researchers generally studied college students, although some managed to work with high school students or recruited "matched" samples of noncollege students from the same geographical area (e.g., DeLamater and MacCorquodale, 1979). The early studies in the 1950s tended to focus on attitudes toward premarital sex; those in the 1960s shifted more specifically to the question of premarital sexual behaviors. This research was primarily driven by concerns about the changing role of sexuality in the (heterosexual) courtship patterns of young people. In contrast to Kinsey's wide-ranging inquiries, post-Kinsey investigators dealt rather delicately with heterosexual issues and not at all with other aspects of the sexual lives of young people.

The 1970 Kinsey Institute study also produced complementary findings for numbers of reported heterosexual partners. Table 2-2[11] shows the number of premarital heterosexual partners reported by gender and decade of birth for ever-married adults in the sample. This table clearly documents the trend over the century of a greater number of sexual relationships for adults prior to marriage. Moreover, the table shows that this trend, although evident to some extent for men, is much more dramatic for women.

Unfortunately, if one wishes to draw inferences about the frequency of particular sexual behaviors in the American population, both Kinsey's data and most later research are restricted either by lack of a sampling design or by sampling from a limited population (e.g., students at the University of Wisconsin in 1973). A number of these studies, however, provide suggestive results and test methodologies that are instructive for further research; estimates of the prevalence of premarital intercourse from selected studies are presented in Appendix B. Although there is considerable variability

[11] Adapted from Klassen and colleagues, Table 1 (in this volume).

TABLE 2-2 Number of Premarital Heterosexual Partners Reported by Ever-Married Men and Women of Different Ages

Number of Premarital Partners	Age in 1969 (and year of birth)					
	21–29 (1940–1948)	30–39 (1930–1939)	40–49 (1920–1929)	50–59 (1910–1919)	60 + (pre-1910)	All
Ever-married men						
None	12.4%	12.8%	20.3%	26.1%	39.2%	23.0%
1 (spouse)[a]	12.4	9.3	7.2	7.4	6.1	8.3
1 (not spouse)[b]	5.1	5.0	2.4	5.3	5.5	4.7
2	7.9	8.2	10.6	5.9	8.5	8.3
3	7.3	7.8	8.2	9.0	6.5	7.7
4	7.3	7.8	5.3	6.9	3.4	6.0
5	6.2	8.9	6.3	7.4	5.8	7.0
6–9	10.7	11.4	10.6	8.0	6.5	9.3
10–14	10.7	12.5	11.1	11.2	10.2	11.2
15–19	6.2	4.6	5.3	2.7	2.4	4.1
20–29	8.5	8.5	9.2	7.4	5.5	7.7
30–39	2.3	1.4	1.4	0.5	0.0	1.0
40–49	1.1	0.7	0.5	0.0	0.0	0.4
50 +	1.7	1.1	1.4	2.1	0.3	1.2
Total	100.0	100.0	100.0	100.0	100.0	100.0
No. of responses	177	281	207	188	293	1,146
No. missing	13	24	40	30	62	169

Ever-married women						
None	37.7%	59.1%	68.6%	71.4%	87.7%	62.7%
1 (spouse)[a]	31.2	18.6	16.6	14.3	6.0	18.4
1 (not spouse)[b]	5.9	5.8	3.0	5.8	3.0	4.8
2	10.1	7.9	6.3	3.6	2.1	6.4
3	8.0	2.7	1.8	1.3	0.0	3.2
4	1.8	2.7	1.5	0.9	0.4	1.5
5	1.2	2.1	1.5	0.9	0.0	1.2
6–9	2.7	0.0	0.0	1.3	0.0	0.9
10–14	1.2	0.7	0.0	0.0	0.4	0.5
15–19	0.3	0.0	0.4	0.0	0.0	0.1
20–29	0.0	0.3	0.4	0.4	0.4	0.3
30 +	0.0	0.0	0.0	0.0	0.0	0.0
Total	100.0	100.0	100.0	100.0	100.0	100.0
No. of responses	337	291	271	224	235	1,358
No. missing	12	17	13	17	10	69

NOTE: Entries labeled "No. missing" indicate the number of cases for a particular age group and gender that were missing information on the number of sexual partners. (Age data were incomplete for 3 persons in the survey; 75 survey respondents who were heads of households but under 21 years of age are excluded from analysis.)

[a]One reported premarital sexual partner who was the future spouse.
[b]One reported premarital sexual partner, but this person was not the future spouse.

SOURCE: Secondary analysis of 1970 Kinsey Institute Survey data. See also the analysis by Klassen and colleagues (in this volume).

among the studies, the data suggest a slow evolution through the late 1960s with increasing proportions of young women engaging in intercourse before marriage, followed by more rapid increases in the early 1970s.

The first national probability sample survey that asked nearly as wide a set of questions on sexual conduct as the Kinsey research was conducted in 1967. It was relatively small (1,177 respondents) and was restricted to college students (Gagnon and Simon, 1987). In a two-stage sample design, 12 schools were first selected from a sample list of accredited four-year colleges and universities; lists of undergraduates in the school directories were then used to sample students. The response rate for the study (counting as nonrespondents those students who could not be located) was 75 percent (Gagnon and Simon, 1987:13). The survey covered masturbation (Atwood and Gagnon, 1987), premarital coital and noncoital sexual activity (Gagnon et al., 1970; Simon et al., 1972), first coital experience (Carnes, 1975), menarche (Gagnon, 1983), sex education (Spanier, 1976), homosexual behavior, sources of sexual arousal (Berger et al., 1973), childhood sexuality, and experiences of women with victimization. The information gathered on specific sexual behaviors included ages, frequencies of conduct, numbers of partners, and sexual practices (Gagnon and Simon, 1987). In addition, data were gathered on contraceptive knowledge and practices. Because one goal of the study was to set sexuality in the context of normal psychosexual development, data on a wide variety of social, psychological, and background variables were also gathered. In general, except for the questions about homosexuality (for which there appeared to be substantial underreporting; see Gebhard [1972:27]), the data from this study were similar to those reported in studies of less representative samples of college students.

A comprehensive national survey of the entire adult population (but covering a more restricted range of sexual behaviors) was conducted in 1970 for the Kinsey Institute by the National Opinion Research Center (NORC) of the University of Chicago. Unfortunately, because of a dispute among the investigators, little has been published from this important survey. (Some of the history of the study can be found in Booth [1988] and Klassen [1988].) At the request of the committee, the original investigators, with the assistance of National Research Council staff, have summarized some of the relevant data on heterosexual behaviors (Klassen et al., in this volume).

The 1970 Kinsey Institute survey, particularly when combined with more recent studies of adolescent experience, provides important insights into temporal trends in heterosexual experience among adolescents and young adults. For example, it is possible to use the retrospective reports of age at first premarital experience from several surveys to reconsider Kinsey and colleagues' (1948, 1953) analyses of temporal trends in premarital sexual behaviors. Figure 2-3a plots the percentages of men and women in the 1970 Kinsey Institute survey who reported a premarital sexual contact in which one partner came to a sexual climax (from Klassen et al., Table 3, in this volume). There is an upward trend from the cohort born at the beginning of the century through the cohort born in 1944–1949 for both men and women. Among ever-married men, the percentage reporting premarital sexual activity to the point of orgasm before age 19 rose from 41 percent for those born prior to 1911 to 79 percent for those born in 1944–1949. Among ever-married women, the rise is more dramatic (although the percentages consistently remain below those for men): the percentage reporting premarital sexual contact to the point of orgasm (by one partner) before age 19 rose from 5.5 percent for those born prior to 1911 to 50 percent for those born in 1944–1949. Similar results are found for sexual activity at younger ages. The percentage of young men reporting such behavior before age 16 rises from 15 percent (pre-1911 birth cohort) to 37 percent (1944–1949 birth cohort), while the corresponding female percentages rise from 2 percent to 15 percent.

It is possible to combine the data from the Kinsey Institute study reported by Klassen and colleagues (in this volume) with more recent data to extend such analyses through time. First, however, issues of data comparability must be considered. The 1970 Kinsey Institute study did not include a direct question on age at first intercourse. Instead, respondents were asked at what age they first had a sexual contact in which one partner (or both partners) came to a sexual climax (see the note to Figure 2-3a). There is no way to estimate what proportion of these activities involved sexual activities other than intercourse. Keeping this difficulty in mind, results from the 1970 Kinsey Institute survey can be compared with those of the 1982 National Survey of Family Growth (NSFG), shown in Figure 2-3b (Hofferth et al., 1987). The NSFG interviewed a national probability sample of women and asked a direct question on intercourse.[12]

[12]Appendix Table B-6 (in this volume) presents data from the two studies for the same birth cohort (1944–1949). The percentage of this cohort in the NSFG who reported premarital intercourse by age 20 (46 percent) was somewhat lower than the percentage in the Kinsey Institute study (Klassen et al., in this volume) who reported sexual activity to the point of orgasm (56 percent). The results suggest that, as expected, the Kinsey

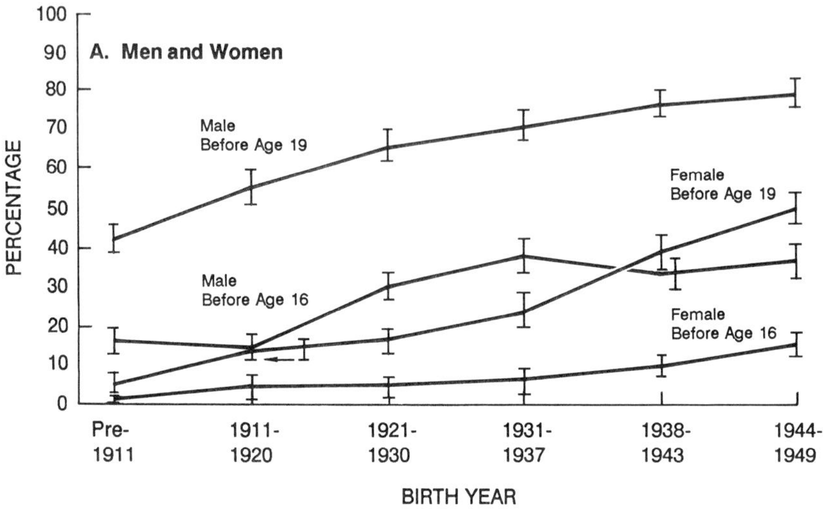

FIGURE 2-3a Percentages of ever-married men and women in the 1970 Kinsey Institute survey who reported a premarital heterosexual sexual contact in which one partner came to a sexual climax before ages 16 and 19. SOURCE: Klassen and colleagues (in this volume). Error bars denote approximately one standard error around estimates. NOTE: The 1970 Kinsey Institute study asked the following question to collect these data: "How old were you the first time you had sexual activity with someone of the opposite sex, when either you or your partner came to a sexual climax? If the first time was when you got married, please give your age at that time. This includes other sexual activity, as well as intercourse, if one of you had a sexual climax (orgasm)." Persons who reported that their first experience was in marriage are counted as having no premarital experience.

One general observation from these figures is inescapable: there has been a massive change in the sexual behavior of American men and women during the twentieth century.[13] The data for women suggest both an increase in the proportion of those who are sexually-active and a decline in the age at which the transition from being

---

Institute data overestimate the incidence of sexual intercourse by a particular age. The trend across birth cohorts, however, appears to be roughly comparable in the two sources.

It is not possible to rule out other sources of variation in these estimates, such as differences in the ages of respondents (and hence the length of recall involved) when they were supplying these data. Respondents in this cohort were 21–26 years old in the 1970 Kinsey Institute survey and 33–38 years old in the 1982 NSFG. Thus, respondents in the NSFG were recalling events 12 years more distant in time than those being reported in the Kinsey Institute survey.

[13]In addition to the well-known issues of reliability and validity of self-reported data on sexual behavior, it should be recognized that the sexual experiences of that fraction of a birth cohort that survives until the survey date may not be representative of the experiences of the entire cohort. For example, men in the pre-1911 cohort would have been 60 years of age or older at the time of the 1970 Kinsey Institute survey.

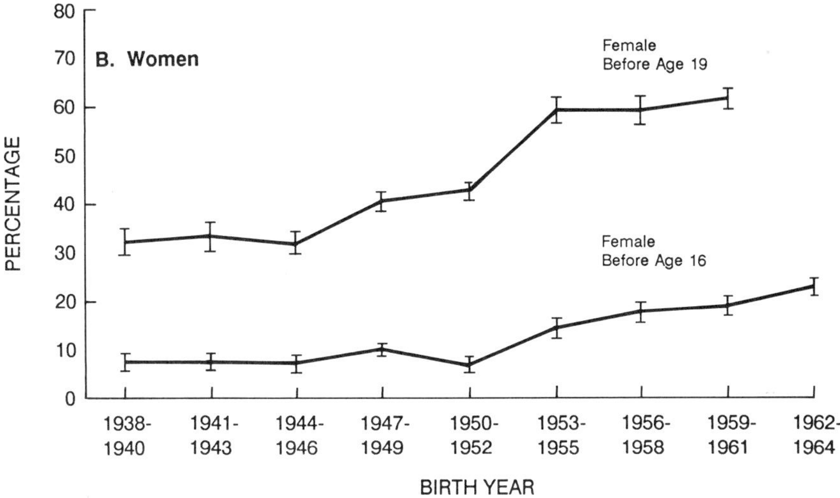

FIGURE 2-3b Percentage of women in the 1982 National Survey of Family Growth who reported premarital heterosexual intercourse before ages 16 and 19. Error bars denote approximately one standard error around estimates. SOURCE: Hofferth and colleagues (1987).

coitally inexperienced to coitally experienced occurs. For adolescent females, marriage has ceased to be strongly tied to sexuality. Thus, fewer than 6 percent of American women born before 1911 reported any premarital sexual activity that led to orgasm by either partner prior to age 19. In contrast, more than 62 percent of women born in 1959–1961 reported premarital sexual intercourse prior to age 19.

Changes in male sexual behavior are harder to track owing to the propensity of fertility studies—the source of much data on sexual behavior—to focus on women. The 1970 Kinsey Institute data (and the earlier observations of Kinsey and his colleagues), however, do suggest a shift in the character of premarital sex. Substantial proportions of young men at every observable point in the century report premarital sexual activity. Yet with the decline in their activity with prostitutes and an increase in the number of young women who were willing to have intercourse before marriage, it has been claimed that young men became increasingly involved in new forms of social negotiation and responsibility in sexual relationships and that these changes led to a rearrangement of the timing, character, and social psychology of sexual life among young people. Thus, P. Y. Miller and Simon (1974) report a convergence between male and female rates of premarital intercourse in a household probability sample of young people in Illinois in 1973, and they argue that, even though there was not a full convergence, there was evidence that young men and young women are now governed by more similar standards of sexual interaction. Young men appear more likely than in earlier decades to talk about love and affection in the context of a sexual encounter, and young women appear more likely to seek intercourse without romantic attachment.

Further Trends During the 1970s

A series of three surveys of probability samples of American adolescents were conducted in 1971, 1976, and 1979 (Kantner and Zelnik, 1983a,b; Zelnik and Kantner, 1985), and they provide additional detail on the changes that occurred during the last decade. Because these surveys were motivated largely by concerns about adolescent pregnancy, they were understandably limited in the scope of information they collected on sexuality. Only a few questions about sexuality were included, and they were limited to heterosexual behavior.[14] Perhaps most revealing of the surveys' focus on fertility is the fact that the survey samples in 1971 and 1976 were exclusively female.

Nonetheless, data from these surveys repeat and extend the basic findings of the previous analyses. Figure 2-4 shows, among women residing in metropolitan areas, a sizable increase in only eight years in the proportions of young people reporting the initiation of sexual intercourse: the percentage reporting intercourse before age 19 rose from 48 percent in 1971 to 71 percent in 1979; the percentage reporting intercourse prior to age 16 rose from 22 percent to 40 percent. These trends differ somewhat for black and white adolescent females.

Along with younger age at onset of sexual activity, the percentage of sexually active females (in metropolitan areas) aged 15 to 19 having more than one partner has increased somewhat. As Figure 2-5 shows, the percentage with multiple partners rose from just under 40 percent in 1971 to just over 50 percent in 1979 (Zelnik, 1983:Table 2-6). Figure 2-6a displays the distribution of the number of sexual partners reported at 17 and 19 years of age by never-married women in the 1979 survey. Although roughly one half of the 17-year-olds

[14] In the 1979 survey, data were collected on feelings about premarital sex; age, location, and planning for first intercourse; timing of second and last premarital intercourse; frequency of intercourse in the last 4 weeks and the last 12 months; total number of premarital partners and number of partners in the last 4 weeks; and the reason for discontinuing premarital sex.

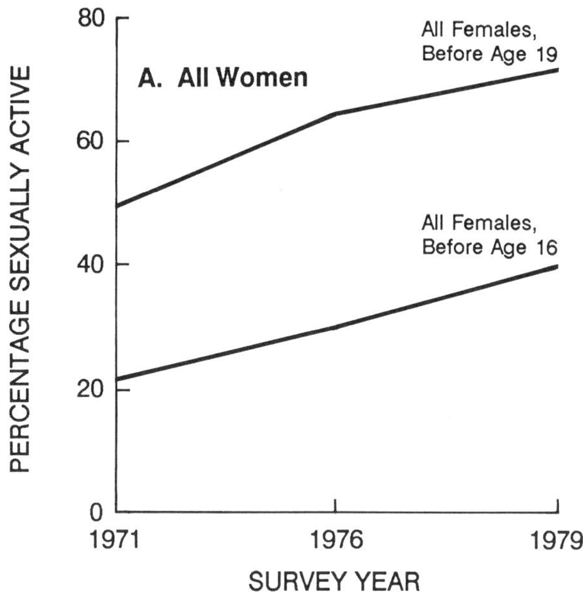

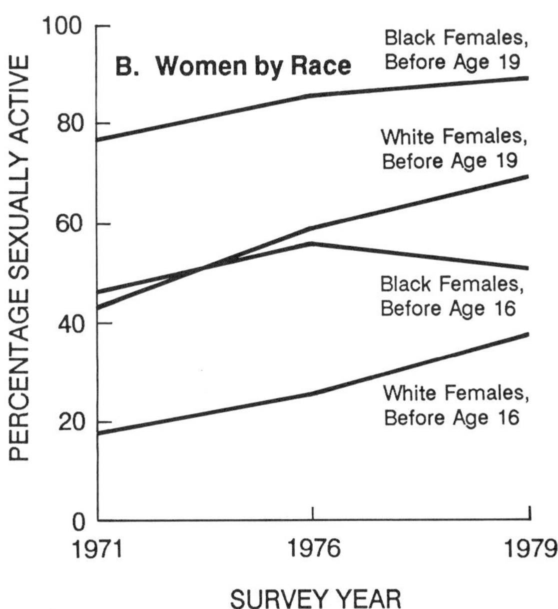

FIGURE 2-4 Percentages of (a) all young women and (b) young white women and young black women residing in metropolitan areas who reported premarital sexual intercourse prior to ages 16 and 19 in surveys conducted in 1971, 1976, and 1979. SOURCE: Zelnik (1983).

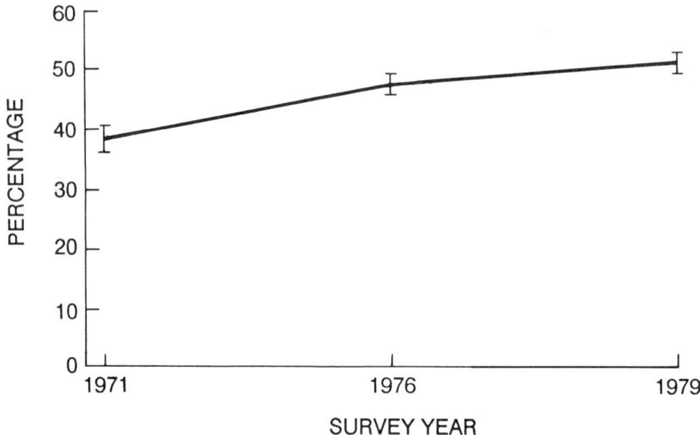

FIGURE 2-5 Percentage of sexually active young women ages 15–19 in the 1979 survey who reported more than one partner. Samples were restricted to women living in metropolitan areas. Error bars denote approximately one standard error around estimates. SOURCE: Zelnik (1983:Table 2-6).

and one third of the 19-year-olds were sexually inexperienced (i.e., had had no partners), a substantial fraction related having several sexual partners. For example, among the 19-year-old women, 15 percent reported having 4 or more sexual partners and 3 percent reported 10 or more partners; for 17-year-olds, the reported numbers were considerably lower, but 5 percent claimed 7 or more partners. Comparing these data for young women born during the 1960s with the 1970 Kinsey Institute data on the number of premarital partners reported by women born during earlier periods of this century provides strong evidence that a major shift had occurred in the social norms governing nonmarital heterosexual sexual behavior among young women.

Unmarried young men declared many more sexual partners than unmarried young women in these surveys. As Figure 2-6b shows, 7 percent of 17-year-olds, 24 percent of 19-year-olds, and 26 percent of 21-year-olds reported 10 or more partners. Even among 17-year-old males, more reported intercourse with 6 or more partners (20 percent) than reported only a single sexual partner (17 percent). Nonetheless, the modal response category for 17-year-old males was no partners: 45 percent of the male sample reported that they had not had intercourse prior to age 17.

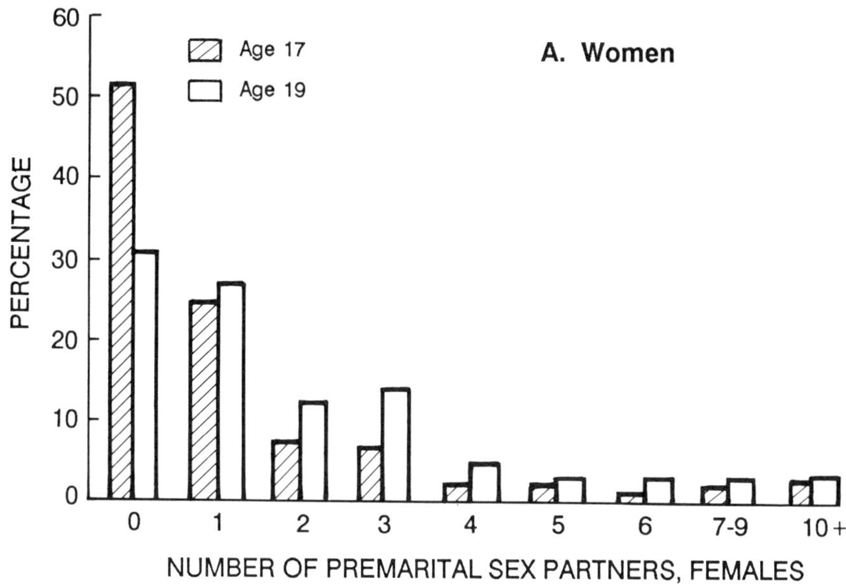

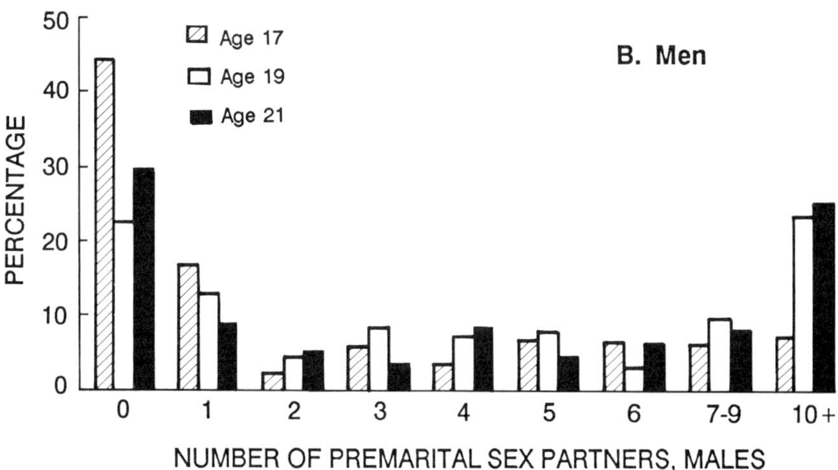

FIGURE 2-6 Number of premarital sexual partners reported by (a) young women at ages 17 and 19, and (b) young men at ages 17, 19, and 21. The survey sample was restricted to persons residing in metropolitan areas. SOURCE: Secondary analysis of 1979 survey of young men and women conducted by Kantner and Zelnik; see Zelnik (1983) for a description of the survey.

ADULT HETEROSEXUAL BEHAVIORS

As was noted earlier, there is a dearth of reliable information on adult sexual behavior of all types. At a late stage in the committee's deliberations, it received preliminary findings from a project that had been conducted by the National Institute of Child Health and Human Development (NICHD) and the National Opinion Research Center (NORC) to develop a rigorous basis from which to infer patterns of sexual behavior in the adult population of the United States. The results of the preliminary stage of the program were reported briefly by Michael and colleagues (1988); the committee received a final data tape from this preliminary effort in October 1988, and we describe some findings in this section. Because of extreme time pressures, however, the committee's analyses of this data set have been restricted in scope.

In addition to this new source of data, there is also some information available from other recent commercial surveys. The intense interest in the AIDS epidemic prior to 1988 spawned a number of opinion polls that asked questions related to AIDS and HIV transmission. The surveys were generally restricted to asking about knowledge and attitudes concerning AIDS, but a few asked explicit questions about sexual behaviors. Although such brief and quixotic forays into behavioral measurement do not ordinarily merit serious attention, some unique data have been obtained in at least one national poll. Because of the paucity of information relevant to HIV transmission, the results of that survey are presented in some detail (despite the committee's reservations about the representativeness of the sample). The results of this poll supplement the early findings of the NICHD/NORC effort.

We begin by briefly reviewing the data collection methods used in the two surveys and then move to a consideration of the results they obtained. Where possible, we have sought to present both individual and combined results from the surveys, although in some cases, this was simply not possible because the two surveys did not ask the same questions. The reader will also note that there are many important substantive areas about which there are simply no data from these or any other reliable sources. For example, although both surveys provide data on the number of sexual partners reported by respondents during the previous 12 months, no information is available on the frequency of sexual activity with different partners or the frequency of particular activities (e.g., anal intercourse) that may pose an elevated risk of HIV transmission. Moreover, there is no direct information on the frequency of condom use (although one of the surveys does provide data on the frequency of condom purchases). Thus, even if the data provided from these surveys were flawlessly derived from large samples, there are substantial gaps in knowledge that seriously compromise our understanding of heterosexual behaviors in the U.S. population that have the potential to transmit HIV. Nevertheless, these data provide the rough beginnings of a body of urgently needed information on the sexual behavior of the U.S. population.

Details of Survey Execution

1988 General Social Survey

The General Social Survey, or GSS, the program conducted by NICHD/NORC, is an annual, full-probability sample survey of noninstitutionalized American adults. Survey respondents are interviewed in person for approximately one hour on a wide range of social and political topics (Davis and Smith, 1988). The 1988 GSS interviewed 1,481 adults between February 14 and April 28, 1988, obtaining a response rate of 77 percent. At the conclusion of the 1988 GSS, respondents were asked to complete a one-page self-administered questionnaire. The questionnaire asked about the number and gender of respondents' sexual partners during the past 12 months and their relationships with these partners. (A preliminary analysis of these data has been reported by Michael and colleagues [1988].)

Los Angeles Times Survey

In July 1987, 2,095 adults were interviewed from a sample that had been designed as a probability sample of telephone-owning households. The survey design incorporated both a national sample and an oversampling of the five cities reporting the greatest numbers of AIDS cases (Los Angeles, Miami, New York City, Newark, and San Francisco).

Because of a low response rate,[15] the estimates produced from the survey cannot confidently be projected to the *entire* adult population

[15]For the entire survey (i.e., 1,208 cases in the national sample and 887 cases in the five-city oversample), we calculated a 33 percent response rate (using a procedure that conforms to the guidelines adopted by the Council of American Survey Research Organizations). However, because the survey drew an 887-case oversample from five urban areas (New York, Newark, Los Angeles, San Francisco, and Miami) in which response rates are traditionally much lower, we believe the effective response rate for the national sample (excluding the oversample) was actually higher than 33 percent. Unfortunately,

of the United States. Rather, the survey results are reflective of a portion of that population: those (one third to one half of adults) who can be reached by telephone (within three call-backs) and who will consent to being interviewed by telephone in what is described as a "public opinion survey" being conducted by a newspaper. It should be noted, however, that most of the nonresponse in this survey was apparently unrelated to the survey's content. The overwhelming majority of persons who refused to be interviewed did so during the household screening (1,279 of the 1,471 refusals), before being asked questions on AIDS or on sexual behaviors.

Turner and coworkers (in press:Table 1) report that the demographic characteristics of respondents in this survey agree roughly with Census Bureau estimates of the age and marital status distributions of the national adult population; there is some underrepresentation of men and blacks, however, and a more substantial underrepresentation of persons with less than a high school education.[16]

The questions asked in the survey elicited information on the following:

- number of sexual partners during the past year,
- frequency of condom purchases during the past year,
- precautions taken against AIDS,
- estimates of personal risk of contracting AIDS, and
- knowledge about the ways in which AIDS is transmitted and attitudes toward various AIDS-related social policies (e.g., school attendance by children with AIDS).

Survey Results

Both surveys asked respondents a question about the number of their sexual partners during the past year.[17] The responses to this question yielded a number of interesting results. Table 2-3 displays

---

the *Los Angeles Times* survey organization could not easily provide information on response rates for different sample strata.

[16]Bias in the education distribution is a well-known deficiency of samples obtained by many commercial and academic telephone surveys (see Turner and Martin, 1984:Vol. 1, Figure 3.1). In the substantive analysis reported by Turner and colleagues (in press) and in the committee's analysis in this chapter, weights encoded in the data set by the survey organization have been used in all tabulations. These weights incorporate adjustments to provide a better match to Census demographics (see Turner et al., in press:Table 1).

[17]The questions posed to respondents were: "About how many sexual partners would you say you have had in the last year?" (*L.A. Times*); and "How many sex partners have you had in the last 12 months?" (NORC).

the results obtained in both surveys, collapsing (for the moment) the top category to three or more partners. This table also presents the overall estimates (and standard errors) derived by combining the two sets of data and estimating a model of the table that fits the 4-way marginal (partners by age by marital status by gender).[18] The combined results of the two surveys indicate several findings of interest.

- Among unmarried men and women aged 18–24, only 19 percent of women and 16 percent of men reported that they had been without a sexual partner during the entire year.
- Forty percent of unmarried men and 15 percent of unmarried women aged 18–24 reported three or more partners in the preceding 12 months.
- For unmarried men, the percentage reporting three or more partners declined with age (although the trends varied between surveys). Even among men aged 65 years and older, however, approximately 4 percent reported three or more sexual partners. In both surveys, no woman in this age group reported more than one sexual partner during the preceding year.
- Approximately 1 percent of unmarried women and 6 percent of unmarried men reported nine or more partners during the previous year. Because the survey did not obtain information on the gender of partners, it is impossible to separate heterosexual and homosexual partnerships.
- Roughly 4 to 6 percent of married men, aged 25–49, reported two or more sexual partners during the preceding 12 months.

[18]Using a stratified jackknife procedure (Fay, 1982) to fit a hierarchical series of log-linear models to the 5-way table, we found that a model that fit the $\{PAGM\}$ and $\{AGMS\}$ marginals (where P = partners, A = age, M = marital status, G = gender, and S = survey) could be improved slightly by also constraining the model to fit the $\{PS\}$ marginal (jackknifed likelihood-ratio chi-square for comparison of two alternate models: $J^2 = 1.49$, $d.f. = 3$, $p = .051$). This improvement is of borderline statistical "significance." An examination of estimates of the λ^{PS} parameters for this "improved" model indicates that the observed intersurvey discrepancy was largely attributable to minor variations between the surveys in the numbers of persons with no sexual partners and with one partner. Estimates of the λ^{PS} parameters (and standard errors) for a log-linear model constrained to fit $\{PAGM\}$ $\{SAGM\}$ $\{PS\}$ were .127 ($s.e.$ = .070) for zero partners; −.123 (.063) for one partner; .035 (.073) for two partners; and −.040 (.072) for the category three or more partners. (Model parameters are [arbitrarily] coded so that positive values indicate an "excess" of NORC cases in the specified category.) With the effects of weighting and the complex sample design in the range of $deff = 1.6$, significant effects were not found for other multivariate parameters involving P and S (e.g., $\{PAS\}$, $\{PGS\}$, $\{PMS\}$, etc.). It should be noted that all model comparisons fit the $\{SAGM\}$ marginals, which allows for intersurvey differences in the demographic composition of the samples drawn by the two surveys.

TABLE 2-3 Number of Sexual Partners in the Last Year by Gender, Marital Status, and Age from the 1987 Telephone Survey Conducted by the *Los Angeles Times* (LAT) and the 1988 Personal Interview Survey Conducted by the National Opinion Research Center (NORC)

		Number of Sexual Partners in Last Year					
		None	1	2	3+	Total	(*N*)
Unmarried men							
18–24	LAT	14.1%	38.6%	8.7%	38.6%	100%	(83)
	NORC	19.6	24.0	12.8	43.6	100	(68)
	Comb. fit	16.5	32.3	10.5	40.7	100	(151)
	(s.e.)	(4.8)	(5.9)	(3.5)	(5.8)		
25–34	LAT	8.1	61.3	8.1	22.5	100	(99)
	NORC	17.9	41.9	7.7	32.5	100	(63)
	Comb. fit	12.4	52.9	7.9	26.9	100	(162)
	(s.e.)	(3.7)	(6.4)	(2.3)	(4.5)		
35–49	LAT	3.7	34.3	22.2	39.9	100	(64)
	NORC	20.3	44.3	15.2	20.3	100	(59)
	Comb. fit	13.5	39.7	18.2	28.5	100	(123)
	(s.e.)	(4.8)	(6.3)	(4.0)	(5.4)		
50–64	LAT	13.9	44.4	6.3	35.4	100	(43)
	NORC	50.0	30.8	11.5	7.7	100	(21)
	Comb. fit	22.3	41.3	7.5	29.0	100	(64)
	(s.e.)	(5.8)	(11.3)	(3.6)	(9.0)		
65+	LAT	80.0	12.2	5.5	2.3	100	(37)
	NORC	61.1	27.8	2.8	8.3	100	(30)
	Comb. fit	74.0	17.2	4.6	4.2	100	(67)
	(s.e.)	(6.4)	(5.3)	(3.0)	(2.1)		
Unmarried women							
18–24	LAT	16.3	56.1	10.4	17.3	100	(112)
	NORC	23.5	47.9	16.8	11.8	100	(50)
	Comb. fit	19.0	52.8	12.7	15.5	100	(162)
	(s.e.)	(3.9)	(5.9)	(4.1)	(5.1)		
25–34	LAT	17.7	69.2	10.6	2.5	100	(108)
	NORC	9.1	62.2	16.1	12.6	100	(90)
	Comb. fit	13.2	65.3	13.6	7.9	100	(198)
	(s.e.)	(3.2)	(4.8)	(3.1)	(2.4)		
35–49	LAT	23.5	57.9	12.0	6.6	100	(107)
	NORC	27.5	51.9	12.2	8.4	100	(94)
	Comb. fit	25.5	54.9	12.1	7.5	100	(201)
	(s.e.)	(4.3)	(4.8)	(3.7)	(2.4)		
50–64	LAT	52.8	32.5	12.8	1.9	100	(85)
	NORC	69.0	25.0	6.0	0.0	100	(60)
	Comb. fit	60.2	29.9	8.8	1.2	100	(145)
	(s.e.)	(5.6)	(5.5)	(3.8)	(0.8)		
65+	LAT	92.7	7.3	0.0	0.0	100	(114)
	NORC	95.0	5.0	0.0	0.0	100	(114)
	Comb. fit	93.7	6.3	0.0	0.0	100	(228)
	(s.e.)	(1.7)	(1.7)	(0.0)	(0.0)		

Continued

TABLE 2-3 *Continued*

		Number of Sexual Partners in Last Year					
		None	1	2	3+	Total	(*N*)
Married men							
18–24	LAT	0.0%	84.3%	3.2%	12.5%	100%	(22)
	NORC	0.0	80.8	0.0	19.2	100	(13)
	Comb. fit	0.0	83.6	2.5	13.9	100	(35)
	(s.e.)	(0.0)	(9.1)	(2.5)	(9.2)		
25–34	LAT	0.1	92.6	2.1	5.2	100	(127)
	NORC	2.8	93.1	2.8	1.4	100	(72)
	Comb. fit	1.0	92.7	2.3	4.0	100	(199)
	(s.e.)	(0.6)	(2.9)	(1.2)	(2.4)		
35–49	LAT	4.1	92.0	0.0	3.8	100	(190)
	NORC	5.1	89.1	3.6	2.2	100	(129)
	Comb. fit	4.6	90.7	1.7	3.1	100	(319)
	(s.e.)	(1.7)	(2.0)	(0.7)	(1.2)		
50–64	LAT	3.4	94.9	0.6	1.1	100	(91)
	NORC	10.9	85.5	1.2	2.4	100	(74)
	Comb. fit	5.9	91.7	0.9	1.6	100	(165)
	(s.e.)	(2.0)	(2.3)	(0.6)	(0.8)		
65+	LAT	11.4	83.4	4.0	1.2	100	(64)
	NORC	25.5	71.5	0.0	2.9	100	(68)
	Comb. fit	17.3	78.4	2.3	1.9	100	(132)
	(s.e.)	(3.0)	(4.8)	(2.3)	(1.0)		
Married women							
18–24	LAT	2.6	97.4	0.0	0.0	100	(44)
	NORC	0.0	86.6	10.4	3.0	100	(32)
	Comb. fit	1.7	93.6	3.7	1.0	100	(76)
	(s.e.)	(1.7)	(2.9)	(2.1)	(1.1)		
25–34	LAT	0.1	97.9	2.0	0.1	100	(156)
	NORC	1.1	97.8	0.0	1.1	100	(87)
	Comb. fit	0.5	97.8	1.2	0.5	100	(243)
	(s.e.)	(0.5)	(1.2)	(0.9)	(0.5)		
35–49	LAT	3.4	92.6	0.7	3.3	100	(235)
	NORC	3.5	96.5	0.0	0.0	100	(125)
	Comb. fit	3.5	94.2	0.4	1.9	100	(360)
	(s.e.)	(1.5)	(1.8)	(0.2)	(1.1)		
50–64	LAT	17.5	82.5	0.0	0.0	100	(125)
	NORC	14.5	83.7	0.6	1.2	100	(78)
	Comb. fit	16.3	83.0	0.2	0.5	100	(203)
	(s.e.)	(5.2)	(5.2)	(0.2)	(0.5)		
65+	LAT	15.9	84.0	0.1	0.0	100	(66)
	NORC	29.0	69.4	0.0	1.6	100	(61)
	Comb. fit	21.7	77.5	0.1	0.7	100	(127)
	(s.e.)	(4.2)	(4.2)	(0.1)	(0.7)		

NOTE: Percentage distributions for the *Los Angeles Times* data set were calculated using weights encoded in the data set by the survey organization. Sample sizes shown are unweighted *N*s. NORC percentages are calculated from weighted tabulations. Combined fit estimates and standard errors were derived using procedures of Fay (1982) to take account of complex sample design and sample weighting. (Weights in each survey were normalized so that the weighted *N* for each survey equaled the unweighted case count.)

Question Wordings. Los Angeles Times: "About how many sexual partners would you say you have had in the last year?" NORC: "How many sex partners have you had in the last 12 months?"

Approximately 1 to 2 percent of married women in this age range reported two or more sexual partners.

- Of unmarried persons who described themselves as "strongly religious" Christians in the *Los Angeles Times* survey, 66 percent of men and 40 percent of women reported at least one sexual partner in the past year; 26 percent of men and 12 percent of women in this group reported two or more partners over the past 12 months (Turner et al., in press:Table 2).

The data from these surveys also contain anomalies that begin to suggest the difficulties of conducting rigorous research on human sexual behaviors. For example, nontrivial proportions of married respondents reported that they had no sexual partners during the preceding year. For some, this may, indeed, be a true statement, and the increase in these proportions with age supports this view. It is also possible, however, that some respondents may not consider their spouses to be "sexual partners"—one example of the many possible ways in which the language and frames of reference researchers and respondents bring to a survey may differ. These differences can have important implications for the interpretation of the resultant data, and they mandate careful pretesting and pilot work for those who would use surveys to learn about sexual behavior in the population.

Condom Use and Risk Perception

Given the high level of awareness in the United States that HIV can be transmitted sexually, condom purchases by persons reporting a large number of sexual partners during the preceding year are of particular interest. In an analysis of the *Los Angeles Times* data set,[19] Turner and colleagues (in press) found that, even though frequency of condom purchases increased with the number of sexual partners (for both men and women), 45 percent of the men reporting nine or more partners during the past year and 65 percent of the women reporting three or more partners stated that they had never purchased condoms during the past year. Although it is possible that condoms were used without being purchased (e.g., they were supplied by the other partner) or that other low-risk sexual practices were employed, this result suggests that sexual intercourse without protection against HIV transmission may be fairly common, even among people who have a large number of sexual partners.

[19]The 1988 GSS did not ask respondents about condom use.

Substantial proportions of those in the *Los Angeles Times* sample who reported many sexual partners also believed they were not at risk of contracting AIDS. Thus, when respondents rated their risk of contracting AIDS on a scale of 1 to 7 (with 1 representing the lowest possible risk and 7 the highest), the majority of those with nine or more sexual partners chose the lowest level (Turner et al., in press:Table 4). Even in urban areas that have experienced the greatest number of AIDS cases (i.e., New York, Newark, San Francisco, Los Angeles, and Miami), almost one half of the respondents with nine or more partners assessed their risk of contracting AIDS at the lowest level offered.[20]

As these analyses begin to suggest, the psychological and social processes that underlie sexual behaviors are complex. Indeed, as Chapter 5 discusses, this complexity poses substantial challenges for the design and implementation of interventions designed to facilitate change in risk-associated sexual behavior (e.g., by decreasing the frequency of sexual behaviors that carry a high risk of transmitting HIV and other sexually transmitted infections).

Special Studies

In addition to the two national studies of adult heterosexual behavior, we discuss below two other research efforts that offer important insights. One of these (Blumstein and Schwartz, 1983) provides comparative information on heterosexual, gay, and lesbian couples. Although this study uses a nonprobability sample, its conclusions are of interest, even though its numerical results cannot be generalized with known margins of sampling error to the population of heterosexual, gay, and lesbian couples. The second research project (Wyatt, 1988a) studied relatively small samples (*N*s = 122 and 126, respectively) of white and Afro-American women in Los Angeles County; this project is of particular value because it collected extensive data on sexual practices from a probability sample of Afro-American women—a population for which there are few data.

[20]Turner and colleagues (in press) also found that high levels of condom use could not account for the optimistic risk assessments of many of these respondents. Thus, among persons reporting five or more sexual partners during the last 12 months, 30 percent of those who rated their risk as low (1 or 2) reported that they never purchased condoms and 25 percent reported only one to four purchases. Indeed, there was no significant association between condom purchasing and perceived risk among persons with five or more sexual partners.

Couples Study Data

Between the spring of 1978 and late 1979, Blumstein and Schwartz (1983) mailed self-administered questionnaires to a large number of couples, including married heterosexuals, cohabiting heterosexuals, gay male couples, and lesbian couples. The majority of these couples requested the questionnaires as a result of hearing appeals for cooperation by the investigators on television and reading reports about the study in the mass media; in the case of the gay male and lesbian couples, people also requested questionnaires as a result of hearing about the study from others who had participated. Some 22,000 questionnaires were mailed to the 11,000 couples who volunteered to participate in the study, and somewhat over one half of those to whom they were mailed returned the two questionnaires as required for inclusion in the study. Of the 7,397 married or cohabiting heterosexual couples who requested questionnaires, 4,314 (58 percent) returned them, as did 969 (52 percent) of the 1,875 gay male couples and 778 (46 percent) of the 1,723 lesbian couples who requested them. All of these volunteer couples completed a long (38 pages), self-administered questionnaire about various aspects of their relationships, and these data provide the statistical base for the study. Of these cases, 320 (129 heterosexual, 98 gay male, and 93 lesbian couples) were purposively selected to be interviewed face to face. The couples were first interviewed apart and then as a couple; they were subsequently asked to solve some couple dilemmas without interviewers present but with a tape recorder running. Finally, a subsample of those who filled out the self-administered questionnaire was mailed a shorter questionnaire 18 months after the interview to determine whether the relationship had remained intact. The response rate for this instrument ranged from 67 percent among cohabitors to 82 percent among married couples.

The sample obtained by Blumstein and Schwartz was skewed in several ways. Although the researchers were seeking a "large and diverse sample of respondents" (Blumstein and Schwartz, 1983:15) that would reflect an array of values and life-styles, the mode of case gathering they used resulted in a case base that was 95 percent white, 85 percent college educated, and centered in three metropolitan regions (Seattle, San Francisco, and New York). The case gathering involved a number of stages of self-selection that seem likely to have produced systematic biases. Respondents had to be aware of appeals made in the mass media, to write for questionnaires, and to fill out (with the partner's knowledge), a long instrument about intimate topics, a task that required substantial literacy and attention.

The published data from the study focus on the roles of money, work, and sexuality in coupled relationships, exploring differences among couple types. The data on sexuality do not differ a great deal from the data gathered by other studies of volunteer populations in which the findings are based on the reports of individuals. Sexual frequency differed among the various types of couples and was patterned in different ways, depending on the duration of the relationship. Married couples were having sex at least once a week, and rates lower than once a month among these couples were rare. However, the rates these couples reported were higher than those of most sampled populations and may represent the volunteer bias of the study. Cohabitor couples had sex more often than married couples, but the cohabitors were also comparatively younger with shorter durations of living together. The pattern for gay men was similar to those found in other studies: much higher rates of sexual activity early in relationships but much lower rates later on. Lesbians reported far less sex in their relationships than did the other groups. Patterns of sexuality outside of the couples followed at least a ranking pattern that is similar to other studies: 26 percent of married heterosexual men, 21 percent of married heterosexual women, 33 percent of male cohabitors, 30 percent of female cohabitors, 92 percent of gay men, and 28 percent of lesbians reported sexual relationships outside of that of the primary couple. These differences in prevalence are reflected in numbers of partners as well (see Table 2-4). The prevalence figures for heterosexual men are somewhat lower than might have been expected from other similar data sources, but the requirement that both persons participate in the study might have reduced these numbers. Differences in the duration of relationships also affected these rates: the longer the relationship, the greater the prevalence of sexuality outside the couple relationship and the larger the number of partners. As noted earlier, however, it is important to interpret these figures cautiously. The numerical estimates from this study cannot be confidently generalized to the population at large because the survey used a convenience sample.

White and Afro-American Women in Los Angeles

In a series of papers, Wyatt and her collaborators have reported on the sexual experiences of 126 Afro-American and 122 white women residing in Los Angeles County. The study (Wyatt, 1985:508–510)

TABLE 2-4 Number of Outside Sexual Partners During Relationship

	Number of Sexual Partners						
Group	0	1	2–5	6–20	20 +	N^a	
Husbands	74%	8%	11%	6%	2%	3,591	(913)
Wives	79	9	8	3	1	3,606	(750)
Male cohabitors	67	12	16	4	1	634	(210)
Female cohabitors	70	13	12	4	0	639	(197)
Gay men	18	6	16	25	35	1,914	(1,513)
Lesbians	72	15	12	1	0	1,554	(368)

NOTE: As described in the text, these distributions cannot be generalized to the national population because the study was based on a convenience sample of couples.

[a]Total *N* is the number of individuals who reported any instances of nonmonogamy since the beginning of the relationship; the parenthetical *N* is the number of individuals who reported how many sexual partners they had outside the relationship. The percentage distribution for the numbers of partners is calculated on the percentage of respondents who reported nonmonogamy.

SOURCE: Blumstein and Schwartz (1983).

enlisted women aged 18–36 using a telephone survey to recruit suitable probability samples. The sample of white women was matched to the sample of Afro-American women on education, marital status, and the presence of children in the household (Wyatt, 1988b:15). All respondents were subsequently interviewed in person at a location of their choice. The interviews, which were usually conducted in two sessions, covered a broad range of topics. The women's sexual histories were obtained using a 478-item structured interview whose topics included sources of sexual education; onset, frequency, and circumstances of various sexual behaviors; frequency and circumstances of any sexual abuse during childhood or adolescence, consequences of sexual abuse; experiences of sexual harassment in school work, or social settings; and sex role stereotypes. The total interview time ranged from three to eight hours, depending on the woman's sexual experiences. The refusal rate for the survey was 45 percent (including women who refused to schedule an interview and women who terminated the telephone recruitment before their eligibility could be determined).[21]

[21]Wyatt (1985:509) reported identifying 1,348 households in which a woman resided. Of these, 709 women met the study's inclusion criteria and agreed to be interviewed, 266 met the inclusion criteria and refused to be interviewed, and 335 women terminated

Wyatt (1988a:9–11) has reported several findings of interest from this study:

- 39 percent of white women and 48 percent of Afro-American women in this study reported that their first experience of sexual intercourse occurred at or before age 16;
- 74 percent of white women and 26 percent of Afro-American women reported 13 or more sexual partners since age 18;
- 43 percent of white women and 21 percent of Afro-American women reported *some* experience with anal intercourse; and
- 5–6 percent of each sample reported engaging in anal intercourse on a regular basis (one or more times a month).

These data suggest, as do the findings of the two national surveys, that there is a sexually active subset of the adult population (that includes both whites and Afro-Americans) that engages in heterosexual behaviors that may carry a significant risk of HIV transmission.

TRENDS IN SEXUAL BEHAVIOR AMONG PERSONS OF THE SAME GENDER

The study of sexual conduct among persons of the same gender—referred to as homosexuality by some and as the sexuality of gay men and lesbians by others—has a number of dimensions that are directly relevant to the AIDS epidemic and to the sexual transmission of HIV. Key aspects of same-gender sexual behavior include

- the number of persons who have sex with persons of the same gender;
- the frequency of such contacts and the number of partners in various periods;
- the sexual techniques used in sexual encounters;
- the number of sexual partners who are of the opposite gender; and
- the social characteristics of the individual and of his or her sexual partners (i.e., the personal sexual network of an individual).

---

the telephone recruitment interview before it could be determined whether they met the study's inclusion criteria.

Equally important to an understanding of behavior is setting these variables into the changing cultural, historical, and social circumstances of sexual conduct with persons of the same gender over the last four decades in the United States. This context is important for an understanding of the complexity of same-gender sexuality, the variety of ways in which it is expressed, and the willingness of different individuals and groups who have sexual partners of the same gender to adopt safer sex practices. Finally, it is important to recognize that the terms used to describe sexual activity among people of the same gender are culturally and politically significant. That is why we have often chosen to use the term *same-gender sexual conduct* and its variants rather than *homosexuality* or *gay men and lesbians*, except when such terms are historically or culturally appropriate.

The Kinsey Research

The general challenge that Kinsey and the Kinsey reports posed to widely held beliefs about sexuality has been discussed earlier in this chapter. It was in the area of what happened sexually between men and men and between women and women, however, that Kinsey's work most clearly diverged from prior scientific and moral perspectives. This divergence occurred in both the survey's empirical findings and in the explanation of those findings. In his studies, Kinsey found that a far larger number of people than expected reported that they had had sex with persons of the same gender. Kinsey's conception of the relation between sexual activity among persons of the same gender and sexual activity with persons of the other gender also differed quite markedly from earlier research.

Prior to the Kinsey studies—and in the period during which they were being conducted—persons who had sex with persons of the same gender were in nearly universal danger of social ostracism of the most severe kinds: criminal prosecution and imprisonment, coerced psychotherapy, blackmail, robbery, and victimization by the criminal justice system.[22] Anyone who was attracted sexually or emotionally to persons of the same gender and admitted this fact to others was treated as perverse or deviant. Even those who kept their sexual

[22]Gagnon and Simon (1973) summarize Kinsey's data on the experiences of men with extensive homosexual histories and with histories of robbery, blackmail, and troubles with the police. Weinberg and Williams (1974) present data on men who experienced trouble in military and civilian life prior to the 1970s, and Kinsey and coworkers (1948) discuss the legal difficulties of men with homosexual experience. Chapter 7 (Figure 7-2) presents contemporary survey data on public prejudice against same-gender sexual experience.

preferences to themselves often experienced severe psychological conflicts. In general, it was believed that the negative psychological and social situations that characterized the lives of persons who were "homosexual" were a simple consequence of their moral or psychological defects rather than the result of social persecution and oppression under which they acquired and expressed their sexual desires.

Kinsey (e.g., Kinsey et al., 1948:616–617) opposed the theoretical belief, which was well established among psychiatrists and psychoanalysts, that persons with substantial amounts of same-gender sexual experience constituted a discrete category of persons whose lives were entirely governed or at least strongly influenced by this sexual preference (Freud, 1905; Bergler, 1956). This conception was very close to the prior folk belief, shared by both "heterosexuals" and "homosexuals," that "homosexuality" was grounded in a gender defect (either constitutional or learned). Homosexual men were somehow insufficiently masculine (and therefore effeminate), and homosexual women were insufficiently feminine (and therefore masculine). More complicated explanations were formulated, but at the center of the theory was the belief that there existed a class of persons whose conduct depended on common pathological origins (Socarides, 1978). From this perspective, there must be a profound psychological or biological division between heterosexuals and homosexuals; consequently, the former were treated as essentially normal and the latter as essentially abnormal.

Kinsey attacked this dichotomy on two levels: sexual theory and individual experience. On the basis of theory, he argued against homosexuality as a discrete social, moral, or psychological "type." He proposed that the relation between heterosexuality and homosexuality be treated as a continuum rather than two discrete categories, and he argued that sexuality could best be understood through the proportion of other-gender and same-gender sexual acts (and fantasies) in which individuals engaged. Kinsey based his view on a distinction he saw between the biological diversity found in unmanaged nature and the limitations on diversity found in civilized societies based on agriculture. Translating this concept into the sexual arena, a contrast was created between the sexual bounty of the natural world and Western cultural selection for a monocrop of procreative heterosexuality. Thus, Kinsey and his coworkers wrote:

> Males do not represent two discrete populations, heterosexual and homosexual. The world is not to be divided into sheep and goats. Not all things are black nor all things white. It is a fundamental of taxonomy that nature rarely deals with discrete categories.

> Only the human mind invents categories and tries to force facts into separated pigeon-holes. The living world is a continuum in each and every one of its aspects. The sooner we learn this concerning human sexual behavior the sooner we shall reach a sound understanding of the realities of sex. (1948:639)

That continua are as much human inventions as dichotomies, and that there is, for certain purposes, a need to distinguish between sheep and goats, are reasonable intellectual responses to Kinsey's view. The important points, however, are Kinsey's decision to make heterosexuality and homosexuality a question of acts rather than of common pathological origins and his proposal of a continuum within which an individual's position can fluctuate over the life course.

To measure an individual's position on this continuum from heterosexuality to homosexuality, Kinsey developed the H–H (or 0–6) scale. Interviewers collected a record of a person's experiences and psychic reactions during the sex history portion of the interview and, on returning from the field, counted up—necessarily in somewhat crude ways—the frequency of sociosexual experiences, with and without orgasm, with partners of the same or different genders (independent of marital status and other factors). The proportion of same-gender experiences was used to place the interviewee on the H–H scale. In addition, estimates were made of the frequency of sexual dreams with and without orgasm and the proportion of masturbation that could be classified as having same-gender or other-gender content. These calculations were less precise than those from sociosexual experience, most significantly because of the weaker attention that was given to fantasy in the interviews. The counts were made for each year of life and then were added together to produce totals both for the life span and for various life periods. There was a good deal of judgment involved in the assignment of scale scores, and the Kinsey researchers often estimated the "importance" of different kinds of sexual activity when assessing their contribution to the final scale number chosen.

By focusing on acts rather than on persons, Kinsey argued that there is no such thing as a homosexual person, only persons with various mixtures of acts. He did not, however, actually propose a specific theory of the acquisition, maintenance, or transformation of either heterosexuality or homosexuality in his 1948 volume. The closest he came was to argue:

> If all persons with any trace of homosexual history, or those who were predominantly homosexual, were eliminated from the population today, there is no reason for believing that the incidence of the homosexual in the next generation would be materially

> reduced. The homosexual has been a significant part of human sexual activity ever since the dawn of history, primarily because *it is an expression of capacities that are basic in the human animal.* (Kinsey et al., 1948:666; emphasis added)

Later, in the volume on women, and largely in response to critics of this argument, Kinsey wrote:

> The data indicate that the factors leading to homosexual behavior are (1) the basic physiologic capacity of every mammal to respond to any sufficient stimulus; (2) the accident which leads an individual into his or her first sexual experience with a person of the same sex; (3) the conditioning effects of such an experience; and (4) the indirect but powerful conditioning which the opinions of other persons and the social codes may have on an individual's decision to accept or reject this type of sexual contact. (Kinsey et al., 1953:447)

The grudging readmission of what is at least a stripped-down version of the roles of psychology and culture in sexual life is an important shift, one that is characteristic of a change in Kinsey's views as he writes about female rather than male sexuality (Gagnon, 1978).

What is problematic for Kinsey's view of people as embodying a mixture of sexual acts is that at the time Kinsey's work was being published, most individuals with same-gender sexual experiences actually lived in terms of the social types Kinsey fought so hard to dissolve. Persons with same-gender sexual experiences often viewed themselves and were viewed by others, whether hostile or friendly, as enacting or resisting the social roles provided in the homosexual culture of the day: "sissy," "queer," "dyke," "fem," "butch," "trade," and "faggot" were experienced as significant cultural labels. On the other hand, Kinsey's theoretical arguments were given additional power by the sheer number of persons in his collection of cases who reported at least some sex with persons of the same gender. In addition, both his supporters and critics considered the number of persons who had reported same-gender sexual experience to be generalizable to the larger population. As was argued earlier, there is no scientific basis for accepting such a generalization, but because Kinsey provides the earliest figures in this area and because these figures have been used as bases for national estimates, they need to be discussed.

In *Sexual Behavior in the Human Male*, Kinsey and his colleagues reported that

> . . . *37 per cent* of the total male population has *at least some overt homosexual* experience to the point of orgasm between adolescence

> and old age . . . *10 per cent* of the males *are more or less exclusively homosexual* (i.e., rate 5 or 6) for at least three years between the ages of 16 and 55. . . . *8 per cent* of the males are *exclusively homosexual* (i.e., rate a 6) for at least three years between the ages of 16 and 55. . . . *4 per cent* of the white males are *exclusively homosexual throughout their lives,* after the onset of adolescence. (1948:650–651; all emphases in the original; the numbers 5 and 6 refer to Kinsey's 0–6 H–H scale noted previously)

There is reason to be cautious about these figures, even when they are not being used to create national estimates. The chapter in the 1948 report on male homosexual behavior was based on 4,301 cases, a group that included a substantial number of persons with current or prior prison experience. The inclusion of large numbers of prisoners biased the resulting figures. Analyzing only the college attenders in the Kinsey collection of cases, Gagnon and Simon (1973:131) found that

> [i]n a reanalysis of the cases of 2,900 young men who were in college between the years 1938 and 1950, the bulk of whom were under thirty at the time they were interviewed, 30 percent had undergone at least one homosexual experience in which either the interviewee *or* his male partner was stimulated to the point of orgasm (note that this differs from the Kinsey definition). Of these 30 percent, however, slightly more than one-half (16% of the total) had shared no such experiences since the age of fifteen, and an additional third (9% of the total) had experienced all of their homosexual acts during adolescence or incidentally in the years before they reached the age of twenty. Thus, for 25 percent of all males who were interviewed, homosexual experience was confined predominantly to adolescence or to isolated experiences in the later adjacent years. The remaining 5 to 6 percent are divided into those men who had only homosexual experiences, comprising some 3% of the 2,900, and the remaining 3% who had substantial homosexual histories as well as heterosexual histories.

Although these figures may offer some insight, they cannot replace data that have been collected from more carefully sampled and equally well-interviewed populations. What this and other reanalyses of the Kinsey data have in common, however, is that the estimates they provide of the extent of male homosexual experience are lower than those of Kinsey.

From Kinsey to the AIDS Epidemic

The Kinsey research findings on same-gender sexuality generated a number of responses in the period from 1955 to 1975. The appeal for understanding and tolerance that was implicit in his scientific views had an effect among several groups interested in the reform of sexual laws. The empirical findings that there were many persons with same-gender sexual lives and the public discussion of the existence of "homosexuality" were taken up by the emergent social and political groups among homosexuals who were campaigning for legal reform and social tolerance (e.g., the Mattachine Society and the Daughters of Bilitis, as well as other, more transitory groups). Slow changes in the actual social and living conditions of persons with same-gender sexual desires and experiences were accompanied by an increase in research interest among social psychologists and sociologists.

Following a line of work initiated by sociological criminologists and later continued by labeling theorists who took for granted the social reality of cultural labels and their consequences, a small number of ethnographic studies of homosexual communities were undertaken in the 1950s and 1960s (e.g., Leznoff and Westley, 1956; Hooker, 1966). Although often influenced by Kinsey, these studies moved away from traditional questions of etiology and focused on issues of life careers and adjustment and of psychological identity and culture among men and women living in same-gender subcultures. They found extraordinary variety. Although the men and women that made up these same-gender subcultures were participating in a common cultural community, they did not appear to have common attributes. As a result, researchers were moved to understand these people not in terms of some common set of psychological characteristics but in terms of their social and cultural origins. In the late 1960s a critique of traditional etiologic and psychiatric studies (Simon and Gagnon, 1967; Gagnon and Simon, 1973) included several major points.

- There was no evidence that same-gender sexual preferences were acquired through special or pathological pathways. There was also no evidence of special or frequent pathology among persons with such preferences that could not be explained by social oppression during the acquisition of and performance of same-gender sexuality.
- The issue of the origins of same-gender sexual preference was overemphasized and extremely difficult, if not impossible, to resolve, given that adult research subjects could offer only retrospective reports that were often compromised by strong cultural pressures to adopt dominant theories of origins or development.
- Same-gender sexual conduct varied substantially according to the current circumstances of the subcommunity

in which persons with such preferences participated and the relation of that subcommunity (especially relations involving sexual oppression) to the larger community in which it was embedded.

- The primary focus of research should be the conditions of social life among those with same-gender sexual preferences, rather than the differences between same-gender and other-gender sexuality.
- The nonsexual aspects of such persons' life-styles were often more important in shaping their sexual lives than vice versa.
- Historical changes in societal tolerance of same-gender sex would be of consequence for the social and psychological adjustment of persons with same-gender sexual desires and experience.
- More generally, it was argued that the sexual life course was relatively discontinuous and that alterations in what appeared to be stable adjustments, including gender preference in sexual partners, were frequent, if not common.

Although agreement was never total on all of these positions among all researchers (e.g., Diamond, 1977; Pillard et al., 1981; Green, 1987), there was substantial movement of the majority of researchers toward a research program built on these ideas.

Nevertheless, biases toward constructing a common "homosexual personality" remained common in psychological circles until strongly challenged in the 1970s (Morin, 1977). Several major studies in the tradition of psychopathology compared "convenience" (nonprobability) samples of heterosexuals and homosexuals (Bieber et al., 1965; Saghir and Robins, 1973). By 1973, however, the psychiatric definitions had changed, and same-gender sexuality was no longer taken as prima facie evidence of psychopathology (American Psychiatric Association, 1973; see also the discussion by Bayer, 1987).

The early small studies were followed by two others, funded by the National Institute of Mental Health, that interviewed larger samples from Chicago during 1967–1968 (Gagnon and Simon, 1973) and from San Francisco during 1970–1972 (A. P. Bell and Weinberg, 1978). The Chicago study interviewed 457 white men; the San Francisco study interviewed more than 900 individuals with same-gender sexual preferences plus a group of controls. Both studies suffered from the defect of using convenience samples of people who were sufficiently open about their sexual preferences to be available to

TABLE 2-5 Number of Sexual Partners of the Same Sex Reported During Lifetime by Homosexual Respondents

Number of Homosexual Partners Ever	Homosexual Respondents			
	White Males	Black Males	White Females	Black Females
1	0%	0%	3%	5%
2	0	0	9	5
3–4	1	2	15	14
5–9	2	4	31	30
10–14	3	5	16	9
15–24	3	6	10	16
25–49	8	6	8	11
50–99	9	18	5	8
100–249	15	15	1	2
250–499	17	11	1	2
500–999	15	14	0	0
1,000 or more	28	19	0	0
N	574	111	227	64

SOURCE: Bell and Weinberg (1978:308).

researchers. Indeed, only one study in this period studied men who were having sex with other men but who did not participate in the gay community (L. Humphreys, 1970).

These studies confirmed what earlier research had indicated: there was wide diversity among members of the gay community in both social background and patterns of social and sexual conduct. Of particular relevance in the San Francisco study were the patterns of coupling found in these communities and the importance of coupled and affectional relations to both gay men and gay women. The patterns of sexual practices did not differ a great deal from the Kinsey period, but there was some evidence of larger numbers of sexual partners in the groups that were recruited exclusively from the homosexual community itself (Table 2-5).

The studies also documented the importance of social networks for psychological adjustment and the importance of gender in structuring the differences found between gay men and lesbians. Again, there was no evidence of a specific set of etiologic origins for homosexuality or for a singular personality type among male or female homosexuals (A. P. Bell and Weinberg, 1978). In a later publication, however, A. P. Bell and colleagues (1981:216) hinted that these data might suggest a possible biological propensity for same-gender sexuality: "[O]ur study provides no basis for rejecting biological explanations outright. It also suggests some more specific implications for the form which such explanations might take." However, these suggestions have proved to be controversial.

1970 Kinsey Institute Data on Same-Gender Sexual Behavior

About this same time (late 1960s, early 1970s), the National Institute of Mental Health also funded the Kinsey Institute study (described earlier), a national probability sample that included questions on same-gender sexuality. Although most of the data have not been published, limited permission was granted to conduct a secondary analysis of the data on same-gender sexual contact among men. A full report of these analyses has been published by Fay and colleagues (in press).

Their analyses were complicated by missing information: approximately one quarter of the male respondents did not complete the items on same-gender sexual experiences. A procedure was devised for imputing missing values; Table 2-6 shows the resultant distribution of reported plus imputed same-gender sexual experiences in the male population by the age at which the last sexual contact took place. It was estimated that 3.3 percent of the adult male population in 1970 had such sexual contact after age 20 and that it occurred (during a specified period) either occasionally (1.9 percent) or fairly often (1.4 percent). When experiences at any age are included, it is estimated that 5.5 percent had some period in their lives when same-gender sexual contact occurred "occasionally" and 2.9 percent had such experiences "fairly often."

There are significant differences, as would be expected, between the reported adult same-gender experiences of men who marry and men who remain unmarried (see Table 2-7). Men who were 30 years of age or older at the time of the 1970 survey and who had never married were two to three times more likely than currently married men to report homosexual contacts after age 20 and also to have had a period in which the frequency of contact was "fairly often"; this category includes 3.5 percent of never-married men 30 years of age or older, 1.2 percent of currently married men, 1.7 percent of formerly married men, and 2.4 percent of single men 21–29 years of age. While there is greater prevalence of same-gender experience among never-married men, these estimates suggest that from 1 to 2

TABLE 2-6 Estimates of Percentage of Adult Male Population with Any Homosexual Experience, by Age at Last Contact and Frequency of Contact

	Level of Activity (as percentage of total sample)					
Age at Last Contact	Once	Twice	Rarely	Occasionally	Fairly Often	Total
Under 15	2.9	1.2	1.4	2.2	0.6	8.4
15–19	0.9	0.8	1.2	1.3	0.9	5.2
20 +	0.8	0.9	1.8	1.9	1.4	6.7
Total	4.6	2.9	4.4	5.5	2.9	20.3

SOURCE: Fay et al. (in press).

percent of married men have had adult homosexual experiences that, in some period in their lives, were fairly frequent.

These estimates diverge from the Kinsey estimate that 4 percent of men are *exclusively* homosexual throughout their lives. Of course, a question remains as to which estimate is closer to the "true value." We are presently unable to answer this question with confidence. There is no doubt that the sample of persons interviewed in the 1970 Kinsey Institute survey was more "representative" of the American adult population than the earlier Kinsey samples. What remains unknown is the nature and extent of the survey's interview biases. (We do not know, for example, whether the personal interviews of Kinsey and colleagues [1948] achieved more [or less] accurate reporting of the experience of respondents than could be obtained with a written questionnaire, the procedure used in the 1970 survey.) However, the sampling methodology of the 1970 survey should eliminate the kind of sample bias that plagued the original Kinsey collection. On the other hand, the level of nonresponse in the 1970 survey reintroduces the possibility of substantial bias in the composition of the sample of men who actually responded to the relevant survey questions. This issue is of particular importance because, as Cochran and coworkers (1953:675) wrote of the Kinsey studies,

> no sex study of a broad human population can expect to present incidence data for reported behavior that are *known* to be correct to within a few percentage points. Even with the best available sampling techniques, there will be a certain percentage of the population who refuse to give histories. If the percentage of refusals is 10% or more, then however large the sample, there are no statistical principles which guarantee that the results are

TABLE 2-7 Estimates of Percentage of Adult Male Population with Homosexual Experience by Marital Status, Age at Last Contact, and Frequency of Contact During Period of Peak Activity (with separate estimates for single males aged 21–29 and 30 +)

Homosexual Experience	Reported and Imputed	(*SE*)	Only Reported	Reported and Imputed	(*SE*)	Only Reported
	Currently Married			Divorced, Widowed, Separated		
Last contact at any age	19.6%	(1.4)	14.1%	19.3%	(3.2)	13.4%
Level 1: One time	4.7	(0.6)	3.8	3.4	(1.3)	1.6
Level 2: Two times	2.5	(0.7)	1.7	3.5	(1.4)	2.4
Level 3: Rarely	4.4	(0.7)	3.1	3.3	(1.0)	2.4
Level 4: Occasionally	5.4	(0.9)	4.0	5.0	(1.6)	3.1
Level 5: Fairly often	2.6	(0.5)	1.6	4.1	(1.6)	3.9
Levels 3–5	12.4	(1.3)	8.7	12.4	(2.8)	9.4
Levels 4, 5	8.0	(1.1)	5.6	9.1	(2.5)	7.1
Last contact at age 15 +	10.9	(0.9)	6.8	13.2	(2.8)	10.2
Levels 3–5	7.7	(0.9)	4.7	10.6	(2.6)	9.4
Levels 4, 5	4.9	(0.8)	2.9	7.8	(2.4)	7.1
Level 5	1.9	(0.5)	1.0	3.9	(1.7)	3.9
Last contact at age 20 +	6.0	(0.8)	3.1	7.2	(2.0)	5.5
Levels 3–5	4.5	(0.7)	2.3	5.6	(1.8)	4.7
Levels 4, 5	2.8	(0.7)	1.4	4.4	(1.4)	3.9
Level 5	1.2	(0.4)	0.6	1.7	(0.9)	1.6
N	1,161		899	154		127

	Single, Age 21–29			Single, Age 30 +		
Last contact at any age	23.7%	(4.1)	16.2%	32.9%	(7.7)	22.0%
Level 1: One time	4.4	(1.9)	2.9	6.4	(2.2)	4.9
Level 2: Two times	5.0	(2.9)	4.4	7.3	(4.3)	7.3
Level 3: Rarely	5.7	(2.2)	4.4	4.7	(2.2)	2.4
Level 4: Occasionally	4.9	(2.1)	2.9	9.0	(4.1)	4.9
Level 5: Fairly often	3.8	(1.9)	1.5	5.5	(2.8)	2.4
Levels 3–5	14.3	(3.6)	8.8	19.2	(5.8)	9.8
Levels 4, 5	8.7	(2.9)	4.4	14.5	(5.2)	7.3
Last contact at age 15 +	15.1	(3.8)	10.3	23.1	(5.7)	17.1
Levels 3–5	9.7	(3.0)	5.9	15.6	(5.1)	9.8
Levels 4, 5	5.9	(2.3)	2.9	12.0	(4.7)	7.3
Level 5	3.2	(1.6)	1.5	4.5	(2.5)	2.4
Last contact at age 20 +	10.1	(2.9)	7.4	15.2	(4.7)	12.2
Levels 3–5	6.6	(2.5)	4.4	12.3	(4.7)	9.8
Levels 4, 5	3.3	(1.7)	1.5	9.3	(4.2)	7.3
Level 5	2.4	(1.5)	1.5	3.5	(2.2)	2.4
N	80		68	55		41

NOTE: Standard errors (*SEs*) were calculated to take account of the complex sample design and the effects of random variation in imputing the missing data.

SOURCE: Fay et al. (in press).

> correct to within 2 or 3 per cent. . . . [A]ny claim that this is true must be based on the undocumented opinion that the behavior of those who refuse to be interviewed is not very different from that of those who are interviewed.

It should be noted, however, that Fay and colleagues (in press) report a reanalysis of newly available data collected by Michael and coworkers (1988) that provides some corroboration of the estimates obtained from the 1970 Kinsey Institute survey. Although coding categories cannot be precisely matched, estimates of rates of same-gender sexual contact during the preceding 12 months appear similar to those obtained in the 1988 NORC General Social Survey.

The difficulties of gathering reliable data on the number of persons with same-gender sexual experience are quite obvious. The behavior remains the object of considerable social hostility, and some people, for various reasons including fear of discrimination (and worse), conceal their experiences, even within important social relationships. In a social survey, this segment of the population may have considerable incentive to refuse to respond or to deny its experience.

It is also important to remember that these studies were conducted during a period in which the earlier reform movements within the "homosexual community" coalesced politically and became the gay liberation movement. In part driven by those who were self-identified as homosexual and in part prompted by other social movements of the period, political activism increased within what was to become the community of gay men and lesbians (R. A. L. Humphreys, 1972; D'Emilio, 1983). This political activism was implemented at a number of levels:

- practical electoral politics in those communities with substantial populations of gay men and lesbians;
- attempts to increase social services in local communities, including services for the young and elderly and improved police–community relations;
- coalitions to foster gay rights at the state and national levels;
- development of gay caucuses within professional and scientific societies; and
- an intellectual ferment about the nature of sexual preference and its relation to the larger social order—including its relation to scientific investigation.

The complex research agenda that characterized the period from the early 1970s to the beginning of the AIDS epidemic reflected major changes within the gay and lesbian communities themselves. The decision by a large number of people to openly label themselves gay men or lesbians changed the experience of same-gender sexuality. From a relatively narrow "homosexual" community based primarily on sexual desire and affectional commitment between lovers and circles of friends, there emerged a community characterized by the building of residential areas, commercial enterprises, health and social services, political clubs, and intellectual movements. This process has been chronicled in the gay and lesbian press, but historical analysis is just beginning (see, e.g., D'Emilio, 1983; Katz, 1976, 1983). Such communities did not emerge everywhere: many people participated primarily as passive members; still others continued to use the community primarily for the sexual access it provided through its increasing number of leisure institutions. Nevertheless, the existence of such communities changed the experience of those with same-gender sexual preferences and their relation to the larger community. Increasingly, gay men and women began to see themselves as a minority similar to other social and ethnic minorities (Weinberg and Williams, 1988).

It is possible to identify a number of research programs begun in the early 1970s that differed substantially from earlier studies. They were often associated with specific reform agendas and openly included gay men and lesbians as full scientific participants. This is one of the most crucial changes in the landscape of research on same-gender sexuality: people who would have been only the subjects of research and barred from participation as researchers because of their "biases" became valued members of research programs. These programs included the following types of endeavors:

- Studies of homophobia and prejudice against gay men and lesbians following the research tradition that asks why majority groups fear and hate minorities (pioneered by studies of anti-Semitism). Such research involves locating persons who seem more likely to express such feelings as a function of their social location or psychological predispositions.
- Applied studies, particularly within professional organizations, that seek to identify sources of discrimination against gay men and lesbians. Within professional societies, this type of study includes discrimination against research on same-gender sexuality or preference.

- Studies of mental health among gay men and lesbians.
- Studies of gay male and lesbian communities, often focusing on political and social issues rather than matters of sexuality or social and psychological adjustment.
- Studies of the possible childhood or biological origins of same-gender sexuality (A. P. Bell et al., 1981), which often provoke fierce political debate, as do discussions of the social construction of gay male or lesbian identities (Dececco, 1988).
- Attempts to recover the history of same-gender desire in various historical periods, including the recent past. Major developments have involved the creation of research archives, oral histories, and the use of previously suppressed materials and archives on earlier periods (e.g., Katz, 1976; Dover, 1978; Boswell, 1980). This is one of the most active current research areas within gay male and lesbian communities.

Research on Same-Gender Male Sex Since the Onset of the AIDS Crisis

The first recognized risk group for AIDS in 1981 was men who reported having sex with other men (CDC, 1981a,b,c; Friedman-Kien, 1981; Gottlieb et al., 1981; Follansbee et al., 1982; Friedman-Kien et al., 1982). The clustering of cases among male same-gender sexual contacts (CDC, 1982) established the fact that AIDS was sexually transmitted. To determine the specific aspects of sexual behavior responsible for transmitting and promoting AIDS, more than 15 major studies of gay male sexual behavior and its relation to AIDS were undertaken in the United States from 1982 to 1984. Research was conducted primarily in San Francisco, Los Angeles, Chicago, Pittsburgh, Baltimore, Washington, D.C., and New York City. Most of these studies employed longitudinal designs and are thus ongoing; however, many interim reports have been published, through which the primary mode of transmission of HIV among homosexual men (unprotected anal intercourse) has been established. In addition, there now exists an extensive and expanding data base on gay male sexual behavior patterns—a source of information that did not exist prior to the AIDS epidemic.

The link between sexual behavior and AIDS was elaborated during the early 1980s. Prior to the discovery of HIV in 1983–1984, two case–control studies on AIDS were conducted. The first study (Marmor et al., 1982) focused on men in New York City and compared AIDS patients who had Kaposi's sarcoma with control subjects who were not ill. In addition to inhaled nitrite use and frequency of sexually transmitted disease, a key difference between AIDS patients and controls was the number of different sexual partners reported by each group. Subjects with AIDS were more likely than control subjects to have had 10 or more different partners in a typical month prior to the onset of symptoms. In an expansion of this study (additional cases and control subjects from other U.S. cities were added to the data set), Jaffe and coworkers (1983) replicated this finding. In their research, subjects with AIDS reported an average of 61 different sexual partners over the year prior to symptom onset, while control subjects reported an average of 25. These investigators also found that, compared with control subjects, significantly more subjects with AIDS met their sexual contacts at gay bath houses. In addition, subjects with AIDS had higher mean scores than control subjects on a measure of fecal exposure during sex.

Using helper T-cell counts as the disease marker of interest, Goedert and coworkers (1985) showed that gay men in Washington, D.C., who had sexual contact with men from New York City were more likely to have low helper T-cell counts than were Washington gay men who did not have contact with men from New York City. The Goedert team also found that the frequency of receptive anal intercourse among these men was associated with a decrease in helper T cells. This association between receptive anal intercourse and reduced helper T cells was also demonstrated by Detels and colleagues (1983) in Los Angeles.

Thus, before the viral cause of AIDS was known or detectable, behavioral research had shown that being sick with AIDS or showing laboratory signs of immune deficiency was associated with (1) a large number of different sexual partners; (2) receptive anal intercourse or other rectal trauma; (3) the use of bath houses for sexual contact; (4) frequent infection with sexually transmitted diseases, particularly gonorrhea, syphilis, and enteric parasites; (5) sexual contact with gay male residents of New York City; and (6) the use of inhaled nitrites. There had been no consensus about a disease model of AIDS prior to 1984, however, and consequently, there was much controversy over whether AIDS was an infectious, transmissible disease or a disease brought on by the immunologic consequences of unhealthy and excessive involvement with sex and drugs (Martin and Vance, 1984). This debate, combined with the emphasis on the extremely large numbers of sexual partners and evidence of drug use among urban homosexual men, had the unfortunate effect of diverting attention away from specific behaviors. A stereotype of the gay person with AIDS had emerged from the scientific work, and this stereotype, which was picked up by the popular media, made it appear that the disease afflicted only the most "reckless" gay men.[23]

The stereotyping of AIDS also resulted in a similar distancing phenomenon in the larger, heterosexual population. AIDS was considered to be an affliction that was limited to gay men. Indeed, prior to the adoption of "acquired immune deficiency syndrome," the disease was referred to as the gay-related immune deficiency or GRID, the gay plague, and gay cancer. The result of such labeling was that AIDS was presented to the public as a disease whose threat was restricted to gay-identified men. Although the early research on AIDS had correctly identified key transmission factors for the disease, the focus on the risk group rather than on specific risky behaviors may have interfered with accurate assessments of personal risk, based on their individual behavior, among gay and nongay persons.

The discovery of HIV in 1983–1984 coincided with the establishment of the Multicenter AIDS Cohort Studies (MACS) by the National Institute on Allergy and Infectious Diseases (see the descriptions in Kaslow and colleagues [1987]). Five centers were awarded contracts: Los Angeles, Baltimore, Pittsburgh, Chicago, and San Francisco/Berkeley. (To conduct their research in an unconstrained fashion, the San Francisco/Berkeley group became independent of the other four centers early in the planning stages of the study.) The purpose of these cooperative studies was to recruit and follow an initially AIDS-free cohort of approximately 5,000 gay men over a three-year period to determine the natural history of AIDS and HIV infection. A key strength of the MACS design lay in the large number of subjects to be recruited and the administration of a common core of assessment instruments regarding sexual behavior and drug use. The limitations of the design for studying future disease transmission lay primarily in the ways in which subjects were recruited. The MACS recruited volunteers who were most often self-identified gay men and members of the local gay communities. They tended to be disproportionately white, well educated, and middle class, and those few who were less educated or less affluent, or who were members of minority groups, were usually attached in some way to members of the majority. This skewing is exactly what has characterized nearly

---

[23]For an example of this view in the popular media, see "Gay America in Transition," *Newsweek*, August 8, 1983:30.

all studies of homosexual men (and lesbians) as far back as the Kinsey studies (Davies, 1986; Schreiner, 1986).

Trends in Same-Gender Sexual Behavior

Anal Intercourse

Published reports based on MACS data established the role of receptive anal intercourse in the transmission of HIV (Chmiel et al., 1987; Kingsley et al., 1987; Polk et al., 1987; Winkelstein et al., 1987a,c). This key finding has been replicated and reported by other research groups involved in major epidemiological work with gay men in Boston (Mayer et al., 1986), New York City (Goedert et al., 1984; Martin, 1986b,c; Stevens et al., 1986), and San Francisco (Darrow et al., 1987b; Moss et al., 1987). Receptive anal intercourse without a condom is the only sexual behavior for which a consistent level of risk can be demonstrated in the epidemiological analyses reported in these studies. In multivariate analyses of HIV risk, unprotected receptive anal intercourse statistically overwhelms all other sexual acts. It is important to note, however, that the lack of detectable statistical risk for sexual acts other than receptive anal intercourse cannot be taken as evidence that no other type of sexual contact carries the risk of transmitting HIV infection. As noted by all of the investigators cited above, sexual behaviors are highly intercorrelated; thus, the unique risk associated with only one particular act can never be accurately evaluated. Two separate case reports[24] indicate that HIV infection occurred in the absence of anal intercourse activity for at least three years. In both of these cases, frequent receptive oral-genital sex was reported. In a review of the evidence on the risk of HIV transmission through homosexual contact among men, a recent IOM/NAS report concluded that "cohort and case-control studies of homosexual men . . . show that the risk of HIV infection is greatest for persons who engage in receptive anal intercourse. The risk of infection is less for partners who engage in insertive anal intercourse, and the risk appears even lower for oral receptive intercourse" (IOM/NAS, 1988:43).

The risk of HIV infection among highly sexually active gay men decreases significantly with the cessation of receptive anal intercourse

[24]Mayer and DeGruttola (1987); J. L. Martin, Columbia University School of Public Health, personal communication based on unpublished data (1988).

(Winkelstein et al., 1987a; Martin et al., in press). The large-scale reduction in the frequency of this particular sexual practice is believed to account for the near elimination of new cases of HIV infection (as of 1987) among participants in gay male cohort studies. Incidence rates of less than 0.5 percent have been observed in San Francisco (Winkelstein et al., 1987a), as well as in New York City.[25]

In addition to the longitudinal MACS studies, a number of other investigators have been following cohorts of gay men to compile detailed behavioral data over time. In a recent review by Becker and Joseph (1988), it was shown that data from San Francisco (McKusick et al., 1985; Winkelstein et al., 1987a,c), New York City (Martin, 1986a, 1987a), and Chicago (Emmons et al., 1986; Joseph et al., 1987) converged on the finding that, beginning in 1986, between 50 and 90 percent of the gay men in these samples had abstained from insertive or receptive anal intercourse. Similar changes have been described among gay men in Boston (McCusker et al., 1988b).

This conclusion cannot be generalized to less populated geographic regions of the United States, however. In a survey of gay men in urban areas of New Mexico (C. C. Jones et al., 1987), it was found that 70 percent of the sample had engaged in receptive anal intercourse in the year prior to the interview (1984–1985), and most did so without condom protection at any time. Similarly, Beeker and Zielinski (1988) reported that gay men in upstate New York engaged in unprotected receptive anal intercourse during 1986 at a rate twice that of gay men in New York City. Such geographic variation in unprotected anal intercourse rates underscores three needed actions: (1) continuation of existing descriptive epidemiological studies of gay male sexual behavior, (2) initiation of new epidemiological studies of gay male sexual behavior in less populated geographic regions of the country, and (3) intensified prevention efforts aimed at reducing rates of unprotected anal intercourse among gay men living outside the major U.S. metropolitan areas.

Condom Use

Safer sex guidelines recommend the use of condoms for both oral sex and anal intercourse, but condom use rarely accompanies oral sex among gay men (Martin, 1987a). Although the incidence of condom use with oral sex has certainly increased from 1981 to 1986, no more than 5 percent of respondents in a New York City sample reported the

---

[25] J. L. Martin, Columbia University School of Public Health, personal communication based on unpublished data (1988); J. L. Martin et al. (in press).

consistent use of condoms for oral sex (Martin, 1987a). Estimating the rates of condom use during anal intercourse has proven more difficult than estimating intercourse activity per se. Condom use tends to be highly variable over time as well as across situations. For example, both Des Jarlais (1988) and Martin and colleagues (in press) report that individuals are less likely to use a condom when they engage in sex with a primary partner than when they engage in sex with a less well-known partner. Even within a particular partner dyad, the relative frequency of condom use varies. There are few data on the rate of condom failure, breakage, or slipping in natural (versus laboratory) settings with regard to homosexual anal intercourse.[26]

Obtaining convergent data across studies is not possible because the time frame (i.e., a week, month, or year) varies from study to study and the particular point in time (i.e., the date) also varies. McKusick and colleagues (1985) found that 8 percent of San Francisco respondents used a condom during anal intercourse (although the frequency was unspecified) during the latter half of 1983. In another study of San Francisco gay men conducted by telephone in 1985 (Research and Decisions Corp., 1985), 7 percent of the sample reported engaging in unprotected anal intercourse outside of a "primary relationship." Some of the clearest data on condom use among gay men come from the study by Martin and coworkers (in press). Using episodes of receptive anal intercourse as the unit of analysis, these investigators found an increase in *protected* episodes from fewer than 1 percent in 1981 to 19 percent in 1985, 60 percent in 1986, and 71 percent in 1987. Shifting the unit of analysis to individual respondents, these investigators found increases (from 2 percent in 1981 to 62 percent in 1987) in the percentage of men who always used a condom during anal intercourse.

Other Sexual Activities

Gay men appear to be highly sensitive to the publicized risk differentials between oral–genital sex (perceived as low-risk activity) and anal intercourse (perceived as higher in risk). Indeed, the perception of high risk associated with all sexual acts involving anal contact or

[26]There is reason to suspect that findings from studies of condom breakage during heterosexual vaginal intercourse (e.g., Free et al., 1980, 1986) may not generalize to anal intercourse. Wigersma and Oud (1987) have reported data from a study of 17 gay couples in the Netherlands who reported their experiences with five brands of condoms (used with different quantities of lubricant). Rates of condom rupture (per "test" session) ranged from 0 percent for the "stiffest" condom to 13 percent for a condom rated among the least "stiff." Condoms were reported to "slip off" in 0–10 percent of test sessions.

the ingestion of semen is clearly reflected in the behavioral trends over time that have been observed in the cohorts studied in Chicago (Joseph et al., 1987), New York City (Martin, 1986a, 1987a; Martin et al., in press), and San Francisco (McKusick et al., 1985). These studies indicate that, in contrast to insertive and receptive anal intercourse, receptive and insertive oral–genital sex—without swallowing semen or ejaculating in the partner's mouth—are still common sexual practices among gay men. For example, the most recent estimates from New York City (Martin et al., in press) suggest that, in 1986, although 80 percent of gay men either abstained entirely from or always used a condom during anal intercourse, approximately 85 percent of gay men engaged in oral–genital sex (without a condom) at least once during the year.

It is important to note that, in the large natural history studies, more esoteric sexual practices (e.g., oral–anal activity [anilingus], fisting, and behavior involving the ingestion of urine and fecal material) have shown no consistent association with HIV infection or AIDS. These practices were the focus of much early speculation about the reason homosexual men were the primary targets for AIDS; yet the descriptive epidemiological studies that have since become available indicate that these practices were relatively rare compared with oral–genital sex and anal intercourse. In addition, current estimates indicate that fewer than 20 percent of gay men engage in oral–anal sexual contact (Joseph et al., 1987; Martin et al., in press), and fewer than 1 percent engage in fisting activities or the ingestion of urine or fecal material.[27] These data suggest that educational messages must underscore the facts that HIV is transmitted through widely practiced sexual activities and that transmission is not limited to those who engage in what might seem to be unusual sexual practices.

Celibacy, Monogamy, and Multiple Partners

Published studies of gay male sexual behavior and its relationship to AIDS and HIV infection have demonstrated significant declines in the average number of sexual partners reported by gay men. Representative findings include the following:

- in San Francisco, from 1984 to 1986, a 60 percent decline was observed in the number of men reporting 10 or more sexual partners in a six-month period (Winkelstein et al., 1987a);

[27] J. L. Martin, Columbia University School of Public Health, personal communication based on unpublished data (1988).

- in Chicago, from 1985 to 1986, the average number of sexual partners declined by 2 percent per month (Joseph et al., 1987); and
- in New York City, from 1981 to 1985, the median number of sexual partners declined by 72 percent (Martin, 1987a).

These dramatic reductions in numbers of partners reflect, in part, a substantial decline in the use of extradomestic locations for sex—in particular, gay bath houses, sex clubs, and the back rooms of bars. McKusick and colleagues (1985) reported a 60 percent decline in 1983–1984 among their San Francisco cohort in the average number of visits to sex clubs or bath houses. In New York City, Martin (1987a) reported a decline from 50 percent to 10 percent in the number of men using a gay bath house for sex between 1981 and 1985. Although the location in which sex occurs is unlikely to be directly related to the transmission of HIV or other diseases, it is important to note that locations such as gay bath houses and sex clubs functioned for gay men in the same way "shooting galleries" (see Chapter 3) have functioned for drug injectors in establishing the AIDS epidemic and the spread of HIV infection. Such locations provide settings that promote transmission-related behavior at a rate far beyond that possible outside these settings. This conclusion is supported by New York data (Martin, 1987a) indicating that in 1981 the median number of (cumulative) sexual partners reported in sexual encounters in extradomestic settings was 36; in contrast, the median number of partners reported in sexual encounters in domestic settings was 5.

Although the average number of sexual partners reported by gay men has declined rapidly since the onset of AIDS, rates of monogamy (i.e., confining sexual relationships to a single partner) and celibacy have increased slowly. A comparison of these rates across studies is difficult because the various investigators did not use a standard time frame. For example, McKusick and colleagues (1985) reported that 41 percent of their San Francisco sample were monogamous for one month in 1983. Joseph and coworkers (1987) reported that, in their Chicago cohort, the rate of monogamy rose from 18 percent to 25 percent over a six-month period in 1984–1985. Martin and colleagues (Martin, 1986a; Martin et al., in press) reported increasing rates of monogamy in New York City over contiguous yearly periods from 1985 through 1987. However, these rates were strongly influenced by whether respondents were involved in a primary relationship[28] with another man. Among those so involved, monogamy increased from 18 percent in 1985 to 25 percent as of 1987; among those gay men not involved in a primary relationship, the rate of monogamy rose from 7 percent in 1985 to 11 percent in 1987.

Yet despite the difficulty in making cross-study comparisons of rates of monogamy, the data clearly converge on the fact that the majority of gay men, whether partnered or single, has not adopted monogamy in the wake of the AIDS epidemic. Neither has there been a dramatic increase in the rate of celibacy among gay men (Martin, 1987a). Taken together, the available data indicate that the primary shifts that have occurred among gay men in response to AIDS/HIV have been in the realm of specific sexual practices, rather than in the adoption of monogamy or the elimination of sexual contact altogether. Eight years into the AIDS epidemic, oral sex without the exchange of semen, abstinence from all types of anal sex, and the use of condoms by the minority who continue to engage in anal intercourse appear to characterize male homosexual sexual behavior in major U.S. metropolitan areas.

FEMALE PROSTITUTION

There is a general belief that female prostitution might play an important role in the spread of HIV infection in Western nations.[29] Indeed, some policy makers in the United States and in other countries have called for or instituted various measures to "control" the potential spread of the disease by controlling the behavior of prostitutes. Such measures range from the punitive (mandatory testing and imprisonment) to the more supportive (the provision of education and condoms). There appears to be some interest in protecting prostitutes from infection, but the more prominent concern of policy makers seems to be the role of prostitutes in spreading the disease into those groups that are currently at low risk of infection.

[28]Martin (1987a:578) operationalized the definition of having a primary relationship with a lover as follows: "A respondent qualified as having a lover if: 1) he said he had a lover; 2) his lover viewed him as his lover (reciprocity); 3) friends viewed the two as a couple (public recognition); and 4) the relationship was extant for six months or more (duration)."

[29]In our review, we focus on female prostitution, not because of its greater epidemiological importance but rather because of the extreme paucity of scientific evidence on patterns of male prostitution. As noted subsequently, the committee recommends that research to fill this gap be given high priority.

Prostitutes' increased risk of becoming infected and transmitting the virus is thought to result from the sexual activities involved in their work and the association between IV drug use and prostitution in some groups. The relevant sexual practices include having a large number of sexual partners with limited ability to discriminate among them; specific sexual practices (i.e., anal sex) that may increase the risk of HIV transmission; and the inability, for whatever reason, to use safer sex techniques. In addition, prostitutes may have a history of other STDs, a factor that may increase the likelihood of transmission. Lending support to these views is the evidence from central African societies showing that prostitution has played an important role in the transmission of the disease among heterosexuals there (Kreiss et al., 1986; Piot et al., 1987a; see also the discussion by Alexander [1987a] on the relevance of the African data to the U.S. situation).

Prostitutes occupy a marginalized social niche that offers the possibility of personal and economic exploitation by other individuals and groups in the society (e.g., the police, pimps, criminals, customers) (Gagnon, 1977; Heyl, 1977). The experiences of exploitation and oppression these women undergo often produce disorderly lives over which they feel they have little control (James, 1980). Their ability to manage their sexual interactions or to engage in safer sex practices may be limited. Customer demands for specialized services and pressure to provide them at higher prices may override any desire to engage in safer sex practices.

In some locales, there is a substantial amount of IV drug use among prostitutes or the frequent association of prostitutes with IV drug users (Goldstein, 1979). The actual proportions of prostitutes who are IV drug users or who associate sexually with IV drug users are uncertain, but there is evidence that such proportions are substantial among minority populations and in certain regions of the United States. For example, a 1987 survey of street prostitutes in the New York City area indicated that approximately one half had injected drugs at least once and one third had injected drugs at some time during the previous two years (Des Jarlais et al., 1987).

Although these factors suggest that female prostitution could play a role in the AIDS epidemic, there is very little actual evidence about the role of prostitution in the transmission of HIV (Alexander, 1987a). Indeed, there is very little evidence about most of the important dimensions of prostitution that are relevant either to disease spread or to the behavioral changes that could limit such spread.

Social Context of Prostitution

Prostitution attracts a great deal of public attention, usually either as a social problem or a moral dilemma, but the research that has been conducted on its internal organization as an occupation or on its actual service relation to the larger social community is relatively meager. Much of the information on prostitution that has been collected in the United States has been motivated by concerns for social control or social change, sometimes provoked by national emergencies (e.g., the health of servicemen during World Wars I and II; see Brandt [1987]) and sometimes by local moral crusades. Such information is often partisan, unsystematic, anecdotal, and alarmist—devoted to "doing something" about prostitution and the prostitute.

All prostitution shares the common characteristic of (and, indeed, is defined by) exchanging sexual activity for payment; as a result, it has a superficial appearance of similarity in all social contexts (as reflected in the modern phrase, "the world's oldest profession"). Yet the actual social organization of prostitution and its meaning in any specific society or culture can be quite different (Gagnon, 1968; James, 1977). In the United States, for example, both the social organization of prostitution as an activity and its relation to the "sexual economy" of the larger society have changed over the past 80 years. In the early years of the century, bordellos and street prostitution (which were the most common ways in which prostitution appeared in large cities) were suppressed as part of the sustained efforts of "health and purity" crusaders (Brandt, 1987; Hobson, 1987). By the end of World War II, even the most recalcitrant of the vice zones in American cities were disappearing. Prostitution was also affected, from the late nineteenth century on, by a decline in steady customers as a result of a reduction in the number of permanently single men in the population and the steady increase in the sexual accessibility of "good" women as part of a changing courtship system (see the discussion earlier in this chapter). The Kinsey data suggest that regular and frequent contact with prostitutes declined between the two world wars, although the incidence of such experience remained high (Kinsey et al., 1948). Thus, female prostitution may play a different role in the lives of men today than it did in the past.

One of the most important forces shaping the organization of female prostitution is the twofold (formal and informal) regulatory apparatus that is devoted to controlling it. (For a careful description and review of the differences among the United States, the Netherlands, and Sweden, see Hobson [1987].) Prostitution is usually managed formally by the state, either through the criminal justice system or through a combination of the criminal justice system, disease control agencies, and welfare activities (Decker, 1979). In the United States, prostitution is a criminal offense in all states except Nevada, which regulates brothels (Alexander, 1987b:195). In practice, this criminalization has resulted in situations in which the local police, prosecutors, and courts have attempted some or all of the following courses of action:

- to suppress prostitution entirely by systematic and aggressive enforcement;
- to suppress prostitution in certain areas of the community and allow it in others, creating informal zones of tolerance or de facto legalization of non-street prostitution (Alexander, 1987b);
- to engage intermittently in widely publicized crusades against prostitutes at the instigation of citizens' or official groups; or
- to arrest at regular intervals a certain number of prostitutes who work in the most exposed locations.

Short of attempts to suppress prostitution entirely, all of these techniques may involve either some corruption of the police or an accommodation between the police and the criminalized populations, which produces irregular enforcement. The way in which prostitution is organized in most communities is usually a response to these social control policies and practices.

Because of the legal and moral status of prostitution, it is difficult to supply answers to a wide variety of questions that are relevant to the role prostitution might play in the epidemic. For example, there is no good estimate of the number of women who work as prostitutes. The usual sources of data are either arrest and imprisonment records, which are known to select primarily those populations most vulnerable to the criminal justice system (the poor, minorities, drug users, the inexperienced, those working on the street), or estimates by various "knowledgeable" observers. Such estimates vary quite widely. In fact, no one knows how many women work full-time, part-time, or only intermittently as prostitutes. Nor does anyone know how many women have ever worked as prostitutes and what their career paths have been—how old they were when they started, how steadily they worked, whether they have left and then returned to the occupation, and the periods involved in these exits and reentries.

There is some information suggesting that the background characteristics, patterns of recruitment, work careers, and departures from the occupation of prostitute vary considerably across cultures and societies; this knowledge is based on ethnographic studies, biographical statements, or expert testimony rather than on fully systematic research (*The Streetwalker*, 1959; Young, 1964; Bryan, 1966; James, 1976; Barrows and Novak, 1986; L. Bell, 1987; Delacoste and Alexander, 1987; Schedlin, 1987). It is also known that women do not move randomly into prostitution and most of them do not remain in it for a lifetime. The sectors from which female prostitutes are recruited vary substantially for different groups within large societies. How a woman manages a life in prostitution will often depend on (1) the resources or skills she brings to the work, (2) the quality of available opportunities to learn the requisite social and sexual skills to maintain her own sense of identity and her relations with the "important people" in a new social world (Bryan, 1965; Heyl, 1977; Silbert and Pines, 1982); and (3) the structural constraints on her ability to work in the most profitable ways (e.g., black prostitutes have difficulty working in gambling casinos). Movement out of prostitution into a more conventional life will also depend on such skills and resources, as well as on a certain degree of luck regarding the woman's original placement in the prostitution system (Delacoste and Alexander, 1987). For some women in some societies, prostitution may be a vehicle for upward social mobility or an alternative to occupations that present an even greater danger to their survival.

The site of a prostitute's work appears to have major effects on her life (Cohen, 1980; Carmen and Moody, 1985). The availability and dangerousness of sites usually depend on the legal status of prostitution in a particular locale and on informal agreements with the police. Women find customers on the street, in bars, and in official or unofficial zones; they work out of cars, in brothels, and over the telephone. The sexual act or acts are carried out in private or semiprivate places such as hotels, vehicles, bedrooms of bordellos, on the streets, and in other semiprivate public spaces. The more public the access to customers and the more public the sexual activity, the greater the risk of involvement with the police and the greater the risk of assault, rape, or robbery by passersby or customers. Those women who are most vulnerable to "trouble" have in fact provided the most information about the psychological and social backgrounds of prostitutes.

The type of clientele a prostitute serves is critical to her economic and personal life. Knowledge is very sketchy about the number of customers served by individual prostitutes working at different sites during specific periods. The social characteristics of these customers are likely to depend on the place of work and its relation to the community. Some studies have asked women to estimate the number of their recent partners, but there is apt to be considerable error in these counts, as well as in their reporting of the social characteristics of clients (in part, these errors rest on both inadequate knowledge and inadequate recall). Although prostitutes are often recruited from lower socioeconomic strata and minority populations, clients come from all social strata. If women work in rural or lower socioeconomic areas, their clients are often from the same social levels. In many urban areas, however, prostitute populations are only partially stratified by the socioeconomic status of their clientele. Women who work the streets may serve somewhat poorer clients while women who work by phone may have a more affluent clientele, but this is not always true. In some cities, brothels are socioeconomically stratified as a function of cost. There appears to be some mobility of the more attractive and more socially skilled prostitutes to client populations of higher socioeconomic status, but the extent of this mobility has not been documented.

Depending on their work sites and on other factors, prostitutes will have varying levels of control over the number of clients they have in a day or week. Women who work in zones or in bordellos that serve working-class men (especially men who are without other women) may have many men each day. Those who work on the telephone will have far fewer. There is evidence that prostitutes who serve working-class clients, at least in Western societies, are more likely to be asked for "straight sex," while middle- and upper-class clients will often ask for more experimental sexual activities (Gagnon, 1977). There is also some evidence that many women attempt to have oral sex rather than intercourse with clients because of the lower level of effort involved and the potentially higher payment. However, women may experience pressure (from "pushers," e.g., pimps and madams, whose income is dependent on their efforts) to increase the number of clients they serve or to accede to all of the sexual desires of clients (including not using condoms).

The incomes of prostitutes vary enormously, as do their expenses. Call girls may charge more per customer, but they must keep up an expensive front. Many prostitutes must pay off officials, even in countries in which prostitution is legally regulated. Many women have men to support, even when they do not have pimps. Still others have children for whom they are responsible. Like all marginal occupations, prostitution must confront the dangers of unemployment, underemployment, illness, or injuries from violence at work (without health insurance or compensation), as well as the risks of arrest and imprisonment and hence the costs of bail bonds, lawyers' fees, loss of employment time, and so forth. This lack of control of important dimensions of life creates psychological burdens for the individual prostitute that cannot be attributed to prior "psychopathology" (Jackman et al., 1963).

Prostitution and AIDS

The role of prostitution in the transmission of sexually transmitted diseases (STDs) other than AIDS has received more attention as a pretext for social control than as a subject of research (Brandt, 1987; Hobson, 1987:Chapter 6). A useful review of research on the role of prostitution in the transmission of STDs prior to the AIDS era can be found in Darrow (1983). Darrow points out that the surge of STDs in the 1960s was probably as much a function of failures of the health care system (e.g., in ignoring the behavioral patterns of disease transmitters) as it was a consequence of the increased use of nonbarrier contraceptives, increased numbers of sexual partners, and other changes in sexual practices. The general belief that prostitutes do not play an important role in the transmission of STDs may be incorrect, particularly for such "new" diseases as herpes and chlamydia (Darrow, 1983).

As a result of the AIDS epidemic, health agencies have shown increased interest in female prostitution, and CDC has thus begun coordinated studies in collaboration with research groups in Las Vegas, Atlanta, Colorado Springs, Los Angeles, San Francisco, Miami, southern New Jersey, and northern New Jersey (Darrow, 1988). The rates of HIV infection found in these convenience samples as of January 1988 are shown in Table 2-8. Perhaps the most important finding of this study is that HIV infection in the prostitutes studied thus far is found predominantly among those with histories of IV drug use. In the total collection of cases (1,456), 727 women showed evidence of IV drug use. Of these women, 150 (20.6 percent) were HIV seropositive. Data reported at the Fourth International Conference on AIDS from this same study suggested that, of one group of women who showed no evidence of IV drug use, only 38 of 729 (about 5 percent) were infected with HIV, and the majority of those infected came from one research site (24 of the 38 were from Miami)

TABLE 2-8 HIV Seroprevalence Among Women Who Reported Engaging in Prostitution (at least once) Since January 1978

Site	Percentage HIV Positive (*N* tested)						Source
	Evidence of IV Drug Use[a]		No Evidence of IV Drug Use		All Women		
Las Vegas	0 %	(10)	0 %	(27)	0 %	(37)	Brothels
Atlanta	1.5	(65)	0	(58)	0.8	(123)	Outreach
Colorado Springs	3.9	(52)	0	(46)	2.0	(98)	STD clinic
Los Angeles	3.7	(164)	4.4	(138)	4.0	(302)	Detention centers
San Francisco	9.7	(103)	0	(110)	4.7	(213)	Outreach
Miami	26.2	(195)	8.2	(292)	15.4	(487)	Detention centers
Southern New Jersey	42.9	(14)	0	(14)	21.4	(28)	Outreach
Northern New Jersey	59.7	(124)	18.2	(44)	48.8	(168)	Methadone clinics
Total	20.6	(727)	5.2	(729)	12.9	(1,456)	

NOTE: STD: sexually transmitted disease.

[a]Evidence of drug use indicated by self-report of ever injecting a drug subcutaneously or intravenously for nonmedical purposes or physical finding of needle marks on arms or legs.

SOURCE: Provisional data reported by Darrow (1988); data provided by the Multicenter Collaborative Study Group (J. B. Cohen and C. Wofsy, University of California/San Francisco; J. French, New Jersey Department of Health; P. Gill, University of Southern California Cancer Center; J. B. Muth and J. Potterat, El Paso County Health Department; O. Ravenholt, Clark County Health Department; R. K. Sikes, Georgia Department of Human Resources; J. J. Witte, Florida Department of Health Rehabilitative Services).

(Darrow et al., 1988).[30] At the same time, there are considerable differences among research sites in the number of drug-using prostitutes who are seropositive for HIV, suggesting that drug-use practices (in particular, needle-sharing) may vary substantially from city to city.

The connection between prostitution and IV drug use is not a simple one (Goldstein, 1979). There is substantial ethnographic and statistical evidence that IV drug use by prostitutes is concentrated among minorities or among women who work on the streets (Schedlin, 1987). In addition, changes in patterns of drug use among prostitutes parallel those of the larger drug-using community. Thus, increases in the use of injected cocaine and crack smoking as substitutes for heroin appear to be occurring among IV drug-using prostitutes in those cities in which similar changes are observed among other drug users.

There is some anecdotal evidence that women who are recruited into prostitution through a drug habit or women who acquire a drug habit after becoming prostitutes may have somewhat different life careers than those who do not use drugs. The use of drugs puts women at far greater risk of arrest (there is both the burden of the work and the habit); it may interfere in adopting prudent patterns of work (including safer sex); and it increases interactions with criminal populations to secure drugs. In some communities, there are different "strolls" (street areas of work) for those who are drug users and those who are not, with the latter viewing themselves as professional sex workers, unlike those who are driven to the occupation by their need for drugs.[31] In the most extreme cases of drug-motivated prostitution, there have been recent anecdotal reports of women becoming semipermanent residents of crack houses and exchanging sex for crack.

The use of condoms by prostitutes has received some attention from researchers. The prevalence of protected intercourse (i.e., the use of condoms) by women in the sex industry appears to vary with the context of the sexual encounter. J. B. Cohen (1987) found that 38 percent of the prostitutes interviewed in this study reported that they "always" used condoms with clients; only 10 percent reported that they "never" used them in professional relationships. However, these women did not view personal relationships as posing HIV-associated risks, and only 14 percent reported using condoms with husbands or

---

[30] A more detailed description of the Atlanta study can be found in Leonard and colleagues (1988).

[31] C. B. Wofsy, Departments of Medicine and Microbiology, University of California at San Francisco, personal communication (1988).

boyfriends. Other studies (e.g., Darrow, 1987b) have confirmed the finding that safer sex is practiced by female prostitutes more often in a professional context than in a personal one.

CDC is currently supporting studies of female prostitutes as part of its continuing concern with the role of prostitution in HIV transmission. One study focuses on the sexual and social networks of prostitutes in Colorado Springs; the other, in San Francisco, is a continuation of an outreach, treatment, and social mobilization program (Project Aware) directed at women sex workers. These studies hold promise for understanding the role of prostitution in HIV transmission and as part of the ongoing sexual life of American society. In addition, the National Institute on Drug Abuse has funded a three-city (Los Angeles, Boston, and Phoenix) outreach and education program that will recruit some 1,500 women who are prostitutes or partners of male IV drug users. This project is aimed primarily at AIDS health intervention and education, but it should also yield some data about prostitution as well.

The AIDS epidemic has heightened public and official concerns about the role of prostitution in disease transmission. These concerns tend to overwhelm the important policy debate, particularly within the feminist movement and between feminists and sex workers, about the stance that women in general, and sex workers and feminists in particular, should take on the issue of prostitution. A range of positions has been debated, from "suppression and rescue" to decriminalization (Snitow et al., 1983; G. Rubin, 1984; L. Bell, 1987; Delacoste and Alexander, 1987). Prostitutes themselves have become increasingly active participants in this debate, and in some locales, they have organized in trade union fashion to protect themselves from exploitation and advance their causes. Research on prostitution and attempts to engage prostitutes in helping to control the AIDS epidemic (as well as other STDs) will have to deal with this debate and with attempts at self-empowerment in organized prostitute groups as one of the important conditions of future research and education.

The Customers of Prostitutes

If data on female prostitution are limited, there is even less available information on their customers (particularly data that have been provided by the customers themselves). It is reasonable to assume that the risk of HIV infection to the male partners of prostitutes will depend on the frequency with which such men have paid contacts, the number of different women with whom contact occurs, the sexual techniques that are paid for, and the men's prior history of other STDs.

In the Kinsey studies, among white, college-educated men, about 30 percent reported sexual contact with a prostitute at least once in their lifetime; only 4 percent reported extensive experience. Among men with less than a college education, the proportion reporting some experience was similar (34 percent), but nearly 12 percent reported extensive experience. This difference by education is reflected in the number of prostitute partners reported in a lifetime: among college-educated men, 21 percent reported 10 or more prostitute partners, and 3 percent reported 51 or more partners. The number of prostitute partners reported by men with less than college educations is much higher: 41 percent reported 10 or more partners, and 14 percent reported 51 or more partners. What may be even more striking is that, of the 918 white college men who were asked if they preferred sex with a prostitute or nonprostitute, 7 percent said they were indifferent, 4 percent said they usually preferred a prostitute, and 6 percent said they always preferred a prostitute (Gebhard and Johnson, 1979:425). However, as noted earlier, these data should be treated with great care, given the problematic procedures used for case collection and the fact that they refer to a much earlier period (40 to 60 years ago).

Two recent studies provide some useful data on the clients of female prostitutes, although neither study could offer conclusive findings on the characteristics of these men. Both studies of men who reported contact with prostitutes (with no other HIV-associated behavior) found that approximately 1.5 percent of the men were infected with HIV (Chaisson et al., 1988; Wallace et al., 1988). In the Wallace research, demographic and behavioral data were collected on 340 men in the New York City area who reported contact with prostitutes. The men had a mean age of 33 and an average of 15 years of education; they had a lifetime average of 94 sexual exposures to prostitutes, with a median of 23 exposures. The most common sexual practice was oral sex. Slightly fewer than one half (45 percent) of the men studied reported that they never used condoms with prostitutes.

The few other studies of the clients of prostitutes suffer from the same kind of sampling difficulties seen in the Kinsey study. Some discuss motivations for using the services of prostitutes (Kinsey et al., 1948; Gibbens and Silberman, 1960; Winick, 1962; G. Pomeroy, 1965; see Gagnon [1977] for a summary). Recent research suggests that power may be important in motivating men to seek sex with prostitutes (Schedlin, 1987; for evidence offered by prostitutes, see Delacoste and Alexander [1987]) because the interaction allows the man to assume that he can do "anything."

It would be difficult, although not impossible, to collect adequate data among men who use the services of prostitutes. Such studies would require household samples in which men are asked about prostitute use; specialized samples of men who are regularly associated with prostitutes but who might not be included in a household sample; studies of men who are particularly likely to use the services of prostitutes (e.g., men in the military and in other all-male occupational groups); and men from cultures in which contacts with prostitutes are considered part of the culturally supported repertoire of sexual life.

METHODOLOGICAL CONSIDERATIONS IN SURVEYS OF SEXUAL BEHAVIOR

Although there are considerable gaps in knowledge about the sexual behavior of the American population, important advances have been made in areas crucial to understanding HIV transmission. In the last eight years, great progress has occurred in understanding gay male sexual behavior in relation to AIDS and HIV infection. Nevertheless, even in this research domain, the accuracy of any given set of estimates is open to question, as most studies employ different assessment methodologies with unknown psychometric properties, different time frames, and different types of samples. Although it is accurate to conclude that particular associations and trends have been replicated, the actual population parameters (e.g., means, covariances, standard errors) have not been replicated across studies; therefore, they are not known with any degree of certainty at this time.

In this section, we briefly review some of the methodological issues that will continue to concern future researchers, including such issues as the accuracy of self-reported data on sexual behavior, methodologies for sampling men who have same-gender sexual contacts, and problems associated with the development of reliable survey instruments.

Accuracy of Self-Reported Data on Sexual Behavior

In dealing with self-reported behavior, there is always concern about the accuracy of responses.[32] Even if a reluctance to answer is overcome with guarantees of anonymity, the question of accuracy remains. This is especially true when self-reports cannot be checked against more objective data. The age at onset of sexual activity is a good example: it is an extremely important variable from the point of view of risk assessment (for both STDs and unplanned conceptions), public policy, and program design. Understanding its range in any given population is essential to determining where, for whom, and at what age interventions are required. The question is whether the age at onset of sexual activity can be accurately determined from survey interview data.

In one school-based study of young urban blacks, approximately 90 percent of the males and 95 percent of the females responded when asked their age at first intercourse (Zabin et al., 1986a). That their answers are credible is supported by two pieces of evidence. First, there are similarities between the overall responses in these groups and responses reported from similar populations elsewhere in the country. Second, there are similarities between the shapes of male and female curves of sexual activity onset and curves representing pubertal markers for each sex—wet dreams for young men and menarche for young women. The two curves peak at the same age for young men; the sexual activity onset curve peaks two years after menarche for young women, which is consistent with observations in similar urban communities. Mott (1985:21–23) has reported, however, that 29 percent of young men and 15 percent of young women in the National Longitudinal Survey[33] stated that they were virgins in the 1983 survey but had previously reported (in 1982) that they had experienced sexual intercourse. This kind of discrepancy suggests that the question of how good self-reported data are depends on the degree of accuracy required. If what is needed is a rough marker of early, normative, and late onset of sexual activity within a group, the data appear good. If the exact year of onset is needed, there is more of a question about accuracy.

---

[32]See also the discussion of this issue in Chapter 3.

[33]The National Longitudinal Survey is a recurring survey; the fifth-round survey of youth (aged 14–22 when first interviewed in 1979) studied a probability sample of 6,143 males and 6,078 females during 1983. One major focus of this round of the survey was the study of the relationships between school leaving, fertility, and employment (Mott, 1985).

As the example of age at onset of sexual activity indicates, one of the most difficult theoretical aspects of the measurement of human sexual behavior using survey techniques is the problem of "validity"; that is, the deviation of the value obtained by a measurement from the presumed "true" value for the underlying trait. Typically, for most behavioral phenomena, researchers assume that there is a true value and that measurements deviate from it (either randomly or systematically). For such characteristics as chronological age, evidence other than self-reports can be sought—for example, in the historical records provided by birth certificates—to validate the self-reported data. Ancillary studies that gather such independent data can be used to estimate the magnitude and direction of bias in the self-reported data and to recalibrate the estimates derived from the self-reports to adjust for reporting bias. Even for many sensitive behaviors, official records may be useful: for example, it is possible to gauge the extent of bias and unreliability in reports of offenses like drunk driving by culling arrest records. However, measures that are inherently subjective, such as reports on attitudes and feelings, are not amenable to this type of approach. If someone reports that he or she is "happy," there is no analogue to a check of official records to determine whether the report is accurate.

All behaviors (including sexual behaviors) are theoretically objective; that is, in theory they could be verified by an observer. Ordinarily, intimate behaviors do not occur in the presence or sight of an observer other than the subject (and the partner, if any). Thus, the validation of self-reported data on human sexual behavior cannot—except in the rarest of circumstances—proceed in ways that are considered to be appropriate for validating data on other behavioral phenomena.[34] Devising alternative procedures to validate measurements that are not amenable to direct verification will require careful thought and investigation—and success is not assured. In this regard, other efforts to validate survey measurements of subjective phenomena may be informative.[35] Clearly, survey estimates of sexual behavior are subject to many of the same nonsampling errors that are well known in other areas of measurement, and some of the models that have been found useful in these areas might also find

---

[34] Masters and Johnson's (1966) laboratory studies of human sexual response are one of the rare exceptions. However, their research was intended to study sexual response in a purposely designed, "artificial" environment, rather than in natural settings using a representative population.

[35] For a summary and review of the literature, see Turner and Martin (1984:Vol. 1, Chaps. 4–6); see also Beniger (1984), MacKuen (1984), and MacKuen and Turner (1984).

application here (e.g., Turner, 1978, 1984; Bradburn and Sudman, 1979; Clogg, 1984; Duncan, 1984; Jabine et al., 1984).

One possible approach is to compare changes in sexual behavior with changes in other related phenomena. It may be possible, for example, to construct a convincing validation by demonstrating that an independent series of measurements of change in the incidence of gonorrhea in a population over time could be predicted from a concurrent time series monitoring the self-reported incidence of unprotected sexual contacts with new partners in the same population. Although there are many potential pitfalls to executing a successful validation in this way, the committee believes that the feasibility of using such indirect procedures should be given further, careful consideration.

Sampling Gay and Bisexual Men

A major problem for research on same-gender sexual contact is the lack of an efficient sampling frame from which to draw random samples of men who have sex with men. Not only are the definitions of "homosexual" and "bisexual" problematic, but the enlistment of community support is a vital first step in any such survey. The approaches taken by various investigative teams confronted with the difficulty of sampling homosexual and bisexual men for surveys on AIDS and HIV are instructive. Before reviewing these approaches, however, it should be noted that practical constraints precluded the use of probability sampling in many of these surveys. Although such constraints are understandable, the committee believes future survey efforts will benefit greatly from the increased use of probability sampling procedures.

A common approach taken in many early investigations was the convenience sample drawn from a narrow source, such as private medical practices (Marmor et al., 1982; Goedert et al., 1985), sexually transmitted disease clinics (Jaffe et al., 1985), or gay bars and bath houses (McKusick et al., 1985). Some of these studies have been useful in dating the introduction of HIV into the gay population and in establishing the associations between specific sexual patterns and AIDS and HIV infection. Others have been helpful in pointing out particular aspects of behavior that should be studied. However, using data from these studies to estimate population parameters is unsound. Any group of individuals drawn from treatment sources such as clinics or private practices will have higher rates of most types of physical disorders compared with individuals who are not found in treatment settings. In addition, those in treatment settings will also have higher rates of the biological and behavioral risk factors associated with illness. Thus, it is impossible to derive valid estimates of, for example, the prevalence of HIV antibody among homosexual men, the incidence of new cases of HIV infection, or the frequency of specific sexual activities from treatment-based study groups or from groups of gay men drawn from locations that promote the type of behavior one is interested in studying.

An approach to sampling gay and bisexual men that moves a step beyond the convenience sample in rigor is to recruit volunteers through print ads and public notices. This approach has been used to develop entire samples (Detels et al., 1987; Fox et al., 1987), as well as to supplement extant samples of gay men assembled in the late 1970s for testing and evaluation of the hepatitis B vaccine (Stevens et al., 1986; Joseph et al., 1987). Although this approach is clearly superior to relying on a single narrow subject source, the samples are not probability samples and numerical results cannot be confidently generalized with known margins of sampling error. It should also be noted that there have not as yet been substantial efforts to systematically assess the differences in subsamples of gay men as a function of their source of recruitment.

One study built systematic differences into the sampling scheme (Martin, 1986a, 1987a; Martin et al., in press). These investigators drew a probability sample of all gay men belonging to at least one gay organization in New York City as of 1985 (response rates were 96 percent for the organizations and 72 percent for recruited individuals). The sample was supplemented by non-probability samples of gay respondents drawn from a public health clinic and face-to-face recruitment efforts and by self-selected volunteers. An additional systematic source of selection involved recruitment into the study group through personal referral by those already enrolled. The rationale for this addition was to move away from individuals who were directly accessible to the study team and to contact and recruit people from networks in the larger gay community that were more difficult to reach (Martin and Dean, 1985).

The only face-to-face interview study in the United States that employs a probability sample of gay and bisexual men is the San Francisco Men's Health Study (Winkelstein et al., 1987a). A clustered probability sampling of the 19 San Francisco census tracts centering on the Castro district (the area of the city that is most densely populated by gay men and that has the highest incidence of AIDS cases) generated a sample of more than 600 gay men. The strength of this approach lies in its ability to derive defensible estimates of population parameters; indeed, it could be argued that this approach represents a standard that should be aspired to by other research in this field. It must be noted, however, that the sample only contains men who live in a particular gay enclave of San Francisco. It is not representative of men with same-gender sexual preferences who live elsewhere and who may choose to live apart from the gay community. Additional restrictions on the generalizability of findings from this sample (involving levels of sexual activity, socioeconomic status, race, and age) are imposed by sampling the Castro district. Such restrictions would apply in any sample of a gay neighborhood, including New York City's Greenwich Village or the city of West Hollywood, California. Even recognizing that a particular type of gay man constitutes the sample, the response rate of 59 percent obtained by Winkelstein and his group suggests that a particular type of gay man living in the gay section of San Francisco may have been willing to identify himself as gay or bisexual to the researchers and to participate in the study. It would be extremely valuable to know more about the 41 percent of the sample who were nonresponders. In sum, although the use of probability samples is scientifically preferable to any other method, it does not guarantee a representative sample: the limitations imposed by the sampling frame itself and by nonresponse must be acknowledged.[36]

The sample from the Castro reported a preponderance of men who stated that their sexual partners were exclusively male. Moreover, Winkelstein and colleagues (1987b) reported a low rate of heterosexual partnering among the men in their sample identified as bisexual (Table 2-9). This result can be usefully contrasted to the finding from the national population surveys, which indicated that a substantial fraction of men with histories of adult homosexual contact was currently or previously married. There are several possible explanations for the apparent divergence. For example, the national population surveys should be finding more "closeted" men than are found in studies focusing on men who reside in gay-identified communities. Similarly, recent contacts may be evidence of a different

---

[36] Although the investigators did not obtain information on nonparticipants, they did compare the demographic characteristics of the survey sample with the characteristics of residents of the tracts as reported in the 1980 census. This analysis indicated a modest underrepresentation (-8.2 percentage points) of men aged 25–29 and an overrepresentation (+8.9 percentage points) of men aged 35–44. The most striking divergence of the sample from the census occurred for education: 89.8 percent of the sample reported one or more years of college; the census estimate for these tracts was 24.6 percentage points lower.

TABLE 2-9 Numbers and Percentages of Male and Female Sexual Partners of Homosexual, Bisexual, and Heterosexual Men Residing in the 19 Census Tracts Centering on the Castro District of San Francisco, January–June 1984

	Homosexual	Bisexual		Heterosexual
No. of Partners	No. (%) of Male Partners	No. (%) of Male Partners	No. (%) of Female Partners	No. (%) of Female Partners
0	46 (7.2)	24 (13.9)	117 (67.6)	12 (5.7)
1	137 (21.4)	36 (20.8)	27 (15.6)	99 (46.7)
2–4	182 (28.4)	44 (25.4)	23 (13.3)	75 (35.4)
5–9	104 (16.2)	32 (18.5)	2 (1.2)	20 (9.4)
10 +	172 (26.8)	37 (21.4)	4 (2.3)	6 (2.8)
Total	641 (100.0)	173 (100.0)	173 (100.0)	212 (100.0)

NOTE: Six subjects were not included because of missing data.

SOURCE: Winkelstein et al. (1987b). Copyright, 1987, American Medical Association.

(and more consistent) pattern than can be determined from lifetime contacts. Clearly, however, more data will be required to determine a plausible interpretation of this apparent divergence in findings.

Developing Reliable Survey Instruments

Measurement Time Frames

Another methodological problem that makes cross-study comparisons nearly meaningless is the lack of consistent time frames associated with particular assessment instruments. In estimating the number of sexual partners of gay men, for example, some studies focused on a "typical" month in a particular year, multiplied that value by 12 (for the yearly total), and then multiplied that value by the number of years of being sexually active to produce a lifetime total (Marmor et al., 1982; Jaffe et al., 1983). Other studies focused on a one-month period, comparing that number to the number reported for the same month in the previous year (McKusick et al., 1985). Still others focused on a one-year period and generated estimates based on 12 months (Martin, 1987a). It is impossible to make direct comparisons of estimates that were derived in such diverse ways, and it should be noted that problems of accurate recall can be substantial when respondents are asked to make estimates covering a 12-month period (see Jabine et al., 1985).

This problem is even more sharply illustrated in estimates of the occurrence or nonoccurrence of a particular behavior (e.g., monogamy, celibacy, abstinence from intercourse). For such analyses, the time frame covered by the assessment is essential to an understanding of the results: clearly, monogamy for one month is quite different from monogamy for one year.

Interviewer Versus Self-Administered Assessments

One reason assessment approaches may vary so greatly is that some studies use interviewer-administered questionnaires (Martin, 1987a; Winkelstein et al., 1987c; Fox et al., 1987; McCusker et al., 1988b) while others use self-administered questionnaires (Marmor et al., 1982; McKusick et al., 1985; Joseph et al., 1987). Given the complexity of sexual behavior and the numerous contingency questions that are required in the event of an affirmative answer, it may be inappropriate to employ self-administered assessment questionnaires. It must be recognized nonetheless that accurate reporting of sexual behaviors in face-to-face interviews may be embarrassing for some respondents. This may in turn cause some respondents to conceal important aspects of their sexual histories. There is some evidence (e.g., Klassen et al., in press) suggesting that respondents are more likely to report sensitive sexual behaviors on self-administered questionnaires, but methodological research on survey measurements of other sensitive topics is equivocal (see, e.g., Bradburn and Sudman, 1979:Table 2). Although no firm conclusions can be drawn, it is clear that further methodological research on the validity and reliability of alternative interview techniques is needed.

Behavioral Specificity

Behavioral specificity is a prerequisite for all research on sexual behavior and AIDS. Use of overly complex constructs such as "safer sex" in assessment protocols or in reporting results can obscure the behavioral phenomena of most interest and risk misunderstandings about the exact meaning of the measurements. The problem is demonstrated in the lack of clarity that emerges with respect to risk taking in reports by Martin (1986a) and Stall and colleagues (1986). These investigators used composite indicators of risk rather than specific sexual behaviors as the outcomes of interest, making interpretation of the findings problematic. Another issue involves specification of sexual behaviors in which an individual may act as the inserter or the receiver (Research and Decisions Corp., 1985). This is an especially important problem with respect to homosexual sex, since men can readily play both receptive and insertive roles during sex. Thus, one needs to know not only the type of sex act but the role that was played (e.g., receptive anal intercourse).

Reliability and Validity of Measures

It should also be noted that very few studies in this field have reported data on the reliability and validity of their sexual behavior measures. Martin (in press) reported test–retest reliability, as did Saltzman and colleagues (1987); however, no such reports can be found in other major epidemiological studies of gay male sexual behavior and AIDS. In the face of the epidemic, conducting and reporting studies has assumed a higher priority than the refinement of methodologies; now, however, it is time to step back and assess the limitations of the studies that have been conducted so that sounder efforts can be mounted in the future.

Sample Coverage

Although many studies have demonstrated declines in risk-associated sexual behaviors among men who have sex with other men, they do so, as noted previously, among only one segment of the total population: self-identified gay men and members of local gay communities. Missing (as they are from most sex research) are men with same-gender sexual preferences who are members of minority ethnic and racial groups, who are from the working class, or who are poor; also missing are men from rural areas and smaller cities who primarily have sex with men, as well as men who have sex with both men and women. By using gay communities as sampling sites, these studies have probably located the areas of the country with the highest levels of sexually transmitted infection, but in doing so, they have missed other populations about which, consequently, very little is known.

Lack of knowledge is particularly acute regarding men with same-gender sexual preferences who belong to racial and minority groups in which different cultural standards may obtain about sex between men. The work of Carrier (1976) suggests that, among Latino groups, sex between men often occurs along strongly stereotyped lines in which one partner is consistently the *activo* (the inserter) and the other the *passivo* (the insertee). The active partner does not consider himself to be homosexual, and anal intercourse may occur both with male and female partners. In other minority communities, casual sex for pay may occur with male or female partners with relative indifference. There is also evidence in minority communities of wholly self-contained pairs and groups of men who practice sex only with men but have little or no contact with visible gay communities.

Also important to a complete assessment of the risk of HIV transmission among people with same-gender sexual preferences are studies of men who have sex with both men and women, following quite different social–psychological scripts to organize their experience (Gagnon, 1977). Many young men have a few sexual experiences with other men for pay; a few have many experiences. The sexual patterns of such "hustlers" are quite varied, ranging from the delinquent boy who has sex primarily with young women while being paid for sex with men, to the young man who has sex exclusively with men for pay (A. J. Reiss, 1961). The "average" hustler probably does not exist, and patterns of sex for pay among men probably vary enormously, depending on the local community. Similarly, men who have secret sexual experiences with other men in addition to a heterosexual marriage are also bisexual but in quite a different sense than are men who have sex with other men only in prison or when in other all-male groups (L. Humphreys, 1970; Gagnon and Simon, 1973). Of course, such men are potential bridges between heterosexual and homosexual partners.

These populations are often quite difficult to locate when networks are sampled starting with gay-identified men, although careful ethnographic studies may find some networks that include them. Work with delinquent boys, studies of "bright-light" areas (e.g., Times Square in New York City), and research efforts in minority communities may uncover examples of these patterns. Other middle-class bisexuals may be found through studies of swingers' clubs. None of these procedures, however, can generate a sample in a way that will allow estimates based on it to be generalized to a larger population.

Little research—even studies of those who identify themselves as gay men and lesbians—has ventured outside of urban communities in which there are concentrations of potential respondents. As a result, understanding of the life of gay men and lesbians is restricted to a few contexts, despite substantial evidence that, even within the United States, the sexual lives and networks of gay men and lesbians differ from community to community (E. White, 1980). As more reliable national samples of persons with same-gender sexual experience become available, they will allow far better judgments to be made about the information that has been gathered on more restricted populations (Davies, 1986). Ultimately, these data may be particularly important in studying the linkages among sexual strata—that is, fitting together the experiences of gay men, lesbians, bisexuals, and heterosexuals—and providing a historical perspective for studying social change in same-gender sexual behaviors.

ANTHROPOLOGY'S PERSPECTIVE ON HUMAN SEXUAL BEHAVIOR

Our discussion thus far has dealt entirely with research carried out through interviews that are usually conducted by means of a survey (and typically with a standard questionnaire). Although the pioneers of this method of sex research were recruited from many different fields (Kinsey, as previously noted, was a biologist), this research tradition has been sustained largely by persons trained in sociology, demography, psychology, and survey research.

A rather different tradition of studying human sexual behavior arises within the field of anthropology. The methods of anthropology, and of ethnography in particular, offer important alternative perspectives for understanding sexual behavior. In circumstances in which other techniques cannot be used because of constraints on resources or the sensitivities of the population being studied, the information provided by ethnographers may be the only information that can be collected.

In this section, we briefly review the anthropological literature on human sexual behavior and discuss ways in which this research approach is being used in contemporary studies of sexual behavior and behavioral change related to AIDS.

From 1929 to the 1970s

When Malinowski published his pioneering work *The Sexual Life of Savages* in 1929, Havelock Ellis, a well-known theorist on sexual behavior, confidently predicted the arrival of a new era in the study of human sexual behavior. Anglo-Saxon puritanism of the nineteenth century was now cast aside, and twentieth-century investigators would no longer consider unfamiliar sexual customs to be shocking, disgusting, or even unspeakable. People were also learning to view their own sex taboos a little less solemnly (Ellis, 1929:xiii). Nonetheless, detailed anthropological research on sexual conduct in non-Western cultures is something of a recent phenomenon. A few anthropologists of European descent had showed an early interest in the field (Schapera, 1941; Layard, 1942, 1959; Elwin, 1947); in addition, an American publication, *Patterns of Sexual Behavior* (Ford and Beach, 1951), provided a compendium of such exotic data as the preferred locations of intercourse, standards of female beauty, and positions of intercourse in various cultures. Anthropologists, however, gave little attention to the expression and meaning of sexuality in different social and historical contexts. As in other branches of the social sciences, there was virtually no research that could contribute to general theories of human sexual development and gender identity.

Yet sex was not an entirely forbidden topic. The fear of "overpopulation" in the so-called underdeveloped countries and the proliferation of birth control studies in the 1950s and 1960s captured the attention of anthropologists who were interested in various aspects of population dynamics. Anthropological studies gave some precision to the debate about whether it is the large size of families that explains their poverty or whether people have large families because they are poor (Mamdani, 1972). Fine-grained research pointed to the economic value of children, especially adolescent sons, as contributors to family income and as protectors of family property and of elderly or widowed parents later in life (B. White, 1975; Cain, 1977). The economic interests in producing children were shown to vary somewhat by class and in different historical periods. These studies gave rise to a research tradition that defined the political and economic contexts of changing sexual practices, a tradition that continues to the present. Studies of the changes in reproductive behavior associated with the recent shift from low to high levels of fertility in Thailand (Knodel et al., 1984) and of the contrasts in the demographic transition experienced by the gentry, artisans, and peasants in Sicily from 1850 to the present (Schneider and Schneider, 1984) are part of that research tradition.

A different research approach was followed by anthropologists with an interest in symbolism. In the 1960s, many anthropologists viewed the body as a metaphor for society (Douglas, 1966). Food taboos, the eating and sharing of food, and rules about sexual activities were thus seen as statements, in each location, about the body politic. Throughout the 1970s, this field of enquiry gained new energy and intellectual direction from feminist scholars who were interested in the power implications of accepted notions of gender and sexuality in Western and non-Western contexts (Reiter, 1975; MacCormack and Strathern, 1980; for a review essay on feminist publications in this period, see Vicinus [1982]). "Male," "female," "sex," and "reproduction" were shown to have different meanings in any given culture and had to be understood within a larger context of cultural beliefs, classifications, and assumptions. Questions about the meaning of sex—as erotic techniques, medical facts, or Freudian psychology—were said to be embedded in matters of rank, prestige, and the economy in kinship-based societies (Ortner and Whitehead, 1981). As Malinowski (1929:xxiii) observed earlier in regard to South Sea Islanders, "sex is not a mere physiological transaction. . . . It dominates in fact almost every aspect of culture. Sex, in its widest meaning . . . is rather a sociological and cultural force than a mere bodily relation of two individuals."

Throughout the 1970s, anthropologists continued to examine theoretical issues related to the social construction of gender, but they paid little attention to actual sexual behavior, viewing gender and sexuality as conceptually linked. Although research in the 1980s initially continued along this path, it has gradually become clear that gender and sexuality should be analytically separated to reflect more accurately their separate social existence (G. Rubin, 1984; Vance, 1984).

The 1980s Prior to AIDS

As Malinowski suggests, in many non-Western cultures, sex provides the template for social life, resulting in the formation of gender identities and psychosexual development that differ from those of the West. In the West, life stages tend to be defined by steps in education, work, or career; yet in Bangladesh, to take one example, there are nine accepted life stages that are closely linked to expectations about sexual behavior and reproduction. Moreover, as might be anticipated in a culture that leans heavily on biological differences to construct distinctions in gender, the expected behavior of Bangladeshi men and women differs greatly. Preadolescence (ages 11–12), for example, is recognized as a distinct stage more for girls than for boys because of the importance of a girl's behavior to her reputation and that of her family. A girl is expected to learn proper female decorum before the end of this period so she can play the female part well once puberty sets in. According to local moral standards, late adolescence (ages 16–20) is a dangerous stage of life, applying more to males than to females because males usually remain unmarried. A boy of this age works to contribute to family income, unless he is at school, but it is considered disgraceful if an adolescent female has to work outside the home, even in the poorest families. Gender role expectations become exaggerated at this time. It is not considered shameful for a young man to look at a young woman with a sensuous eye; on the contrary—the young woman bears the blame. Moreover, boys have a period of some years to establish their identity before marriage, while girls are thrust into a quasi-adult—and subservient—role in their teens (Aziz and Maloney, 1985:48–60).

The Bangladeshi life scheme, like those of other cultures in South Asia, is constructed without reference to Freud and thus lacks a concept of infantile sexuality or an analysis of prepubertal sexual socialization. In such an environment, Erikson's (1964) eight-stage development cycle, with its two opposing qualities to be resolved in each stage, emerges as quaintly Eurocentric. South Asian life schemes are not premised on conflict resolution within life stages but proceed ladder-like, bidding the individual to find his or her place in the total universe (Aziz and Maloney, 1985).

The sexual "revolution" of the 1970s and the continued deconstruction of gender assumptions provoked a new wave of enquiry into the sexual behavior of "others." This research further confirmed the fact that sexuality is astonishingly plastic and variable in its expression from culture to culture. As Gregor (1985:3) notes in his study of sexuality among an Amazonian group, the Mehinaku, " [n]o purported universals of sexual behavior are unquestioned, and only a few seem reasonably well documented. Among the best established of these is that males have a higher level of sexual interest than do females."

Evidence for the plasticity of sexual behaviors came especially from studies in New Guinea. Institutionalized same-gender relationships among men, reported by earlier investigators, were now examined in light of contemporary psychoanalytic and psychosocial theories of human development. Ritualized homosexual behavior among men, reliably reported from perhaps 10–20 percent of all Melanesian groups (Herdt, 1984), indicated that these activities were not a deviant form of cultural behavior. (Suggestions of same-gender relationships among women have been glancingly reported for the region, but the female–female erotic relationship remains a historically underinvestigated topic.)

The organization of sexual practices and the formation of gender identities in the small "homosexual" societies of New Guinea are integral to the systems of production and reproduction in these societies. Among the Sambia of Papua New Guinea, for example, homosexual practices begin at ages 7–10, when all young boys are taken from their mothers to be initiated into the male cult. For some

10–15 years, they engage in erotic practices, first as fellator, ingesting the semen of an older bachelor, and then as fellated or semen donor. At the same time, the boys and youths must avoid women or be punished, as elders teach them that semen is the sole physical and psychic path to manhood. The cultural gift of semen is said to be the only way older men can ensure the growth, development, and masculinity of members of their sex. In the Sambian culture, there is much talk of growth, physical attractiveness, and the formation of the intellect but no word that translates as "homosexual." The pattern of same-gender sexual activity and avoidance of women continues until marriage, after which the young men may follow "bisexual" behaviors for some years. With fatherhood, however, all same-gender activity is expected to cease. The final outcome, exclusive heterosexual activity, brings Sambia males to the endpoint of a prescribed erotic path to adulthood (Herdt, 1981).

Descriptions of the cultural life of the Sambia and of other "homosexual" groups in Papua New Guinea challenge Westerners to reevaluate standard generalizations about adolescence and sexual development. Socially sanctioned sexual behaviors in these non-Western cultures differ across the region and include oral sex, anal intercourse, and the application of semen (which is considered to be a life force and is rubbed into incisions on the initiates' bodies) (Lindenbaum, 1987). Because different groups have generally disparaging views about the sexual activities of their neighbors, variations in these practices involve the creation of ethnic identity within a regional complex. As Kelly (1977:16) comments about the peoples of the Great Papuan Plateau: "Inasmuch as the members of each tribe become men in different ways, they are predominantly different kinds of men, culturally distinct beings at the most fundamental level." Like speech, religion, race, food habits, and clothing, then, sexual conduct appears to provide a highly charged basis for ethnic division and discrimination.

Although the expressions of homosexual behavior in Papua New Guinea vary across the region, they do not belong to a separate sphere of cultural activity. Differing among themselves, they nevertheless display a profile of shared symbolic themes, a sense of variation and permutation on a common Melanesian fund of sociosexual behavior and social organization (Lindenbaum, 1984). Within and beyond the geographic regions in which ritualized "homosexuality" occurs, men give ritual attention to body fluids (the expulsion of blood and the infusion of semen), the injection of various substances to promote masculine growth, the life-draining dangers of heterosexual intercourse, and the fear of women who are menstruating. The Melanesian data indicate that "homosexuality" and "heterosexuality" are related cultural constructs.

Anthropological Research Since AIDS

Continued attention to gender relations, a resurgence of interest in psychoanalysis, and a focus within medical anthropology on sexually transmitted disease—especially AIDS—have directed anthropologists to ask new questions.[37] Many research projects are now concerned with the cultural construction of sexual practices relevant to HIV transmission. For example, a preliminary study among Mexicans of rural origin in northern Mexico describes transvestite "homosexuals" who are symbolically construed as women in numerous contexts. On festive occasions, they dress as women, adopt female names, and use female pronouns to refer to each other. As symbolic women, they have sexual relations with other men who are often married and who in local terms are considered heterosexual. The married men view the transvestites as sexual surrogates for "real" women. Women themselves demonstrate greater tolerance for male sexual encounters with transvestites than with female prostitutes or concubines because there is less risk of desertion or of diminished economic support for the family. Standard interviews and questionnaires that are insensitive to such culturally constructed sexual practices would overlook a form of male "bisexuality" that is normalized and rendered socially invisible but that may be an important avenue for HIV transmission (Alonso and Koreck, 1988).

Recent enquiries into the meaning of same-gender sexual behaviors among Afro-American men in Baltimore (Pounds, 1987), Chicanos in Texas and Arizona (Mata and Jorquez, 1988), men in Nicaragua (Lancaster, 1988) and urban Brazil (Parker, 1987), and "closeted" homosexuals and gay men in New York City (Kochems, 1987b) reveal a range of male identities, differing from community to community. Each study emphasizes that self-identification must be taken into account so that key differences in the cultural construction and experience of sexual practice are not obscured. In many

---

[37] For an account of the feminist shift in focus during this period, see Rich (1988). Rich points to the broad range of factors reshaping female sexuality in the 1980s: reactions to AIDS, which have revived homophobia; the "second wave" of feminists becoming mothers in the 1980s (leading to the notional rejoining of sexuality and reproduction); and the implications of conservative/liberal political skirmishes over the control of sexuality (the attacks on abortion, day-care centers, and civil rights).

accounts, for example, men who have intercourse with other men do not consider themselves to be bisexual. In addition, as Alonso and Koreck (1988) suggest, groups of different national and regional origins, as well as ethnic and class affiliations, should not be subsumed into an inclusive category (e.g., "Hispanic"). The same might also be true for other population categories (e.g., women, blacks, and Asians).

Another line of current investigation centers on the knowledge, beliefs, and attitudes about AIDS and the perception of risk in various populations—for example, in Rwanda (Feldman et al., 1987), among gay and lesbian teenagers in Chicago (Herdt, n.d.), and in a midwestern college population.[38] Also under investigation are gender differences in knowledge about AIDS and sexual behaviors (Strunin and Hingson, 1987). In addition, the cultural impact of AIDS testing has been evaluated (McCombie, 1986).

The studies that have been discussed thus far are a natural extension of the symbolic anthropology of the 1970s and early 1980s with its emphasis on meaning and interpretation. The shape of the research, however, is molded by current knowledge of the spread of AIDS and HIV infection and by the value of anthropological findings to epidemiology or to health administration. Ethnographies published before the advent of AIDS have also been culled for descriptions of the social factors that are relevant to the spread of the virus. The African literature provides detailed accounts of sexual relations and marriage, ritual and therapeutic activities involving blood (clitoridectomy, circumcision, scarification, incisions for protection, tooth removal, injections from indigenous and nonindigenous practitioners), as well as descriptions of the migration of populations toward urban centers or across regions (see Brokensha et al. [1987], for a survey of relevant studies; see also Hrdy [1987]). This material can inform future epidemiological research, but the accounts need updating as well as enhancement through the inclusion of material about such key behaviors as "homosexuality," "bisexuality," multiple sexual partnerships, drug use, and the use of health care, none of which has been well studied in the past.

AIDS has also drawn some anthropologists into the field of medical anthropology, in which theories are tested and applied. A number of anthropologists are now working in outreach education programs with gay men's advocacy groups (Kochems, 1987a), in programs for

[38] M. D. Quam, Department of Sociology and Anthropology, Sangamon State University, personal communication (1988).

self-help intervention with female IV drug users or female sexual partners of IV drug users (Worth, 1988), in the evaluation of community education programs (Harder et al., 1987), in programs serving male prostitutes (Fisher et al., 1982)[39] and female prostitutes (Schedlin, 1987; Sterk and Leonard, 1988) in the United States, and in studies of multiple-partner relationships in Central Africa (Schoepf, 1988). In addition, anthropologists continue to provide information about beliefs and behaviors that have not been elicited by other research methods and to work more closely with epidemiologists to describe and analyze the spread of illness, which is a cultural and social phenomenon (Feldman and Johnson, 1986; Gorman, 1986; Stall et al., 1986; Flowers, 1988). In studying the effects of the disease on specific populations, anthropologists and historians also point to epidemics as a time of testing for political, economic, social, and cultural institutions (Hartwig and Patterson, 1978; Lindenbaum, 1979; Brandt, 1987).

CONCLUSIONS AND RECOMMENDATIONS

The AIDS epidemic has forced American society to examine itself and its behaviors, institutions, and practices. In no area has that examination been more tortuous than in the realm of sexual behavior. The links between HIV transmission and sexual behavior have focused attention on current knowledge of sexual practices, which has been found to be fragmentary and unreliable. The changes that have occurred in the last few decades in the way Americans conduct their sexual lives are not reflected in what little research there is on sex. Consequently, attempts are being made to alter the course of what is mainly an STD epidemic without the benefit of a sound understanding of the behaviors that spread it—an understanding that is essential to the design of educational efforts and intervention strategies.

To correct this situation and slow the further spread of HIV infection, the committee believes it is imperative to extend and improve the quality of information available on sexual behavior. Basic behavioral research has not received strong support in this country; at present, sex research is barely represented as an activity in federal research agencies. In the past, some sex research was conducted by the government, but it was oriented toward the achievement of a

[39]T. Marotta, Urban and Rural Systems Associates, San Francisco, personal communication (1988).

specific goal (generally, preventing teenage pregnancies) rather than the collection of basic behavioral data.

Although the committee finds the past mission-oriented research efforts of the government to be a valuable and necessary part of the federal research portfolio, there are substantial gaps in basic knowledge that need to be filled if the country is to contain the spread of the AIDS epidemic. **The committee recommends that the Public Health Service support vigorous programs of basic social and behavioral research on human sexual behavior, particularly through such agencies as the National Institutes of Health; the Alcohol, Drug Abuse, and Mental Health Administration; and the Centers for Disease Control.**

If AIDS prevention programs are to be targeted in a more effective and efficient manner, more must be known about those people who are at risk: who they are, where to reach them, and the behaviors they engage in that put them at risk. **The committee recommends that data be collected to estimate the prevalence of the sexual risk-taking behaviors associated with the acquisition and spread of HIV infection in various populations, including those at higher and lower risk.** Similar data are needed to understand the variability of these behaviors across subpopulations and among individuals.

Another element of the sexual behavior equation must also be considered. Sexual conduct is influenced by a variety of factors, including cultural norms and values, physical capabilities, and opportunity. Therefore, **the committee recommends that high priority be given to studies of the social and societal contexts of sexual behaviors.** Furthermore, because sexual behavior is dynamic—evolving and changing over the course of history and throughout the sexually active period of an individual's life—a "snapshot" of risk-associated behaviors will not be sufficient. **The committee recommends that funding be provided (and continued over time) to support prospective longitudinal studies of sexual behavior.** Such studies will enrich our understanding of changes in behavior and help to detect emerging problems.

The committee recognizes that a request for more basic behavioral research will require a heretofore absent long-term commitment to this type of research. Sexually transmitted diseases, unwanted and unplanned pregnancies, and the medical and social consequences of drug use are long-standing, serious problems in our society that require and deserve a long-term commitment. The country is now paying the costs that result when prospective studies are interrupted and research programs are subject to "feast-or-famine" cycles of support. At the moment of crisis, the United States lacks critically important prospective studies and well-trained cadres of researchers.

In addition to basic behavioral studies, the revised set of research priorities the committee endorses includes more targeted investigations. Thus, **the committee recommends that the Public Health Service support research in those subsets of the population that are at increased risk of HIV infection.** Such research should include prostitutes and their clients, minorities (minority women and minority gay men and lesbians), lesbians of all ages, young gay men, gay men living outside the epicenters of the epidemic, socially vulnerable adolescents, the different groups that make up the heterogeneous IV drug-using population, and non-IV drug-using sexual partners of IV drug users.

Female prostitutes are a population of particular interest. Prostitutes are at great risk of HIV infection because of their large numbers of sexual partners, their increased likelihood of contracting another STD (a potential cofactor in the spread of HIV), their association with IV drug users, and their own use of IV drugs. Studies of the recruitment, working conditions, social relations, sexual practices, drug-use patterns, condom usage, fertility patterns, and personal lives of female prostitutes are quite rare, particularly studies that yield quantifiable results. Research on these factors needs to be undertaken—in various locations and with women who function in different kinds of prostitution. One important reason for such studies is that customers of prostitutes are a potential bridge for HIV infection into the general heterosexual female population, a group that may currently be at relatively low risk. The social backgrounds and social networks of male clients should be carefully examined, in addition to seeking answers to the obvious questions about their frequency of prostitute contact, the types of sexual behaviors in which they engage with prostitutes, and their use of condoms.

The AIDS epidemic has also revealed the intricate relationship that exists between sexual behavior and drug use. The committee notes that alcohol and drug use have been linked to increases in sexual behaviors that risk HIV transmission. **The committee recommends immediate steps to close the vast gaps in our knowledge of the relationship of sexual behavior and drug and alcohol use.** Such steps should include developing a better understanding of the variation in drug and alcohol use within subgroups of the population, the effect of alcohol and drug use on the initiation of sexual behaviors that risk HIV transmission, the conditions and antecedents surrounding their initiation, and the actions that might be taken to interrupt such a dangerous chain of events.

Success in carrying out many of the committee's recommendations hinges on knowing far more than is now known about how to identify and elicit information from prostitutes, IV drug users, and other groups that currently exist at the margins of our society. Knowledge is needed about how to follow these individuals over time in the interests of better evidence and about effective data collection methodologies. **The committee recommends that resources be invested in methodological research to develop better procedures to obtain information from hard-to-reach groups.** In particular, support is needed to study appropriate methods for counting the hard to count, to elicit their cooperation in data collection and randomized experimental intervention programs, and to study mechanisms for obtaining valid information about sensitive (and sometimes illicit) behaviors that occur in the contexts of different cultural and language groups.

An area of interest related to information on the spread of HIV and AIDS is the somewhat fragmentary state of statistics on STDs. Underreporting is known to be quite common (particularly for cases diagnosed by private physicians), and this situation may have been exacerbated in recent years by the diversion of public health resources from tracking syphilis and gonorrhea to AIDS (thereby reducing the numbers of new cases of gonorrhea and syphillis that are counted).

A reliable system of statistics on STDs other than AIDS could play an important role in improving our understanding of the course of the AIDS epidemic. Other things being equal, transmission rates for other STDs should respond to the same behavioral interventions that are being designed to reduce the transmission of HIV infection. Because other STDs produce reportable infection rapidly, they might provide a leading indicator for HIV incidence rates. Data on STDs might also be useful for validating time-series measurements derived from surveys of individual sexual behavior. **The committee recommends that an independent review of STD data collection systems be undertaken and sufficient resources provided to undertake any improvements that may be required.**

One intervention strategy whose implementation is efficacious in the prevention of both STDs and HIV infection is the use of condoms (and spermicides), a practice that is regularly recommended to reduce the risk of HIV transmission. Little is known, however, about the effectiveness of these methods in actual use. Condom failure rates for contraception are known to vary, with some subsets of users experiencing high failure rates. The committee believes that research is needed to understand the barriers to the use of condoms and spermicides and the factors associated with their improper use. **The committee recommends that the Public Health Service immediately begin a research program to determine the extent to which the use of condoms and spermicides reduces the risk of HIV transmission. This program should include investigations of the current use of these products, how that use might be modified, and—equally important—how these products themselves may be modified to encourage uses compatible with human skills and dispositions.** One part of this research program should determine whether men and women know how to use condoms effectively and the extent to which they are used regularly. The results of this research should be made available in a timely fashion to those who are designing and implementing AIDS prevention programs.

Biomedical research on HIV infection and AIDS often requires gathering behavioral data from populations that are both hard to reach and from whom it is difficult to gather reliable, valid data. Careful attention needs to be paid to the difficulties of gathering such data, both for the sake of the behavioral data themselves (and the uses made of this information) and because the interpretation of biomedical data often depends on them. **The committee recommends a concerted effort to upgrade and standardize (when possible and desirable) the procedures used to gather behavioral data in clinical and biomedical research settings.** Resources should be made available to ensure that the best social and behavioral science practices and instrumentation are widely available to all scientists conducting relevant research, including those who are studying biomedical topics such as the natural history of HIV infection. **The committee also recommends that funding agencies, both public and private, encourage the sharing of data relevant to HIV infection and AIDS that have been gathered by federal and extramural researchers, within the limits set by scientific priority and confidentiality. To facilitate such sharing, the committee recommends that a data archive be established to support secondary analyses of these data.**

Finally, the committee observes that two of the important components of any strategy for containment of the AIDS epidemic no longer require more research but should be acted on immediately. Simply put, in the face of the spread of a deadly infectious disease that is transmitted by sexual behaviors, there should be no barriers in the way of persons seeking treatment for any sexually transmitted disease or seeking condoms. **The committee recommends that local public health authorities ensure that treatment for all sexually transmitted diseases is readily available to all persons who may seek such treatment. In addition, the committee recommends that local public health authories ensure that condoms are readily available to all sexually active persons.** Promotion of condom use might be facilitated if condoms were sold in a wider variety of retail outlets, including supermarkets, convenience stores, and vending machines placed in diverse locales.

BIBLIOGRAPHY

Aberle, S. D., and Corner, G. W. (1953) *Twenty-five Years of Sex Research: History of the National Research Council Committee for Research in Problems of Sex, 1922–1947.* Philadelphia: W. B. Saunders.

Alexander, P. (1987a) Prostitutes are being scapegoated for heterosexual AIDS. In F. Delacoste and P. Alexander, eds., *Sex Work: Writings by Women in the Sex Industry.* Pittsburgh, Pa.: The Cleis Press.

Alexander, P. (1987b) Prostitution: A difficult issue for feminists. In F. Delacoste and P. Alexander, eds., *Sex Work: Writings by Women in the Sex Industry.* Pittsburg, Pa.: The Cleis Press.

Alonso, A. M., and Koreck, M. T. (1988) Sexuality and AIDS Transmission in the "Hispanic" Community: A Research Note. Pembroke Center for Teaching and Research on Women, Brown University.

American Psychiatric Association. (1973) *Diagnostic and Statistical Manual of Psychiatric Disorders (DSM III).* Washington, D.C.: American Psychiatric Association.

Anderson, R. M., and May, R. M. (1988) Epidemiological parameters of HIV transmission. *Nature* 333:514–519.

Atwood, J., and Gagnon, J. H. (1987) Masturbatory behavior in college youth. *Journal of Sex Education and Therapy* 3:35–42.

Aziz, K. M. A., and Maloney, C. (1985) *Life Stages, Gender and Fertility in Bangladesh.* Dacca, Bangladesh: International Center for Diarrhoeal Research.

Barrows, S., and Novak, W. (1986) *Mayflower Madam: The Secret Life of Sidney Biddle Barrows.* New York: Arbor House.

Bauman, K. E., and Wilson, R. R. (1974) Sexual behavior of unmarried university students in 1968 and 1972. *Journal of Sex Research* 10:327–333.

Bayer, R. (1987) *Homosexuality and American Psychiatry: The Politics of Diagnosis.* Princeton, N.J.: Princeton University Press.

Becker, M. H., and Joseph, J. G. (1988) AIDS and behavioral change to reduce risk: A review. *American Journal of Public Health* 78:394–410.

Beeker, C., and Zielinski, M. (1988) Drugs, Alcohol, and Risky Sex Among Gay and Bisexual Men in a Low Incidence Area for AIDS. Presented at the 116th annual meeting of the American Public Health Association, Boston, Mass., November.

Bell, A. P., and Weinberg, M. S. (1978) *Homosexualities: A Study of Diversity Among Men and Women.* New York: Simon and Schuster.

Bell, A. P., Weinberg, M. S., and Keifer-Hammersmith, S. (1981) *Sexual Preference: Its Development in Men and Women.* Bloomington: Indiana University Press.

Bell, L., ed. (1987) *Good Girls/Bad Girls: Feminists and Sex Trade Workers Face to Face.* Toronto: The Seal Press.

Beniger, J. (1984) Mass media, contraceptive behavior, and attitudes on abortion. In C. F. Turner and E. Martin, eds., *Surveying Subjective Phenomena,* vol. 2. New York: Russell Sage and Basic Books.

Berger, A., Gagnon, J. H., and Simon, W. (1973) Youth and pornography in social context. *Archives of Sexual Behavior* 2:279–308.

Bergler, E. (1948) The myth of a new national disease: Homosexuality and the Kinsey report. *Psychiatric Quarterly* 22:68–88.

Bergler, E. (1951) *Neurotic Counterfeit Sex.* New York: Grune & Stratton.

Bergler, E. (1956) *Homosexuality: Disease or Way of Life.* New York: Hill and Wang.

Bergler, E. (1959) *One Thousand Homosexuals.* Paterson, N.J.: Pageant Books.

Bieber, I., Pain, H. J., Dince, P. Z., Drellich, M. G, Grand, H. G., Grundlach, R. H., Kremer, M. W., Rifkin, A. H., Wilbur, C. B., and Beiber, T. B. (1965) *Homosexuality: A Psychoanalytic Study.* New York: Basic Books.

Billy, J. O. G., and Udry, J. R. (1985) Patterns of adolescent friendship and effects on sexual behavior. *Social Psychology Quarterly* 48:27–41.

Blumstein, P. W., and Schwartz, P. (1977) Bisexuality: Some social psychological issues. *Journal of Social Issues* 33:30–45.

Blumstein, P. W., and Schwartz, P. (1983) *American Couples: Money, Work, and Sex.* New York: Morrow.

Bolling, D. R. (1976) Heterosexual anal intercourse—an illustrative case history. *Journal of Family Practice* 3:557.

Booth, W. (1988) The long, lost survey on sex (News and Comment). *Science* 270:1084–1085.

Boswell, J. (1980) *Christianity, Social Tolerance, and Homosexuality: Gay People in Western Europe from the Beginning of the Christian Era to the Fourteenth Century.* Chicago: University of Chicago Press.

Bradburn, N., and Sudman, S. (1979) *Improving Interview Methods and Questionnaire Design.* San Francisco: Jossey-Bass.

Brady, J. P., and Levitt, E. E. (1965) The scalability of sexual experiences. *Psychological Record* 15:275–279.

Brandt, A. (1987) *No Magic Bullet: A Social History of Venereal Disease in the United States Since 1880.* New York: Oxford University Press.

Brokensha, D., MacQueen, K. M., Stess, L., Patton J., and Conant, F. (1987) Social Factors in the Transmission and Control of AIDS in Africa. Report prepared for the Directorate of Health, Bureau of Science and Technology, Agency for International Development. Institute for Developmental Anthropology, Binghamton, New York.

Bryan, J. H. (1965) Apprenticeships in prostitution. *Social Problems* 12:287–297.

Bryan, J. H. (1966) Occupational ideologies of call girls. *Social Problems* 13:441–450.

Cain, M. (1977) The economic activities of children in a Bangladesh village. *Population and Development Review* 3:201–227.

Cannon, K. L., and Long, R. (1971) Premarital sexual behavior in the sixties. *Journal of Marriage and the Family* 33:36–49.

Carmen, A., and Moody, H. (1985) *Working Women: The Subterranean World of Street Prostitution.* New York: Harper and Row.

Carnes, D. E. (1975) Talking about sex: Notes on first coitus and the double sexual standard. *Journal of Marriage and the Family* 35:677–688.

Carrier, J. M. (1976) Cultural factors affecting urban Mexican male homosexual behavior. *Archives of Sexual Behavior* 5:103–124.

Centers for Disease Control (CDC). (1979) Nonreported sexually transmissible diseases, United States. *Morbidity and Mortality Weekly Report* 28:61–63.

Centers for Disease Control (CDC). (1981a) Follow-up on Kaposi's sarcoma and *Pneumocystis* pneumonia. *Morbidity and Mortality Weekly Report* 30:409–410.

Centers for Disease Control (CDC). (1981b) Kaposi's sarcoma and *Pneumocystis* pneumonia among homosexual men. New York City and California. *Morbidity and Mortality Weekly Report* 30:305–308.

Centers for Disease Control (CDC). (1981c) *Pneumocystis* pneumonia. Los Angeles. *Morbidity and Mortality Weekly Report* 30:250–252.

Centers for Disease Control (CDC). (1982) A cluster of Kaposi's sarcoma and *Pneumocystis carinii* pneumonia among homosexual male residents of Los Angeles and Orange Counties, California. *Morbidity and Mortality Weekly Report* 31:305–307.

Centers for Disease Control (CDC). (1987) Human Immunodeficiency Virus Infections in the United States: A Review of Current Knowledge and Plans for Expansion of HIV Surveillance Activities. Report to the Domestic Policy Council. Washington, D.C.: Department of Health and Human Services. November 30.

Chaisson, R. E., Osmond, D., Bacchetti, P., Brodiek, B., Sande, M. A., and Moss, A. R. (1988) Cocaine, Race, and HIV Infection in IV Drug Users. Presented at the Fourth International AIDS Conference, Stockholm, June 12–16.

Chilman, C. S. (1978) *Adolescent Sexuality in a Changing American Society: Social and Psychological Perspectives.* Bethesda, Md.: U.S. Department of Health, Education, and Welfare.

Chmiel, J. S., Detels, R., Kaslow, R. A., Van Raden, M., Kingsley, L. A., and Brookmeyer, R. (1987). Factors associated with prevalent human immunodeficiency virus (HIV) infection in the Multicenter AIDS Cohort Study. *American Journal of Epidemiology* 126:568–577.

Christensen, H. T., and Gregg, C. F. (1970) Changing sex norms in America and Scandinavia. *Journal of Marriage and the Family* 32:616–627.

Clayton, R. R., and Bokemeier, J. L. (1980) Premarital sex in the seventies. *Journal of Marriage and the Family* 42:759–775.

Clogg, C. C. (1984) Some statistical models for analyzing why surveys disagree. In C. F. Turner and E. Martin, eds., *Surveying Subjective Phenomena*, vol. 2. New York: Russell Sage and Basic Books.

Cochran, W. G., Mosteller, F., and Tukey, J. W. (1953) Statistical problems of the Kinsey report. *Journal of the American Statistical Association* 48:673–716.

Cohen, B. (1980) *Deviant Street Networks: Prostitution in New York City.* Lexington, Mass.: Lexington Books.

Cohen, J. B. (1987) Condom Promotion Among Prostitutes. Department of Epidemiology and General Medicine, University of California at San Francisco.

Coxon, A. P. M. (1986) Report of a Pilot Study: Project on Sexual Lifestyles of Non-Heterosexual Males. Social Research Unit, University College, Cardiff, Wales.

Curran, J. W., Morgan, W. M., Hardy, A. M., Jaffe, H. W., Darrow, W. W., and Dowdle, W. R. (1985) The epidemiology of AIDS: Current status and future prospects. *Science* 229:1352–1357.

Curran, J. W., Morgan, W. M., Hardy, A. M., Jaffe, H. W., Darrow, W. W., and Dowdle, W. R. (1985) The epidemiology of AIDS: Current status and future prospects. *Science* 229:1352–1357.

Darrow, W. W. (1983) Prostitution and sexually transmitted diseases. In K. K. Holmes et al., eds., *Sexually Transmitted Diseases.* New York: McGraw-Hill.

Darrow, W. W. (1986) Sexual behavior in America: Implications for the control of sexually transmitted diseases. In Y. M. Felman, ed., *Sexually Transmitted Diseases*. New York: Churchill Livingstone.

Darrow, W. W. (1987a) Behavioral Changes in Response to AIDS. Presented at the Symposium International de Réflexion sur le Sida, Paris, October 22–23.

Darrow, W. W. (1987b) Condom Use and Use-Effectiveness in High-Risk Populations. Presented at the Conference on Condoms in the Prevention of Sexually Transmitted Diseases, Centers for Disease Control, Atlanta, Ga., February.

Darrow, W. W. (1988) The Potential Spread of HIV Infection in Female Prostitutes. Presented at the annual meeting of the American Psychological Association, August.

Darrow, W. W., Cohen, J. B., French, J., Gill, P., Sikes, R. K., Witte, J., et al. (1987a) Multicenter Study of HIV Antibody in U.S. Prostitutes. Presented at the Third International AIDS Conference, Washington, D.C., June 1–5.

Darrow, W. W., Echenberg, D. F., Jaffe, H. W., O'Malley, P. M., Byers, R. H., Getchell, J. P., and Curran, J. W. (1987b) Risk factors for human immunodeficiency virus (HIV) infections in homosexual men. *American Journal of Public Health* 77:479–483.

Darrow, W. W., Bigler, W., Deppe, D., French, J., Gill, P., Potterat, J., Ravenholt, O., Schable, C., Sikes, R. K., and Wofsy, C. (1988) HIV Antibody in 640 U.S. Prostitutes with No Evidence of Intravenous (IV)-Drug Abuse. Presented at the Fourth International AIDS Conference, Stockholm, June 12–16.

Davies, P. M. (1986) Some Problems in Defining and Sampling Non-Heterosexual Males. Working Paper No. 21. Social Research Unit, University College, Cardiff, Wales.

Davis, D. L., and Whitten, R. G. (1987) The cross-cultural study of human sexuality. *Annual Review of Anthropology* 16:69–98.

Davis, J. A., and Smith, T. W. (1988) *General Social Surveys, 1972–1988.* Chicago: National Opinion Research Center, University of Chicago.

Dececco, J. P. (1988) *Obligation Versus Aspiration.* New York: The Haworth Press.

Decker, J. F. (1979) *Prostitution: Regulation and Control.* Littleton, Colo.: Fred B. Rothman and Company.

Delacoste, F., and Alexander, P., eds. (1987) *Sex Work: Writings by Women in the Sex Industry.* Pittsburgh, Pa.: The Cleis Press.

DeLamater, J., and MacCorquodale, P. (1975) The effects of interview schedule variations on reported sexual behavior. *Sociological Methods and Research* 4:215–236.

DeLamater, J., and MacCorquodale, P. (1979) *Premarital Sexuality: Attitudes, Relationships, Behavior.* Madison: University of Wisconsin Press.

D'Emilio, J. D. (1983) *Sexual Politics, Sexual Communities: The Making of a Homosexual Minority in the United States.* Chicago: University of Chicago Press.

Des Jarlais, D. C. (1988) HIV Infection Among Persons Who Inject Illicit Drugs: Problems and Progress. Presented at the Fourth International AIDS Conference, Stockholm, June 12–16.

Des Jarlais, D. C., Wish, E., Friedman, S. R., Stoneburner, R. L., Yancovitz, F., Mildban, D., El-Sadr, W., Brady, E., and Cuadrado, M. (1987) Intravenous drug users and the heterosexual transmission of the acquired immunodeficiency syndrome. *New York State Journal of Medicine* 87:283–286.

Des Jarlais, D. C., Friedman, S. R., and Stoneburner, R. L. (1988) HIV infection and intravenous drug use: Critical issues in transmission dynamics, infection outcomes, and prevention. *Reviews of Infectious Diseases* 10:151–158.

Detels, R., Fahey, J. L., Schwartz, K., Greene, R. S., Visscher, B. R., and Gottlieb, M. S. (1983) Relation between sexual practices and T-cell subsets in homosexually active men. *Lancet* 1:609–611.

Detels, R., Visscher, B. R., Fahey, J. L., Sever, J. L., Gravell, M., Madden, D. L., Schwartz, K., et al. (1987) Predictors of clinical AIDS in young homosexual men in a high-risk area. *International Journal of Epidemiology* 16:271–276.

Diamond, L. (1977) Human sexual development: Biological foundations for social development. Pp. 22–61 in F. A. Beach, ed., *Human Sexuality in Four Perspectives.* Baltimore, Md.: Johns Hopkins University Press.

Doll, L. S., and Bye, L. L. (1987) AIDS: Where reason prevails. *World Health Forum* 8:484–488.

Douglas, M. (1966) *Purity and Danger: An Analysis of Concepts of Pollution and Taboo.* New York: Praeger.

Dover, K. J. (1978) *Greek Homosexuality.* Cambridge, Mass.: Harvard University Press.

Duberman, M. (1974) The bisexual debate. *New York Times Magazine*, June 28:199–209.

Duncan, O. D. (1984) Rasch measurement in survey research. In C. F. Turner and E. Martin, eds., *Surveying Subjective Phenomena,* vol. 2. New York: Russell Sage and Basic Books.

Ellis, H. (1929) Preface. In B. Malinowski, *The Sexual Life of Savages.* New York: Harcourt Brace Jovanovich.

Elwin, V. (1947) *The Muria and Their Ghotal.* London: Oxford University Press.

Emmons, C. A., Joseph, J. G., Kessler, R. C., Wortman, C. B., Montgomery, S. B., and Ostrow, D. G. (1986) Psychosocial predictors of reported behavior change in homosexual men at risk for AIDS. *Health Education Quarterly* 13:331–345.

Erikson, E. H. (1964) *Childhood and Society.* New York: W. W. Norton.

Fay, R. E. (1982) Contingency Table Analysis for Complex Sample Designs (CPLX): Program Documentation. Statistical Methods Division, Bureau of the Census, Washington, D.C.

Fay, R. E., Turner, C. F., Klassen, A., and Gagnon, J. H. (In press) Prevalence and patterns of same-gender sexual contact among men. *Science* 239.

Feldman, D. A., and Johnson, T. M., eds. (1986) *The Social Dimensions of AIDS: Method and Theory.* New York: Praeger.

Feldman, D. A., Friedman, S. R., and Des Jarlais, D. C. (1987) Public awareness of AIDS in Rwanda. *Social Science and Medicine* 24:97-100.

Fischl, M. A., Dickinson, G. M., Scott, G. B., Klimas, N., Fletcher, M. A., and Parks, W. (1987) Evaluation of heterosexual partners, children, and household contacts of adults with AIDS. *Journal of the American Medical Association* 257:640–644.

Fisher, B., et al. (1982) Report on Adolescent Male Prostitution. Urban and Rural Systems Associates, San Francisco.

Flowers, M. N. (1988) Factors Affecting the Spread of AIDS in Rural Brazil. Workshop on Cultural Factors in AIDS Overseas. Presented at meetings of the American Association for the Advancement of Science, Boston, February 11–15.

Follansbee, S. E., Busch, D. F., Wofsy, C. B., Coleman, D. L., Gullet, J., Aurigemma, G. P., Ross, T., Hadley, W. K., and Draw, L. (1982) An outbreak of *Pneumocystis carinii* pneumonia in homosexual men. *Annals of Internal Medicine* 96:705–713.

Ford, C. S., and Beach, F. A. (1951) *Patterns of Sexual Behavior.* New York: Harper.

Fox, R., Odaka, N. J., Brookmeyer, R., and Polk, B. F. (1987) Effect of HIV antibody disclosure on subsequent sexual activity in homosexual men. AIDS 1:241–246.

France, J. J., Skidmore, C. A., Robertson, J. R., Brettle, R. P., Roberts, J. J. K., Burns, S. M., Foster, C. A., Inglis, J. M., Galloway, W. B. F., and Davidson, S. J. (1988) Heterosexual spread of human immunodeficiency virus in Edinburgh. *British Medical Journal* 296:526–529.

Free, M. J., et al. (1980) Relationship between condom strength and failure during use. *Conception* 22:31.

Free, M. J., Huthings, J., Lubis, F., and Natakusumah, R. (1986) An assessment of burst strength distribution data for monitoring quality of condom stocks in developing countries. *Conception* 33:285–299.

Freud, S. (1905) *Three Essays on the Theory of Sexuality.* New York: Basic Books, 1962.

Friedman-Kien, A. E. (1981) Disseminated Kaposi's sarcoma syndrome in young homosexual men. *American Academy of Dermatology* 5:468–471.

Friedman-Kien, A. E., Laubenstein, L. J., Rubinstein, P., Burniovici-Klien, E., Marmor, M., Stahl, R., Spigland, I., Kim, K. S., and Zolla-Pasner, S. (1982) Disseminated Kaposi's sarcoma in homosexual men. *Annals of Internal Medicine* 96:693–700.

Furth, P. A. (1987) Heterosexual transmission of AIDS by male drug users. *Nature* 327:193.

Gagnon, J. H. (1968) Prostitution. Pp. 209–215 in *The International Encyclopedia of the Social Sciences,* vol. 14. New York: Crowell-Collier.

Gagnon, J. H. (1975) Sex research and social change. *Archives of Sexual Behavior* 4:111–141.

Gagnon, J. H. (1977) *Human Sexualities.* Glenview, Ill.: Scott Foresman.

Gagnon, J. H. (1978) Reconsiderations: A. C. Kinsey et al., *Sexual Behavior in the Human Male*, Philadelphia, Saunders, 1948, 804 pp., and A. C. Kinsey et al., *Sexual Behavior in the Human Female*, Philadelphia, Saunders, 1953, 832 pp. Review essay. *Human Nature* 1:92–95.

Gagnon, J. H. (1983) Age at menarche and sexual conduct in adolescence and young adulthood. In S. Golub, ed., *Menarche.* Lexington, Mass.: D.C. Heath.

Gagnon, J. H., and Simon, W. (1973) *Sexual Conduct: The Social Sources of Human Sexuality.* Chicago: Aldine.

Gagnon, J. H., and Simon, W. (1987) The scripting of oral genital sexual conduct. *Archives of Sexual Behavior* 16:1–25.

Gagnon, J. H., Berger, A., and Simon, W. (1970) Some aspects of sexual adjustment in early and later adolescence. In J. Zubin and A. M. Freedman, eds., *Psychopathology of Adolescence.* New York: Grune & Stratton.

Gebhard, P. H. (1972) Incidence of overt homosexuality in the United States and Western Europe. In National Institute of Mental Health Task Force on Homosexuality, *Final Report and Background Papers.* Washington, D.C.: Government Printing Office.

Gebhard, P. H., and Johnson, A. B. (1979) *The Kinsey Data: Marginal Tabulations of 1938–1963 Interviews Conducted by the Institute for Sex Research.* Philadelphia: W. B. Saunders.

Gebhard, P. H., Pomeroy, W. B., Martin, C. E., and Christension, C. V. (1958) *Pregnancy, Birth and Abortion.* New York: Harper and Row.

Gebhard, P. H., Gagnon, J. H., Pomeroy, W. B., and Christension, C. V. (1965) *Sex Offenders: An Analysis of Types.* New York: Harper and Row.

Gibbens, T. C. N., and Silberman, M. (1960) The clients of prostitutes. *British Journal of Venereal Diseases* 36:113–117.

Goedert, J. J., Sarngadharan, M. G., Biggar, R. J., Weiss, S. H., Winn, D. M., Grossman, R. J., Greene, M. H., Bodner, A. J., Mann, D. L., Strong, D. M., Gallo, R. C., and Blattner, W. A. (1984) Determinants of retrovirus (HTLV-III) antibody and immunodeficiency conditions in homosexual men. *Lancet* 2:711–715.

Goedert, J. J., Biggar, R. J., Winn, D. M., Mann, D. L., Byar, D. P., Strong, D. M., DiGioia, R. A., Grossman, R. J., Sanchez, W. C., Kase, R. R. G., Greene, M. H., Hoover, R. H., and Blattner, W. A. (1985) Decreased helper T-lymphocytes in homosexual men. I. Sexual contact in high-incidence areas for the acquired immunodeficiency syndrome. *American Journal of Epidemiology* 121:629–636.

Goldstein, P. J. (1979) *Prostitution and Drugs.* Lexington, Mass.: Lexington Books.

Gorman, E. M. (1986) The AIDS epidemic in San Francisco: Epidemiological and anthropological perspectives. In C. R. Janes, R. Stall, and S. Gifford, eds., *Anthropology and Epidemiology.* Boston: Dordrect, Reidel, a division of Kluwer Academic Publishers.

Gottlieb, M. S., Schroff, R., Schanker, H. M., Weisman, J. D., Thim Fan, P., Wolf, R. A., and Saxon, A. (1981) *Pneumocystis carinii* pneumonia and mucosal candidiasis in previously healthy homosexual men. *New England Journal of Medicine* 305:1425–1431.

Green, R. (1987) *The "Sissy Boy Syndrome" and the Development of Homosexuality.* New Haven, Conn.: Yale University Press.

Gregersen, E. (1983) *Sexual Practices: The Story of Human Sexuality.* New York: Franklin Watts.

Gregor, T. (1985) *Anxious Pleasures.* Chicago: University of Chicago Press.

Harder, P., Wexler, S., Marotta, T., Murphy, T. S., and Houston-Hamilton, A. (1987) Evaluation of California's AIDS Community Education Program. AIDS Office, California Department of Health Services, Sacramento.

Harris, M. (1983) *Cultural Anthropology.* New York: Harper and Row.

Hartwig, G., and Patterson, K. D., eds. (1978) *Disease in African History.* Durham, N.C.: Duke University Press.

Hayes, C. D., ed. (1987) *Risking the Future: Adolescent Sexuality, Pregnancy, and Childbearing,* vol. 1. Washington, D.C.: National Academy Press.

Hein, K., Cohen, M. I., Marks, A., Schonberg, S. K., Meyer, M., and McBride, A. (1978) Age at first intercourse among homeless adolescent females. *Journal of Pediatrics* 93:147–154.

Herdt, G., ed. (1981) *Guardians of the Flutes.* New York: McGraw-Hill.

Herdt, G., ed. (1984) *Ritualized Homosexuality in Melanesia.* Berkeley: University of California Press.

Herdt, G., ed. (In press) *Homosexuality and Adolescence.* New York: Haworth Press.

Herdt, G. (N.d.) Gay and Lesbian Teenagers. Committee on Human Development, University of Chicago.

Heyl, B. S. (1974) The madam as entrepreneur. *Sociological Symposium* 11:61–82.

Heyl, B. S. (1977) The madam as teacher: The training of house prostitutes. *Social Problems* 24:545–555.

Hite, S. (1987) *Women and Love: A Cultural Revolution in Progress.* New York: Knopf.

Hobson, B. M. (1987) *Uneasy Virtue: The Politics of Prostitution and the American Reform Tradition.* New York: Basic Books.

Hofferth, S. L., and Hayes, C. D., eds. (1987) *Risking the Future: Adolescent Sexuality, Pregnancy, and Childbearing.* Volume 2, *Working Papers and Statistical Appendixes.* Washington, D.C.: National Academy Press.

Hofferth, S. L., and Upchurch, D. M. (1988) Breaking Up: Dissolving Non-Marital Unions. Presented at the annual meeting of the Population Association of America, New Orleans, April 19–23.

Hofferth, S. L., Kahn, J. R., and Baldwin, W. (1987) Premarital sexual activity among U.S. teenage women over the past three decades. *Family Planning Perspectives* 19:46–53.

Hooker, E. (1957) The adjustment of the male overt homosexual. *Journal of Projective Techniques* 21:18–31.

Hooker, E. (1958) Male homosexuality in the Rorschach. *Journal of Projective Techniques* 22:33–54.

Hooker, E. (1966) The homosexual community. Pp. 354–364 in J. C. Palmer and M. J. Goldstein, eds., *Perspectives in Psychopathology.* New York: Oxford University Press.

Hrdy, D. B. (1987) Cultural practices contributing to the transmission of human immunodeficiency virus in Africa. *Reviews of Infectious Diseases* 9:1109–1119.

Humphreys, L. (1970) *Tearoom Trade: Impersonal Sex in Public Places.* Chicago: Aldine.

Humphreys, R. A. L. (1971) New styles in homosexual manliness. *Transaction* (March/April):38–46, 64, 66.

Humphreys, R. A. L. (1972) *Out of the Closets: The Sociology of Homosexual Liberation.* Englewood Cliffs, N.J.: Prentice-Hall.

Institute of Medicine/National Academy of Sciences (IOM/NAS). (1986) *Confronting AIDS: Directions for Public Health, Health Care, and Research.* Washington, D.C.: National Academy Press.

Institute of Medicine/National Academy of Sciences (IOM/NAS). (1988) *Confronting AIDS: Update 1988.* Washington, D.C.: National Academy Press.

Jabine, T. B., Straf, M. L., Tanur, J. M., and Tourangeau, R., eds. (1984) *Cognitive Aspects of Survey Methodology: Building a Bridge Between Disciplines.* Washington, D.C.: National Academy Press.

Jackman, N. H., O'Toole, R., and Geis, G. (1963) The self image of the prostitute. *Sociological Quarterly* 4:150–161.

Jaffe, H. W., Choi, K., Thomas, P. A., Haverkos, H. W., Auerbach, D. M., Guinan, M. E., Rogers, M. F., Spira, T. J., Darrow, W. W., Kramer, M. A., et al. (1983) National case-control study of Kaposi's sarcoma and *Pneumocystis carinii* pneumonia in homosexual men. Part 1. Epidemiologic results. *Annals of Internal Medicine* 99:145–151.

Jaffe, H. W., Darrow, W. W., Echenberg, D. F., O'Malley, P. M., Getchell, J. P., Kalyanaraman, V. S., Byers, R. H., Drennan, D. P., Braff, E. H., Curran, J. W., and Francis, D. (1985). The acquired immunodeficiency syndrome in a cohort of homosexual men: A six year follow-up study. *Annals of Internal Medicine* 103:210–214.

James, J. (1976) Motivations for entrance into prostitution. In L. Crites, ed., *The Female Offender.* Lexington, Mass.: Lexington Books.

James, J. (1977) Prostitutes and prostitution. In E. Sagarin and F. Montanino, eds., *Deviants: Voluntary Actors in a Hostile World.* Glenview, Ill.: Scott Foresman.

James, J. (1980) Self-destructive behavior and adaptive strategies in female prostitutes. In N. L. Farberow, ed., *The Many Faces of Suicide.* New York: McGraw-Hill.

Jessor, S. L., and Jessor, R. (1975) Transition from virginity to non-virginity among youth: A social-psychological study over time. *Developmental Psychology* 11:473–484.

Jones, C. C., Waskin, H., Gerety, B., Skipper, B. J., Hull, H. F., and Mertz, G. J. (1987) Persistence of high risk sexual activity among homosexual men in an area of low incidence of the acquired immunodeficiency syndrome. *Sexually Transmitted Diseases* 14:79–82.

Jones, E. F., Forrest, J. D., Goldman, N., Henshaw, S. K., Lincoln, R., Rosoff, J. I., Westoff, C. F., and Wulf, D. (1985) Teenage pregnancy in developed countries: Determinants and policy implications. *Family Planning Perspectives* 17:53–63.

Joseph, J. G., Montgomery, S. B., Emmons, C. A., Kessler, R. C., Ostrow, D. G., Wortman, C. B., O'Brien, K., Eller, M., and Eshleman, S. (1987) Magnitude and determinants of behavioral risk reduction: Longitudinal analysis of a cohort at risk for AIDS. *Psychological Health* 1:73–96.

Kantner, J. F., and Zelnik, M. (1972) Sexual experience of young unmarried women in the United States. *Family Planning Perspectives* 4:9–18.

Kantner, J. F., and Zelnik, M. (1983a) 1971 U.S. National Survey of Young Women: Selected Variables (machine-readable data file). Data Archive on Adolescent Pregnancy and Pregnancy Prevention, Sociometrics Corporation, Palo Alto, Calif.

Kantner, J. F., and Zelnik, M. (1983b) 1976 U.S. National Survey of Young Women: Selected Variables (machine-readable data file). Data Archive on Adolescent Pregnancy and Pregnancy Prevention, Sociometrics Corporation, Palo Alto, Calif.

Kaslow, R. W., Ostrow, D. G., Detels, R., Phair, J. P., Polk, B. F., and Rinaldo, C. R., Jr. (1987) The Multicenter AIDS Cohort Study: Rationale, organization, and selected characteristics of the participants. *American Journal of Epidemiology* 126:310–318.

Katz, J. N. (1976) *Gay American History: Lesbians and Gay Men in the U.S.A.* New York: Thomas Y. Crowell.

Katz, J. N. (1983) *Gay/Lesbian Almanac: A New Documentary.* New York: Harper and Row.

Kelly, R. (1977) *Etoro Social Structure.* Ann Arbor: University of Michigan Press.

Kingsley, L. A., Kaslow, R., Rinaldo, C. R., Jr., Detre, K., Odaka, N., Van Raden, M., Detels, R., Polk, B. F., Chmiel, J., Kelsey, S. F., Ostrow, D., and Visscher, B. (1987) Risk factors for sero-conversion to human immunodeficiency virus among male homosexuals. *Lancet* 1:345–349.

Kinsey, A. C., Pomeroy, W. B., and Martin, C. E. (1948) *Sexual Behavior in the Human Male.* Philadelphia: W. B. Saunders.

Kinsey, A. C., Pomeroy, W. B., Martin, C. E., and Gebhard, P. H. (1953) *Sexual Behavior in the Human Female.* Philadelphia: W. B. Saunders.

Klassen, A. D. (1988) "Lost" sex survey (correspondence). *Science* 240:375–376.

Klassen, A. D., Williams, C. J., and Levitt, E. E. (In press) *Sex and Morality in the United States*, edited by H. J. O'Gorman. Middleton, Conn.: Wesleyan University Press.

Knodel, J., Havanon, N., and Pramulratana, A. (1984) Fertility transition in Thailand: A qualitative analysis. *Population and Development Review* 10:297–328.

Kochems, L. M. (1987a) Advocacy as Anthropology: A Gay Anthropologist in the Time of AIDS. Presented at the American Anthropological Association meetings, Chicago, November 21.

Kochems, L. M. (1987b) Meanings and Health Implications: Gay Men's Sexuality. Presented at the American Anthropological Association meetings, Chicago, November 21.

Kramer, M. A., Aral, S. O., and Curran, J. W. (1980) Self-reported behavior patterns of patients attending a sexually transmitted disease clinic. *American Journal of Public Health* 70:997–1000.

Kreiss, J. K., Koech, D., Plummer, F. A., Holmes, K. K., Lightfoote, M., Piot, P., Ronald, A. R., Ndinya-Achola, J. O., D'Costa, L. J., Roberts, P., Mgugi, E. N., and Quinn, T. C. (1986) AIDS infection in Nairobi prostitutes: Spread of the epidemic to East Africa. *New England Journal of Medicine* 314:414–418.

Lancaster, R. N. (1988) Subject honor and object shame: The cochon and the milieu-specific construction of stigma and sexuality in Nicaragua. *Ethnology* 27:111–125.

Landrum, S., Beck-Sague, C., and Kraus, S. (1988) Racial trends in syphilis among men with same-sex partners in Atlanta, Georgia. *American Journal of Public Health* 78:66–67.

Layard, J. (1942) *Stone Men of Malekula.* London: Chatto and Windus.

Layard, J. (1959) Homoeroticism in primitive society as a function of the self. *Journal of Analytical Psychology* 4:101–115.

Lederer, L., ed. (1980) *Take Back the Night: Women on Pornography.* New York: Morrow.

Leonard, T. L., Sacks, J. J., Franks, A. L., and Sikes, R. K. (1988) The prevalence of human immunodeficiency virus, hepatitis B, and syphilis among female prostitutes in Atlanta. *Journal of the Medical Association of Georgia* 77:162–164.

Levitt, E. E., and Klassen, A. D. (1974) Public attitudes toward homosexuality: Part of the 1970 national survey by the Institute for Sex Research. *Journal of Homosexuality* 1:29–43.

Leznoff, M., and Westley, W. A. (1956) The homosexual community. *Social Problems* 3:257–263.

Lindenbaum, S. (1979) *Kuru Sorcery.* Palo Alto, Calif.: Mayfield.

Lindenbaum, S. (1984) Variations on a sociosexual theme in Melanesia. Pp. 337–361 in G. Herdt, ed., *Ritualized Homosexuality in Melanesia.* Berkeley: University of California Press.

Lindenbaum, S. (1987) The mystification of female labors. In J. F. Collier and S. J. Yanagisako, eds., *Gender and Kinship.* Stanford, Calif.: Stanford University Press.

Lui, K., Darrow, W. W., and Rutherford, G. W. (1988) A model based estimate of the mean incubation period for AIDS in homosexual men. *Science* 240:1333–1335.

MacCormack, C. P., and Strathern, M. (1980) *Nature, Culture and Gender.* New York: Cambridge University Press.

MacKuen, M. (1984) Reality, the press, and citizens' political agendas. In C. F. Turner and E. Martin, eds., *Surveying Subjective Phenomena,* vol. 2. New York: Russell Sage and Basic Books.

MacKuen, M., and Turner, C. F. (1984) The popularity of presidents, 1963–80 (an empirical attempt to gauge the accuracy of measurements made in 513 national polls). In C. F. Turner and E. Martin, eds., *Surveying Subjective Phenomena,* vol. 2. New York: Russell Sage and Basic Books.

Malinowski, B. (1927) *Sex and Repression in Savage Society.* New York: Harcourt, Brace.

Malinowski, B. (1929) *The Sexual Life of Savages.* New York: Harcourt Brace Jovanovich.

Mamdani, M. (1972) *The Myth of Population Control.* New York: Monthly Review Press.

Marmor, M., Laubenstein, L., William, D. C., Friedman-Kien, A. E., Byrum, R. D., D'Onofrio, S., and Dubin, N. (1982) Risk factors for Kaposi's sarcoma in homosexual men. *Lancet* 1:1083–1087.

Martin, J. L. (1986a) AIDS risk reduction recommendations and sexual behavior patterns among gay men: A multifactorial categorical approach to assessing change. *Health Education Quarterly* 13:347–358.

Martin, J. L. (1986b) Demographic Factors, Sexual Behavior Patterns, and HIV Antibody Status Among New York City Gay Men. Presented at the 94th annual convention of the American Psychological Association, Washington, D.C., August.

Martin, J. L. (1986c) Sexual Behavior Patterns, Behavior Change, and Occurrence of Antibody to LAV/HTLV-III Among New York City Gay Men. Presented at the Second International AIDS Conference, Paris, June 23–25.

Martin, J. L. (1987a) The impact of AIDS on gay male sexual behavior patterns in New York City. *American Journal of Public Health* 77:578–581.

Martin, J. L. (1987b) Psychosocial Determinants and Sexual Behavior Consequences of Knowledge of HIV Antibody Status. Presented at the Centers for Disease Control Conference on HIV Testing Policy, Atlanta, Ga.

Martin, J. L. (1988) The Impact of Knowledge of HIV Antibody Status on Subsequent Sexual Behavior among Gay Men. Presented at the Fourth International AIDS Conference, Stockholm, June 12–16.

Martin, J. L. (In press) The psychological consequences of AIDS-related bereavement. *Journal of Clinical and Consulting Psychology.*

Martin, J. L., and Dean, L. (1985) The Impact of AIDS on New York City Gay Men: Development of a Community Sample. Presented at the 113th annual meeting of the American Public Health Association, Washington, D.C., November.

Martin, J. L., and Dean, L. (In press) Risk factors for AIDS related bereavement in a cohort of homosexual men in New York City. In B. Cooper and T. Helgason, eds., *Epidemiology and the Prevention of Mental Disorders.* London: Routledge & Kegan Paul.

Martin, J. L., and Vance, C. S. (1984) Behavioral and psychosocial factors in AIDS: Methodological and substantive issues. *American Psychologist* 39:1303–1308.

Martin, J. L., Dean, L., Garcia, M., and Hall, W. (In press) The impact of AIDS on a gay community: Changes in sexual behavior, substance use and mental health. *American Journal of Community Psychology.*

Masters, W. H., and Johnson, V. E. (1966) *Human Sexual Response.* Boston: Little, Brown and Company.

Mata, A. G., and Jorquez, J. S. (1988) Mexican-American intravenous drug users' needle-sharing practices: Implications for AIDS prevention. In R. J. Battjes and R. W. Pickens, eds., *Needle Sharing Among Intravenous Drug Abusers: National and International Perspectives.* NIDA Research Monograph Series No. 80. Rockville, Md.: National Institute on Drug Abuse.

May, R. M., and Anderson, R. M. (1987) Transmission dynamics of HIV infection. *Nature* 326:137–142.

May, R. M., and Anderson, R. M. (In press) The transmission dynamics of human immunodeficiency virus (HIV). *Philosophical Transactions of the Royal Society.*

Mayer, K. H., and DeGruttola, V. (1987) Human immunodeficiency virus and oral intercourse. *Annals of Internal Medicine* 107:428–429.

Mayer, K. H., Ayotte, D., Groopman, J. E., Stoddard, A., Sarngadharan, M., and Gallo, R. C. (1986) Association of human T-lymphotropic virus type III antibodies with sexual and other behaviors in a cohort of homosexual men from Boston with and without generalized lymphadenopathy. *American Journal of Medicine* 80:357–363.

McCauley, E. A., and Ehrhardt, A. A. (1980) Sexual behavior in female transsexuals and lesbians. *Journal of Sex Research* 16:202–211.

McCombie, S. C. (1986) The cultural impact of the AIDS test: The American experience. *Social Science and Medicine* 23:455–459.

McCusker, J., Stoddard, A. M., Mayer, K. H., Cowan, D. N., and Groopman, J. E. (1988a) Behavioral risk factors for HIV infection among homosexual men at a Boston community health center. *American Journal of Public Health* 78:68–71.

McCusker, J., Stoddard, A. M., Mayer, K. H., Zapka, J., Morrison, C., and Saltzman, S. P. (1988b) Effects of HIV antibody test knowledge on subsequent sexual behaviors in a cohort of homosexually active men. *American Journal of Public Health* 78:462–467.

McKusick, L., Horstman, W., and Coates, T. J. (1985) AIDS and sexual behavior reported by gay men in San Francisco. *American Journal of Public Health* 75:493–496.

Menken, J. (1988) Fertility Research and AIDS: Does the Knowledge Transfer? Presented at the annual meeting of the Population Association of America, New Orleans, April 19–23.

Michael, R. T., Laumann, E. O., Gagnon, J. H., and Smith, T. W. (1988) Number of sex partners and potential risk of sexual exposure to human immunodeficiency virus. *Morbidity and Mortality Weekly Report* 37:565–568.

Miller, E. F. (1986) *Street Women.* Philadelphia: Temple University Press.

Miller, P. Y., and Simon, W. (1974) Adolescent sexual behavior: Context and change. *Social Problems* 22:58–76.

Morin, S. F. (1977) Heterosexual bias in research on lesbianism and male homosexuality. *American Psychologist* 32:629–637.

Morin, S. F., Charles, K. A., and Malyon, A. (1984) The psychological impact of AIDS on gay men. *American Psychologist* 39:1288–1293.

Moss, A. R., Osmond, D., Bacchetti, P., Chermann, J. C., Barre-Sinoussi, F., and Carlson, J. (1987). Risk factors for AIDS and HIV seropositivity in homosexual men. *American Journal of Epidemiology* 125:1035–1047.

Mott, F. (1985) Evaluation of Fertility Data and Preliminary Analytical Results from the 1983 (5th Round) Survey of the National Longitudinal Surveys of Work Experience of Youth. Technical Report, Center for Human Resource Research, Ohio State University. January.

National Institute of Mental Health Task Force on Homosexuality. (1972) *Final Report and Background Papers.* Washington, D.C.: Government Printing Office.

Nestle, J. (1987) Lesbians and prostitutes: A historical sisterhood. In L. Bell, ed., *Good Girls/Bad Girls: Feminists and Sex Trade Workers Face to Face.* Toronto: The Seal Press.

Newcomer, S. F., and Udry, J. R. (1985) Oral sex in an adolescent population. *Archives of Sexual Behavior* 14:41–46.

O'Campo, M. (1987) Pornography and prostitution in the Philippines. In L. Bell, ed., *Good Girls/Bad Girls: Feminists and Sex Trade Workers Face to Face.* Toronto: The Seal Press.

Ortner, S. B., and Whitehead, H., eds. (1981) *Sexual Meanings: The Cultural Construction of Gender and Sexuality.* New York: Cambridge University Press.

Parker, R. G. (1987) Acquired immunodeficiency syndrome in urban Brazil. *Medical Anthropology Quarterly* 1:155–175.

Parker, R. G. (N.d.) Sexual Culture and AIDS Education in Urban Brazil. Department of Anthropology, University of California.

Peterman, T. A., Stoneburner, R. L., Allen, J. R., Jaffe, H. W., and Curran, J. W. (1988) Risk of human immunodeficiency virus transmission from heterosexual adults with transfusion-associated infections. *Journal of the American Medical Association* 259:55–58.

Pheterson, G. (1987) The social consequences of unchastity. In F. Delacoste and P. Alexander, eds., *Sex Work: Writings by Women in the Sex Industry*. Pittsburgh, Pa.: The Cleis Press.

Pillard, R. C., Poumadere, J., and Carretta, R. A. (1981) Is homosexuality familial? A review, some data and a suggestion. *Archives of Sexual Behavior* 10:465–475.

Piot, P., Kreiss, J. K., Ndinya-Achola, O., Ngugi, E. N., Simonsen, J. N., Cameron, D. W., Taelman, H., and Plummer, F. A. (1987a) Heterosexual transmission of HIV. *AIDS* 1:199–206.

Piot, P., Plummer, F. A., Rey, M. A., Ngugi, E. N., Rouzioux, C., Ndinya-Achola, J. O., Veracautere, G., D'Costa, L. J., Brunham, M., Ronald, A. R., and Brun-Veziner, F. (1987b) Retrospective seroepidemiology of AIDS virus infections in Nairobi populations. *Journal of Infectious Diseases* 155:1108–1112.

Polk, B. F., Fox, R., Brookmeyer, R., Kanchanaraksa, S., Kaslow, R., Visscher, B., Rinaldo, C., and Phair, J. (1987) Predictors of the acquired immunodeficiency syndrome developing in a cohort of seropositive homosexual men. *New England Journal of Medicine* 316:63–66.

Pomeroy, G. (1965) Some aspects of prostitution. *Journal of Sex Research* 1:177–187.

Pomeroy, W. B. (1972) *Dr. Kinsey and the Institute for Sex Research*. New York: Harper and Row.

Pounds, M. B. (1987) Sexual Meanings, Behavior, and Identity Among Afro-American Men in Baltimore. Presented at the American Anthropological Association meetings, Chicago, November 17.

Public Health Service. (1986) The Coolfont report: Public Health Service plan for combating AIDS. *Public Health Reports* 101:341–349.

Read, K. E. (1980) *Other Voices: The Style of a Male Homosexual Tavern*. Novato, Calif.: Chandler and Sharp Publishers.

Reinisch, J. M. (1981) Prenatal exposure to synthetic progestins increases potential for aggression in humans. *Science* 211:1171–1173.

Reiss, A. J. (1961) The social integration of queers and peers. *Social Problems* 9:102–120.

Reiss, I. (1960) *Premarital Sexual Standards in America*. Glencoe, Ill.: The Free Press.

Reiss, I. (1967) *The Social Context of Sexual Permissiveness*. New York: Holt, Rinehart and Winston.

Reiter, R. R., ed. (1975) *Toward an Anthropology of Women*. New York: Monthly Review Press.

Research and Decisions Corporation. (1985) Designing an Effective AIDS Prevention Campaign Strategy for San Francisco: Results from the Second Probability Sample of an Urban Gay Male Community. Prepared for the San Francisco AIDS Foundation.

Rich, R. (1988) Feminism and sexuality in the 1980's. *Feminist Studies* 12:525–561.

Rolph, C. H. (1955) *Women of the Streets*. London: Secker and Warburg.

Ross, M. W. (1987) Problems associated with condom use in homosexual men (correspondence). *American Journal of Public Health* 77:877.

Rubin, G. (1975) The traffic in women. In R. R. Reiter, ed., *Toward an Anthropology of Women*. New York: Monthly Review.

Rubin, G. (1984) Thinking sex. In C. Vance, ed., *Pleasure and Danger*. London: Routledge & Kegan Paul.

Rubin, R. T., Reinisch, J. M., and Haskett, R. F. (1981) Postnatal gonadal steroid effects on human behavior. *Science* 211:1318–1324.

Saghir, M. T., and Robins, E. (1973) *Male and Female Homosexuality: A Comprehensive Investigation.* Baltimore, Md.: Williams and Wilkins.

Saltzman, S. P., Stoddard, A. M., McCusker, J., Moon, M. W., and Mayer, K. H. (1987) Reliability of self-reported sexual behavior risk factors for HIV infection in homosexual men. *Public Health Reports* 102:692–697.

Schapera, I. (1941) *Married Life in an African Tribe.* New York: Sheridan House.

Schedlin, M. G. (1987) If You Wanna Kiss, Go Home To Your Wife: Sexual Meanings for the Prostitute and Implications for AIDS Prevention Activities. Presented at meetings of the American Anthropological Association, November 21.

Schmid, G. P., Sanders, L. L., Blount, J. H., and Alexander, E. R. (1987) Chancroid in the United States. *Journal of the American Medical Association* 258:3265–3268.

Schneider, J., and Schneider, P. (1984) Demographic transitions in a Sicilian rural town. *Journal of Family History* 9:245–272.

Schoepf, B. G. (1988) AIDS, Women and Society in Central Africa. Workshop on Cultural Factors in AIDS Overseas. Presented at meetings of the American Association for the Advancement of Science, Boston, February 11–15.

Schreiner, J. (1986) Measuring the Gay and Lesbian Population. National Organization of Gay and Lesbian Scientists and Technical Professionals, Chicago, Ill.

Shah, F., Zelnik, M., and Kantner, J. F. (1975) Unprotected intercourse among unwed teenagers. *Family Planning Perspectives* 7:39–44.

Siegel, K., and Bauman, L. J. (1986) Sexual Practices Among Gay Men in New York City. Presented at the annual meeting of the American Sociological Association, New York City, August.

Silbert, M. H., and Pines, M. P. (1982) Entrance into prostitution. *Youth and Society* 13:471–500.

Simon, W., and Gagnon, J. (1967) Homosexuality: The formulation of a sociological perspective. *Journal of Health and Social Behavior* 8:177–185.

Simon, W., Berger, A., and Gagnon, J. (1972) Beyond anxiety and fantasy: The coital experience of college youth. *Journal of Youth and Adolescence* 1:203–222.

Smith, E. A., and Udry, J. R. (1985) Coital and non-coital sexual behaviors of white and black adolescents. *American Journal of Public Health* 75:1200–1203.

Snitow, A., Stansell, C., and Thompson, S., eds. (1983) *Powers of Desire: The Politics of Sexuality.* New York: Monthly Review Press.

Socarides, C. W. (1978) *Homosexuality.* New York: J. Aronson.

Spanier, G. B. (1976) Formal and informal sex education as determinants of premarital sexual behavior. *Archives of Sexual Behavior* 5:39–67.

Stall, R., McKusick, L., Wiley, J., Coates, T. J., and Ostrow, D. G. (1986) Alcohol and drug use during sexual activity and compliance with safe sex guidelines for AIDS: The AIDS behavioral research project. *Health Education Quarterly* 13:359–371.

Sterk, C., and Leonard, T. (1988) If You Want to Know, Talk With Us! Narcotic and Drug Research, Inc., New York City.

Stevens, C. E., Taylor, P. E., Zang, E. A., Morrison, J. M., Harley, E. J., de Cordoba, S. R., Bacino, C., Ting, R. C. Y., Bodner, A. J., Sarngadharan, M. G., Gallo, R. C., and Rubinstein, P. (1986) Human T-cell lymphotropic virus type III infection in a cohort of homosexual men in New York City. *Journal of the American Medical Association* 265:2267–2272.

Strunin, L., and Hingson, R. (1987) Acquired immunodeficiency syndrome and adolescents: Knowledge, beliefs, attitudes, and behaviors. *Pediatrics* 79:825–828.

Tanfer, K., and Horn, M. C. (1985) Contraceptive use, pregnancy and fertility patterns among single American women in their 20s. *Family Planning Perspectives* 17:10–19.

Terman, L. M. (1948) Kinsey's "Sexual Behavior in the Human Male": Some comments and criticisms. *Psychological Bulletin* 45:443–459.

The Streetwalker. (1959) London: The Bodley Head.

Thornton, A. (1988) Cohabitation and Marriage in the 1980s. Presented at the annual meeting of the Population Association of America, New Orleans, April 19–23.

Trussell, J., and Kost, K. (1987) Contraceptive failure in the United States: A critical review of the literature. *Studies in Family Planning* 18:237–283.

Turner, C. F. (1978) Fallible indicators of the subjective state of the nation. *American Psychologist* 33:456–470.

Turner, C. F. (1984) Why do surveys disagree? Some preliminary hypotheses and some disagreeable examples. In C. F. Turner and E. Martin, eds., *Surveying Subjective Phenomena,* vol. 2. New York: Russell Sage and Basic Books.

Turner, C. F., and Martin, E., eds. (1984) *Surveying Subjective Phenomena,* 2 vols. New York: Russell Sage and Basic Books.

Turner, C. F., Miller, H. G., and Barker, L. (In press) AIDS research and the behavioral and social sciences. In R. Kulstad, ed., *AIDS, 1988.* Washington, D.C.: American Association for the Advancement of Science.

Udry, J. R., Bauman, K. E., and Morris, N. M. (1975) Changes in premarital coital experience of recent decade-of-birth cohorts of urban American women. *Journal of Marriage and the Family* 37:783–787.

Udry, J. R., Talbert, L. M., and Morris, N. M. (1986) Biosocial foundations for adolescent female sexuality. *Demography* 23:217–230.

Vance, C. (1984) *Pleasure and Danger.* London: Routledge & Kegan Paul.

van Greinsven, G. J. P., Tielman, R. A. P., Goudsmit, J., van der Noordaa, J., de Wolf, F., de Vroome, E. M. M., and Coutinho, R. A.. (1987) Risk factors and prevalence of HIV antibodies in homosexual men in the Netherlands. *American Journal of Epidemiology* 125:1048–1057.

Vener, A. M., and Stewart, C. S. (1974) Adolescent sexual behavior in middle America revisited: 1970–1973. *Journal of Marriage and the Family* 36:728–735.

Vener, A. M., Stewart, C. S., and Hager, D. L. (1972) The sexual behavior of adolescents in middle America: Generational and American-British comparisons. *Journal of Marriage and the Family* 34:696–705.

Vicinus, M. (1982) Sexuality and power: A review of current work in the history of sexuality. *Feminist Studies* 8:133–156.

Wallace, J. I., Mann, J., and Beatrice, S. (1988) HIV-1 Exposure Among Clients of Prostitutes. Presented at the Fourth International AIDS Conference, Stockholm, June 12–16.

Wallis, W. A. (1948) Statistics of the Kinsey report. *Journal of the American Statistical Association* 44:463–484.

Weinberg, M. S., and Williams, C. J. (1974) *Male Homosexuals: Problems and Adaptations.* New York: Oxford University Press.

Weinberg, M. S., and Williams, C. J. (1988) Black sexuality: A test of two theories. *Journal of Sex Research* 25:197–218.

Werdegar, D., O'Malley, P., Bodecker, T., Hessol, N., and Echenberg, D. (1987) Self-reported changes in sexual behaviors among homosexual and bisexual men from the San Francisco City Clinic cohort. *Morbidity and Mortality Weekly Report* 36:187–189.

White, B. (1975) The economic importance of children in a Javanese village. In M. Nag, ed., *Population and Social Organization.* The Hague: Mouton.

White, E. (1980) *States of Desire: Travels in Gay America.* New York: E.P. Dutton, Inc.

Wigersma, L., and Oud, R. (1987) Safety and acceptability of condoms for use by homosexual men as a prophylactic against transmission of HIV during anogenital sexual intercourse. *British Medical Journal* 295:94.

Willis, R. J., and Michael, R. T. (1988) Innovation in Family Formation: Evidence on Cohabitation in the 1986 Follow-up Survey of the NLS/72 Sample. Presented at the annual meeting of the Population Association of America, New Orleans, April 19–23.

Winick, C. (1962) Prostitutes clients' perception of the prostitutes and of themselves. *International Journal of Social Psychiatry* 8:289–297.

Winkelstein, W., Jr., Samuel, M., Padian, N. S., Wiley, J. A., Lang, W., Anderson, R. E., and Levy, J. A. (1987a). The San Francisco Men's Health Study. III. Reduction in human immunodeficiency virus transmission among homosexual/bisexual men. *American Journal of Public Health* 77:685–689.

Winkelstein, W., Jr., Samuel, M., Padian, N. S., and Wiley, J. A. (1987b) Selected sexual practices of San Francisco heterosexual men and risk of infection by the human immunodeficiency virus. *Journal of the American Medical Association* 257:1470–1471.

Winkelstein, W., Jr., Lyman, D. M., and Padian, N. S. (1987c). Sexual practices and risk of infection by the AIDS-associated retrovirus: The San Francisco Men's Health Study. *Journal of the American Medical Association* 257:321–325.

Worth, D. (1988) Self-Help Interventions with Women at High Risk. Montefiore Medical Center, New York City.

Wyatt, G. E. (1985) The sexual abuse of Afro-American and white American women in childhood. *Child Abuse and Neglect* 9:507–519.

Wyatt, G. E. (1988a) Ethnic and cultural differences in women's sexual behavior. In S. J. Blumenthal and A. Eichler, chairpersons, NIMH/NIDA [National Institute of Mental Health/National Institute on Drug Abuse] *Workshop on Women and AIDS: Promoting Healthy Behaviors.* [Volume of background papers for the workshop held in Bethesda, Md., September 27–29.] Rockville, Md.: National Institute of Mental Health.

Wyatt, G. E. (1988b) Re-examining Factors Predicting Afro-American and White-American Women's Age of First Coitus. School of Medicine, University of California at Los Angeles.

Wyatt, G. E. (In press) The relationship between child sexual abuse and adolescent sexual functioning in Afro-American and White-American women. *Annals of the New York Academy of Sciences.*

Wyatt, G. E., Peters, S. D., and Guthrie, D. (1988a) Kinsey revisited. Part 1. Comparisons of the sexual socialization and sexual behavior of white women over 33 years. *Archives of Sexual Behavior* 17:201–239.

Wyatt, G. E., Peters, S. D., and Guthrie, D. (1988b) Kinsey revisited. Part 2. Comparisons of the sexual socialization and sexual behavior of black women over 33 years. *Archives of Sexual Behavior* 17:289–332.

Young, W. (1964) *Eros Denied.* New York: Grove Press.

Zabin, L. S., and Clark, S. D. (1981) Why they delay: A study of teenage family planning clinic patients. *Family Planning Perspectives* 13:205–217.

Zabin, L. S., and Clark, S. D. (1983) Institutional factors affecting teenagers' choice and reasons for delay in attending a family planning clinic. *Family Planning Perspectives* 15:25–29.

Zabin, L. S., Hirsch, M. B., Smith, E. A., and Hardy, J. B. (1984) Adolescent sexual attitudes and behavior: Are they consistent? *Family Planning Perspectives* 16:181–185.

Zabin, L. S., Smith E. A., Hirsch, M. B., and Hardy, J. B. (1986a) Ages of physical maturation and first intercourse in black teenage males and females. *Demography* 23:595–605.

Zabin, L. S., Hirsch, M. B., Smith, E. A., Streett, R., and Hardy, J. B. (1986b) Evaluation of a pregnancy prevention program for urban teenagers. *Family Planning Perspectives* 18:119–126.

Zelnik, M. (1980) Second pregnancies to premaritally pregnant teenagers, 1976 and 1971. *Family Planning Perspectives* 12:69–76.

Zelnik, M. (1983) Sexual activity among adolescents: Perspective of a decade. Pp. 21–33 in E. R. McAnarney, ed., *Premature Adolescent Pregnancy and Parenthood.* New York: Grune & Stratton.

Zelnik, M., and Kantner, J. F. (1972) The probability of premarital intercourse. *Social Science Research* 1:335–341.

Zelnik, M., and Kantner, J. F. (1980) Sexual activity, contraceptive use and pregnancy among metropolitan-area teenagers: 1971–1979. *Family Planning Perspectives* 12:230–237.

Zelnik, M., and Kantner, J. F. (1985) 1979 U.S. National Survey of Young Women and Young Men (machine-readable files and documentation): Data Set Nos. 44 and 45. Data Archive on Adolescent Pregnancy and Pregnancy Prevention, Sociometrics Corporation, Palo Alto, Calif.

Zelnik, M., and Shah, F. K. (1983) First intercourse among young Americans. *Family Planning Perspectives* 15:64–70.

3

AIDS and IV Drug Use

Intravenous (IV) drug users occupy a unique position in the transmission chain of HIV: they pose risks not only for each other but also for their sexual partners and offspring. Although it is not possible at present to predict with certainty the future pattern of heterosexual transmission of HIV in the United States, one aspect of that pattern is gaining sharper focus: it is likely that if heterosexual transmission of the virus becomes self-sustaining, IV drug users will have been the initial source of infection for continued sexual transmission to heterosexuals who do not inject drugs (Newmeyer, 1986; Des Jarlais, 1987a; Des Jarlais et al., 1987).

The threat posed by IV drug use has focused attention on the extent of existing HIV infection among IV drug users; on the current state of knowledge concerning the drug-use and sexual behaviors of this population, including childbearing; and on the number of individuals at risk of acquiring infection through behaviors associated directly or indirectly with IV drug use. Unfortunately, information is scanty in many relevant areas. In the United States and Europe, the majority of the cases of heterosexually transmitted AIDS has occurred in IV drug users' sexual partners, who themselves may not be using drugs (Harris et al., 1983; Des Jarlais et al., 1985; Friedman et al., 1986; Newmeyer, 1986). The majority of cases of AIDS among children has occurred as a result of perinatal transmission from HIV-infected mothers who acquired the infection through drug use (Newmeyer, 1986; Ginzburg et al., 1987; Macks, 1988).

In this chapter the committee reviews what is known about the behaviors associated with HIV transmission among people who inject illicit drugs; these include needle-sharing, sexual behavior, and child-bearing. To highlight data gaps and the research needed to fill them, the chapter also examines the current state of research methodology and the quality of existing data on risk-associated behaviors and on the size of the IV drug-using population.

The AIDS epidemic and the role of IV drug use in the transmission of HIV have also focused the nation's attention on the prevention of drug use and the efficacy of drug treatment programs. These issues are of great concern to the Academy complex[1] and to the nation; yet it is not possible to review the extensive literatures of these topics here. The committee believes that primary prevention of drug use is an important national goal, but questions remain as to whether even substantial improvement in primary prevention would reduce *injection* behavior. Because many people report smoking marijuana and relatively few go on to inject heroin or other injectable drugs, the efficiency of attempts to stop marijuana use as a way to prevent IV drug use is questionable. Nevertheless, primary prevention of *IV drug use* is critical in the light of HIV infection; such prevention requires a better understanding of the complex behaviors and conditions that surround the injection of illicit drugs.

Illicit drug use has been a long-standing social problem in this country, and public policies to deal with it have resulted in drug treatment and law enforcement programs. Yet many of the policies established in the past are inadequate for the problems presented by the AIDS epidemic today. For example, much of what is known about IV drug use comes from studies that used samples recruited from heroin treatment programs; little is known about individuals who inject cocaine or amphetamines, about the more prevalent patterns of multiple and concurrent drug use, or about those who have never sought treatment.

To make rational decisions about the kinds and amounts of resources to be directed toward drug-use problems, the government needs quantitative information on the size of those problems. As of November 14, 1988, 20,752 cases of AIDS had been diagnosed in individuals who reported IV drug use (CDC, 1988). Although the number of HIV-infected IV drug users is not known, seroprevalence data from local convenience samples show rapid growth in infection rates once the virus is introduced into an IV drug-using community

---

[1]The Academy complex comprises the National Academy of Sciences, the National Academy of Engineering, and the Institute of Medicine. Studies of the efficacy of drug treatment and the capability of existing programs to prevent primary drug use are currently under consideration at the Institute of Medicine.

(Angarano et al., 1985; D. M. Novick et al., 1986; Robertson et al., 1986; Moss, 1987; L. F. Novick et al., 1988). However, estimates of the total number of individuals at risk of HIV infection from injecting illicit drugs are subject to considerable error; this problem is treated in detail in the last section of this chapter.

The quality of existing data is not adequate to answer the difficult questions AIDS poses because the current data collection system is only designed to measure crude trends. In the past, law enforcement and other governmental agencies have been more concerned about trends in the number of drug users than about absolute levels. For these agencies, increases in the numbers justified calling for more public resources; decreases allowed policy makers to direct resources elsewhere. Unfortunately, resources to meet drug program needs have been persistently scarce. Treatment programs have been so desperately starved for resources that they could not meet the demand for their services. The total number of drug users was a moot issue in many cities; whatever that number was, it exceeded the number who could be served.

Controlling the spread of the AIDS epidemic demands more knowledge about the size of the IV drug-using population and the dynamics of viral transmission in this group. Efforts to control the spread of other viral infections have not produced information on the dynamics of infection that would be helpful in preventing the spread of HIV. The transmission of other blood-borne viral infections among IV drug users, most notably, hepatitis B virus, occurred rapidly and pervasively (Kreek et al., 1987); in some communities, in fact, the hepatitis B virus saturated the IV drug-using population before transmission studies could be initiated (Louria et al., 1967; Hessol et al., 1987; Lettau et al., 1987). Data are still needed on the distribution and variation of behaviors that transmit HIV, the number of IV drug users, and the proportion of users infected with the virus. Such data are critical to planning for future health care needs, targeting prevention programs, counseling the infected, and protecting the uninfected.

Yet despite the gaps in the current state of knowledge about IV drug use, enough is now known to slow the spread of infection in this population. As discussed later in this chapter, increasing the capacity to treat IV drug use, expanding innovative programs to provide for safer injection, and creating a system to monitor the efficacy of AIDS prevention efforts should be undertaken now. The severity of the AIDS epidemic does not permit a "business-as-usual" approach to the problems associated with IV drug use. These problems call for innovative solutions that take into account the relevant risk-associated behaviors and the complex social networks in which they occur.

Because the material included in this chapter is presented in some detail, the committee highlights below some major points about IV drug use and HIV infection:

- The IV drug-using population is heterogeneous with respect to drug use, life-style, and risk-associated behaviors.
- Although the lay press has expressed some skepticism about IV drug users' capacity and motivation for behavioral change, existing data indicate that, indeed, much change has already occurred in some groups.
- Targeting prevention programs to specific at-risk populations will increase the probability of successfully halting the spread of infection while conserving scarce resources.
- A clearer understanding of the dynamics of viral transmission and the prevalence of HIV infection and risk-associated behaviors is needed.
- HIV seroprevalence data show tremendous geographical variation. Therefore, considerable opportunities remain to halt the spread of HIV infection in many parts of the country and even in uninfected groups that reside in areas with high rates of infection.

The committee has divided its discussion of these issues into four major sections: (1) drug-use behaviors that transmit HIV, (2) risk reduction among IV drug users, (3) conducting research on IV drug use, and (4) measuring the scope of the problem.

DRUG-USE BEHAVIORS THAT TRANSMIT HIV

Two types of behavior are important in examining the problem of AIDS among IV drug users: (1) sharing contaminated injection equipment and (2) sexual behaviors that are known to transmit HIV.

Sharing Drug Injection Equipment

The use of nonsterile injection equipment may account for a range of infections in IV drug users, including bacterial endocarditis, hepatitis, malaria, and cellulitis or soft tissue infections (Louria et al., 1967). As the number of people with whom injection equipment is shared increases, so does the risk of HIV infection (Chaisson et al., 1987b). As with other blood-borne infections to which IV drug users are prone, HIV spreads from the infected to the uninfected user primarily by the sharing of blood-contaminated injection equipment, which serves as the vector of the virus.

IV drug users share injection equipment for a variety of reasons: pragmatically, clean "works" (the collective term for injection paraphernalia) are scarce; legally, the possession of injection equipment is a criminal offense in many states; socially, sharing represents a form of social bonding among IV drug users (Friedman et al., 1986). Before describing the injection behaviors associated with transmission, we discuss the setting in which drug use occurs.

Social Context of Needle-Sharing

Sharing injection equipment is common among IV drug users (Black et al., 1986; Brown et al., 1987). Indeed, some studies have shown that essentially all IV drug users report needle-sharing during some period of their drug-use careers (Black et al., 1986). People are not born injectors; they learn this behavior in the presence of others who have already been initiated (Powell, 1973; Harding and Zinberg, 1977). As discussed below, a lack of equipment and injection skills, together with certain social and physiological factors that surround IV drug use, affect the likelihood of needle-sharing.

Initiation into Drug Use. Much like the first sexual experience, the first injection experience may be anticipated or expected but not planned for (Des Jarlais et al., 1986c). Curiosity about IV drug use, whether sudden or long-standing, and association with people who inject drugs often lead to a moment when the uninitiated is present while drugs are being injected. The desire to join in can result in sharing both drugs and injection equipment. Few people have hypodermic injection equipment "around the house," and few are inclined to pierce their own skin with a needle. Therefore, newcomers to the IV drug-use world are likely to arrive without the proper equipment and to require help in executing the first injection. These circumstances make it highly probable that a novice will begin injecting in the presence of others and will share the equipment of those teaching the "art" of injection. The sharing of drugs and equipment that occurs during initial and subsequent drug-use episodes leads to the notion that communal or joint use is as natural as sharing alcohol, ice, and glasses at a cocktail party.

Contrary to popular myth, the first injection of heroin does not necessarily lead to addiction, and not all heroin users are addicts (Powell, 1973; Robins et al., 1975; Gerstein, 1976). Some individuals experiment with it for a period of time and then quit; others are intermittent users, injecting only on weekends (so-called "weekend warriors") or on isolated occasions ("chippies") (Zinberg et al., 1977). Indeed, initial IV drug-use experiences are not necessarily pleasurable. Heroin use involves a combination of pleasure and discomfort. Continued use over time involves both an acquired sense of pleasure and a differential tolerance for heroin's various effects.

Popular lore about heroin users holds that, once they are "hooked," their appetite for the drug is so great that they will run any risk to obtain it. In contrast, research has shown that users adjust their consumption to such external factors as price and availability (Waldorf, 1970; Hanson et al., 1985). This ability to adapt to various social and market forces also sustains the belief among many users that they are not addicts but merely visitors to the heroin scene who are still in control of their lives (Fields and Walters, 1985).

Adolescent IV Drug Use. To understand more clearly the process of initiation into heroin use,[2] it is helpful to consider the factors that are associated with adolescent drug use. Although studies of drug use among adolescents have not focused on IV use specifically, there are some data indicating that IV drug use among teens is rare. In 1982, adolescents made up only 12 percent of those entering treatment programs, most of which focus on heroin addiction; opiate use accounted for less than 2 percent of adolescents seeking admission to treatment (Polich et al., 1984). Nevertheless, more information is needed on how this behavior is distributed within the adolescent population.

Early initiation into drug use and higher levels of use have been associated with problems in the family environment, including structural factors (e.g., separation, divorce, and single-parent households) and functional factors (e.g., poor communication and the absence of harmony and warmth in the home) (Anhalt and Klein, 1976; Brook et al., 1982; Evans and Raines, 1982; Rachal et al., 1986; Zarek et al., 1987). In most studies, however, the influence of peers, especially older siblings and early sexual partners, was found to be even more powerful than family influences in predicting adolescent drug use, although the effects of each kind of influence were nevertheless

[2] There has been much less research on initiation into the injection of other illicit drugs (e.g., cocaine or amphetamines) than on initiation into heroin use.

significant and independent (Kandel et al., 1978; Brook et al., 1982, 1986). The impact of peers was also found to be related to the type of drug used and was more closely tied to behavior than to attitudes (Huba and Bentler, 1980; Krosnick and Judd, 1982; Kandel et al., 1986; R. E. Johnson et al., 1987). An ethnographic study (Lourie, 1986, 1988) of male and female working-class adolescents in Lowell, Massachusetts, reported that drugs, sex, and violence were sources of physical stimulation and escape for those teenagers, and became central themes of the peer group-associated life-style. The respondents in this study perceived society as offering them no access to legitimate work and pleasure.

Friendship Networks and Intimate Relationships. Once initiated, the IV drug user may continue to inject with those who provided an entree into the drug scene. Needle-sharing is reportedly an integral part of injection and can provide a social bond within the group (Des Jarlais, 1988). Over time, the ties that bind group members may loosen, and individuals may move on to inject with other groups or with another individual in the context of a personal relationship (that may also involve sex); other injection patterns include drug use in more anonymous situations (e.g., "shooting galleries," the communal injection sites often found in large cities) or alone. Pragmatic issues foster injection groups: individuals can pool scarce resources, such as money, drugs, and injection equipment, and the group provides some protection against the violence associated with illicit drug use and the threat of discovery by law enforcement officials. Prior to AIDS, sharing was reported to provide "a sense of successful cooperation within a hostile environment" (Des Jarlais, 1988).

The proportion of IV drug users who have an intimate sexual relationship with another drug user is not known. However, Des Jarlais and colleagues (1986c) suggest that male and female "running buddies" are likely to share injection equipment and have sexual relations. Sharing injection equipment among friends and injecting each other appear to have strong sexual connotations. Male "running buddies" may share needles and the same women in serial sexual relationships.

Shooting Galleries. Once they have been initiated, regular users have to secure both drugs and injection equipment. Because of legal sanctions against the possession of either, many users may be inclined to "shoot up" shortly after a drug purchase. Those who are addicted and suffering drug hunger or withdrawal symptoms may also want to inject promptly. Even if they are not addicted, some users, out of a classical type of conditioning, will feel the urge to inject the drug immediately after purchasing it (Wikler, 1973; Des Jarlais et al., 1985). All of these conditions can increase the likelihood of injection with used equipment.

In large cities, "shooting galleries" have flourished as communal injection sites, often in apartments or abandoned buildings. The operators of the shooting galleries charge a small fee for use of the site, injection water, and rental of injection equipment. Often, the equipment has been used by other addicts and inadequately sterilized or cleaned to remove contaminating blood and infectious pathogens, including HIV (Des Jarlais et al., 1986a).

In cities with relatively few IV drug users, the equivalent of a shooting gallery may be the dealer's apartment, a rented room, or a hotel room in which the dealer makes "house works" available to inject drugs at the time of purchase. The house works are borrowed, used to inject the drugs, and returned to the dealer for the next user—again, often without adequate cleaning or sterilization. Renting or borrowing works reduces the risk of arrest for possession of drug-related paraphernalia. The use of injection equipment provided in shooting galleries and of house works provided by drug dealers results in syringe- and needle-sharing that involve unknown numbers of addicts. The blood exchanged in these situations is likely to cut across existing friendship groups.

Mechanics of Drug Use and Sources of Contamination

Although "needle-sharing" is a convenient shorthand for the practice under discussion, there are at least five elements of the IV drug user's paraphernalia that carry the potential for contamination: the syringe, needle, "cooker," cotton, and rinse water. Collectively, these are known as the "works" (Newmeyer, 1988).

The Syringe. One possible mode of contamination is through infected blood that remains in the syringe between uses. This condition frequently occurs when users "boot," that is, when they draw blood back and forth into a syringe multiple times while it is inserted into a vein to ensure that all traces of the drug are removed from the syringe. (Booting does not occur when users practice intramuscular or subcutaneous injection, also referred to as "skin popping.")

Decontamination—by bleach, alcohol, liquid dish detergent, or hydrogen peroxide—is more likely to be effective if the syringe is flushed to at least the highest level reached by the infected user's injection. Bleach, alcohol, and hydrogen peroxide have been shown to inactivate the virus in vitro (Resnick et al., 1986; Flynn et al., 1988b). However, the sterilization of injection equipment is not without problems, as some disinfectants may dissolve the silicone lubricant of the syringe plunger, thus making its operation quite stiff.

The Needle. Contamination can also occur when a droplet of infected blood remains inside or outside the needle. Decontamination is likely to be effective if the disinfectant is flushed through the needle and the needle is dipped into the disinfectant.

The Cooker. A cooker is the small container (e.g., a spoon, a bottle cap) that is used to dissolve the injectable drug, which is usually a powder. Infected blood can be pushed out of the needle or syringe and into the cooker in the process of drawing up a new shot of the drug. Effective sterilization of the needle and syringe would obviate the possibility of contaminating the cooker. Heating the cooker between shots could also kill the virus, but this is not the usual procedure among heroin users; even if the cooker is heated, the temperature may not be high enough to sterilize it and its contents. There is some anecdotal evidence that, in the post-AIDS era, passing the cooker over the flame a few more times may now be more common. (However, amphetamine users generally dissolve their drug in cold water, often simply using the small bag that originally contained the drug and saving this "washbag" for an extra shot.)

The Cotton. A small piece of cotton is sometimes used to strain out undissolved impurities from the solution in the cooker as it is drawn up into the syringe. Instead of disposing of the cotton after each use, an IV drug user will often "beat the cotton" with a small amount of water to extract one more bit of the drug. The cotton thus can become contaminated with the blood of infected users. If the needle and syringe have been sterilized, however, the cotton is less likely to be a source of infection.

The Rinse Water. Water is used to rinse out syringes and needles before they are reused—not necessarily to decontaminate the equipment but to prevent clotting and therefore unusable works. If there is no effective decontamination step (e.g., multiple rinses with a bleach solution), the use or reuse of a common rinse water supply can be a source of contamination.

The details of injection practices related to sharing, booting, rinsing, and heating the cooker vary greatly; in addition, these behaviors are constantly evolving in light of the awareness of the risk of HIV transmission. It is difficult to assess the impact of these behavioral changes on stemming the spread of HIV. An interesting variation in injection behavior described recently in Baltimore (J. Newmeyer, Haight-Ashbury Free Medical Clinic, San Francisco, personal communication, May 25, 1988) enables users to share drugs without sharing the needle or syringe. To ensure that a drug is split equally between users, half of the contents of a single syringe is injected into a second syringe. In fact, there might still be an HIV transmission risk if either syringe were contaminated before the drug-sharing procedure, but the likelihood of contamination is much less because the drug—rather than the needle—is shared.

Frequency of Injection

Another factor associated with HIV infection is the frequency of injection: those who inject drugs frequently are more likely to be seropositive than those who inject less often (Blattner et al., 1985; Des Jarlais, 1987b). Some IV drug users are hard-core addicts who inject drugs many times every day; some are otherwise successful middle-class users who inject less frequently. Still other IV drug users inject many times a day for a few months and then stop; some others inject only a few times a year.[3]

The sharing of injection equipment appears to be common behavior in both IV drug users who inject frequently and in those who inject less often (Friedland et al., 1985). However, more frequent injections are likely to mean more episodes with shared equipment, thus increasing the likelihood of HIV infection. In addition, for IV drug users who are addicted, the symptoms of drug withdrawal can heighten the sense of urgency or desire for the drug and decrease the likelihood that safer injection practices will be used. Finally, whether an IV drug user did most of his or her injecting prior to 1975 or later will greatly affect his or her risk of HIV infection. Other important

[3]Data from the Client-Oriented Data Acquisition Process (CODAP; see also footnote 8 in this chapter) indicate a wide range of variability in the frequency of drug use prior to admission to drug treatment (NIDA, 1981). The range is from no use in the past month to three or more times daily in the past month. Gerstein (1976) also distinguishes between different types of IV drug users, ranging from the hard-core "strung-out" users who inject frequently to situational users who inject only occasionally.

variables in determining the risk of HIV infection include the prevalence of infection in the local population, the number of people who practice needle-sharing, the number and frequency of injections, and the injection route (intravenous, intramuscular, or subcutaneous).

Polydrug Use

One consistent finding with significant implications for treatment and prevention efforts is that of multiple drug use among those who inject drugs. Studies of treatment populations (B. D. Johnson et al., 1985; Ball et al., 1986) suggest that a majority (60–90 percent) of IV heroin users report regular use of at least one other nonopiate. (A survey of approximately 100 former heroin users enrolled in methadone maintenance clinics in the New York City area found that 91 percent also reported IV cocaine use [Brown and Primm, 1988].) The choice of drugs for injection varies among different drug subcultures and over time. Heroin was the dominant injected drug a few years ago, but today, IV drug users may also inject cocaine, heroin and cocaine in combination, or a variety of other drugs, including amphetamines (Black et al., 1986).

Cocaine has been linked to HIV infection in New York City and San Francisco (Chaisson et al., 1988; Friedman et al., 1988). Among 673 IV drug users surveyed in San Francisco, IV cocaine use significantly increased the risk of HIV infection (Chaisson et al., 1988). Unfortunately, to date, some forms of drug treatment, including methadone, have not been effective for cocaine dependency. Indeed, Chaisson and colleagues (1988) found that 26 percent of cocaine users who were already in long-term methadone treatment began injecting cocaine *after* they entered treatment. Injection practices also appear to vary for different drugs. With cocaine's shorter-lived "high," IV drug users who shoot cocaine may inject themselves repeatedly until their supply is exhausted—thus injecting themselves more frequently than if they were using heroin alone.[4]

Cocaine is associated with HIV infection in several ways. When cocaine is injected with nonsterile injection equipment, it poses the risk of blood-borne HIV infection. When it is smoked (as "crack"), it can be associated with high-risk sexual activity because crack frequently heightens perceptions of sexual arousal (Friedman et al., 1988). Like heroin, it can be used at or near the site of purchase

[4]Gold and coworkers (1986) report that cocaine's desired subjective effects are so rapid and short-lived that administration must be repeated every 20–30 minutes to maintain the high. Siegel (1984) describes individuals who use cocaine 3–20 times per day.

in so-called "crack houses." Unlike heroin, however, crack is cheap and relatively easy to use, and any evidence of its possession is easily obliterated—factors that have probably contributed to its popularity (Inciardi, 1987). The use of crack can result in increased risk of HIV infection owing to decreased sexual inhibitions and an increased desire for drugs. Outreach workers in Harlem report finding women and girls (some only in their early teens) who are engaging in unprotected intercourse in exchange for either money or crack (Friedman et al., 1988). Moreover, ethnographic data reported by Friedman and colleagues (1988) indicate that crack use among women can lead to prostitution, which in turn can lead to heroin use, thus amplifying among these women the risk of acquiring and spreading HIV infection.

Sexual Behaviors and IV Drug Use

As of November 14, 1988, CDC (1988) reported 3,359 cases of AIDS that were attributed to heterosexual transmission. Of the total cases, 2,154 (64 percent) were people who reported heterosexual contact with a person with AIDS or a person at risk of AIDS. The other 1,205 (36 percent) were people who reported no other risk-associated behavior but were born in countries in which heterosexual transmission has played a key role in the spread of the virus. The vast majority of the cases that have been diagnosed among those born in this country is thought to be associated directly with IV drug use or with sexual contact with an IV drug user (Brown, 1988).[5] Yet less is known about the dynamics of heterosexual HIV transmission from IV drug users than about transmission from index cases in hemophiliac, transfusion recipient, or bisexual male populations. The general efficiency of heterosexual HIV transmission is not known, but it seems likely that the prospects for understanding this dimension of the epidemic would be improved if attention were directed toward the most frequent occurrence of the phenomenon: sexual transmission related to the IV drug-using population.

In the past, drug-use behaviors in the IV drug-using population received more attention than sexual behaviors; now, however, sexual

[5]Substance use may be associated with sexually acquired AIDS aside from any direct role played by IV injection equipment as a vector for HIV. The use of mood-altering drugs may have a disinhibiting effect, whether for pharmacological or cultural reasons (Reinarman and Leigh, 1987), and may result in unsafe sex practices that otherwise might not have occurred. Recent studies point to strong noncompliance with safer sex techniques when alcohol and other drugs have been used (Stall et al., 1986; Faltz and Madover, 1987; Flavin and Frances, 1987).

behaviors have become the focus of recent studies, which are providing some insight into the range of behaviors that occurs. Surveys of IV drug users who had recently entered methadone treatment programs (in New York City; northern New Jersey; San Antonio, Texas; and Los Angeles, California) found that more AIDS prevention measures were being taken with respect to drug use than with respect to sexual activity: only 14 percent of the respondents in these studies reported that they had begun or increased condom use (Battjes and Pickens, 1988). In another study (Primm et al., 1988), more than half (60 percent) of the IV drug users' sexual partners did not inject drugs; however, male respondents were more likely than female respondents to report a noninjecting sex partner. Only 5 percent of the study participants reported condom use; among this 5 percent, condoms were used in only 35 percent of all sexual encounters.

Sexual behavior and drug use are topics that are often investigated separately by researchers whose careers have focused on one or the other activity. Yet sex and drug use are apt to be inextricably linked, and the nexus between these two most private activities is a critical area for AIDS research. In certain contexts, sexual behavior cannot be separated from drug use. For example, among female IV drug users who are the sexual partners of male IV drug users, sex is often used to obtain drugs or is an aspect of a relationship based on drug use. A social structure that supports male dominance may make it difficult for women to propose behavioral changes (to say "no" to sex, to use condoms, or to refrain from certain types of sex). Women who are financially dependent on men or who exchange sex for money or other necessities of life may face the dilemma of choosing between economic survival and unsafe sex (Worth, 1988).

Data from samples recruited through drug treatment programs, such as the Treatment Outcome Prospective Study or TOPS (see foonote 19 in this chapter), find that the bulk of the active drug-using population consists of young men (Ginzburg, 1984). Indeed, men constitute 74 percent of treatment admissions for heroin use. Women constitute a proportionately smaller group, although over the last decade the problem of drug addiction among women "is one of large and growing proportions" (Cuskey and Wathey, 1982). Nevertheless, women are often omitted or seen as peripheral in ethnographic accounts of the heroin world, and studies of female IV drug users are rare (Rosenbaum, 1979a). The links among IV drug use, heterosexual transmission, and perinatal infection may bring further attention to women who are at risk of AIDS through IV drug-related behavior. A review of the 1,819 women who were diagnosed as having

AIDS between 1981 and 1986 (Guinan and Hardy, 1987) found that the majority of these women reported IV drug use. The second most common AIDS risk factor for women is heterosexual contact with a person at risk for AIDS. Indeed, Wofsy (1987) has estimated that as many as 20,000 women whose sexual partners are IV drug users may be infected with HIV.

According to Des Jarlais and colleagues (1984), as many as 80 percent of male IV drug users are in a primary relationship with women who do not themselves use drugs; female IV drug users, on the other hand, are apt to be partnered with male drug users. Thus, women are at risk of HIV infection that is both directly and indirectly associated with IV drug use. While some information on female IV drug use is available from women entering drug treatment, little is known about women who are involved in intimate relationships with male IV drug users.

Ethnographic studies of female IV drug users at the Stuyvesant Polyclinic and the Montefiore Medical Center in New York City (Wofsy, 1987; Worth, 1988) have found that proposals to change sexual practices (including the use of condoms) require redressing the balance of power within intimate relationships. For these women, asking a man to use a condom provokes the fear of breaching relations that may fulfill the woman's sexual, personal, financial, and drug needs.

As discussed in Chapter 2, prostitutes are at risk of acquiring HIV infection through both sexual and drug-use behaviors. A 1987 survey of street prostitutes in the New York City area indicated that approximately one half had injected drugs at least once and one third had injected drugs at some time during the previous two years (Des Jarlais et al., 1987). The prevalence of unprotected intercourse among prostitutes varies with the context of the sexual encounter; safer sex is practiced by female prostitutes in professional relationships more often than in personal ones (Cohen, 1987; Darrow et al., 1988). The prostitute population is worthy of further attention, as male and female prostitutes are at risk of being infected by and of spreading infection to their sexual partners, both professional and personal, as well as to their offspring.

Because of the link between IV drug use and perinatal transmission of HIV, information is needed about contraceptive and childbearing behaviors in the IV drug-using population. Unfortunately, currently available data permit only a rudimentary picture of these behaviors. Despite heroin's capacity to suppress fertility to a certain extent in women, Cuskey and Wathey (1982) found that, in New

York City, birth rates for addicted women were higher than those for nonaddicted women. Others (Densen-Gerber et al., 1972; E. M. Johnson, 1987) have reported an association between drug use and promiscuity and prostitution. Women who use intravenous drugs may also be poor users of contraception. In a study that matched women on age, ethnicity, and marital status, Ralph and Spigner (1986) noted that contraception was less frequent among female addicts than among nonaddicted women. The importance of these data becomes apparent in view of the fact that perinatal HIV transmission can occur if the mother is infected. With the majority of women with AIDS in their childbearing years (CDC, 1987a), offspring of IV drug users may constitute a growing proportion of future cases of HIV infection.

Toward a Better Understanding of Risk-Associated Behaviors

Intravenous drug use comprises a complex set of behaviors that are enacted in diverse social situations. Drug use is a social problem that is rooted in a network of other problems; most students of drug use believe that only complex, far-reaching solutions that take into account all aspects of that network will ultimately be effective. Such solutions require the attention of a range of agencies—law enforcement, social service, health, housing, and education. Programs that address the individual in the context of peers, family, and community and those that focus on the multiple factors that influence drug use hold the most promise. Solutions to the problems of drug use will also require the attention of a range of disciplines. Many questions that will arise can best be answered by the social and behavioral sciences; others will require the expertise of pharmacology, toxicology, and other biomedical sciences. In addition, knowledge is needed on how addiction occurs and on the biological factors that influence drug use, addiction, cessation, and relapse. Finally, mechanisms to improve collaboration and coordination among those seeking solutions will be required for effective action. **The committee thus recommends that high priority be given to studies of the social and societal contexts of IV drug use and IV drug-use prevention efforts.**

The dynamics of IV drug use—injection behaviors, drugs of choice, and sexual and contraceptive behaviors—vary over time for each drug user. They also vary across cultures and geographic locations, as well as by age, race, gender, and ethnicity. These variations have important implications for the spread of HIV that cannot be captured by or understood through cross-sectional studies that provide only a "snapshot" view of evolutionary and variable behaviors. It will be necessary to make a long-term commitment to a diversified behavioral research portfolio on IV drug use with sufficient support to sustain these efforts. Multiple, prospective longitudinal studies are needed to keep abreast of problems and changes as they occur.

Studies that seek to understand sensitive, private behaviors pose formidable but not insurmountable challenges. That it is worthwhile to devote the necessary resources to meet these challenges is indisputable: the public health benefits to be gained, particularly for ethnic and racial minority populations, are great. As discussed in the final section of this chapter, research has consistently shown that racial and ethnic minorities bear a disproportionately large burden of morbidity and mortality associated with HIV infection.

Information is urgently needed about IV drug-use patterns and how injection behaviors vary by age, race, sex, ethnicity, sexual orientation, and other demographically significant variables. (For example, women and men report quite different reasons for initiating drug use, and they also report different patterns of use [Burt et al., 1979; Rosenbaum, 1981; E. M. Johnson, 1987].) Knowledge is also needed about how people enter and exit the IV drug-using population, the conditions under which individuals progress from sniffing or smoking injectable drugs to shooting them, how needle-sharing behaviors are initiated and sustained, and how to intervene effectively in these dangerous practices. **The committee recommends that high priority be given to research on the natural history of IV drug use, with an emphasis on prospective longitudinal studies of the factors associated with initiation into and cessation of IV drug use.**

As stated earlier, IV drug-use behaviors convey the risk of HIV infection to sexual partners and offspring. Unfortunately, how sexual and contraceptive behaviors vary and are distributed within the heterogeneous IV drug-using population are incompletely understood. Although projected estimates of future HIV infection rates are subject to considerable variation, it is likely that a significant proportion of heterosexually and perinatally acquired infection will come from the IV drug-using population. Therefore, **the committee recommends that high priority be given to studies of the sexual and procreative behavior of IV drug users, including methods to reduce sexual and perinatal (mother–infant) transmission of HIV.**

Implementing the recommendations offered in the preceding paragraphs will provide the information necessary to understand some of the drug-use behaviors that transmit HIV. Yet understanding is only the first step in controlling the spread of disease. Collecting data on dynamic, risk-associated behaviors requires a long-term commitment; thus, research should proceed as efforts are being made to facilitate HIV risk reduction among IV drug users.

RISK REDUCTION AMONG IV DRUG USERS

Although the area of research on risk reduction to prevent HIV transmission among IV drug users is only a few years old, there is already a rapidly accumulating body of knowledge that contradicts the common assumption that IV drug users are incapable of changing their behavior. This section traces the history of those studies, summarizes the current state of knowledge, and indicates directions for future research.

Changes in Injection Behavior

The first risk reduction studies among IV drug users were conducted in New York City, where signs of infection were noted early in the epidemic and where the greatest number of AIDS cases has occurred. Ethnographic interviews conducted in New York in the fall of 1983 among IV drug users who were not in treatment indicated that these drug users were aware of AIDS. Data from this study also indicated that many people knew the virus was transmitted through shared injection equipment, and many recognized the potential benefit of behavioral change in this practice (Des Jarlais et al., 1986b). This awareness of AIDS and knowledge of the routes of transmission developed prior to any AIDS prevention programs for IV drug users in New York. It reportedly arose from information transmitted through the mass media and through the informal communication networks among IV drug users in the city.

Formal interviews of methadone patients from the New York City area were conducted in the fall of 1984 (Friedman et al., 1987b). In a similar study, individuals in methadone treatment and prison detoxification programs were interviewed in 1985 and 1986 (Selwyn et al., 1987). In all of the samples, the majority of respondents reported some form of AIDS risk reduction. The most commonly reported means taken to avoid HIV infection were the increased use of illicit sterile injection equipment, reduction in the number of persons with whom the respondent was willing to share equipment, and reduction or cessation of IV drug use.

In the spring of 1985, field studies of persons selling drug injection equipment in New York showed that there had been a large-scale expansion of the illicit market for sterile injection equipment, and at least part of the expansion was attributed to concerns about AIDS (Des Jarlais et al., 1985). The demand for sterile injection equipment was so great, in fact, that counterfeit sterile needles and syringes were being sold: needles and syringes that had been used were rinsed out and replaced in their original packages, which were then resealed and sold as unused.

The state of New Jersey began an ex-addict outreach program in the fall of 1985 (Jackson and Neshin, 1986; Jackson and Rotkiewicz, 1987). The program trained ex-addicts as AIDS educators, who then went into the IV drug-using community and taught current IV drug users about AIDS: how it is transmitted and how to decontaminate used injection equipment by boiling the equipment in water or soaking it in bleach or alcohol. Many IV drug users reported that they found instruction in sterilizing injection equipment to be useful. However, somewhat to the surprise of the designers of the program, a common response of those users reached by the ex-addicts was a desire to reduce the risk of AIDS by entering drug treatment and reducing or eliminating drug injection behavior. The state responded by establishing a program in which the ex-addict outreach workers distributed vouchers that could be redeemed for a period of free detoxification treatment. (Normally, this treatment would have cost the IV drug user $50–$75.) More than 85 percent of the vouchers were redeemed by IV drug users for detoxification treatment.

In 1987 reports were published on the increasing use of the syringe exchange program in Amsterdam (van den Hoek et al., 1987; Buning et al., in press) and the bleach distribution program in San Francisco (Chaisson et al., 1987a; Watters, 1987a). The Amsterdam program had actually been established prior to concerns about AIDS, but it was greatly expanded when AIDS cases were diagnosed in the city. Contrary to popular belief, the expansion of the program—from the distribution of 25,000 sterile needles and syringes in 1984 to 700,000 sterile needles and syringes distributed in 1987—did not lead to an increase in the number of IV drug users in the city or to a decrease in the number of IV drug users entering drug treatment (Buning et al., 1988, in press). In another study conducted in Amsterdam (van den Hoek et al., 1987), increased use of the needle exchange program occurred simultaneously with reductions in the reported frequency of drug injection among the respondents.

The bleach distribution program in San Francisco involved community health outreach workers who distributed small bottles of full-strength household bleach. The instructions on the bottle stated that needles and syringes should be rinsed twice with the bleach and then twice with clean water. This procedure could be carried out very quickly (as compared with the previously recommended 10- to 15-minute procedure of soaking a needle and syringe in a 10 percent bleach solution). A large number of IV drug users in San Francisco—one half of the subjects in one study (Chaisson et al., 1987a) and two thirds of the respondents in another (Watters, 1987a)—rapidly adopted use of the small bottles of bleach. A large-scale program of antibody testing and counseling was also being conducted at the same time as the bleach distribution campaign. Either one or both of the programs together may have caused behavioral change or at least sensitized IV drug users to the need for such change (Moss and Chaisson, 1988).

Other studies reported in 1987 indicate some limitations on the AIDS prevention efforts aimed at IV drug users. An evaluation of an ex-addict outreach program in Baltimore showed that IV drug users in the city were changing their behavior to reduce the risk of AIDS; however, the change could not be attributed to the efforts of the outreach workers (McAuliffe et al., 1987). A study in Sacramento, California, found that knowledge of AIDS by itself did little to change the risk behavior of IV drug users in that city; most continued to engage in high-risk behavior, even though they were aware of how AIDS is transmitted and believed that they would become exposed if they continued the behavior (Flynn et al., 1987). In this sample, information and even perceived self-susceptibility were insufficient to alter behavior.

A number of studies of AIDS risk reduction have been reported in 1988. Table 3-1 notes these efforts, as well as other recent AIDS risk reduction research. The topics of these studies include risk reduction associated with entry into methadone maintenance treatment (Abdul-Quader et al., 1987; Ball et al., 1988; Blix and Gronbladh, 1988; Hartel et al., 1988; Yancovitz et al., 1988), syringe exchange programs (Alldritt et al., 1988; Buning et al., 1988, in press; Hart et al., 1988; Ljungberg et al., 1988; van den Hoek et al., 1988b), purchasing sterile injection equipment at pharmacies (Espinoza et al., 1988; Fuchs et al., 1988; Goldberg et al., 1988), information campaigns (Bortolotti et al., 1988; de la Loma et al., 1988), and counseling with antibody testing (Hemdal, 1986; Bottiger et al., 1988; Casadonte et al., 1988; Gibson et al., 1988; Moss et al., 1988a; Olin and Kall, 1988; van den Hoek et al., 1988a), as well as many studies in which the mechanism of change was not specified.

There are now enough studies of AIDS risk reduction among IV drug users to derive some generalizations that describe the current state of knowledge. First, it is quite clear that IV drug users will modify their behavior to reduce their risk of AIDS. Although the studies that support this conclusion tend to rely heavily on self-reported behavioral modifications, there are enough studies in which there is some independent evidence of change to conclude that the self-reports reflect what has actually occurred. Examples of the independent confirmation of change include the increased demand for sterile injection equipment in New York City, increased use of syringe exchange programs, and acceptance of bottles of bleach for decontamination of used injection equipment.

The second generalization that can be made is that there is wide variation in the percentage of drug users that reported AIDS risk reduction in the different studies. Percentages ranged from 85 percent in two studies in New York (Ball et al., 1988; Battjes and Pickens, 1988; Yancovitz et al., 1988) to what researchers termed "poor" in Madrid, Spain (de la Loma et al., 1988). Interpreting this variation is difficult for several reasons. The studies use different outcome measures that range from the increased use of sterile injection equipment to entrance into drug treatment to any self-reported change in behavior. Even when the "same" outcome measure is used in different studies, the wording of the study questionnaires may be sufficiently different as to make comparisons across studies quite difficult. Problems in interpreting the behavioral change data also arise from a lack of specification of the mechanism or "cause" of the behavioral change. Most of the studies that have been conducted did not identify causal factors; of those that did, different analytic frameworks were used to describe the mechanisms of change, which appeared to vary according to the local environment. For example, the potential effects of an AIDS education campaign in an area in which sterile injection equipment may be lawfully purchased in pharmacies cannot be compared easily with a similar campaign in an area in which legal access to and possession of sterile injection equipment are prohibited. Nevertheless, despite the problems in assessing the extent and causes of AIDS risk reduction in different geographical areas, it is still possible to conclude from the data that risk reduction has occurred,

TABLE 3-1 Recent Studies of AIDS Risk Reduction and the Prevention of HIV Transmission Among IV Drug Users

Location	Possible Mechanism of Behavioral Change	Study Report
New York City	Increased marketing of illicit syringes	Des Jarlais et al. (1985)
		Des Jarlais and Hopkins (1985)
	Media coverage, social support	Friedman et al. (1987b)
	Unspecified	Selwyn et al. (1987)
		Friedman and Des Jarlais (1988)
	Counseling/testing	Hemdal (1986)
		Casadonte et al. (1988)
	Methadone treatment	Abdul-Quader et al. (1987)
		Hartel et al. (1988)
		Yancovitz et al. (1988)
	Outreach/bleach distribution	Serrano and Goldsmith (1988)
New Jersey	Outreach/increased treatment	Jackson and Rotkiewicz (1987)
	Education programs	Jackson and Baxter (1988)
San Francisco	Counseling/testing	Gibson et al. (1988)
	Outreach/bleach distribution	Moss et al. (1988a)
		Chaisson et al. (1987a)
		Watters et al. (1988)

Sacramento, California	Bleach/other disinfectants	Flynn et al. (1988b)
Multiple sites—United States	Methadone treatment	Ball et al. (1988)
	Outreach/bleach distribution	Wiebel and Altman (1988)
	Unspecified	Battjes and Pickens (1988)
Amsterdam	Counseling/testing	van den Hoek et al. (1988a)
	Increased syringe exchange program	Buning et al. (1988)
		Buning et al. (in press)
		van den Hoek et al. (1988b)
London	Syringe exchange	Hart et al. (1988)
Multiple sites—United Kingdom	Syringe exchange	Alldritt et al. (1988)
Lund, Sweden	Syringe exchange	Ljungberg et al. (1988)
Edinburgh, Scotland	Unspecified	Robertson et al. (in press)
Glasgow	Legal sale of syringes	Goldberg et al. (1988)
Paris	Legal sale of syringes	Espinoza et al. (1988)
Madrid	Information campaign	de la Loma et al. (1988)
Innsbruck, Austria	Counseling/legal sale of syringes	Fuchs et al. (1988)
Padua, Italy	Information campaign	Bortolotti et al. (1988)
Multiple sites—Italy	Education, methadone	Rezza et al. (1988)
Uppsala, Sweden	Methadone treatment	Blix and Gronbladh (1988)
Stockholm	Counseling/testing	Bottiger et al. (1988)
		Olin and Kall (1988)

although it is highly variable. Unfortunately, researchers simply are not yet proficient at measuring and conceptualizing that variation.

The third generalization concerning risk reduction among IV drug users is an apparently counterintuitive and synergistic relationship between "safer" injection programs and drug treatment to reduce or eliminate injection behavior. The common assumption that providing the means for safer injection will encourage drug use and undermine drug treatment is contradicted by the data collected to date. The Amsterdam syringe exchange program has been collecting data longer than any other program; its results clearly show that syringe exchange has not encouraged drug use. As noted earlier, the program was begun in 1984, during which 25,000 sterile needles and syringes were distributed. The number distributed rose to 700,000 in 1987; it is estimated that 750,000 sterile needles and syringes will be distributed in 1988. During this expansion period, there was no decrease in the number of persons entering either methadone maintenance or drug-free treatment programs. Moreover, there appeared to be no increase in the number of heroin users in the city, which remained constant at approximately 7,000–8,000. Approximately 25–30 percent of these users (or 1,750–2,400) report current injection behavior (van den Hoek et al., 1988b). During this period, the average age of IV drug users in the city increased, indicating that the group is an aging cohort with little influx of new users.

Two studies from Amsterdam indicate that the syringe exchange program might actually be associated with reductions in IV drug use rather than increases. In a study conducted by van den Hoek and colleagues (1988b), the number of subjects who were injecting on a daily basis decreased during the time the syringe exchanges increased. Buning and colleagues (1986, 1988) compared IV drug users in Amsterdam who participated in the syringe exchange program with IV drug users who did not participate. These researchers found higher rates of needle-sharing and an increased frequency of injection (both of which are associated with HIV infection) among drug users who did not use the exchange program.

Although syringe exchange programs in other locations abroad are still in the preliminary stages of development, none so far has reported any increase in drug use among clients. Similarly, there have been no reports from these programs of increases in the number of IV drug users in the early phases of drug-use careers. It appears that the programs provide needed services to IV drug users and facilitate their entry into drug treatment without being coercive (Hart et al., 1988; Ljungberg et al., 1988). Maintaining a nonjudgmental attitude toward participants and providing a range of risk-reducing options from which the IV drug user can choose may be two of the factors that are critical to the success of syringe exchange programs (Alldritt et al., 1988).

In the United States, there has been a similar complementarity between programs that provide the means for safer injection and drug treatment programs. As noted earlier, the first ex-addict outreach program in New Jersey evolved from one that taught sterilization methods into one with expanded treatment capacity (Jackson and Rotkiewicz, 1987; Jackson and Baxter, 1988). The outreach programs in New York and San Francisco that distribute bleach have had to develop referral-to-treatment programs and street counseling components to keep up with the demand for these services (Des Jarlais, 1987b).

Because of the well-known difficulty of ending drug use without any relapse (see Chapter 4), many treatment programs have seen the promotion of safer injection practices as complementary to their efforts to reduce or eliminate drug injection. A number of methadone programs in Amsterdam are also sites for the syringe exchange program (Buning et al., 1986; Buning, 1987b). At least one treatment program in San Francisco is a site for bleach distribution, and several programs in New York are teaching IV drug users how to use bleach to disinfect injection equipment (D. C. Des Jarlais, New York State Division of Substance Abuse Services, personal communication, August 1988).

Although there are as yet no data from long-term studies, current data suggest that safer injection programs and drug treatment can be complementary means to reduce the risk of HIV transmission among IV drug users. However, more research is needed to understand the mechanisms that link safer injection programs with the actual reduction of risk-associated behavior. To successfully implement innovative programs in this country, researchers and program operators must also understand how, in the absence of supporting data, people maintain beliefs about what does and does not encourage drug use.

Changes in Sexual Behavior

Although there is evidence of large-scale changes in injection behavior among IV drug users from many different geographic areas, there is little encouraging news with respect to the sexual transmission of HIV in this population. Early studies show that relatively few IV

TABLE 3-2 Studies of Sexual Behavior Change in IV Drug Users

Location	Reference
New York City	Casadonte et al. (1988)
	Mosely et al. (1988)
	Primm et al. (1988)
Sacramento, California	Flynn et al. (1988a)
Multiple cities	Battjes and Pickens (1988)
Paris	Espinoza et al. (1988)
	Lowenstein et al. (1988)
Padua, Italy	Bortolotti et al. (1988)

drug users are practicing safer sex (Friedman et al., 1987b; Watters, 1987a; van den Hoek et al., 1988b). Typically, for every two to three IV drug users who report changes in injection behavior, only one reports any change in sexual behavior. More recent studies support these findings. Table 3-2 lists the studies presented at the Fourth International AIDS Conference that were related to heterosexual transmission among IV drug users. All of them found less reduction of risk-associated sexual behaviors than of risk-associated injection behaviors: typically, only one quarter of those surveyed reported condom use. No one yet knows why sexual behaviors in this population resist change. There appear to be many potential reasons, including a realistic fear that introducing safer sex will lead to a break-up of the relationship (Casadonte et al., 1988) and difficulty in initiating a discussion of sexual topics (Mosely et al., 1988). As noted earlier, the typical sexual relationship of an IV drug user involves a male who injects drugs and a female who does not (Des Jarlais et al., 1984; Primm et al., 1988). The asymmetries of risk and power may thus contribute to difficulties in initiating safer sex practices.

In a consideration of the reasons why IV drug users are not practicing safer sex, researchers should not neglect the reasons why the heterosexual population in general is not doing so. IV drug users are often treated by researchers as a population that is separate and discrete from the general public. Yet among the public are many subgroups that may share some beliefs, attitudes, and values with IV drug users. Among respondents to a recent national telephone survey who reported five or more sexual partners in the past year, more than 30 percent indicated that they had never purchased condoms during that time (Turner et al., in press). Intravenous drug users may simply be conforming to their community norms with regard to their sexual practices. In fact, deviation from those norms might call attention to their drug use and increase stigmatization. Moreover, it is important not to underestimate the potential for public confusion surrounding the dangers of heterosexual transmission and the negative impact of such confusion on behavioral change. Mixed messages have been given concerning the risks associated with heterosexual behavior.[6]

As noted earlier, there is an important exception to the lack of risk reduction in sexual behavior. Prostitutes have shown a willingness to use condoms with clients, although they report safer sexual practices less often in the context of personal relationships.

As discussed in Chapter 2, the determinants of patterns of sexual behavior are quite complex. It is unlikely that there is any single reason for the difficulties involved in facilitating change in the sexual behavior of most IV drug users. It will take careful research to elucidate these difficulties and their causes and to devise prevention strategies for helping individuals in this group change risk-associated behavior. Sudden breakthroughs in this area are not likely.

Toward Reducing Risk-Associated Behavior Among IV Drug Users

The problem of HIV infection among IV drug users and its transmission to their sexual partners and offspring requires both immediate action and long-term research. Immediate action is necessary because of the potential for the rapid spread of HIV among IV drug users within short periods. Although the current state of knowledge does not permit permanent or long-term solutions to drug-use problems and HIV infection in this population, enough is known now, on the basis of existing research and sound management techniques, to slow the spread of disease. In June 1988, the report issued by the IOM/NAS AIDS committee concluded that federal efforts to reduce HIV transmission among IV drug users were grossly inadequate. This committee concurs with that finding and **recommends that the appropriate government authorities take immediate action to (1) provide drug treatment upon request for IV drug users throughout the country; and (2) sustain and expand current programs that provide for "safer injection" to reach all current IV drug users in the nation on a continuing basis and with appropriate research evaluation.** From a public

[6]See Masters et al. (1988) and R. E. Gould's article in the January 1988 issue of *Cosmopolitan* magazine ("Reassuring News About AIDS: A Doctor Tells Why You May Not Be At Risk").

health perspective, it is unacceptable that persons who want to stop injecting drugs cannot receive immediate treatment. Furthermore, there is consensus among people who work in the area of drug use that treatment can produce a dramatic reduction in drug injection, even though relapse after treatment is a continuing problem (Des Jarlais, 1987a; Hubbard et al., 1988).

Preventing the spread of HIV infection requires more than additional treatment slots, however. Problems associated with drug-use relapse and with retaining individuals in treatment need to be solved; in addition, support is needed to maintain newly developed skills associated with positive treatment outcomes, such as job training, employment, and interpersonal skills. Preventing further infection also requires programs to alter those behaviors that are known to transmit HIV. Admittedly, there are insufficient data on how to provide the most effective AIDS prevention programs for those who inject drugs. Still, intervention programs cannot wait to implement findings that may take some time to generate.

As discussed in detail in Chapters 4 and 5, prevention programs should include planned variations of intervention strategies accompanied by sound evaluations to determine what is likely to be successful in preventing further infection and what is less likely to be helpful. Currently, however, there is no national system for monitoring ongoing prevention activities for IV drug users. **The committee recommends that the appropriate government authorities take immediate action to establish data collection systems for monitoring present AIDS prevention efforts for IV drug users.** At a minimum, a system is needed that provides data on the AIDS prevention services being offered throughout the country to IV drug users and their sexual partners, the rates of participation in these programs, and the characteristics of participants. Additional means must be used to reach those vulnerable members of the IV drug-using population who do not come into contact with the treatment system and to assess and serve their needs.

Reaching and serving these hard-to-reach IV drug users will require innovative methods and additional resources. Mobile vans and a cadre of outreach workers familiar with the IV drug culture, who can go into shooting galleries and other settings in which risky behaviors are occurring, have proven helpful in reaching individuals who have not been in touch with other services or agencies that deal with drug users. In short, services, whether education, information, or primary medical or social services, must be brought to IV drug users; it cannot be assumed that IV drug users will seek them out.

The committee finds that the severity of the AIDS epidemic does not permit a business-as-usual approach to the problems associated with IV drug use. All opportunities for halting the spread of HIV infection should be seized, intelligently and quickly.

Obviously, primary prevention of IV drug use would be an effective prevention strategy for HIV transmission associated with the injection of illicit drugs. Yet IV drug use is a long-standing problem in American society and has withstood many prevention efforts to date. All previous research indicates that, despite prevention and intervention efforts, a substantial number of persons will continue to inject drugs, at least over the short term. Some of these will be persons who refuse to accept treatment; others will be persons for whom current forms of treatment are not effective. Those already using drugs should be helped to modify risk-associated behaviors. If abstinence from drug use is not achievable, it should not detract from the pursuit of other goals related to stopping the spread of HIV.

A pluralistic, multitiered approach to HIV prevention is called for among IV drug users. Current studies indicate that safer injection programs are not associated with increases in IV drug use and do lead to large-scale risk reduction among IV drug users. The existing data on legal access to sterile injection equipment or the use of bleach as a disinfectant do not show which is the "best" type of safer injection program. Planned variations of these programs with appropriate evaluations are needed to learn more about designing and implementing more effective programs while simultaneously preventing further infection. These variations and the evaluation of safer injection programs should include both equipment sterilization efforts and needle exchange programs.

As detailed in Chapter 4, achieving and sustaining behavioral change is frequently difficult. The change that can reasonably be expected will not be perfect. For example, IV drug users may reduce the number of persons with whom they share injection equipment, but they may continue to share with a close personal friend or sexual partner. Indeed, as described later in this chapter, the use of the same injection equipment within a close relationship is sometimes not even thought of as "sharing" (Des Jarlais and Friedman, 1988). In addition, although IV drug users may exchange syringes "regularly" or decontaminate injection equipment "regularly," such "regular" risk-reducing activity may not occur 100 percent of the time. In the throes of narcotic withdrawal, almost all IV drug users report using whatever injection equipment is available (Des Jarlais et al., 1986a; Selwyn et al., 1987).

Given the high relapse rates of drug users after they leave drug treatment programs and the ineffectiveness of currently available treatment for some injectable drugs, the complete elimination of injection behavior is not a realistic goal. Change should be conceptualized as risk reduction rather than complete risk elimination. Moving toward a more moderate, more realistic set of goals will broaden the possible approaches to risk reduction programs; these efforts should include mechanisms to prevent relapse. **The committee recommends that high priority be given to research that will lead to improved drug-use treatment, including studies of relapse prevention and of treatment for cocaine dependence. Applied research should include planned variation and evaluation of experimental programs.**

Recent research indicates that HIV seroprevalence among IV drug users may have stabilized in several areas, including New York City (Brown et al., 1988; Des Jarlais, 1988), Stockholm (Bottiger et al., 1988), and Innsbruck (Fuchs et al., 1988). Although these developments are certainly encouraging, it is important to note that stabilization in a seroprevalence rate is also compatible with the introduction of new cases of HIV infection. Stabilization can result from the simultaneous loss of seropositive individuals (owing to migration, lack of participation in antibody testing programs after an initial positive test, and so forth) and the entry of seronegative persons into the local IV drug-using population. Modest rates of new infection could be sustained indefinitely and would not necessarily be detected by current survey strategies. The committee wishes to emphasize that the data indicating relative stabilization in HIV seroprevalence rates in these areas should not be construed to mean that the problems of HIV infection among IV drug users in those locales have been solved. Rather, these findings should be viewed as evidence of a capacity and willingness to change risk-associated behaviors in a population that has been characterized in the past as uncooperative and self-destructive.

CONDUCTING RESEARCH ON IV DRUG USE

The difficulties involved in conducting research on IV drug use, some of which were discussed in the preceding sections, are only part of the challenge researchers face in this area. There are several additional policy-related and methodological issues that must be addressed to permit the development of intervention programs to interrupt the spread of HIV.

Research Traditions

Research on illicit substance use has suffered from a disciplinary and topical balkanization, with scholars from various disciplines working independently, often with a discrete focus on a single substance. For example, biobehavioral research on IV drug use has had a twofold focus: explaining how illicit drugs can reinforce behavior and describing the mechanisms of tolerance that develop after repeated administration of certain drugs. Psychiatric and psychological research, on the other hand, has tended to define substance use as a form of mental illness. This tradition has sought to identify the precursors of illicit drug use and to assess the effectiveness of different types of psychotherapy for treatment. Sociological and anthropological research in the area has focused on drug use as a form of social behavior and thus has explored drug-user subcultures—their norms, beliefs, and values. This research has also examined the relationships between drug use and other deviant behavior, particularly criminal activity, and the relationships among race, social class, and IV drug use. Research into the causes and cures of drug use has also been complicated by competing views of drug use as a medical (and public health) or moral (and criminal law) problem (Drew, 1986).

Most of what is currently known about drug users comes from users who have been involved in treatment programs and users who have come into contact with law enforcement agencies (Ginzburg, 1984). Little is known about those users who are not in touch with these systems. (Some of the problems of using such circumscribed data soon become apparent when this information indicates that ethnic and racial minorities are overrepresented in public treatment programs [Ginzburg et al., 1987] and there are few data on individuals who seek treatment in private health care settings.) In addition, data have been collected primarily to satisfy policy needs related to treatment and criminal justice, uses that determine what kinds of data are collected. Individuals who make plans for treatment programs need to know how many people will require their services and how to make their programs culturally sensitive to the populations they serve; criminal justice agencies require information about the role of drugs in crime. The data that serve these purposes are not necessarily adequate or appropriate for infectious disease containment efforts.

Researchers are only now beginning to collect data on the behaviors associated with HIV transmission in the IV drug-using population. The Heroin Lifestyle Study (Hanson et al., 1985), which was conducted in the early 1980s in the inner cities of Chicago, New York, Philadelphia, and Washington, D.C., cast some of the first rays of light on IV drug-use behaviors that are relevant to AIDS. What emerges from these studies is a more detailed description of behaviors that show variability by race, ethnic group, gender, age, and geographic location.[7] To understand more about this variability and gather more subgroup-specific information, field workers who are often ex-addicts and ex-offenders are being recruited to locate active IV drug users in shooting galleries, after-hours clubs, and the like. In these attempts, they gather data on daily drug-use and related behaviors, take life histories, and make observations.

Despite these promising beginnings, however, there remain certain logistical hurdles and methodological problems that need to be cleared away before we can move more effectively toward the goal of reducing risk-associated behavior among IV drug users.

Tied as it has been to policy needs, research on drug use in the past suffered the vicissitudes of shifting policies and resource availability. For example, the Client-Oriented Data Acquisition Process (CODAP)[8] collected demographic data and drug-use histories on all individuals entering federally and state-funded drug treatment programs. In the early 1980s, however, what had previously been direct federal support for this and other drug-related programs was superseded by a block grant program that shifted control from federal agencies to the states. When the total funds allocated to these efforts were cut, many states, exercising their discretionary powers over the design and management of drug programs, unfortunately chose not to continue collecting CODAP data.

Still, significant research has been conducted and data of variable quality have been collected, but topics remain that are either underexplored or that have not been investigated at all. Most studies on IV drug use have investigated the injection of heroin; much less is known about the injection of cocaine or other drugs. In addition, methodological limitations persist. The methodological problems are as diverse as the population to which drug researchers wish to apply

[7]It should be pointed out that survey data do not support the hypothesis that race, sex, or age explain heroin use in cities (Greenberg and Roberson, 1978).

[8]CODAP was supported by NIDA from 1973 to 1981 to collect basic drug-related information on clients of treatment programs receiving federal or state funds. These data included information on prior treatment and the use of primary, secondary, and tertiary drugs of abuse, as well as client demographic data. CODAP also created a census of drug users in publicly funded treatment programs and provided useful indicators of trends in demographic characteristics of drug users. However, CODAP data were not sufficiently detailed to be of use to researchers or clinicians (NIDA, 1981).

methodologies. Drug users do not necessarily cooperate as research subjects by restricting their behavior to forms that can be studied using simple questionnaires. For example, single-substance drug use lends itself relatively easily to research design; the polydrug use that a significant portion of IV drug users actually report is much more difficult to measure (B. D. Johnson et al., 1985). To investigate these topics properly, old methodologies must be improved and new ones devised. The next section discusses some of the challenges inherent in these tasks.

Investigating Risk-Associated Drug Behaviors

Researchers use two basic methods to understand the nature of drug use and the extent of consumption patterns: (1) statistical surveys of defined populations and (2) ethnographic studies. Each approach focuses on quite different populations (the overlap of which is unknown) and uses very different methodologies. Analyses of the drug-using population also rely on self-reported data and on indirect indicator data, which are provided by institutional sources (e.g., treatment programs, emergency rooms, medical examiners, the criminal justice system). Some of the ways in which these approaches can be used in research on IV drug use are discussed below.

Methods

Data on drug-use behaviors have been derived from ethnographic studies and from surveys. Each method has its strengths and weaknesses; both approaches are needed to improve understanding of the nature and scope of the drug-use problem. Surveys, which are used in efforts to quantify drug-related behavior, tend to be costly and are difficult to conduct among people who have good reason to hide from those who are trying to identify them. Moreover, they are limited to samples of particular groups (e.g., individuals living in households, arrestees, or people admitted to drug treatment programs). Nevertheless, surveys are needed to ascertain the dimensions of the problem: such studies can provide critically needed and statistically sound data on IV drug-using populations. Of course, data derived from surveys will have limitations (Hubbard et al., 1978): there is a proportion of identified drug users that cannot be located for interviews; in addition, those who can be located may refuse to answer specific questions or may provide erroneous information. The nature and extent of the bias generated by such responses must be considered in interpreting survey results.

Ethnographic research may be the more appropriate method of obtaining critical information about such topics as the dynamics of IV drug use, including the initiation and continuation of drug-use behaviors (Waldorf, 1980). Often, trained ethnographers are permitted access to otherwise clandestine groups and can describe variations and patterns of behavior in rich detail. They are frequently able to reach the most active drug users and dealers, those who in general are the most criminally involved and the most likely to suffer from a broad spectrum of health problems. Moreover, unlike other research strategies whose findings often lag months and even years behind the actual events, ethnographic studies can yield timely results that may act as an early warning of emerging problems.

Ethnographic field research can also help larger scale research efforts to ask relevant questions using appropriate language and to refine survey instruments and interview procedures so as to reduce recall problems and avoid misunderstanding.[9] For example, "needle" and "sharing" are two words that can be misunderstood by researchers and respondents alike. Because some needles separate from their syringes, it is possible to share needles without sharing syringes or to share syringes without sharing needles. If the research interview does not ask about sharing syringes as well as needles, the respondent's answer to the question may be technically accurate, but it may not be a good measure of the potential for HIV transmission.

"Sharing" can also be understood differently by researchers and respondents. There are several ways in which IV drug users can use the same injection equipment and not think of themselves as sharing. First, a drug user may purchase or rent equipment that has already been used by another IV drug user. Because the identity of the previous user is not known, because there is money involved, and because considerable time may have elapsed between the first and second use, a drug user may not consider this type of multiple use to be sharing. If the injection equipment is new or sterilized, the first person using it is not at risk for HIV infection because it has not yet been shared; who goes first in the multiple use of injection equipment complicates the definition of sharing. Finally, two IV drug users, particularly if they are sexual partners or have a very close personal relationship, may consider a single needle and syringe set to be theirs together. Both may use the set without thinking of it as sharing, which for them may refer to letting someone other than one of the joint owners use the equipment.

---

[9] See Iglehart (1985) for a discussion of the use of vernacular language among black street addicts.

As these examples show, the descriptive information that ethnographers gather about drug-use practices can be helpful in improving the wording of survey questions and the data they provide. Institutions such as drug treatment programs, emergency rooms, medical examiners, and the criminal justice system can also provide information on different segments of the user population. The major indicator data that are available on injectable illicit drugs primarily cover heroin use; they include the Drug Abuse Warning Network (DAWN) emergency room data,[10] medical examiner autopsy reports, state treatment admission reports, and U.S. Drug Enforcement Agency price purity information.[11] Each data source is an indirect indicator of heroin use prevalence. Although the indicators clearly span a range of populations, detailed information on the community or ecological characteristics of the area from which the individual or data came is rare. The other major limitation of indicator data is the unknown relationship of the data to the actual prevalence of heroin use.

No single approach to or study of a limited segment of the drug user population can provide the complete, accurate information needed for useful estimates. Consequently, efforts should be made to bridge the gulfs between survey research, which is traditionally conducted by sociologists and psychologists, and ethnographic research, which largely falls within the domain of anthropology. Moreover, steps should be taken to strengthen the links between investigators with expertise in these areas.

In addition, two other issues must be considered in studying the IV drug-using population: the reliance of many studies on convenience samples and the use of self-reported information.

Convenience Samples

Many studies have obtained data on groups of heroin users that are "convenient" to study. (Regrettably, there are far fewer data on individuals who inject other drugs, such as amphetamines or cocaine.) One of the main sources of heroin users from which to draw research

[10]Established in 1973, DAWN abstracts information on drug-related medical emergencies from the emergency room records of nonfederal hospitals in 26 metropolitan areas. The data that are collected include demographic characteristics of patients and selected details on reportable drug-use episodes. DAWN is also used to acquire information on currently used drugs that may be creating a local epidemic or local health problems.

[11]The U.S. Drug Enforcement Agency began a systematic review of heroin and cocaine prices and degrees of purity in 1971. Price purity index data are presented in dollars per pure milligram of drug. The cost is a weighted average of retail purchases and seizures.

samples is the treatment client population (i.e., those drug users who participate in treatment programs). The most accessible members of the drug-using population, treatment clients can be divided into three groups: (1) new admissions or readmissions, (these clients have the most recent experience in the drug "market" and therefore may provide the most accurate firsthand reports), (2) clients currently in treatment, and (3) former treatment clients. Research samples have been recruited from detoxification, methadone maintenance, and residential drug-free treatment programs. In the past, a type of sampling frame (from which treatment samples have been selected) was available on a monthly basis in the lists of newly admitted clients compiled by the states under the CODAP program (NIDA, 1981). These lists lent themselves to randomly selected samples of treatment clients. As noted earlier, however, many states no longer collect such data, and a complete census of the treatment population is no longer available to researchers or policy makers. It is also important to recognize that, because the initial assignment of a client to a treatment program is not random, samples drawn from the treatment population may not be representative of the larger IV drug-using population or even of the population of those in treatment.

Arrestees are another "convenient" population of particular interest because 15–50 percent can be identified as drug users (Eckerman et al., 1976) and only 20–25 percent of those arrested users have ever been in treatment (Collins et al., 1988). Nevertheless, there are significant problems in selecting a sample from this population. Some type of screening interview must be used to identify IV drug users. Without urinalysis, self-reported levels of injectable drugs may underestimate actual use in this population (Eckerman et al., 1976; Toborg and Kirby, 1984; Wish et al., 1984).

Studies of street drug users employ a somewhat different type of convenience sample in that subjects are not selected from a program mounted by an organization or agency but are recruited "off the street." It is extremely difficult to apply survey methods to this group; ethnographic studies, on the other hand, can reach elements of the drug-using population that are rarely captured by other research strategies. Studies of this subpopulation of IV drug users are particularly important because this group includes those drug users who are the most active, the most criminally involved, the most involved in the drug-dealing network, and the most vulnerable to a broad spectrum of health problems.

Although useful, studies based on convenience samples are limited in their utility because their findings cannot be generalized to the total population of IV drug users. To estimate accurately the prevalence of heroin consumption at a particular time or in different types of users, a comprehensive understanding of heroin use for all types of users is necessary. Yet the IV drug-using population is heterogeneous, encompassing a variety of users who differ by age, race, sex, and socioeconomic status and who change their drug-use patterns over time. Clearly, relying on generalizations to describe this diverse population would not achieve the level of understanding needed to design intervention programs to interrupt HIV risk-associated behaviors. No one method or data source will be sufficient to tap the diversity of the IV drug-using population. A partial picture is provided by studies of particular groups—drug treatment clients, criminals who use drugs, and users who seek help in emergency rooms or die. What must also be known are (1) the degree to which these groups overlap and (2) the extent to which other groups within the population are not captured through these data sources. For example, an unknown portion of the heroin-using population will be absent from these institutional populations; on the other hand, some drug users will be part of both treatment and prison populations in a given year.

Attempts are being made to move away from exclusive reliance on convenience samples in studies of IV drug users. Several researchers have attempted to collect data from probability samples of the street population (Des Jarlais et al., 1985; McAuliffe et al., 1987). An important element of being able to conduct such studies is the identification of "major copping" (i.e., active drug sales) areas and systematic mapping of drug-related activity. Once such determinations have been made, enumeration and identification of actions and individuals, as well as the selection of potential informants, can be accomplished in ways that approach the rigor of a random sample survey method, which offers the possibility of results that can be more confidently generalized to a larger population. However, there may be variation by geographic area that will continue to limit the capacity to generalize these findings beyond the local population.

Self-Reported Information

The manner in which a sample is selected is but one of the factors that affects data quality in studies of IV drug users. Another important issue is the heavy dependence in these studies on interviews or other sources of self-reported data. Such dependence arises as a result of a number of constraints that affect the collection of data relevant to HIV transmission. For instance, the behaviors of interest can be observed, but ethical limitations affect such observations (and subsequent reporting), owing to the illicit nature of the behaviors involved. There are also no readily available biological markers for indirectly measuring risk-associated behaviors (e.g., needle-sharing). Urinalysis can validate self-reports of very recent use of specific drugs, but it does not provide any information on the route of administration. Interviews or questionnaires are the only feasible means to collect data for large-scale quantitative studies, although ethnographic participant–observation methods can provide another type of useful data. Given the centrality of self-reported data to understanding and facilitating change in risky behavior among IV drug users, it is worthwhile to examine briefly what is known about factors that affect the validity and reliability of this form of data collection.

One important factor involves the level of understanding a respondent brings to the interview or questionnaire. Many IV drug users are not well educated; some are functionally illiterate. In addition, for many, English is not their first language (Friedman et al., 1986).[12] Thus, using questionnaires that are self-administered, that have complex structures or wording, or that are available only in English can hardly serve a study of this population well. Moreover, because respondents may be considerably embarrassed to admit that they cannot read or do not understand a question, researchers cannot expect them to bring these difficulties to the attention of the person collecting the data.

A standard threat to valid self-reported data is whether or not the subject is deliberately providing false information (Harrell, 1985; Rouse et al., 1985). In a society in which IV drug use is both illegal and highly stigmatized, IV drug users will often have many practical reasons for not admitting that they use drugs. This denial may well include their unwillingness to admit that they are still injecting drugs while in treatment or after they have left treatment. Consequently, it is critical that interviewers not be perceived as people who can have an effect on drug treatment, legal proceedings, or other such interventions. Care must be taken to allow researchers to collect the

[12]CODAP data for 1981 indicated that 15.6 percent of the drug treatment population had a 9th grade education or less and that an additional 27.8 percent had only a 10th or 11th grade education. The large percentage of Hispanics in the IV drug-using population that seeks treatment suggests that many IV drug users may not have English as a first language. In a study of 200 New York City female addicts (Cuskey and Wathey, 1982), 52 percent were high school dropouts and 60 percent had not held a job for more than six months during the preceding year.

best possible data while still protecting IV drug users' privacy and maintaining the confidentiality of the information they provide.

Even if a respondent is motivated to be truthful with a researcher, however, it is possible that the stigmatization and illegal nature of drug injection will bias his or her memory of drug injection behavior (Maddux and Desmond, 1975; Bale et al., 1981). Such psychological denial has been observed with a variety of behaviors that are negatively valued in society. Alternatively, drug users may take pride in their ability to obtain and use illicit drugs and may exaggerate their use of drugs to others, either consciously or through biasing effects on memory.

Remembering the details of drug injection—for example, what equipment was used and how many people used it—over periods of days to years can be quite difficult, even if a respondent is motivated to remember the behavior in question "properly." A person who is using IV drugs heavily may be injecting heroin 3–4 times daily or cocaine 10 or more times per day. Human recall in this type of situation is often based on a mental averaging of what was done most or some of the time (Bradburn et al., 1987).

Yet, despite the potential problems in obtaining valid self-reported data from IV drug users, a body of findings is emerging that is consistent across studies. As noted earlier in this chapter, the frequency of illicit drug injection over time and the frequency of sharing drug injection equipment across friendship groups have been associated with the risk of HIV infection in a number of studies (Robertson et al., 1986; Des Jarlais and Friedman, 1987b). Thus, the consistency of association among frequency of injection, use of shared injection equipment, and infection supports the perception that researchers can obtain valid self-reported data from IV drug users with respect to illicit drug-use behaviors (Maddux and Desmond, 1975).

Toward Better Quality Data

The need for better information about IV drug users has prompted the committee to recommend that high priority be given to studies of this population. Little is known about variations in the injection patterns of adolescents, minorities, women, and other IV drug users who do not come into contact with organizations and agencies that serve the drug-using population. Studies are also needed of those IV drug users who are not being captured by current sampling strategies. These "invisible" drug users are apt to include individuals in the mainstream of society (i.e., from upper and middle socioeconomic classes) who are more likely to seek treatment in private health care facilities.

The status of IV drug users as members of the heroin community is often secret. These users may or may not be identified on the street as addicts, depending on their means of obtaining the drug and the stage of their drug-use careers. Their drug use may be hidden even from family and friends. **The committee recommends that high priority be given to studies of IV drug users who are not in contact with health care, drug-use treatment, or criminal justice systems.**

Reaching the relevant groups to collect data and deliver intervention programs and services will not be easy. The successful recruitment of IV drug users into drug treatment and intervention programs and into research protocols, and their subsequent retention in such efforts, will require careful management of those procedures and practices that could identify participants. Intravenous drug users often view the identifiers required in some research as an invasion of privacy and a means of uncovering issues and behaviors that they do not want uncovered. Yet these same identification practices can improve the quality and richness of data and facilitate the evaluation of programs. A careful balance must be struck between serving the need to collect useful data and respecting the sensitivities of study respondents.

Also needed are methodological studies of how to obtain better self-reported information and how to determine when a particular subject is not providing valid data. It is critical to understand under what conditions IV drug users are more or less likely to disclose information and to remember past events accurately, particularly those events that may involve complex and variable patterns of behavior such as needle-sharing. Techniques that have been tried in other areas (e.g., varying the setting of the interview or asking the respondent to record sensitive information without being observed by the interviewer) deserve further investigation. **The committee recommends that high priority be given to methodological studies to determine ways of improving the quality of self-reports of sexual and drug-use behavior.** Conducting such studies, however, will require a long-term commitment to research on illicit drug use; the benefits of methodological research, including a better understanding of how to maximize the validity of self-reported data from persons who use illicit drugs, will be evident as the findings from such research are incorporated into future studies.

Sampling IV drug users is difficult, both theoretically and operationally. Typical statistical sampling procedures may not yield useful estimates, and even procedures that have been designed to sample rare and elusive populations (Sudman et al., 1988) are problematic. Using such techniques as geographically clustered samples and network samples can help inform the estimation process. Regardless of the method or combination of methods used, the estimation process will continue to rest more on judgment than on formal statistical inference.

MEASURING THE SCOPE OF THE PROBLEM

Prevalence of IV Drug Use

Estimates of the number of IV drug users and the rates of seroprevalence among them are an essential feature of overall attempts to gauge the spread of AIDS, to target intervention programs, and to plan for the health care resources that are likely to be needed in the future. Inaccurate estimates of the nature and scope of the IV drug-use problem may hinder the formulation of appropriately targeted AIDS prevention policies. Moreover, inadequate data can stymie efforts to refine understanding of the relative degree of peril associated with the behaviors that are known to transmit HIV.

Currently, the accurate estimation of the prevalence of IV drug use is hindered by (1) the lack of a sound conceptual model of the dynamic nature of IV drug use, (2) the lack of appropriate statistical models, and (3) the limitations of existing data and data collection systems. Any attempt to improve the estimation process will require major efforts in each of these areas. Without such efforts, the basic assumptions underlying HIV seroprevalence estimates and other rates that require a sound denominator will continue to be questioned.

Estimates of the total number of IV drug users were published in the November 1987 report prepared by the Public Health Service for the White House Domestic Policy Council and in a special supplement to CDC's *Morbidity and Mortality Weekly Report* (CDC, 1987a,b). One of the background papers commissioned by the committee (see Spencer, in this volume) contains a critique of the estimates generated in that report to illustrate the lack of data and models for assessing the extent of IV drug use in the United States. The deconstruction of current estimates (i.e., breaking down the totals into the components on which they are based) indicates that these estimates may be subject to substantial error. One possible source of error is the lack of agreement among those providing data on who should be counted in the ranks of the IV drug-using population.

Definition of an IV Drug User

A basic problem in constructing estimates of drug use is the difficulty of defining the term *IV drug user.* The types and combination of drugs injected and the frequency of needle use vary considerably among users, as do individual drug-use "careers." Hard-core or addicted users may inject many times daily; other IV drug users may inject less frequently and may never become addicted (Gerstein, 1976; Zinberg, 1984; Hanson et al., 1985). Indeed, during their drug-use careers, individuals may move through phases of regular and intermittent use (Simpson et al., 1986). However, all phases that involve needle-sharing carry some level of risk (albeit a variable one) of contracting HIV infection. Furthermore, those ex-users who are now asymptomatic may already be infected from prior needle-sharing.

When using multiple data sources to estimate the total number of IV drug users, it is important to keep the drug user definition constant across all sources. The level of precision of this definition for any given study will depend on the study's purpose. To study the transmission of HIV infection, for example, researchers will need to estimate seroprevalence for IV drug users classified by frequency of injection, how long they have been injecting, whether they share needles and with whom, as well as other relevant dimensions of drug use.

In its 1987 report, CDC (1987a) distinguished between two types of IV drug users: regular users, who inject at least once a week, and less frequent or occasional users, who inject less often than regular users but who have used drugs more than just once or twice. Two sets of national estimates were produced for each type of IV drug user: the original Public Health Service estimates for 1986 and revised estimates for 1987 (see Table 3-3).

To assess the accuracy of these estimates, it is necessary to know the population definitions that were used in estimating the total number of each type of IV drug user and the seroprevalence rates. How different are the operational definitions? How accurate are the estimates for the populations as operationally defined?

TABLE 3-3 Estimated Number of IV Drug Users and Their HIV Status

Type of IV Drug Use	Estimated Number of IV Drug Users	Approximate Seroprevalence Rate (percentage)	Estimated Number of HIV-Infected Users
Original estimate (1986)			
Regular users	750,000	30	225,000
Occasional users	750,000	10	75,000
Total	1,500,000		300,000
Revised estimate (1987)			
Regular users	900,000	25	225,000
Occasional users	200,000	5	10,000
Total	1,100,000		235,000

SOURCE: CDC (1987a).

Techniques for Estimating the Total Number of IV Drug Users

In general, three kinds of techniques are used to estimate the total number of IV drug users in the United States: (1) indirect estimates, (2) informed "guesstimates," and (3) direct estimates (Butynski et al., 1987).

Indirect estimates are based on regression models that attempt to relate indicator data (e.g., the number of burglaries or heroin-related deaths) to the prevalence of IV drug use. Estimates of the total population are obtained by substituting observed (or predicted) values of the indicators in the regression model.

Informed guesstimates are produced by looking at any available indicators or other correlates of IV drug-use prevalence and making an informed guess about the number of IV drug users. The accuracy of indirect estimation or informed "guesstimation" can be no greater than the accuracy of the direct estimates on which they depend.

Direct estimates are based on surveys (e.g., the National Household Survey on Drug Abuse, conducted by NIDA), on back-extrapolation methods, or on dual-systems estimates.

The National Household Survey attempts to measure the prevalence of drug use in the general population (age 12 and older) through a household survey (see Miller et al., 1983). While this is a reasonable way to understand the scope of the problem, the method has its limitations. The sampling frame excludes persons living in transient households or in institutions (e.g., university dormitories and prisons), persons in the military, and persons with no fixed residence.

In addition to sampling limitations, there are problems with nonrespondents and those who underreport drug use. The extent of bias in the survey results is unknown, but it is potentially large.

Back-extrapolation methods have used AIDS mortality and HIV seroprevalence data to estimate the number of IV drug users. The total number of IV drug users is a function of the estimated number of AIDS cases among IV drug users divided by the probability that an IV drug user will have had AIDS. This method carries difficulties in determining both the numerator and the denominator. For example, the numerator must be corrected for underreporting,[13] and the denominator must take into account the uncertainties concerning the probability of progressing from HIV infection to AIDS.

Dual-systems estimates, also known as capture–recapture or tag–recapture estimates, are perhaps the most widely used method for making direct estimates. The capture–recapture method assumes that only a small fraction of the addict population would ever be reported to authorities. Two independent lists of IV drug users are generated—for example, a list of persons in heroin treatment programs and a list of persons treated in emergency rooms for adverse reactions to heroin use. If a treatment sample is identified (tagged) and the tagged individuals subsequently turn up in a second sample (for example, among emergency room admissions related to drug use), the proportion of tagged to untagged individuals in the second sample allows an estimate to be made for the larger population. The total number of IV drug users is a function of the size of each list and the number of "matches" or names found on both lists. Some of the problems known to occur with dual-systems estimates include errors in the construction of the lists, variability in the selection probabilities for different types of individuals (some IV drug users are more likely than others to appear on a list, and those in treatment may be less likely to be treated in emergency rooms), and missed matches owing to the use of assumed names.

National Aggregates of State Estimates

The second set of CDC estimates of the total number of IV drug users in the United States (CDC, 1987a) indicates that more than 1 million people inject illicit drugs. National estimates of this kind

[13] A recent study of the outcome of HIV infection among IV drug users in New York City found that, of 31 deaths, 6 were attributable to infectious agents that are not categorized as opportunistic agents associated with an AIDS diagnosis (Des Jarlais et al., 1988b). These deaths were associated with pneumonia not caused by *Pneumocystis carinii*, with endocarditis, and with tuberculosis. (See also Des Jarlais and colleagues [1988a], as discussed in Chapter 1, footnote 2.)

are developed by aggregating estimates of the number of IV drug users in each state. Two organizations that have combined state data to produce such estimates are the National Association of State Alcohol and Drug Abuse Directors, Inc. (NASADAD), and NIDA.

NASADAD asked each state alcohol and drug agency to provide estimates of the total number of IV drug users in their state for fiscal year 1986, as well as the methods used to arrive at that estimate. Of the 17 states that reported data, the highest estimate was provided by New York, followed by California and Texas. Ten states reported that their estimates were based on indirect measures or indicators. Three states reported that only guesstimates were used; four states indicated they used a combination of methods. The total number of IV drug users reported for the 17 states was 1,067,000. Adding the state-plan estimates for the other 33 states, Puerto Rico, and the District of Columbia produces an estimated total of 1,447,000 IV drug users.

NIDA's national estimate of 1.1 million IV drug users in the United States[14] is based on the following:

500,000	Estimated heroin addicts in 1982
+250,000	IV heroin users who are not addicted
+475,000	Heavy users of cocaine with a previous history of IV drug use
−150,000	Overlap in cocaine/heroin use
+25,000	IV drug users who do not inject heroin or cocaine
1,100,000	Total estimate of IV drug users

In reporting its estimates, NIDA verifies that the numbers were reported correctly, but it does not assess the accuracy of the estimates. The national estimates described here can be no better than the individual state estimates on which they are based, and those estimates are subject to variation from forces other than statistical or methodological limitations. Political motivations may also color the numbers: the desire to obtain funds might cause higher estimates; the desire to show success in the war against drugs might produce lower estimates.

---

[14]Spencer (in this volume) presents a detailed discussion of these estimates. Sources cited for these estimates are (a) Estimated heroin addicts in 1982: Shreckengost (1983); (b) IV heroin users who are not addicted: NIDA estimate from analysis of unpublished data; (c) Overlap in cocaine/heroin use: NIDA, *"Demographic Characteristics and Patterns of Drug Use of Clients Admitted to Drug Abuse Treatment Programs in Selected States: Annual Data 1985,"* analysis of unpublished data; (d) Heavy users of cocaine with a previous history of IV drug use *and* IV drug users who do not inject heroin or cocaine: NIDA, *"National Household Survey on Drug Abuse: Main Findings 1985,"* analysis of unpublished data.

The accuracy of the estimates of the number of IV drug users is not objectively ascertainable; nevertheless, based on a review of the estimation methods (see Spencer, in this volume), it is not unreasonable to believe that the error could be on the order of 100 percent. That is to say, the true number of IV drug users could be as few as half a million or as great as 2 million.

Consumption and Turnover Rates Among IV Drug Users

A comprehensive, accurate assessment of the prevalence of IV drug use is largely dependent on an adequate understanding of the development, maintenance, and cessation of heroin consumption patterns, the diversity of drug-related behaviors, and the movement in and out of the IV drug-using population (turnover). Such understanding is not easy to achieve, however. The use of multiple drugs and increased cocaine consumption have made the description of drug-use patterns quite difficult (Fishburne et al., 1980; Johnston et al., 1981; Bray et al., 1982; B. D. Johnson and Goldstein, 1984). Patterns of illicit drug use in general, and heroin use in particular, have changed markedly over the past decade (Bray et al., 1982; Hubbard et al., 1985b). Illicit drugs and their markets also vary from city to city (Person et al., 1976; Schlenger and Greenberg, 1978) and from neighborhood to neighborhood (Greenberg and Roberson, 1978). In addition, different ethnic groups have very different patterns of use (Austin et al., 1977; Hubbard et al., 1983) and obtain drugs from different sources.

Much of what is known about IV drug use comes from studies of heroin use. That literature in turn focuses far more on the maintenance of usage patterns than on turnover, an important factor in gauging both the prevalence of IV drug use at specific points in time and the likelihood of exposure to HIV.

Treatment populations provide the major source of data on heroin consumption. However, because the patterns of drug use prior to treatment may differ from patterns seen during other phases of the drug career, using these populations as the major source of data may give a somewhat distorted picture of heroin use. For example, data from the Treatment Outcome Prospective Study (TOPS)[15] indicated that heroin use was common among clients entering all

[15]TOPS is a long-term longitudinal study of drug users who receive treatment from publicly funded programs. Begun in 1979 and supported by NIDA, the study seeks to understand the natural history of drug users before, during, and after treatment. More than 11,000 subjects who entered treatment between 1979 and 1981 were interviewed at the point of intake into the treatment system; a subset of 4,600 has been followed after discharge from treatment through 1986.

treatment modalities: 85 percent of the detoxification clients, 93 percent of the methadone outpatients, 55 percent of the residential clients, and 31 percent of the outpatient drug-free clients had a history of daily heroin use (Hubbard et al., 1986). Yet a large proportion of the clients entering TOPS programs was already in treatment during the year prior to entry, and many were incarcerated.

A composite measure or index that fully describes the risk associated with IV drug use must include some information on past use. Hubbard and colleagues (1985b) developed an index that combined information on current and former use of heroin. Former daily users were separated from those who used heroin weekly or daily for a limited, recent time period. Recent users were also divided into those who used heroin as their principal illicit drug and those who frequently used other opioids as well.

Heroin and other narcotics users report the most complex patterns of use during the year prior to treatment. Weekly or daily use of other drugs is commonly reported, including other narcotics, tranquilizers, barbiturates or sedatives, cocaine, and amphetamines. These complex patterns suggest that users may differ greatly in the course of the development of addiction and the movement into and out of heroin use. Some may be more likely to substitute other drugs for heroin, and some may be more likely to relapse after treatment. Improved prevalence estimates require open-systems models that can accommodate substantial movements into and out of the IV drug-using population. To refine modeling efforts, detailed information is needed on the complex dynamics of patterns of drug use.

Modeling the IV Drug-Using Population: Constraints and Limitations

There are a number of models to predict drug-use prevalence and drug consumption that attempt to reflect the complex dynamics of drug use. These models are based on sound statistical principles; yet because they require extensive and often elaborate assumptions, for which, unfortunately, there are generally limited supporting data, they do not always produce accurate estimates that can be used with confidence.

Valid assumptions and accurate data are crucial to a model's ability to predict future trends. In a study to determine the effects of differing levels of accuracy of key assumptions, Glenn and Hartwell (1975) reviewed various applications of two approaches to estimating drug-use prevalence: the capture–recapture method and direct estimation. In a comparison of Greenwood's (1970) use of U.S. Drug Enforcement Agency records with Andima and coworkers' (1973) use of the New York City narcotics register, Glenn and Hartwell noted that very different estimates were developed. Their conclusion was that, although both methods were theoretically sound, the data bases and key assumptions of the approaches were subject to substantial error. Recent advances in methodology (Woodward and Bentler, 1978; Doscher and Woodward, 1983) and the availability of data from the CODAP system have allowed estimates to be made with a greater degree of precision (Woodward et al., 1984). Even now, however, the confidence intervals for these estimates are quite large.

Efforts are under way to test model assumptions concerning the dynamics of drug use and to generate better data for more accurate predictions. For example, analysis of the drug treatment careers of TOPS clients and the estimation of transitional functions of treatment entry and reentry using events-based analysis have provided data to increase the validity of a number of the techniques (Hubbard et al., 1985a). Direct estimation techniques have been used with the NIDA National Household Survey data (Miller et al., 1983), drug treatment population demographic data, and hepatitis reports (Minichiello, 1974). These approaches are limited, however, by the rarity of some types of behavior and the scant research on such transitional functions as episodic drug use and return to treatment.

Although a number of studies have focused on the characteristics of drug users, few have examined the characteristics of the community environment. Clearly, any study of the drug consumption patterns of individual users should also include information on the community context, preferably at the census tract level. Some attempts have been made to combine data on community and individual characteristics. For example, Schlenger and Greenberg (1978) investigated the correlation of the Heroin Problem Index (HPI) with characteristics of the DAWN (Drug Abuse Warning Network) standard metropolitan statistical areas (SMSAs) available from the 1970 census.[16] A similar study conducted for the U.S. Drug Enforcement Agency (Greenberg and Roberson, 1978) included an analysis of characteristics at the census tract and SMSA levels in five cities. Longitudinal studies that will measure changes in local environments are also needed.

[16]Schlenger and Greenberg (1978) found that cities with high levels of heroin use did not differ from cities with low levels of use on such variables as racial composition, proportion of young men, violent crime rate, median income, and proportion of households headed by a woman. Greenberg and Roberson's (1978) study found no support for the notion that the composition of race, sex, and age in cities and neighborhoods is correlated with heroin use.

In the past, modeling techniques have been applied to a number of different drug problems, for reasons ranging from the need for greater understanding of the dynamics of drug demand and supply to assessing the impact of alternative policies for dealing with drug use at the community level. Several models based on systems dynamics have been developed in the drug-use area (O'Brien, 1973; Levin et al., 1975). Yet each of the available models is limited by some key problems in the underlying assumption or assumptions. The capture–recapture model depends on the questionable assumptions that the population is stable, that each capture is an independent event and is not dependent on previous capture, and that a complete capture history is available. For the systems dynamics models, the choice of variables limits the utility of any model. For example, market models tend to exclude social and psychological factors, a gap that results in the inability of the model to explain changes in consumption levels caused by the voluntary cessation of use by individual users.

In general, synthetic estimation models rely on indirect estimates of the prevalence of heroin use, which are drawn from indicators of representative geographical areas; the data are then weighted for national estimates. Within this two-stage estimation procedure, the assumptions that are made greatly influence the final results and warrant close scrutiny. Such assumptions include the following: (1) linear relationships exist between indicators and prevalence; (2) confirmed, reliable estimates are available in at least one community; and (3) areas for which data are available are representative of the national population.

As is the case with most mathematical models, models of heroin consumption could benefit from further elaboration and the use of other mechanisms to improve their predictive powers. There are several strategies for proceeding. For example, existing models could be tested with new data or new assumptions concerning the dynamics of drug use. Alternatively, new models could be constructed. Also necessary to continued model development and improvement are the enhanced coordination of data collection for indicator data, surveys of key populations, and systematic ethnographic studies.

The committee recognizes the problems inherent in collecting data on IV drug users for modeling efforts. It is difficult to study illicit behavior and to count those who wish to elude the attention of representatives of authority. Nevertheless, such studies must be undertaken; vague estimates and trends in IV drug use will no longer suffice. The committee finds the current estimates of the prevalence of IV drug use to be seriously flawed. Coping with the AIDS epidemic requires more precise estimates of the total number of IV drug users at a particular point in time, as well as estimates of the number of individuals moving into and out of IV drug use in this country. To construct such estimates, more information is required about the turnover in this population and how to measure it. It is also crucial to overcome shortcomings in the conceptualization of models and of IV drug use, as well as the limitations posed by existing data and data collection systems. The committee is particularly troubled by the destruction of important data archives as a result of a lack of continuous support[17] and finds such short-sighted planning regrettable. It also deems it especially important to improve the knowledge that is derived from convenience samples: more needs to be known about the direction and extent of bias in such samples. Improving the quality of data will require basic methodological research that has not been supported in the past.

Prevalence of AIDS and HIV Infection Among IV Drug Users

Approximately one quarter of all AIDS cases diagnosed in this country among adults and adolescents is related to IV drug use (Schuster, 1988). However, because of the very strict definition of AIDS that has been established for surveillance purposes, it is thought that the number of reported cases underestimates the size of the problem. A review of death certificates in 1985 found reporting to be 90 percent complete. Still, Hardy and coworkers (1987) have suggested that an additional 13 percent of deaths among IV drug users were related to HIV but did not meet the CDC criteria for AIDS. The number of non-AIDS deaths among IV drug users in New York City increased from 257 in 1978 to 1,607 in 1985 (Des Jarlais et al., 1988b). This increase is presumed to reflect fatal consequences of HIV infection that did not meet the CDC surveillance definition for AIDS, including infections from nonopportunistic pathogens (see Table 3-4). Other factors, such as better record-keeping or better surveillance, can also result in increases in the number of reported deaths; however, one study of narcotic-related deaths in New York (Stoneburner et al., 1988) ruled out improved recognition and reporting in explaining increased mortality.

---

[17] Lack of funding forced the closure of a data archive that was a valuable repository of data sets from previous research on drug use. This archive, which was funded by NIDA, was located at Texas Christian University from November 1973 until December 1981.

TABLE 3-4 Selected Causes of Non-AIDS Deaths Among New York City IV Drug Users in 1981 and 1985

Cause	1981	1985
Pneumonia (not *Pneumocystis carinii*)	15	193
Tuberculosis	3	35
Endocarditis	4	64

SOURCE: Des Jarlais et al. (1988a).

Unfortunately, less is known about the rates of HIV infection among IV drug users than is known about the prevalence of AIDS. Much of the data on HIV infection in this group has been collected from small samples of convenience recruited from methadone maintenance programs, drug-free treatment programs, detoxification programs, prisons, and the street. With such limited data, it is not possible to know the prevalence of HIV infection among IV drug users in the United States at this time. What researchers are beginning to suspect, however, is that the number of AIDS cases may not accurately reflect the disease burden of this population. What is known is that there is great variability in rates of infection across the country (Table 3-5). Geographic variation in the number of AIDS cases indicates that there are still important opportunities to prevent the further spread of the disease. The following paragraphs discuss what is known about HIV infection and describe the patterns that have been seen to date.

Reviews of HIV seroprevalence studies of IV drug users show persistent associations of seroprevalence rates with geography and ethnicity (CDC, 1987a; Des Jarlais and Friedman, 1987b; Curran, 1988; Hahn et al., 1988). In the United States, there are wide variations in HIV seroprevalence by region of the country. As shown in Table 3-6, for individuals reporting IV drug use, the rates of HIV infection are highest in the New York City area (typically, 50 percent or higher); intermediate (15–35 percent) in other urban areas (e.g., Baltimore, Hartford, and San Francisco); and very low (5 percent or lower) in some western cities (e.g., Los Angeles).

Several factors contribute to the geographic variability of HIV seroprevalence rates among IV drug users in the United States. First, most IV drug users do not appear to travel extensively. In addition to limited economic resources, the need for a constant supply of drugs probably reduces their mobility, although they appear to travel some,

TABLE 3-5 Percentage of All Reported AIDS Cases Among IV Drug Users in the United States

State/District	Total AIDS Cases[a]	Percentage of AIDS Cases Among IV Drug Users[b]
New York	12,103	32.7
California	9,981	2.5
Florida	3,169	15.1
Texas	2,919	3.0
New Jersey	2,555	47.7
Illinois	1,176	6.0
Pennsylvania	1,084	9.9
Georgia	957	7.6
Massachusetts	915	13.7
Washington, D.C.	885	6.8
United States	44,129	16.6

[a]The total includes cases reported through October 31, 1987.
[b]IV drug users include only heterosexual men and women with a history of IV drug use.

SOURCE: Allen and Curran (1988).

especially to locations where friends can help them obtain drugs. Other IV drug users—for example, prostitutes or those who sell drugs—may be induced to travel by their ability to earn money in new cities. Data on the life-styles of IV drug users include little information on physical mobility. Clearly, additional research in this area will be needed to target prevention strategies and to model the future course of the AIDS epidemic.

The second factor influencing the great geographic variation in HIV seroprevalence is the potential for the rapid transmission of infection within a particular locale. As is seen with other infectious diseases, a self-sustaining epidemic occurs when one infected individual produces new infection in more than one other person (see Chapter 1). Using blood samples collected and stored from previous investigations, researchers have reported increases (from approximately 10–50 percent or greater) in seroprevalence over a period of 3–4 years in New York (D. M. Novick et al., 1986; L. F. Novick et al., 1988); Edinburgh, Scotland (Robertson et al., 1986); and Milan, Italy (Angarano et al., 1985; Moss, 1987). The committee wishes to point out, however, that these rapid increases occurred prior to widespread awareness of AIDS. Given current knowledge of HIV transmission and of behavioral change associated with prevention activities, the rapid spread of HIV infection among IV drug users should not be seen as inevitable.

Geographic variation in rates of infection may also reflect the disproportionate burden of disease borne by racial and ethnic minority groups. Chaisson and coworkers (1987b) found HIV infection among IV drug users in San Francisco to be significantly more prevalent among blacks and Hispanics than among whites. Weiss and colleagues (1985) reported similar findings in New Jersey. As of November 14, 1988, of all reported AIDS cases, 26 percent were diagnosed among blacks and 15 percent were diagnosed among Hispanics (CDC, 1988). Of the cases attributed to IV drug use, blacks accounted for 50 percent and Hispanics accounted for 30 percent.[18]

Although consistently higher seroprevalence rates have been found among minority IV drug users, more complete interpretations of the data raise questions about factors that may differentially predispose minorities to HIV infection. In some studies (e.g., Marmor et al., 1987b), racial and ethnic differences do not retain statistical significance after controlling for drug use and needle-sharing. However, in the study of IV drug users from San Francisco, both blacks and Latinos were found to have a greater prevalence of HIV infection than whites, a finding that persisted after adjusting for reported needle-sharing (Chaisson et al., 1987b). The reasons for these differences are not yet understood. There may be behavioral differences in IV drug-use and needle-sharing behaviors across ethnic groups that are actually more accurately measured by questions on ethnicity than by questions on the behaviors themselves. Clearly, the amount of error in measuring ethnicity is likely to be much less than the error in measuring complex behavior over long periods of time. In other studies (e.g., Schoenbaum et al., 1986), racial and ethnic differences may be due to the recruitment of subjects from different areas within a single city, thus reflecting residential segregation and perhaps multiple epidemics of HIV within one city.

The frequency of ethnic differences in seroprevalence rates clearly indicates a need for additional research to explain these differences and the careful development of prevention strategies to reduce the chances of becoming infected, as well as the stigmatization and scapegoating of subpopulations. **The committee recommends that high priority be given to research on the estimation of the current number of IV drug users in the United States and**

[18] These data exclude individuals who report both IV drug use and homosexual behavior.

TABLE 3-6 Seroprevalence Among IV Drug Users Tested in Various Settings in Selected U.S. Cities and States

State	City/Area	Year	Setting	Number Tested	Percentage Positive
Arkansas	Statewide	1987	STD clinic	56	0
California	Los Angeles	1986	Methadone/detoxification	728	2
	San Francisco	1985	Methadone	128	5
		1987	Detoxification	229	11
		1987	Street	232	24
Colorado	Denver	1985	Methadone/drug-free	263	2
		1986	Drug treatment	100	5
Connecticut	Hartford	1985	Drug treatment	45	7
		1986/1987	Drug treatment	83	13
		1986/1987	Hospital	50	44
Delaware	Statewide	1987	Drug treatment	52	8
Florida	Miami	1986	Methadone	186	5
Georgia	Atlanta	1987	Drug treatment	100	10
Louisiana	New Orleans	1985	Drug treatment	230	1
Massachusetts	New Bedford	1986	Methadone	114	24
Maryland	Baltimore	1986	Drug treatment	184	29
		1986/1987	Prenatal clinic	115	30

Minnesota	Minneapolis	1985	Methadone	32	0
		1987	Drug treatment	231	1
New Jersey	Newark/Jersey City	1984	Drug treatment	NA[a]	50
	New York City region	1984[b]	Drug treatment	1,300	2–59[c]
New Mexico	Albuquerque	1986/1987	Drug treatment	419	1
New York	Bronx	1985/1986	Methadone	493	34
	Brooklyn/Harlem	1985	Drug treatment	553	54
		1986	Drug treatment	280	61
		1987	Drug treatment	237	57
	Manhattan	1984	Methadone/detoxification	290	51
		1986	Methadone	165	49
Ohio	Cleveland	1986	Methadone	250	2
Puerto Rico	Caguas	1986[b]	Drug treatment	88	59
	San Juan	1987	Methadone	74	45
Texas	San Antonio	1986	Drug treatment	106	2
		1987	Drug treatment	97	0
Washington	Tacoma	1985–1987	Methadone	247	1
Wisconsin	Milwaukee	1986	Drug treatment	264	2

NOTE: Some samples include individuals who report other risk factors in addition to IV drug use (e.g., prostitution, homosexual/bisexual contacts). STD: sexually transmitted disease.

[a]NA indicates that data were not available.
[b]There is some uncertainty in this case about the dates on which data were collected.
[c]The results of several studies conducted in a specific area and in a given year were consulted to produce this figure.

SOURCE: CDC (1987a).

of seroprevalence rates among different groups of IV drug users.

CONCLUSION

Having reviewed a number of the obstacles to behavioral research, disease prevention, and health promotion efforts for IV drug users, the reader may be left with the perception that these are monumental roadblocks to understanding and intervening in the behaviors associated with HIV transmission in this group. While the committee does not wish to deny the existing impediments to an understanding of the problem, it finds that the formidable challenges described in this chapter are not insurmountable. Changes in risk-associated behavior have already been reported by IV drug users. An awareness of the risks of HIV infection and a willingness to change behavior in the face of those risks are great among both infected and uninfected individuals.

Now, innovative approaches and carefully planned variations of intervention strategies, accompanied by sound evaluation, are the order of the day. Despite major gaps in current knowledge and understanding of drug use and the limitations imposed by imperfect methods for gathering data, the committee finds that considerable valuable information has already been acquired. Moreover, the knowledge base needed to design, implement, and evaluate measures to change high-risk behavior in IV drug users continues to grow.

Opportunities remain to halt the spread of HIV infection among IV drug users. There are data that describe the IV drug-using population as considerably smaller than the population of gay men at risk. The population of IV drug users that has already been infected with HIV is still concentrated in relatively few urban areas, such as New York City and northern New Jersey. Enough data are now available to formulate rational plans for preventive action. Combining the results of research and improved understanding with the principles of intervention and evaluation presented in the next part of this report can bring the progress we seek in interrupting the spread of HIV among IV drug users and other at-risk groups.

BIBLIOGRAPHY

Abdul-Quader, A. S., Friedman, S. R., Des Jarlais, D. C., Marmor, M. M., Maslansky, R., and Bartelme, S. (1987) Methadone maintenance and behavior by intravenous drug users that can transmit HIV. *Contemporary Drug Problems* 14:425–434.

Adler, P. A. (1985) *Wheeling and Dealing.* New York: Columbia University Press.

Agar, M. (1973) *Ripping and Running.* New York: Seminar Press.

Akins, C., and Beschner, G. (1980) *Ethnography: A Research Tool for Policymakers in the Drug and Alcohol Fields.* Washington, D.C.: National Institute on Drug Abuse.

Alldritt, L., Dolan, K., Donoghoe, M., and Stimson, G. V. (1988) HIV and the Injecting Drug User: Clients of Syringe Exchange Schemes in England and Scotland. Presented at the Fourth International AIDS Conference, Stockholm, June 12–16.

Allen, J. R., and Curran, J. W. (1988) Prevention of AIDS and HIV infection: Needs and priorities for epidemiologic research. *American Journal of Public Health* 78:381–384.

Andima, H., Bergner, L., Krug, D., Patrick, S., and Whitman, S. (1973) A prevalence estimation model of narcotics addiction in New York City. *American Journal of Epidemiology* 98:56–62.

Angarano, G., Pastore, G., Monno, L., Santantonio, F., Luchena, N., and Schiraldi, O. (1985) Rapid spread of HTLV-III infection among drug addicts in Italy. *Lancet* 2:1302.

Anhalt, N. S., and Klein, M. (1976) Drug abuse in junior high school populations. *American Journal of Drug and Alcohol Abuse* 3:589–603.

Austin, G. A., Johnson, B. D., Carroll, E. E., and Lettieri, D. J. (1977) *Drugs and Minorities.* NIDA Research Issues No. 21. Rockville, Md.: National Institute on Drug Abuse.

Bale, R. N., Van Stone, W. W., Engelsing, T. M. J., and Zarcone, V. P. (1981) The validity of self-reported heroin use. *International Journal of the Addictions* 16:1387–1398.

Ball, J. C., Corty, E., Erdlen, D., and Nurco, D. (1986) Major patterns of polydrug abuse among heroin addicts. In *Problems of Drug Dependence.* Proceedings of the 47th Annual Scientific Meeting, Committee on Problems of Drug Dependence. NIDA Research Monograph No. 67. Rockville, Md.: National Institute on Drug Abuse.

Ball, J. C., Lange, W. R., Myers, C. P., and Friedman, S. R. (1988) The Effectiveness of Methadone Maintenance Treatment in Reducing IV Drug Use and Needle Sharing Among Heroin Addicts at Risk for AIDS. Presented at the Fourth International AIDS Conference, Stockholm, June 12–16.

Battjes, R. J., and Pickens, R. (1988) AIDS Transmission Risk Behaviors Among Intravenous Drug Abusers (IVDAs). Presented at the Fourth International AIDS Conference, Stockholm, June 12–16.

Becker, H. S. (1953) Becoming a marijuana user. *American Journal of Sociology* 59:235–242.

Black, J. L., Dolan, M. P., DeFord, H. A., Rubenstein, J. A., Penk, W. E., Robinowitz, R., and Skinner, J. R. (1986) Sharing of needles among users of IV drugs (letter). *New England Journal of Medicine* 314:446–447.

Blattner, W., Biggar, R. J., Weiss, S. H., Melbye, M., and Goedert, J. J. (1985) Epidemiology of human T-lymphotropic virus type III and the risk of acquired immunodeficiency syndrome. *Annals of Internal Medicine* 103:665–670.

Blix, O., and Gronbladh, L. (1988) AIDS and IV Heroin Addicts: The Preventive Effect of Methadone Maintenance in Sweden. Presented at the Fourth International AIDS Conference, Stockholm, June 12–16.

Bortolotti, F., Stivanello, A., Carraro, L., and LaGrasta, F. (1988) Effect of AIDS Prevention Campaign on the Behavior of Drug Abusers in Italy. Presented at the Fourth International AIDS Conference, Stockholm, June 12–16.

Bottiger, M., Forsgren, M., Grillner, L., Biberfeld, G., Eriksson, G., and Jonzon, R. (1988) Monitoring of HIV Infection Among IV Drug Users in Stockholm. Presented at the Fourth International AIDS Conference, Stockholm, June 12–16.

Bradburn, N. M., Rips, L. J., and Shevell, S. V. (1987) Answering autobiographic questions: The impact of memory and inference on surveys. *Science* 263:157–161.

Bray, R. M., Schlenger, W. E., Craddock, S. G., Hubbard, R. L., and Rachal, J. V. (1982) Approaches to the Assessment of Drug Use in the Treatment Outcome Prospective Study. RTI/1901/01-05S. Research Triangle Institute, Research Triangle Park, N.C.

Brook, J. S., Whiteman, M., and Gordon, A. S. (1982) Qualitative and quantitative aspects of adolescent drug use: Interplay of personality, family, and peer correlates. *Psychological Reports* 51:1151–1163.

Brook, J. S., Whiteman, M., Gordon, A. S., Namura, C., and Brook, D. (1986) Onset of adolescent drinking: A longitudinal study of intrapersonal and interpersonal antecedents. *Advances in Alcohol and Substance Abuse* 5:91–110.

Brown, L. S., Jr. (1981) Substance abuse and America: Historical perspective on the federal response to a social phenomenon. *Journal of the National Medical Association* 73:497–506.

Brown, L. S., Jr. (1988) IV Drug Use and HIV Disease. Paper prepared for the CBASSE Committee on AIDS Research and the Behavioral, Social, and Statistical Sciences.

Brown, L. S., Jr., and Primm, B. J. (1988) Sexual contacts of intravenous drug abusers: Implications for the next spread of the AIDS epidemic. *Journal of the National Medical Association* 80:651–656.

Brown, L. S., Jr., Murphy, D. L., and Primm, B. J. (1987) Needle sharing and AIDS in minorities. *Journal of the American Medical Association* 258:1474–1475.

Brown, L. S., Jr., Battjes, R., Primm, B. J., Foster, K., and Chu, A. (1988) Trends in HIV Infection Among Intravenous Drug Abusers (IVDAs). Presented at the Fourth International AIDS Conference, Stockholm, June 12–16.

Buning, E. (1987a) Amsterdam's Drug Policy and the Prevention of AIDS. Presented at the Conference on AIDS in the Drug Abuse Community and Heterosexual Transmission, Newark, N.J., March.

Buning, E. (1987b) Prevention Policy on AIDS Among Drug Addicts in Amsterdam. Presented at the Third International AIDS Conference, Washington, D.C., June 1–5.

Buning, E., Coutinho, R. A., and van Brussel, G. H. A. (1986) Preventing AIDS in drug addicts in Amsterdam. *Lancet* 1:1435–1436.

Buning, E., Hartgers, C., Verster, A. D., van Santen, G. W., and Coutinho, R. A. (1988) The Evaluation of the Needle/Syringe Exchange in Amsterdam. Presented at the Fourth International AIDS Conference, Stockholm, June 12–16.

Buning, E., van Brussel, G. H. A., and van Santen, G. W. (In press) Amsterdam's drug policy and its implication for controlling needle sharing. In R. Battjes and R. Pickens, eds., *Needle Sharing Among Intravenous Drug Abusers: National and International Perspectives.* NIDA Research Monograph. Rockville, Md.: National Institute on Drug Abuse.

Burt, M. P., Glynn, T. J., and Sowder, B. J. (1979) *Psychosocial Characteristics of Drug-Abusing Women.* NIDA Publ. ADM80-917. Rockville, Md.: National Institute on Drug Abuse.

Butynski, W., Record, N., Bruhn, P., and Canova, D. (1987) State Resources and Services Related to Alcohol and Drug Abuse Problems, FY 1986. National Association of State Alcohol and Drug Abuse Directors, Inc., Washington, D.C.

Casadonte, P. P., Des Jarlais, D. C., Friedman, S. R., and Rotrosen, J. (1988) Psychological and Behavioral Impact of Learning HIV Test Results in IV Drug Users. Presented at the Fourth International AIDS Conference, Stockholm, June 12–16.

Casavantes, E. J. (1976) *El Tecato: Cultural and Sociologic Factors Affecting Drug Use Among Chicanos,* 2d ed. Washington, D.C.: National Coalition of Spanish Speaking Mental Health Organizations.

Centers for Disease Control (CDC). (1987a) Human immunodeficiency virus infection in the United States: A review of current knowledge. *Morbidity and Mortality Weekly Report* 36(Suppl. S-6):1–48.

Centers for Disease Control (CDC). (1987b) Human Immunodeficiency Virus Infections in the United States: A Review of Current Knowledge and Plans for Expansion of HIV Surveillance Activities. Report to the Domestic Policy Council. Centers for Disease Control, Atlanta, Ga. November 30.

Centers for Disease Control (CDC). (1988) *AIDS Weekly Surveillance Report for November 14, 1988.* Atlanta, Ga.: Centers for Disease Control.

Chaisson, R. E., Osmond, D., Moss, A., Feldman, H., and Bernacki, P. (1987a) HIV, bleach, and needle sharing (letter). *Lancet* 1:1430.

Chaisson, R. E., Moss, A. R., Onishi, R., Osmond, D., and Carlson, J. R. (1987b) Human immunodeficiency virus infection in heterosexual intravenous drug users in San Francisco. *American Journal of Public Health* 77:169–172.

Chaisson, R. E., Osmond, D., Bacchetti, P., Brodiek, B., Sande, M. A., and Moss, A. R. (1988) Cocaine, Race, and HIV Infection in IV Drug Users. Presented at the Fourth International AIDS Conference, Stockholm, June 12–16.

Chiasson, M. A., Stoneburner, R. L., Lifson, A. E., Hildebrandt, D., and Jaffee, H. W. (1988) No Association Between HIV-1 Seropositivity and Prostitute Contact in New York City. Presented at the Fourth International AIDS Conference, Stockholm, June 12–16.

Coates, T. J., Stall, R., Mandel, J. S., Boccellari, A., Sorensen, J., Morales, E. F., Morin, S. F., Wiley, J. A., and McKusick, L. (1987) AIDS: A psychosocial research agenda. *Annals of Behavioral Medicine* 9:21–28.

Cohen, J. B. (1987) Condom Promotion Among Prostitutes. Department of Epidemiology and General Medicine, University of California at San Francisco.

Cohen, J. B., Poole, L. E., Lyons, C. A., Lockett, G. J., Alexander, P., and Wofsy, C. B. (1988) Sexual Behavior and HIV Infection Risk Among 354 Sex Industry Women in a Participant Based Research and Prevention Program. Presented at the Fourth International AIDS Conference, Stockholm, June 12–16.

Cohen, J. B., Hauer, L. B., and Wofsy, C. B. (In press) Women and IV drugs: Parenteral and heterosexual transmission of human immunodeficiency virus. *Journal of Drug Issues.*

Collins, J. J., McCalla, M. E., and Powers, L. L. (1988) Drug Use and Serious Crime in Three Cities. Presented at the 40th Annual Meeting of the Society of Criminology, Chicago, November 9–12.

Collins, J. J., Rachal, J. V., Hubbard, R. L., Cavanaugh, E. R., Craddock, S. G., and Kristiansen, P. L. (1982) Criminality in a Drug Treatment Sample: Measurement Issues and Initial Findings. RTI/1901/01-07S. Research Triangle Institute, Research Triangle Park, N.C.

Curran, J. W. (1988) The Epidemiology of HIV Infection and AIDS in the United States. Presented at the Fourth International AIDS Conference, Stockholm, June 12–16.

Cuskey, W. R., and Wathey, R. B. (1982) *Female Addiction: A Longitudinal Study.* Lexington, Mass.: Lexington Books.

Darrow, W. W. (1987) Condom Use and Use-Effectiveness in High-Risk Populations. Presented at the Conference on Condoms in the Prevention of Sexually Transmitted Diseases, Centers for Disease Control, Atlanta, Ga., February.

Darrow, W. W., Bigler, W., Deppe, D., French, J., Gill, P., and Wofsy, C. (1988) HIV Antibody in 640 U.S. Prostitutes with No Evidence of Intravenous (IV)-Drug Abuse. Presented at the Fourth International AIDS Conference, Stockholm, June 12–16.

de la Loma, A., Garcia, S., Ramos, P., and Neila, M. A. (1988) Poor Lifestyle Modification Among IV Drug Users Assisted at an STD Clinic for HIV Infection Diagnosis. Presented at the Fourth International AIDS Conference, Stockholm, June 12–16.

Densen-Gerber, J., Wiener, M., and Hichstedler, R. (1972) Sexual behavior, abortion and birth control in heroin addicts: Legal and psychiatric considerations. *Contemporary Drug Problems* 1:783–793.

Des Jarlais, D. C. (1987a) Effectiveness of AIDS educational programs for intravenous drug users. Background paper prepared for the Health Program, Office of Technology Assessment, U.S. Congress, Washington, D.C.

Des Jarlais, D. C. (1987b) Research on HIV Infection Among Intravenous Drug Users: State of the Art and State of the Epidemic. Presented at the Third International AIDS Conference, Washington, D.C., June 1–5.

Des Jarlais, D. C. (1988) HIV Infection Among Persons Who Inject Illicit Drugs: Problems and Progress. Presented at the Fourth International AIDS Conference, Stockholm, June 12–16.

Des Jarlais, D. C., and Friedman, S. R. (1987a) AIDS and the Sharing of Equipment for Illicit Drug Injection: A Review of Current Data. Prepared for the National Institute on Drug Abuse. New York State Division of Substance Abuse, New York City.

Des Jarlais, D. C., and Friedman, S. R. (1987b) HIV infection among intravenous drug users: Epidemiology and risk reduction. *AIDS* 1:67–76.

Des Jarlais, D. C., and Friedman, S. R. (1988) Gender differences in response to HIV infection. Pp. 159–163 in T. P. Bridge, A. F. Mirsky, and F. K. Goodwin, eds., *Psychological, Neuropsychiatric, and Substance Abuse Aspects of AIDS*. New York: Raven Press.

Des Jarlais, D. C., and Hopkins, W. (1985) Free needles for intravenous drug users at risk for AIDS: Current developments in New York City (letter). *New England Journal of Medicine* 313:1476.

Des Jarlais, D. C., Chamberland, M. E., Yancovitz, S. R., Weinberg, P., and Friedman, S. R. (1984) Heterosexual partners: A large risk group for AIDS. *Lancet* 2:1346–1347.

Des Jarlais, D. C., Friedman, S. R., and Hopkins, W. (1985) Risk reduction for the acquired immunodeficiency syndrome among intravenous drug users. *Annals of Internal Medicine* 313:755–759.

Des Jarlais, D. C., Friedman, S. R., and Strug, D. (1986a) Acquired immunodeficiency syndrome among intravenous drug users: A sociocultural perspective. In D. A. Feldman and T. M. Johnson, eds., *The Social Dimensions of AIDS: Method and Theory*. New York: Praeger.

Des Jarlais, D. C., Friedman, S. R., and Strug, D. (1986b) AIDS and needle sharing within the IV-drug use subculture. In D. A. Feldman and T. M. Johnson, eds., *The Social Dimensions of AIDS: Method and Theory*. New York: Praeger.

Des Jarlais, D. C., Friedman, S. R., Spira, T. J., et al. (1986c) A stage model of HTLV-III LAV infection in intravenous drug users. Pp. 328–334 in *Problems of Drug Dependence*. Proceedings of the 47th Annual Scientific Meeting, Committee on Problems of Drug Dependence. NIDA Research Monograph No. 67. Rockville, Md.: National Institute on Drug Abuse.

Des Jarlais, D. C., Wish, E., Friedman, S. R., Stoneburner, R. L., Yancovitz, F., Mildban, D., El-Sadr, W., Brady, E., and Cuadrado, M. (1987) Intravenous drug users and the heterosexual transmission of the acquired immunodeficiency syndrome. *New York State Journal of Medicine* 87:283–286.

Des Jarlais, D. C., Friedman, S. R., and Stoneburner, R. L. (1988a) HIV infection and intravenous drug use: Critical issues in transmission dynamics, infection outcomes, and prevention. *Reviews of Infectious Diseases* 10:155.

Des Jarlais, D. C., Sotheran, J., Stoneburner, R. L., Friedman, S. R., Marmor, M., and Maslansky, R. (1988b) HIV-1 is associated with fatal infectious diseases other than AIDS among intravenous drug users. Presented at the Fourth International AIDS Conference, Stockholm, June 12–16.

Dolan, M. P., Black, J. L., Deford, H. A., Skinner, J. R., and Rabinowitz, R. (1987) Characteristics of drug abusers that discriminate needle sharers. *Public Health Reports* 102:395–398.

Doscher, M. L., and Woodward, J. A. (1983) Estimating the size of subpopulations of heroin users: Applications of log-linear models to capture/recapture sampling. *International Journal of the Addictions* 18:167–182.

Drew, L. R. (1986) Beyond the disease concept of addiction: Drug use as a way of life leading to predicaments. *Journal of Drug Issues* 16:263–274.

Eckerman, W. C., Rachal, J. V., Hubbard, R. L., and Poole, W. K. (1976) Methodological issues in identifying drug users. In *Drug Use and Crime*. Report of the Panel on Drug Use and Criminal Behavior (Appendix). Research Triangle Park, N.C.: Research Triangle Institute.

Espinoza, P., Bouchard, I., Ballian, P., and Pelo DeVoto, J. (1988) Has the Open Sale of Syringes Modified the Syringe Exchange Habits of Drug Addicts. Presented at the Fourth International AIDS Conference, Stockholm, June 12–16.

Evans, R. I., and Raines, B. E. (1982) Control and prevention of smoking in adolescents: A psychosocial perspective. Pp. 101–129 in T. Coates, A. Petersen, and C. Perry, eds., *Promoting Adolescent Health: A Dialogue on Research and Practice*. New York: Academic Press.

Faltz, B., and Madover, S. (1987) Substance abuse as a co-factor for AIDS. In *Women and AIDS Clinical Resource Guide,* 2d ed. San Francisco: San Francisco AIDS Foundation.

Feldman, H. W. (1977) A neighborhood history of drug switching. Pp. 249–278 in R. S. Weppner, ed., *Street Ethnography: Selected Studies of Crime and Drug Use in Natural Settings*. Beverly Hills, Calif.: Sage Publications.

Feldman, H. W., and Biernacki, P. (1987) The Ethnography of Needle Sharing Among Intravenous Drug Users and Implications for Public Policies and Intervention Strategies. Presented at the Technical Review Meeting, National Institute on Drug Abuse, Bethesda, Md., May 18–19.

Fields, A., and Walters, J. M. (1985) Hustling: Supporting a heroin habit. In B. Hanson, G. Beschner, J. M. Walters, and E. Bovelle, eds., *Life with Heroin*. Lexington, Mass.: Lexington Books.

Fishburne, P. M., Abelson, H. I., and Cisin, I. (1980) *National Survey on Drug Abuse: Main Findings, 1979*. Rockville, Md.: National Institute on Drug Abuse.

Flavin, D. K., and Frances, R. J. (1987) Risk taking behavior, substance abuse disorders, and the acquired immunodeficiency syndrome. *Advances in Alcohol and Substance Abuse* 6:23–31.

Flynn, N. M., Jain, S., Harper, S., Bailey, V., Anderson, R., Acuna, G., et al. (1987) Sharing of Paraphernalia in Intravenous Drug Users (IVDU): Knowledge of AIDS Is Incomplete and Doesn't Affect Behavior. Presented at the Third International AIDS Conference, Washington, D.C., June 1–5.

Flynn, N. M., Jain, S., Bailey, V., Siegal, B., Bank, V., Nassar, N., Lindo, J., Harper, S., and Ding, D. (1988a) Characteristics and Stated AIDS Risk Behavior of IV Drug Users Attending Drug Treatment Programs in a Medium-Sized U.S. City. Presented at the Fourth International AIDS Conference, Stockholm, June 12–16.

Flynn, N. M., Jain, S., Keddie, E., Harper, S., Carlson, J., and Bailey, V. (1988b) Cleaning IV Paraphernalia: Bleach Was Just the Beginning. Presented at the Fourth International AIDS Conference, Stockholm, June 12–16.

Friedland, G. H., and Klein, R. S. (1987) Transmission of the human immunodeficiency virus. *New England Journal of Medicine* 347:1125–1135.

Friedland, G. H., Harris, C., Butkus-Small, C., Shine, D., Moll, B., Darrow, W., and Klein, R. S. (1985) Intravenous drug users and the acquired immunodeficiency syndrome: Demographic, drug use, and needle sharing patterns. *Archives of Internal Medicine* 145:1413–1417.

Friedman, S. R., and Des Jarlais, D. C. (1988) Dimensions of Prevention Programs Among Intravenous Drug Users. Presented at the Fourth International AIDS Conference, Stockholm, June 12–16.

Friedman, S. R., Des Jarlais, D. C., and Sotheran, J. (1986) AIDS health education for intravenous drug users. *Health Education Quarterly* 13:383–393.

Friedman, S. R., Sotheran, J. L., Abdul-Quader, A., Primm, B. J., Des Jarlais, D. C., Kleinman, P., Mauge, C., Goldsmith, D. S., El-Sadr, W., and Maslansky, R. (1987a) The AIDS epidemic among blacks and Hispanics. *Milbank Quarterly* 65(Suppl. 2):455–499.

Friedman, S. R., Des Jarlais, D. C., Sotheran, J., Garber, J., Cohen, H., and Smith, D. (1987b) AIDS and self-organization among intravenous drug users. *International Journal of the Addictions* 22:201–219.

Friedman, S. R., Dozier, C., Sterk, C., Williams, T., Sotheran, J. L., Des Jarlais, D. C., et al. (1988) Crack Use Puts Women at Risk for Heterosexual Transmission of HIV from Intravenous Drug Users. Presented at the Fourth International AIDS Conference, Stockholm, June 12–16.

Fuchs, D., Unterweger, B., Hinterhuber, H., Dierich, M. P., Weiss, S. H., Wachter, H., et al. (1988) Successful Preventive Measures in a Community of IV Drug Addicts. Presented at the Fourth International AIDS Conference, Stockholm, June 12–16.

Gerstein, D. R. (1976) The structure of heroin communities in relation to methadone maintenance. *American Journal of Drug and Alcohol Abuse* 3:571–587.

Gibson, D. R., Wermuth, L., Lovelle-Drache, J., Ergas, B., Ham, J., and Sorenson, J. L. (1988) Brief Psychoeducational Counseling to Reduce AIDS Risk in IV Drug Users and Sexual Partners. Presented at the Fourth International AIDS Conference, Stockholm, June 12–16.

Ginzburg, H. M. (1984) Intravenous drug users and the acquired immunodeficiency syndrome. *Public Health Reports* 99:206–212.

Ginzburg, H. M., and MacDonald, M. G. (1986) The epidemiology of human T-cell lymphotropic virus, type-III (HTLV-III diseases). *Psychiatric Annals* 16:153–157.

Ginzburg, H. M., MacDonald, M. G., and Glass, J. W. (1987) AIDS, HTLV-III diseases, minorities, and intravenous drug use. *Advances in Alcohol and Substance Abuse* 6:7–21.

Glenn, W. A., and Hartwell, T. D. (1975) Review of Methods of Estimating Number of Narcotic Addicts. Research Triangle Institute, Research Triangle Park, N.C.

Gold, M. S., Dackis, C. A., Pottash, A., Extein, I., and Washton, A. (1986) Cocaine update: From bench to bedside. *Advances in Alcohol and Substance Abuse* 5:35–60.

Goldberg, D., Watson, H., Stuart, F., Miller, M., Gruer, L., and Follett, E. (1988) Pharmacy Supply of Needles and Syringes–The Effect on Spread of HIV in Intravenous Drug Misusers. Presented at the Fourth International AIDS Conference, Stockholm, June 12–16.

Goldsmith, D., Hunt, D. E., Strug, D., and Lipton, D. S. (1984) Methadone folklore: Beliefs about side effects and their impact on treatment. *Human Organization* 43:330–340.

Goldstein, P. J., Bellucci, P. A., Spunt, B. J., Miller, T., Cortez, N., Khan, M., Durrance, R., and Vega, A. (1988) *Female Drug Related Involvement in Violent Episodes.* New York: Narcotic and Drug Research, Inc.

Greenberg, S. W., and Roberson, C. B. (1978) Analysis of Drug Abuse Correlates—Final Report. Research Triangle Institute, Research Triangle Park, N.C.

Greenwood, J. A. (1970) Estimate of Number of Chronic Narcotic Abusers in New York City. Cited in background material prepared for the committee by R. L. Hubbard, Research Triangle Institute, Research Triangle Park, N.C.

Guinan, M. E., and Hardy, A. (1987) Epidemiology of AIDS in women in the U.S., 1981–1986. *Journal of the American Medical Association* 257:2039–2042.

Hahn, R. A., Onorato, I. M., Jones, T. S., and Dougherty, J. (1988) Infection with Human Immunodeficiency Virus (HIV) Among Intravenous Drug Users (IVDUs) in the U.S. Presented at the Fourth International AIDS Conference, Stockholm, June 12–16.

Hanson, B., Beschner, G., Walters, J. M., and Bovelle, E., eds. (1985) *Life with Heroin.* Lexington, Mass.: Lexington Books.

Harding, W., and Zinberg, N. (1977) The effectiveness of the subculture in developing rituals and sanctions for controlled drug use. In B. DuToit, ed., *Drugs, Rituals, and Altered States of Consciousness.* Rotterdam: A. A. Balkena.

Hardy, A. M., Starcher, E. T., Morgan, W. M., Drucker, J., Kristal, A., Day, J. M., Kelly, C., Ewing, E., and Curran, J. W. (1987) Review of death certificates to assess completeness of AIDS case reporting. *Public Health Reports* 102:386–390.

Harrell, A. (1985) Validation of self-report: The research records. In *Self-Report Methods of Estimating Drug Use: Meeting Current Challenges to Validity.* NIDA Research Monograph No. 57. Rockville, Md.: National Institute on Drug Abuse.

Harris, C., Butkus-Small, C., Klein, R., Friedland, G. H., Moll, B., Emerson, E. E., Spigland, I., and Steigbigel, N. (1983) Immunodeficiency in female sexual partners of men with AIDS. *New England Journal of Medicine* 308:1181–1184.

Hart, G. J., Carvell, A., Johnson, A. M., Feinmann, C., Woodward, N., and Adler, M. W. (1988) Needle Exchange in Central London. Presented at the Fourth International AIDS Conference, Stockholm, June 12–16.

Hartel, D., Selwyn, P. A., Schoenbaum, E. E., Klein, R. S., and Friedland, G. H. (1988) Methadone Maintenance Treatment (MMTP) and Reduced Risk of AIDS and AIDS-Specific Mortality in Intravenous Drug Users (IVDUs). Presented at the Fourth International AIDS Conference, Stockholm, June 12–16.

Hemdal, P. (1986) Psychological and Behavioral Impact of Learning HTLV-III/LAV Antibody Test Results. Presented at the Second International AIDS Conference, Paris, June 25–26.

Hessol, N. A., O'Malley, P. M., Rutherford, G. W., Darrow, W. W., et al. (1987) Sexual Transmission of Human Immunodeficiency Virus Infection in Homosexual and Bisexual Men Who Participated in Hepatitis B Vaccine Trials. Presented at the Twentieth Annual Meeting of the Society for Epidemiologic Research, Amherst, Mass., June 17.

Hopkins, D. R. (1987) AIDS in minority populations in the U.S. *Public Health Reports* 102:677–681.

Huba, G. J., and Bentler, P. M. (1980) The role of peer and adult models for drug taking at different stages of adolescence. *Journal of Youth and Adolescence* 9:449–465.

Hubbard, R. L., Eckerman, W. C., Rachal, J. V., and William, J. R. (1978) Factors affecting the validity of self-reports of drug use: An overview. In *Proceedings of the American Statistical Association, 1977.* Washington, D.C.: American Statistical Association.

Hubbard, R. L., Schlenger, W. E., Rachal, J. V., Bray, R. M., Craddock, S. G., Cavanaugh, E. R., and Ginzburg, H. M. (1983) Patterns of Alcohol and Drug Abuse of Drug Treatment Clients with Different Ethnic Backgrounds. Presented at the Conference on Alcohol and Culture: Comparative Perspectives from Europe and America, Research Triangle Park Institute, Research Triangle Park, N.C., May 5–7.

Hubbard, R. L., Marsden, M. E., Cavanaugh, E., and Rachal, J. V. (1985a) *Drug Use After Drug Abuse Treatment: Followup of 1979–1980 TOPS Admission Cohorts.* NIDA Treatment Research Monograph Series. Rockville, Md.: National Institute on Drug Abuse.

Hubbard, R. L., Bray, R. M., and Craddock, S. G. (1985b) Issues in the assessment of multiple drug use among drug treatment clients. In M. Baude and H. M. Ginzburg, eds., *Strategies for Research on Drugs of Abuse.* NIDA Research Monograph Series. Rockville, Md.: National Institute on Drug Abuse.

Hubbard, R. L., Marsden, M. E., Cavanaugh, E., and Rachal, J. V. (1986) Drug Use After Drug Treatment. Background paper prepared for the IOM/NAS Committee on a National Strategy for AIDS. April.

Hubbard, R. L., Marsden, M. E., Cavanaugh, E., Rachal, J. V., and Ginzburg, H. M. (1988) Role of drug-abuse treatment in limiting the spread of AIDS. *Reviews of Infectious Diseases* 10:377–384.

Hunt, D. E., Strug, D. L., Goldsmith, D. S., Lipton, D. S., Spunt, B., Truitt, L., and Robertson, K. A. (1984a) An instant shot of aah: Cocaine use among methadone clients. *Journal of Psychoactive Drugs* 16:217–227.

Hunt, D. E., Lipton, D. S., Goldsmith, D., and Strug, D. (1984b) Street pharmacology: Uses of cocaine and heroin in the treatment of addiction. *Drug and Alcohol Dependence* 13:375–387.

Iglehart, A. (1985) Brickin' it and going to the pan: Vernacular in the black inner-city heroin lifestyle. In B. Hanson, G. Beschner, J. M. Walters, and E. Bovelle, eds., *Life with Heroin.* Lexington, Mass.: Lexington Books.

Inciardi, J. A. (1987) Beyond cocaine: Basuco, crack, and other coca products. *Contemporary Drug Problems* 14:461–492.

Institute of Medicine/National Academy of Sciences (IOM/NAS). (1988) *Confronting AIDS: Update 1988.* Washington, D.C.: National Academy Press.

Jackson, J., and Baxter, B. (1988) AIDS Coordinators in Drug Treatment Programs. Presented at the Fourth International AIDS Conference, Stockholm, June 12–16.

Jackson, J., and Neshin, S. (1986) New Jersey Community Health Project: Impact of Using Ex-Addict Education to Disseminate Information on AIDS to Intravenous Users. Presented at the Second International AIDS Conference, Paris, June 25–26.

Jackson, J., and Rotkiewicz, L. (1987) A Coupon Program: AIDS Education and Drug Treatment. Presented at the Third International AIDS Conference, Washington, D.C., June 1–5.

Jacobs, S. E., Kleyn, J., Osborne, O., Clay, C., and Freeman, C. (1988) Intervention Ethnography in Two Communities at High Risk for AIDS. Presented at a meeting of the Society for Applied Anthropology, Tampa, Fla., April 20–23.

Johnson, B. D., and Goldstein, P. J. (1984) Highlights from the Final Report: Economic Behavior of Street Opiate Users. Narcotic and Drug Research, Inc., and the New York State Division of Substance Abuse Services, New York City.

Johnson, B. D., Goldstein, P. J., Preble, E., Schmeidler, J., Lipton, D., Spunt, B., and Miller, T. (1985) *Taking Care of Business: The Economics of Crime by Heroin Abusers.* Lexington, Mass.: Lexington Books.

Johnson, E. M. (1987) Substance abuse and women's health. *Public Health Reports* 1(Suppl.):42–48.

Johnson, R. E., Marcos, A., and Bahr, S. (1987) The role of peers in the complex ideology of adolescent drug use. *Criminology* 25:323–339.

Johnston, L. D., Bachman, J. G., and O'Malley, P. M. (1981) *Student Drug Use in America, 1975–1981.* DHHS Publ. No. ADM 82-1221. Rockville, Md.: National Institute on Drug Abuse.

Jorquez, J. S. (1983) The retirement phase of heroin using careers. *Journal of Drug Issues* 13:343–365.

Jorquez, J. S. (1984) Heroin use in the barrio: Solving the problem of relapse or keeping the *tecato gusano* asleep. *American Journal of Drug and Alcohol Abuse* 10:63–75.

Kandel, D., Kessler, R., and Margulies, R. (1978) Adolescent initiation into stages of drug use: A developmental analysis. In D. Kandel, ed., *Longitudinal Research on Drug Use: Empirical Findings and Methodological Issues.* Washington, D.C.: Hemisphere Publishing Corporation.

Kandel, D., Simcha-Fagen, O., and Davies, M. (1986) Risk factors for delinquency and illicit drug use from adolescence to young adulthood. *Journal of Drug Issues* 16:67–90.

Kreek, M. J., Des Jarlais, D. C., Trepo, C., Novick, D., Quader, A., and Raghunath, J. (1987) Hepatitis Delta Anigenemia in Intravenous Drug Abusers with AIDS: Potential Risk for Health Care Workers. Presented at the Third International AIDS Conference, Washington, D.C., June 1–5.

Krosnick, J. A., and Judd, C. M. (1982) Transitions in social influence and adolescence: Who induces cigarette smoking? *Developmental Psychology* 18:359-368.

Lange, W. R., Snyder, F. R., Lozovsky, D., Kaistha, V., Kaczaniuk, M. A., and Jaffe, J. H. (1987) HIV infection in Baltimore: Antibody seroprevalence rates among parenteral drug abusers and prostitutes. *Maryland Medical Journal* 36:757–761.

Lange, W. R., Snyder, F. R., Lozovsky, D., Kaistha, V., Kaczaniuk, M. A., Jaffe, J. H., and the ARD Epidemiology Collaborating Group. (1988) Geographic distribution of human immunodeficiency virus markers in parenteral drug abusers. *American Journal of Public Health* 78:443–446.

Lettau, L. A., Smith, M. H., Morse, L. J., Bessette, R., Irvine, W. G., Grady, G. F., McCarthy, J. G., Hadler, S. C., Ukena, T., Gurwitz, A., Fields, H. A., and Maynard, J. E. (1987) Outbreak of severe hepatitis due to delta and hepatitis B viruses in parenteral drug abusers and their contacts. *New England Journal of Medicine* 317:1256–1262.

Levin, G., Roberts, E. B., and Hirsch, G. B. (1975) *The Persistent Poppy: A Computer-Aided Search for Heroin Policy.* Cambridge, Mass.: Ballinger.

Ljungberg, B., Andersson, B., Christensson, B., Hugo-Persson, M., Tunving, K., and Ursing, B. (1988) Distribution of Sterile Equipment to IV Drug Abusers as Part of an HIV Prevention Program. Presented at the Fourth International AIDS Conference, Stockholm, June 12–16.

Louria, D., Hensle, T., and Rose, J. (1967) The major medical complications of heroin addiction. *Annals of Internal Medicine* 67:1–22.

Lourie, K. (1986) On the Contradictions of Working Class Drug Subcultures: A Comparative Ethnography. Master's thesis, Brown University.

Lourie, K. (1988) Working Class Youth Drug Subculture: An Anthropological Approach to Sexual Meaning. Cited in background material prepared for the CBASSE Committee on AIDS Research and the Behavioral, Social, and Statistical Sciences by S. Lindenbaum, New School for Social Research, New York.

Lowenstein, W. A., Durand, H., Stern, M., and Tourani, J. M. (1988) Changes of Behavior in French IV Drug Addicts (IVDA). Presented at the Fourth International AIDS Conference, Stockholm, June 12–16.

Macks, J. (1988) Women and AIDS: Countertransference issues. *Social Casework* 69:340–347.

Maddux, J., and Desmond, B. (1975) Reliability and validity of information from chronic heroin users. *Psychiatric Research* 12:87–95.

Marmor, M., Sanchez, M., Krasinski, K., Cohen, H., Bartelme, S., Weiss, L. R., et al. (1987a) Risk Factors for Human Immunodeficiency Virus Infection Among Heterosexuals in New York City. Presented at the Third International AIDS Conference, Washington, D.C., June 1–5.

Marmor, M., Des Jarlais, D. C., Cohen, H., Friedman, S. R., Beatrice, S. T., Dubin, N., El-Sadr, W., Mildvan, D., Yancovitz, S., Mathur, U., and Holzman, R. (1987b) Risk factors for infection with human immunodeficiency virus among intravenous drug abusers in New York City. *AIDS* 1:39–44.

Masters, W. H., Johnson, V. E., and Kolodny, R. C. (1988) *Crisis: Heterosexual Behavior in the Age of AIDS.* New York: Grove Press.

Mata, A. G., and Jorquez, J. S. (In press) Mexican-American Intravenous Drug Users' Needle-Sharing Practices: Implications for AIDS Prevention. NIDA Research Monograph Series. Rockville, Md.: National Institute on Drug Abuse.

Mays, V., and Cochran, S. (1987) AIDS and black Americans: Special psychosocial issues. *Public Health Reports* 102:224–231.

McAuliffe, W. E., Doering, S., Breer, P., Silverman, H., Branson, B., and Williams, K. (1987) An Evaluation of Using Ex-Addict Outreach Workers to Educate Intravenous Drug Users About AIDS Prevention. Presented at the Third International AIDS Conference, Washington, D.C., June 1–5.

Miller, J. D., Cisin, I. H., Gardner-Keaton, H., Harrell, A. V., Wirtz, P. W., Abelson, H. I., and Fishburne, P. M. (1983) National Survey on Drug Abuse. Prepared for the National Institute on Drug Abuse by George Washington University, Washington, D.C., and the Response Analysis Corporation, Princeton, N.J. National Institute on Drug Abuse, Rockville, Md.

Minichiello, L. (1974) Indicators of Intravenous Drug Use in the United States, 1966–1973. Cited in background material prepared for the CBASSE Committee on AIDS Research and the Behavioral, Social, and Statistical Sciences by R. L. Hubbard, Research Triangle Institute, Research Triangle Park, N.C.

Mondanaro, J. (1987) Strategies for AIDS prevention: Motivating health behavior in drug dependent women. *Journal of Psychoactive Drugs* 19:143–149.

Moore, J. W., and Mata, A. G. (1982) *Women and Heroin in a Chicano Community: A Final Report.* Los Angeles: Chicano Pinto Research Project.

Morales, A. (1984) Substance abuse and Mexican-American youth: An overview. *Journal of Drug Issues* 14:297–311.

Mosely, J., Kramer, T. H., Cancellieri, F., and Ottomenelli, G. (1988) Survey of Condom Use in Substance Abusers. Presented at the Fourth International AIDS Conference, Stockholm, June 12–16.

Moss, A. R. (1987) AIDS and intravenous drug use: The real heterosexual epidemic. *British Medical Journal* 294:389–390.

Moss, A. R., and Chaisson, R. E. (1988) AIDS and intravenous drug use in San Francisco. *AIDS and Public Policy Journal* 3:37–41.

Moss, A. R., Chaisson, R. E., Osmond, D., Bacchetti, P., and Meakin, R. (1988a) Control of HIV Infection in Intravenous Drug Users in San Francisco. Presented at the Fourth International AIDS Conference, Stockholm, June 12–16.

Moss, A. R., Bacchetti, P., Osmond, D., Krampf, W., Chaisson, R., Stites, D., Wilber, J., Allain, J. P., and Carlson, J. (1988b) Seropositivity for HIV and the development of AIDS or AIDS related condition: 3 year followup of the San Francisco General Hospital cohort. *British Medical Journal* 296:745–750.

Murphy, S. (1988) Intravenous drug use and AIDS: Notes on the social economy of needle sharing. *Contemporary Drug Problems* 14:373–395.

National Institute on Drug Abuse (NIDA). (1981) *CODAP 1981: Data from the Client-Oriented Data Acquisition Process.* NIDA Statistical Series E, No. 25. Rockville, Md.: National Institute on Drug Abuse.

National Institute on Drug Abuse (NIDA). (1985a) Demographic Characteristics and Patterns of Drug Use of Clients Admitted to Drug Abuse Treatment Programs in Selected States: Annual Data, 1985 (analyses of unpublished data). National Institute on Drug Abuse, Rockville, Md.

National Institute on Drug Abuse (NIDA). (1985b) *Epidemiology of Heroin: 1964–1984.* Rockville, Md.: National Institute on Drug Abuse.

National Institute on Drug Abuse (NIDA). (1985c) National Household Survey on Drug Abuse: Main Findings, 1985 (analyses of unpublished data). National Institute on Drug Abuse, Rockville, Md.

Newmeyer, J. A. (1986) The IV Drug User and Secondary Spread of AIDS. Background paper prepared for the IOM/NAS Committee on a National Strategy for AIDS. December.

Newmeyer, J. A. (1988) The Micro-World of Needle Sharing. Paper prepared for the CBASSE Committee on AIDS Research and the Behavioral, Social, and Statistical Sciences.

Novick, D. M., Kreek, M. J., Des Jarlais, D. C., Spira, T. J., et al. (1986) Antibody to LAV in parenteral drug abusers and methadone-maintained patients: Therapeutic, historical, and ethical aspects. In *Problems of Drug Dependence.* Proceedings of the 47th Annual Scientific Meeting, Committee on Problems of Drug Dependence. NIDA Research Monograph No. 67. Rockville, Md.: National Institute on Drug Abuse.

Novick, L. F., Truman, B. I., and Lehman, J. S. (1988) The epidemiology of HIV in New York State. *New York State Journal of Medicine* 88:242–246.

O'Brien, J. F. (1973) Motivation Aspects of Regular Drug Use: A System Simulation. Doctoral dissertation, North Carolina State University.

Olin, R., and Kall, K. (1988) HIV Status and Risk Behavior Among Imprisoned Intravenous Drug Abusers in Stockholm. Presented at the Fourth International AIDS Conference, Stockholm, June 12–16.

Page, J. B., Chitwood, D. D., and Smith, P. C. (1988) What You Know and Who You Shoot With: Parenteral Drug Use and Risk of HIV Infection. Presented at a meeting of the Society for Applied Anthropology, Tampa, Fla., April 20–23.

Person, P., Retka, R. L., and Woodward, J. A. (1976) *Toward a Heroin Problem Index: An Analytic Model for Drug Indicators.* DHEW Publ. No. ADM 76-367. Washington, D.C.: U.S. Department of Health, Education, and Welfare.

Polich, J. M., Ellickson, P. L., Reuter, P., and Kahan, J. P. (1984) *Strategies for Controlling Adolescent Drug Use.* Santa Monica, Calif.: The Rand Corporation.

Powell, D. H. (1973) A pilot study of occasional heroin users. *Archives of General Psychiatry* 28:586–594.

Preble, E., and Miller, T. (1977) Methadone, wine and welfare. Pp. 229–249 in R. Weppner, ed., *Street Ethnography: Selected Studies of Crime and Drug Use in Natural Settings.* Beverly Hills, Calif.: Sage Publications.

Primm, B. J., Brown, L. S., Gibson, B. S., and Chu, A. (1988) The Range of Sexual Behaviors of Intravenous Drug Abusers. Presented at the Fourth International AIDS Conference, Stockholm, June 12–16.

Rachal, J. V., Guess, L. L., and Marsden, M. E. (1986) Living Arrangements, Ethnicity, and Young Adult Drinking Patterns. Presented at the annual meeting of the American Public Health Association, Las Vegas, September 30.

Ralph, N., and Spigner, C. (1986) Contraceptive practices among female heroin addicts. *American Journal of Public Health* 76:1016–1017.

Raymond, C. A. (1988) First needle-exchange program approved; other cities await results. *Journal of the American Medical Association* 259:1289–1290.

Reinarman, C., and Leigh, B. C. (1987) Culture, cognition, and disinhibition: Notes on sexuality and alcohol in the age of AIDS. *Contemporary Drug Problems* 14:435–460.

Resnick, L., Veren, K., Salahuddin, S. Z., Tondreau, S., and Markham, P. D. (1986) Stability and inactivation of HTLV-III/LAV under clinical and laboratory environments. *Journal of the American Medical Association* 255:1887–1891.

Rezza, G., Oliva, C., and Sasse, H. (1988) Preventing AIDS Among Italian Drug Addicts—Evaluation of Treatment Programs and Informative Strategies. Presented at the Fourth International AIDS Conference, Stockholm, June 12–16.

Robertson, J. R., Bucknall, A. B., and Welsby, P. D. (1986) Epidemic of AIDS related virus (HTLV-III/LAV) infection among IV drug abusers. *British Medical Journal* 292:527–529.

Robertson, J. R., Skidmore, C. A., and Roberts, J. J. K. (In press) HIV infection in intravenous drug users: A follow-up study indicating changes in risk taking behavior. *British Journal of Addiction.*

Robins, L., Helzer, J., and Davis, D. (1975) Narcotic use in Southeast Asia and afterward. *Archives of General Psychiatry* 23:955–961.

Rosenbaum, M. (1979a) Becoming addicted: The woman addict. *Contemporary Drug Problems* 8:141–166.

Rosenbaum, M. (1979b) Funneling Options: The Career of the Woman Addict. Ph.D. dissertation, University of California Medical Center, San Francisco.

Rosenbaum, M. (1981) Sex roles among deviants: The woman addict. *International Journal of the Addictions* 16:859–877.

Rosenbaum, M. (1985) *Women on Heroin.* New Brunswick, N.J.: Rutgers University Press.

Rosenbaum, M., Murphy, S., and Beck, J. (1987) Money for methadone: Preliminary findings from a study of Alameda County's new maintenance policy. *Journal of Psychoactive Drugs* 19:13–19.

Rouse, B. A., Kozel, N. J., and Richards, L. G., eds. (1985) Self-Report Methods of Estimating Drug Use: Meeting Current Challenges to Validity. NIDA Research Monograph No. 57. Rockville, Md.: National Institute on Drug Abuse.

Schlenger, W. E., and Greenberg, S. W. (1978) Characteristics of Cities and Their Relationship to Heroin Use: An Analysis of Heroin Use Correlates in Metropolitan Areas. Research Triangle Institute, Research Triangle Park, N.C.

Schoenbaum, E. E., Selwyn, P. A., Klein, R. S., et al. (1986) Prevalence of and Risk Factors Associated with HTLV-III/LAV Antibodies Among Intravenous Drug Abusers in Methadone Programs in New York City. Presented at the Second International AIDS Conference, Paris, June 25–26.

Schuster, C. R. (1988) Intravenous drug users and AIDS prevention. *Public Health Reports* 103:261–266.

Selwyn, P. A., Feiner, C., Cox, C. P., Lipshutz, C., and Cohen, R. L. (1987) Knowledge about AIDS and high-risk behavior among intravenous drug users in New York City. *AIDS* 1:247–254.

Serrano, Y., and Goldsmith, D. (1988) Adapt: A Response to HIV Infection in Intravenous Drug Users in New York. Presented at the Fourth International AIDS Conference, Stockholm, June 12–16.

Sharff, J. (1987) The underground economy of a poor neighborhood. In L. Mullings, ed., *Cities of the United States: Studies in Urban Anthropology.* New York: Columbia University Press.

Shaw, N., ed. (1987) *Women and AIDS Clinical Resource Guide,* 2d ed. San Francisco: San Francisco AIDS Foundation.

Shreckengost, R. C. (1983) *Heroin: A New View.* Washington, D.C.: Central Intelligence Agency.

Siegel, R. (1984) Changing patterns of cocaine use: Longitudinal observations, consequences, and treatment. In J. Grabowski, ed., *Cocaine: Pharmacology, Effects and Treatment of Abuse.* NIDA Research Monograph No. 50. Rockville, Md.: National Institute on Drug Abuse.

Simpson, D., Joe, G., and Lehman, W. (1986) *Addiction Careers: Summary of Studies Based on the DARP 12 Year Followup.* NIDA Treatment Research Report No. ADM86–1420. Rockville, Md.: National Institute on Drug Abuse.

Speck, R. V., Barr, J., Eisenman, R., Foulks, E., Goldman, A., and Lincoln, J. (1972) *The New Families: Youth, Communes, and the Politics of Drugs.* New York: Basic Books, Inc.

Stall, R., and Biernacki, P. (1986) Spontaneous remission from the problematic use of substances: An inductive model derived from a comparative analysis of the alcohol, opiate, tobacco, and food/obesity literatures. *International Journal of the Addictions* 21:1–23.

Stall, R., McKusick, L., Wiley, J., Coates, T. J., and Ostrow, D. G. (1986) Alcohol and drug use during sexual activity and compliance with safe sex guidelines for AIDS. *Health Education Quarterly* 13:359–371.

Sterk, C. (1988) Cocaine and seropositivity. *Lancet* 1:1052–1053.

Stimson, J. V. (1988) HIV and the Injecting Drug User: Syringe Exchange Schemes in England and Scotland. University of London, Goldsmiths' College.

Stoneburner, R. L., Des Jarlais, D. C., Benezra, D., Gorelkin, L., Sotheran, J. L., Friedman, S. R., Schultz, S., Marmor, M., Mildvan, D., and Maslansky, R. (1988) A larger spectrum of severe HIV-1-related disease in intravenous drug users in New York City. *Science* 242:916–919.

Sudman, S., Sirken, M., and Cowan, C. (1988) Sampling rare and elusive populations. *Science* 249:991–996.

Toborg, M. A., and Kirby, M. P. (1984) Drug Use and Pretrial Crime in the District of Columbia (preliminary findings). National Institute of Justice, Washington, D.C.

Turner, C. F., Miller, H. G., and Barker, L. (In press) AIDS research and the behavioral and social sciences. In R. Kulstad, ed., *AIDS 1988: A Symposium.* Washington, D.C.: American Association for the Advancement of Science.

van den Hoek, J. A. R., Coutinho, R. A., Zadelhoff, A. W., van Haastrecht, H. J. A., and Goudsmit, J. (1987) Prevalence, Incidence, and Risk Factors of HIV Infection Among Drug Addicts in Amsterdam. Presented at the Third International AIDS Conference, Washington, D.C., June 1–5.

van den Hoek, J. A. R., van Haastrecht, H. J. A., Goudsmit, J., and Coutinho, R. A. (1988a) Influence of HIV-AB Testing on the Risk Behavior of IV Drug Users in Amsterdam. Presented at the Fourth International AIDS Conference, Stockholm, June 12–16.

van den Hoek, J. A. R., Coutinho, R. A., van Haastrecht, H. J. A., van Zadelhoff, A. W., and Goudsmit, J. (1988b) Prevalence and risk factors of HIV infections among drug users and drug using prostitutes in Amsterdam. *AIDS* 2:55–60.

Waldorf, D. (1970) Life without heroin: Some social adjustments during long-term periods of voluntary abstention. *Social Problems* 18:228–242.

Waldorf, D. (1980) A brief history of illicit drug ethnographies. In C. Akins and G. Beschner, eds., *Ethnography: A Research Tool for Policymakers in the Drug and Alcohol Fields.* Rockville, Md.: National Institute on Drug Abuse.

Waldorf, D., Murphy, S., and Reinarman, C. (1977) *Doing Coke: An Ethnography of Cocaine Users and Sellers.* Washington, D.C.: Drug Abuse Council.

Wallace, J. I., Mann, J., and Beatrice, S. (1988) HIV-1 Exposure Among Clients of Prostitutes. Presented at the Fourth International AIDS Conference, Stockholm, June 12–16.

Watters, J. K. (1987a) Preventing Human Immunodeficiency Virus Contagion Among Intravenous Drug Users: The Impact of Street-Based Education on Risk-Behavior. Presented at the Third International AIDS Conference, Washington, D.C., June 1–5.

Watters, J. K. (1987b) A street-based outreach model of AIDS prevention for intravenous drug users: Preliminary evaluation. *Contemporary Drug Problems* 14:411–423.

Watters, J. K., Lewis, D., Cheng, Y.-T., Jang, M., and Carlson, J. (1988) Drug-Use Profile, Risk Participation, and HIV Exposure Among Intravenous Drug Users in San Francisco. Presented at the Fourth International AIDS Conference, Stockholm, June 12–16.

Weiss, S. H., and Biggar, B. J. (1986) The epidemiology of human retrovirus-associated illness. *Mt. Sinai Journal of Medicine* 53:579–591.

Weiss, S. H., Ginzburg, H. M., and Goeddert, J. J. (1985) Risk of HTLV-III exposure and AIDS among parenteral drug abusers in New Jersey. Presented at the International Conference on AIDS, Atlanta, Ga., April.

Weppner, R. S., ed. (1977) *Street Ethnography: Selected Studies of Crime and Drug Use in Natural Settings.* Beverly Hills, Calif.: Sage Publications.

Weppner, R. S. (1983) *The Untherapeutic Community: Organizational Behavior in a Failed Addiction Treatment Program.* Lincoln: University of Nebraska Press.

Wiebel, W. W. (In press) Combining ethnography and epidemiologic methods in targeted AIDS interventions: The Chicago model. In R. Battjes and R. Pickens, eds., *Needle Sharing Among Intravenous Drug Abusers: National and International Perspectives.* NIDA Research Monograph. Rockville, Md.: National Institute on Drug Abuse.

Wiebel, W. W., and Altman, N. (1988) AIDS Prevention Outreach to IVDUs in Four U.S. Cities. Presented at the Fourth International AIDS Conference, Stockholm, June 12–16.

Wikler, A. (1973) Dynamics of drug dependence: Implications of a conditioning theory for research and treatment. *Archives of General Psychiatry* 28:611–616.

Wish, E. D., Brady, E., Cuadrado, M., and Sears, A. (1984) Preliminary Findings from the Drug Use as a Pretrial Behavior in Arrestees Project. New York State Division of Substance Abuse Services and Narcotic and Drug Research, Inc., New York City.

Wofsy, C. B. (1987) Human immunodeficiency virus infection in women. *Journal of the American Medical Association* 257:2074–2076.

Woodward, J. A., and Bentler, P. N. (1978) Statistical lower bounds to population reliability. *Psychological Bulletin* 85:1323–1326.

Woodward, J. A., Retka, R. L., and Nig, L. (1984) Construct validity of heroin abuse estimators. *International Journal of the Addictions* 19:93–117.

Worth, D. (1988) Self-help Interventions with Women at High Risk of HIV Infection. Montefiore Medical Center, New York City.

Wyatt, G. E. (1987) Ethnic and Cultural Differences in Women's Sexual Behavior. Department of Psychiatry and Biobehavioral Sciences, University of California at Los Angeles.

Yancovitz, S., Des Jarlais, D. C., Peyser, N., Senie, R., Drew, E., Mildvan, D., et al. (1988) Innovative AIDS Risk Reduction Project: Interim Methadone Clinic. Presented at the Fourth International AIDS Conference, Stockholm, June 12–16.

Zarek, D., Hawkins, J. D., and Rogers, P. D. (1987) Risk factors for adolescent substance abuse: Implications for pediatric practice. *Pediatric Clinics of North America* 34:481–493.

Zinberg, N. E. (1984) *Drug, Set and Setting: The Basis for Controlled Intoxicant Use.* New Haven, Conn.: Yale University Press.

Zinberg, N. E., Harding, W., and Winkeller, M. (1977) A study of social regulatory mechanisms in controlled illicit drug users. *Journal of Drug Issues* 7:117–133.

Part II

Intervening to Limit the Spread of HIV Infection

In Part II, we review strategies that hold promise for halting the spread of HIV infection. Unfortunately, because few of the AIDS intervention programs conducted to date have been evaluated, there is little basis for determining the best way to facilitate change in risk-associated behavior. Therefore, in Chapter 4, the committee has enumerated principles of human behavior that are known to influence health behavior, principles that form the cornerstone for the design and implementation of intervention programs. Chapter 5 then discusses the purpose, processes, and problems of conducting evaluations to determine the effects of intervention programs. Rigorous evaluation is the key to determining which AIDS intervention efforts are working and which are not, knowledge that is essential to monitor performance and improve future efforts to halt the spread of HIV infection.

4

Facilitating Change in Health Behaviors

This chapter summarizes some of the major findings of research that has been undertaken to understand how to facilitate change in human behavior to prevent disease and promote health.[1] Special attention has been given to the way this research relates to altering the behaviors associated with the transmission of HIV infection.

At the beginning of its study, the committee had hoped that factors clearly associated with altering HIV-related behaviors could be identified by examining evaluations of existing AIDS prevention programs. Unfortunately, although considerable behavioral change has been documented among the individuals who reported engaging in high-risk behavior, much less attention has been paid to understanding how and why those changes occurred. There has been little useful evaluation of the few major intervention programs that have been undertaken, and there have been even fewer studies that compared the efficacy of alternative interventions (Office of Technology Assessment, 1988). Consequently, the committee has had to rely on a more basic analysis of intervention strategies, using principles of human behavior established through empirical research in the social and behavioral sciences, to suggest useful programs to prevent the spread of HIV infection.

[1]There are many literatures that report empirical findings of behavioral studies that have attempted to modify individuals' health-related behaviors (e.g., promotion of seat belt use, participation in screening and immunization programs, compliance with prescribed regimens). However, because of the many unique features surrounding the behaviors involved in the transmission of HIV, this chapter emphasizes only those principles of behavior and research findings that appear to be most directly related to the behaviors that can transmit HIV.

AIDS intervention programs have been established out of the need and desire to act quickly. The tremendous effort that has already been expended to halt the spread of infection is laudable; nevertheless, the committee has concluded that much more could be accomplished. Well-designed research programs and effective intervention strategies are needed to maximize the likelihood of progress. Furthermore, the design of such activities must take into consideration a wide range of conceptual and empirical research approaches, derived from the various fields that make up the social and behavioral sciences. There are also methodological issues that must be addressed. (These are discussed in detail in the next chapter.) Much is understood about human behavioral change and about messages and their effectiveness. Yet the application of these ideas to specific groups typically can be undertaken in more than one way, and rarely is theory strong enough to tell us in advance which method will be the more effective. This state of knowledge leads to two central methodological principles: (1) the practice of using planned variations in messages, programs, and campaigns should be standard in AIDS intervention programs, and (2) a plan for evaluating the comparative success of the variations should be a critical component of any intervention. Only in this manner can the most effective interventions be rapidly and reliably determined. To "streamline" the preparation of educational materials and intervention programs by choosing a single, "best-we-think-we-can-do" product is to delay the identification of effective intervention strategies.

Two fundamental themes can be seen in the principles of behavior presented in the following pages:

1. For behavior to change, individuals must recognize the problem, be motivated to act, and have the knowledge and skills necessary to perform the action.
2. To increase the likelihood of action, impediments in the social environment must be removed or weakened and inducements for change provided whenever possible.

By focusing on facilitating change in risk-associated behavior, the committee does not wish to impute a diminished importance to maintaining those behaviors that are *not* associated with risk. Clearly, the best way to prevent IV drug-associated HIV transmission is to prevent the use of drugs. However, intravenous use of illicit drugs is a long-standing problem in U.S. society; it has resisted prevention efforts to date and is unlikely to disappear in the foreseeable future. Sexual behavior must also be considered in realistic terms.

Although social norms present sexual abstinence as a laudable goal for the adolescent population and monogamy as an appropriate status for adults, the data presented in Chapter 2 clearly show that the realities of sexual behavior are not always consistent with the norms. Changing the behavior of individuals is important in the management of many health problems; it is critical in the prevention of AIDS.

Motivating and sustaining change in risk-associated intimate and addictive behaviors are not easy; they will require a continued commitment to diverse and, at times, innovative approaches. Yet there is much reason to be hopeful about the potential for success of behavioral interventions to prevent the spread of HIV infection. A wealth of research on health behavior indicates that individuals are certainly capable of undertaking changes in important areas of conduct; indeed, substantial changes in individual behavior have already been reported among homosexual men and IV drug users in response to the AIDS epidemic (Becker and Joseph, 1988; Office of Technology Assessment, 1988). Surveys of IV drug users from the New York City area indicate high levels of awareness and knowledge about AIDS, increased demand for treatment, and substantial changes in needle-sharing practices and the sterilization of injection equipment (Des Jarlais, 1987). The variations in the amount and types of change that have been reported across groups and by geographic location should not detract from the substantial modifications made by those at greatest risk of this fatal disease. As Becker and Joseph have noted, "in some populations of homosexual/bisexual men, this may be the most rapid and profound response to a health threat which has ever been documented" (1988:407).

In this chapter the committee identifies factors that are likely to help an individual alter risk-associated behaviors and sustain healthy ones. Providing accurate, appropriate, and effective information is the logical starting point for any health program. Education plays an important role in facilitating behavioral change, allaying unnecessary fears, and reducing discrimination. However, as the committee's discussion of education programs indicates, information alone is generally insufficient to alter behavior. Therefore, the chapter also provides an analysis of the strategies needed to motivate individuals to change unhealthy behaviors and to sustain healthy ones. Because the behaviors of interest are enacted in social situations, the final sections of the chapter include discussions of the social support needed to facilitate health behavior and the existing social impediments that hinder change in individual behavior and the implementation of HIV prevention programs.

EDUCATION PROGRAMS

For behavior to change, individuals must understand the risks they incur by engaging in that behavior. In this section, the committee reviews the role of education programs in preventing HIV infection, including the behavioral modifications that increased knowledge can reasonably be expected to accomplish. The remainder of the section focuses on three aspects of such programs that have particular relevance for AIDS prevention: (1) the content of health messages and, especially, the level of fear evoked by the message; (2) the role of the media in purveying health messages and the effect of risk perception on taking appropriate action; and (3) the problems associated with the introduction and adoption of new ideas and technologies, including antibody testing.

The Role of Education and Knowledge in Preventing the Spread of HIV Infection

Information is necessary but often insufficient by itself to effect behavioral change. Consequently, the association between knowledge and facilitating behavioral change is of particular interest to intervention planners. Empirical studies have found knowledge about HIV and its transmission to be of varying importance in effecting and sustaining behavioral change (Emmons et al., 1986; Kelly et al., 1987b). Becker and Joseph (1988) postulate that there may be a "threshold" effect: beyond a certain level, increases in knowledge or changes in attitude may not increase changes in behavior. Alternatively, an indirect relationship may exist between knowledge and attitudes, on the one hand, and behavior, on the other; another possibility is that intervening variables may link these factors. Yet the uncertainties surrounding the role of information in behavioral change do not obviate the need for this basic element of health programs: it would be unconscionable not to provide accurate, comprehensible information about HIV and AIDS.

Thus, the logical starting point for any AIDS education program is the provision of information. General information about AIDS, including facts about the causative virus and routes of transmission, has been successfully disseminated through posters, pamphlets, radio and television, word-of-mouth, community communications networks, and, recently, a brochure from the Public Health Service, which was mailed to every household in the United States. AIDS is very much on the public's mind. In national surveys, approximately 90 percent of respondents reported seeing, hearing, or reading something about AIDS within the last week (Dawson et al., 1988); in public opinion polls, almost all respondents knew that AIDS is caused by a virus that is transmitted through sexual behaviors or shared injection equipment (Turner et al., in press). The public also holds numerous erroneous beliefs, however, and questions persist about the role of kissing and toilet seats in the transmission of HIV. It is important, therefore, to understand how to provide additional information.

As AIDS education efforts continue, more attention must be directed toward how the material is presented. Print and broadcast media offer the economy of reaching many people with a unified message. However, face-to-face communication for hard-to-reach individuals (e.g., IV drug users) is also needed to clarify questions, deal with fear or inertia, and facilitate access to needed goods and services. It must be recognized by those designing education programs that access to mainstream sources of information for minority groups and others may be limited by lower levels of educational achievement and a limited capacity to comprehend messages in English. Information must be delivered in a manner that is comprehensible and relevant to the audience it is intended to reach. Clearly, this requirement will entail providing written and spoken messages in the different languages and idioms of the various ethnic, racial, social, age, and sexual orientation groups that make up the national population. Much of the currently available information on AIDS and HIV transmission does not fulfill these criteria. An analysis of 16 educational brochures on AIDS prevention found that, on the average, they were written at a 14th-grade (second year of college) reading level (Hochhauser, 1987). This is clearly unsatisfactory.

There is also a need in AIDS education for frank exchange that allows no misunderstanding. Clear, explicit language is required; yet its use in AIDS education continues to be impeded by the pervasive American reticence about discussing sexual behavior (see Chapter 7). The results of such reticence and the lack of straightforward communication are seen in the misconceptions that remain about HIV transmission. For example, the use of the expression "exchange of bodily fluids" in early information campaigns left many people with unsubstantiated concerns about the risk associated with kissing; others may not have understood this term to include the preseminal and vaginal fluids present during foreplay. Many adolescents continue to believe that HIV infection can be acquired through casual contact, such as shaking hands or simply being near someone with AIDS (DiClemente et al., 1986, 1988; Reuben et al., 1988). In some instances, the lack of clear information encourages continued risk-associated behavior. Some IV drug users, for example, still believe that water is sufficient for sterilizing injection equipment; others believe infected individuals can be identified by their appearance. Moreover, homosexual men who believed they had successfully "fought off" the virus (as one would fight off the flu by mounting an antibody response) were more likely to report continued participation in high-risk sexual activities than men who had a clearer, more accurate sense of whether or not they were infected (Coates et al., 1985). In other instances, misinformation impedes desirable behavior. Among the general population, more than one quarter of a national sample (26 percent) believed that a person could get AIDS from donating blood (Dawson et al., 1988).

Modes of information dissemination are another aspect to be considered in providing AIDS education. An example of the use of a spectrum of networks to disseminate AIDS messages is the program created by the San Francisco AIDS Foundation in the early years of the epidemic (Communication Technologies, 1987). One component involved advertising campaigns that were designed to reach large numbers of people: ads urging safer sexual practices and providing information about AIDS were placed in newspapers and magazines, on billboards, and in buses and other forms of public transportation. They were also carried on television and radio. To achieve greater visibility and acceptability in the local gay population, a widely distributed and controversial poster featured two nude men embracing with the caption, "You Can Have Fun and Be Safe, Too" (Communication Technologies, 1987:11). Later communications used the theme, "The Best Defense Against AIDS Is Information" and targeted a broader population. Pamphlets published in the languages spoken in the community were distributed through the mail, in the streets, at public forums, and through health care facilities. (These materials included "Can We Talk?," a brochure for homosexual men that has been translated and copied around the world.) A project to provide anonymous antibody testing with counseling was also implemented, and appeals to provide protection through antidiscrimination legislation were promoted.

The program also attempted to teach safer sex skills and enhance the erotic attractiveness of safer sex. One project, called

"Bartenders Against AIDS," provided information on AIDS prevention to local bartenders and included training on how to support safer sex among customers (Communication Technologies, 1987:17). Small group meetings were held in individuals' homes and elsewhere (the Stop AIDS Project) to clarify the guidelines of safer sex practices and produce commitment to their use through face-to-face interaction and discussions. Over time, the design of the campaign was altered, based on the findings of marketing research. In addition, pamphlets and flyers were updated regularly to reflect new material and epidemiological findings and to reach new audiences. Foundation personnel collaborated with journalists to assist in the process of creating informative, accurate articles.

The community-level programs noted above are supported and complemented by educational efforts at the federal level. CDC is the lead agency for AIDS prevention programs in the Public Health Service. It supports a range of extramural information and education activities and selected intramural efforts, including

- a multimillion-dollar school education program;
- a national hot line;
- a multimedia advertising campaign whose slogan is "America Responds to AIDS";
- a national clearinghouse for printed AIDS information available to the public on request;
- multimillion-dollar cooperative agreements with the 50 states, 5 territories, and 4 other locales to support community task forces, hot lines, and antibody testing and counseling; and
- community demonstration projects to disseminate information, promote change in social norms and risk-associated behavior, and provide antibody testing and counseling.

As detailed later in this chapter, there is clearly more to influencing health behavior than the provision of information, as has certainly been seen in smoking and drug prevention campaigns. To change behavior, at a minimum, individuals need to perceive that they are personally at risk of acquiring a serious condition, that efficacious preventive actions can be undertaken, and that barriers to initiating or continuing these preventive practices can be minimized or overcome (Janz and Becker, 1984). Supportive environments ensure a quicker adoption and more consistent maintenance of behavioral change. Education, however, is the beginning. Various agencies in the public and private sectors have been making considerable efforts to provide information on the AIDS epidemic to the public. Federal efforts have been hampered by constraints on the use of language that can convey the AIDS prevention message frankly and explicitly. The committee finds that the gravity of this epidemic allows no room for misunderstanding. **The committee recommends making information available in clear, explicit language in the idiom of the target audience.**

The Function of Fear in Health Messages

Information, prevention, and treatment programs for sexually transmitted diseases (STDs) for both the military and civilian populations have relied to varying extents on threatening messages that evoke high levels of fear. Similar tactics have been used in programs to prevent AIDS. (For example, such messages as "Bang Bang You're Dead" have been used to call attention to the fatal consequences of sexually transmitted HIV infection.) Whether these messages have been effective in changing behavior is not known because there have been no controlled studies or evaluations of their impact. Research suggests, however, that the efficacy of such a frightening and uninforming message is doubtful.

Messages designed to evoke high levels of fear or those that rely exclusively on threats may be intuitively appealing in the case of preventing a deadly disease, but they have been shown to be effective for most people only if coupled with advice about how behavioral change can reduce the threat (Sutton, 1982; Becker, 1985). Anxiety alone does not necessarily lead to behavioral change. For example, in the syphilis campaign undertaken early in this century, the educational messages crafted for the military sought to arouse fear in the troops (Brandt, 1987). Knowledge about STDs was measured in military inductees before and after STD prevention films (e.g., "Fit to Fight" and "Fit to Win"). Premovie and postmovie measurements revealed that these strategies changed general impressions about STDs (e.g., horror and fear were increased and persisted for weeks after the viewing), but knowledge and behavior did not change (Lashley and Watson, 1922). During World War II, however, when a prophylaxis program based on condoms and treatment was initiated, soldiers responded favorably. As many as 50 million condoms were accepted by soldiers each month, and rates of syphilis declined in this population over that time (Brandt, 1987). Nevertheless, the lack of a systematic evaluation of the message and prophylaxis programs (a shortcoming of most STD programs) foils any attempt to draw conclusions as to what factor(s) did or did not work in reducing syphilis in this population.

Like the military STD prevention programs, early drug prevention programs for youths were largely aimed at providing information and evoking fear (Polich et al., 1984). The content of the message and the time devoted to the presentation of information varied greatly across the programs, making it difficult to compare their relative effectiveness. Yet general trends in the findings that have been produced indicate that knowledge alone does not change drug-associated behaviors, nor do messages with high threat content. School-based programs that rely heavily on fear have not been successful, apparently because the fear is associated with a low-probability event and because there is a substantial time lag between risk-associated behavior and adverse outcome (Des Jarlais and Friedman, 1987). The assumption that teenagers would not use drugs if they were informed about the inherent dangers of drug use did not take into account the social factors involved in initiating and sustaining drug-use behavior.

Ideally, health promotion messages should heighten an individual's perceptions of threat and his or her capacity to respond to that threat, thus modulating the level of fear. Job (1988) has proposed five prescriptions for the role of fear in health education messages:

1. Messages containing elements of fear should be introduced before discussing the desired behavior.
2. The behavior or event that is associated with the risk should be perceived as real and likely to occur to the audience targeted for that message.
3. A reasonable, desirable alternative behavior that protects against the undesired health problem should be offered. Attention to short-term benefits is desirable and can reinforce long-term behavioral change.
4. The level of fear invoked should be sufficient to create awareness of a potential problem but not so high as to evoke denial. Similarly, the fear level should be low enough that it can be effectively managed by the adoption of the desired behavior.
5. The resulting reduction in fear should be of such magnitude that it will reinforce the desired behavior and confirm its effectiveness.

What is not yet known is how to introduce fear in the right way in a particular message intended for a particular audience. Acquiring that knowledge will require planned variations of AIDS education programs that are carefully executed and then carefully evaluated.

The committee recommends that AIDS prevention messages strike a balance in the level of threat that is conveyed. The level should be sufficiently high to motivate individuals to take action. However, it should not be so high that it paralyzes individuals with fear or causes them to deny their susceptibility. Fear-arousing health promotion messages must also provide specific information on steps that can be taken to protect the individual from the threat to his or her well-being.

The Role of the Media

The media play an important role in informing individuals about and alerting them to health risks. They can also help people develop relevant protective social skills (e.g., how to resist peer pressure without losing face, how to ask questions, how to receive information from authority figures) and technical skills (e.g., how to use a condom, how to sterilize a needle). In addition, the media influence and are influenced by the norms of the community. This committee concurs with the findings of the IOM/NAS AIDS committee (IOM/NAS, 1988) and the Presidential Commission on the Human Immunodeficiency Virus Epidemic (1988); both of these bodies found that the gravity of HIV infection calls for an expanded use of the media in educational activities.

Because of a lack of evaluation of AIDS media campaigns in the United States, little can be said about their impact on risk-associated behaviors. Yet there can be little doubt that the media play important roles in transmitting factual information and in helping to create a social climate conducive to the successful change of health-related conduct. An obvious example is the use of the mass media in antismoking campaigns. Since 1973, adult per capita tobacco consumption has fallen every year; it is presently at its lowest point in a century. There is general agreement that extensive, sustained mass media health promotion programs played an important role in this achievement (Flay, 1987).[2]

---

[2]To date, evaluations have been conducted of 40 mass media campaigns that attempted to influence smoking behavior through broadcast information on health risks posed by cigarettes, printed information to promote smoking cessation (fact sheets, self-help manuals, and hot lines), and self-help clinics. At follow-up intervals ranging from 3 to 12 months, the following mean percentages of participants had continued success in quitting smoking (the data are presented by type of cessation program): American Lung Association cessation manual, 3–4 percent; American Lung Association manual and

The media can arouse interest, transmit information, demonstrate skills, and assist in the process of diffusing new ideas. In the 1987 National Health Interview Survey (Dawson et al., 1988), 82 percent of the sample reported getting information on AIDS from television, 60 percent indicated that newspapers were an important source of knowledge, 28 percent acquired information from magazines, and 8 percent heard about AIDS on the radio. IV drug users reported learning about AIDS from the media and from existing communication networks within the drug-using community (Office of Technology Assessment, 1988). Media messages can influence the ideas of individuals both directly and indirectly—that is, through their effects on opinion leaders and by legitimation of the message. To maximize media effects, the media should be linked to local public health resources to ensure that appropriate messages are crafted for the local targeted audiences and that well-designed evaluations of media efforts are conducted. Of course, the media are not meant to replace one-on-one communication or face-to-face interactions that permit the clarification of issues and answering of questions.

Limitations and conventions in print and broadcast journalism constrain the extent to which media material can influence behavioral change (Check, 1987). For example, the media are not a scientific institution; they have to popularize news topics to make them appeal to a mainstream audience. Nevertheless, despite the somewhat constrained role of the mass media, they have made significant contributions to efforts to prevent the spread of HIV infection.

Theories of social learning (e.g., Bandura, 1977; N. M. Clark, 1987) and social modeling (e.g., Green and McAlister, 1984) and models of information processing suggest how people adopt ideas proffered by the media. Some learning occurs through observation and imitation. There are certain attributes of the role models portrayed by the media that encourage imitation. These include attractiveness, perceived social competence, expertise, and trustworthiness, qualities that are essential in changing attitudes, beliefs, decision making, and behavior. After presenting a scenario that includes these attributes, the learning process approaches completion when the individual perceives herself or himself to be similar to (i.e., identifies with) these models. However, additional skills may be needed in order to imitate the behaviors. The acquisition of these skills may be a more gradual process, requiring specific demonstrations and guidelines that are repeated (Green and McAlister, 1984).

---

maintenance, 5–6 percent; media alone, 5 percent; media plus printed material, 8 percent; media plus self-help clinics, 16 percent (Flay, 1987).

The individual goes through a series of psychological processes that range from being exposed to information, paying attention to it, comprehending the message, developing beliefs, making decisions, repeating and learning from the process of developing beliefs and making decisions, and, finally, acting. Most media campaigns focus on information transmission rather than on decision making or action.

Several other social learning principles must be considered in crafting media material to effect behavioral change. Because belief is influenced by the perceived trustworthiness of the source of information, source credibility is particularly important when the ideas being presented are new or controversial (Green and McAlister, 1984). Decisions to act can be influenced by displays of incentives, by the values attached to proposed actions, and by messages that enhance self-confidence. At the community level, program goals are more likely to be adopted if their presentation is preceded by messages that arouse awareness and interest among members of that community. Again, experimentation will be necessary to find the best strategies for implementing these theories.

Social marketing (the application of marketing techniques to social problems) provides tools[3] that will influence the acceptability of new ideas and products. An ideal strategy would be one that develops the right product, uses the right promotions strategy, puts the product in the right place for the right audience, and makes it available at the right price (Kotler and Zaltman, 1971). Several community-based programs, including the San Francisco AIDS Foundation program, have used such approaches for AIDS prevention campaigns. In the San Francisco case, an advertising agency was hired to conduct focus groups and prepare newspaper advertisements promoting safer sex among gay men. The themes stressed by the agency were the effectiveness of safer sex practices, individual and community responsibility for appropriate action, and the recent changes in the community's norms and values to support safer sex. One poster promoted condom use: a photograph of a condom, watch, and pocket change was accompanied by the message, "It takes nine cents and twenty seconds to save a life" (Communication Technologies, 1987:Appendix C). At the same time, condoms were being promoted and distributed at gay events, workshops on safer sex, bars, and checkout counters at gay department stores (Pappas,

[3]For example, condoms packaged for women and available in stores on the same shelves as feminine hygiene products.

1987). Questions remain, however, about the effectiveness of social marketing tools in solving problems of health promotion; many studies have used them in combination with other intervention techniques, and there have been few careful studies that have been able to isolate the effects of social marketing techniques on individual health behavior.

The IOM/NAS AIDS committee recommended "continued attention to the development of policies to foster the use of condoms" (IOM/NAS, 1988:8). Unquestionably a highly desirable outcome, increasing the acceptability of condoms in this country is nevertheless an objective that offers some interesting marketing problems. Policies regarding condom advertisements vary. As discussed in Chapter 7, television executives have been reluctant to air condom advertisements, although public health announcements that include information about condoms have been accepted and aired. The networks say they are afraid their audiences will be offended by such commercial presentations. Yet there is an apparent lack of consistency in this concern for viewers' sensibilities, as ads for feminine hygiene products have been accepted, and several popular television series have included fairly explicit sexual scenes. Moreover, public opinion polls do not indicate that the public would be more offended by condom ads than they are by other advertisements.

The broadcast media are an important tool that should be mobilized (to the extent that it is reasonable and feasible) to assist in preventing the further spread of HIV infection. With their unparalleled capacity to reach and influence individuals, the media should be encouraged and helped in whatever ways are necessary to play their unique, vital role in halting this epidemic.

The committee recommends that television networks present more public service messages on those behaviors associated with HIV transmission and practical measures for interrupting the spread of infection. The committee also recommends that television networks accept condom advertisements.

Risk Perception

For an individual to be motivated to take action against AIDS (or any other disease), the disease must be perceived as a personal risk with serious consequences (Rosenstock, 1960; Janz and Becker, 1984). A person who does not believe that the disease in question is serious or that he or she could contract it is unlikely to undertake preventive action.

There is a large body of information on risk perception and risk analysis that could be brought to bear on the design and implementation of AIDS information and education campaigns.[4] How statements of risk are interpreted depends on an individual's perceptions of the value associated with avoiding the health problem in question, the quality of information about intervention strategies, and the available incentives and preferences for action (Lave, 1987). Programs that do not attend to variations in risk perception are less likely to be successful in motivating individuals to act.

Researchers have seen an association between knowledge about AIDS and perceived risk (DiClemente et al., 1988). Thus, the awareness of HIV infection in a local IV drug-using population may increase the perception of risk among drug users and therefore the likelihood of appropriate action. However, it should be noted that *very* high rates of local infection could reinforce the notion that a single episode of sharing would inevitably lead to infection. An individual who strongly suspects that he or she is already infected may be less willing to undertake difficult changes in behavior. Such a fatalistic perspective could undermine behavioral modification efforts.

The subjective assessment of personal risk levels does not always correlate with more objective assessments. A 1983 survey of homosexual men from the San Francisco area recruited subjects from bathhouses (before they were closed) and bars, and through advertisements and professional organizations (McKusick et al., 1985). The bathhouse and bar groups had a very high level of awareness of AIDS, and there was extensive knowledge of risk factors reported throughout this sample; these groups also reported the highest rates of sexually transmitted diseases and had more evidence of HIV infection than did other groups. Yet despite their knowledge of risk factors, many respondents continued anonymous sexual contacts and other high-risk sexual behavior. Indeed, 65 percent of those in the bathhouse group said they had already made all the changes in their lives necessary to adapt to the threat of AIDS, and half believed they were less susceptible to AIDS than were (unspecified) others. Empirical studies of other health problems confirm the notion that people tend to report themselves to be less at risk than their peers for a variety of threats (Weinstein, 1987).

---

[4]For more information, see the forthcoming National Academy of Sciences report, *Improving Risk Communication,* which summarizes the complex literature and research experience in risk perception and risk management.

It appears that people estimate future risk by extrapolating from past events in their life (Weinstein, 1987). Under this system, if a problem has not yet occurred, it is unlikely to be a future threat. This optimistic bias (the notion that "it can't happen to me") is particularly strong in adolescence, as illustrated by teenagers' responses to learning that they are pregnant (Brooks-Gunn and Furstenberg, in press). However, adults are also unrealistically positive in their assessment of future risk.

There are several possible reasons for such optimistic outlooks. One is denial (in the case of serious risk). For example, 45 percent of heterosexual men and 65 percent of heterosexual women from a national sample who reported nine or more sexual partners in the past year indicated that they had never purchased condoms. Almost 60 percent rated their personal risk of contracting AIDS at the lowest possible level of the interview's risk scale (Turner et al., in press). Other possible reasons for unrealistically optimistic assessments of risk are the enhancement of self-esteem or the avoidance of embarrassment or stigma (in the case of a preventable risk). For instance, it may be so difficult for men who engage in same-gender sex to recognize it as gay or homosexual behavior that they deny the HIV-associated risks. In addition, cognitive error (for low-frequency risk) or lack of experience among adolescents and immature adults may account for unfounded optimism about risks. Many adolescent females underestimate the risk of pregnancy; presumably, they would also underestimate the likelihood of contracting a disease such as AIDS. For these reasons, and the others noted above, **the committee recommends that programs to initiate and sustain changes in risk-associated behavior take into account how the targeted population perceives and understands risk.**

Adoption and Diffusion of Innovations

Empirical applications of the concepts of adoption and diffusion of innovations have identified certain factors that influence the likelihood that individuals will accept new ideas, technologies, products, recommended practices, and other innovations. These factors include individuals' characteristics (e.g., membership in communication networks, the influence of opinion leaders), the characteristics of the innovation itself, and the social climate into which the innovation is to be introduced (Rogers, 1962). The planned introduction of a new idea, program, or policy (i.e., an innovation) must take these factors into account prior to communicating or spreading (i.e., the process of diffusion) the innovation to members of a social system over time (Rogers and Adhikarya, 1980).

Some new tools and ideas are more likely than others to be acceptable to particular groups. If alternative approaches are available, the one that is most consistent with ongoing, accepted practices in a group should be emphasized. If no alternatives exist, steps should be taken to modify any negative perceptions of the proposed strategy on the parts of opinion leaders and the target audience. Organizational and social impediments to adoption should be identified and removed, whenever possible. To facilitate the adoption of innovations, adequate funding, staff, and expertise should be provided, and representatives from the broad spectrum of the groups that make up the target population should be encouraged to participate in the design and implementation of the program.

The literature on the characteristics of adopters emphasizes the critical role of "opinion leaders." These are individuals who occupy central positions in communication networks and are recognized as expert (having knowledge and experience) and trustworthy in areas that are relevant to the particular innovation in question. In general, they tend to be younger and better educated than their peers; they tend to be more "cosmopolitan" (i.e., they regularly look beyond their local interests and groups to learn what is new, they read more magazines and newspapers, etc.); and they are often consulted for advice about new things. Finally, they are usually among the first individuals to try the innovation and thus are in a unique position either to recommend or discourage its further diffusion among their friends and colleagues (Becker, 1970). Rogers (1962) finds that in assessing an intervention, individuals are more likely to take into account the opinion of those of their peers who have already adopted it than they are to accept the research findings of experts. Peers serve as models of behavior that can be imitated by others from the same social network.

Diffusion can be viewed as a multistep process—new information influences opinion leaders, who then go on to influence others who, in turn, influence still others, and so forth. Consequently, it may be important to identify opinion leaders and concentrate on them the available resources for change.[5] A more dynamic process suggests that individuals are affected directly (e.g., by the mass media) and

[5]Opinion leaders can be identified with sociometric techniques—for example, asking a sample of individuals from the group to be influenced to name two or three persons to whom they would turn for advice and information about the relevant innovation.

by opinion leaders at the same time. This model would require addressing both the external sources of messages as well as the opinion leaders.

There are at least two approaches that individuals who introduced new concepts and products (so-called change agents) can employ to increase the likelihood of an innovation's adoption: (1) use resources that will actually improve the innovation or (2) use persuasion that will change the perceptions of it (Becker, 1970). In a number of instances, successful campaigns in the past have changed both the physical characteristics and the perceptions of interventions. For example, alarming increases in gonorrhea rates in Sweden led to a massive multifaceted campaign to promote condom use. Information and statistics on the disease were provided to the general public in a comprehensible manner while posters, brochures, and T-shirts hailed the arrival of new styles of condoms in bright colors and attractive containers. Condom sales subsequently increased by more than 2 million in two years, and gonorrhea rates declined precipitously in Sweden at the same time they were increasing in other European countries. Consumer attitudes about condoms moved rapidly toward more acceptability among a variety of consumers, including young people and women (Ajax, 1974; Darrow, 1987; Potts, no date).

The failure to act to prevent the acquisition or spread of HIV infection cannot be blamed exclusively on individuals. Communication problems, cultural and religious barriers, poor access to health resources and prevention services, community-level embarrassment, apathy, and misunderstanding have all contributed to the spread of HIV infection among some groups, especially minorities.[6] The tragic increase in the prevalence of infection within minority groups illustrates some of the problems that are associated with the introduction, acceptance, and use of new concepts and techniques to prevent disease. The design and implementation of successful programs to facilitate behavioral change should take into account existing organizations in minority communities and prevailing social environments.

Finally, those who promote change should become aware of the organizational and social environments that might impede the adoption and diffusion of ideas or practices (Greer, 1977). For example, it may be necessary to provide existing organizations with increased resources (money, staff, or expertise) or to create new organizations. At the community level, it may be important to involve a wide variety of interest groups in the persuasive efforts to achieve a broad

[6]See S. G. Boodman, "Hispanic Culture Redefines AIDS Fight: Communication Problems, Moral Traditions Hinder Efforts," *The Washington Post,* December 28, 1987:A1.

base of acceptance for a new practice. Various types of people may be needed: those who are different from the community may be helpful in teaching (being perceived as competent); those who are like the community may be better at persuading (being perceived as trustworthy) or serving as models for new behaviors (being perceived as alike).

The committee recommends that innovative approaches to AIDS prevention programs be introduced in a planned manner that reflects well-established principles about the adoption and diffusion of new ideas. Specifically, (1) opinion leaders of target populations should be identified and incorporated into the flow of influence to maximize credibility and persuasiveness in the target audience; (2) a new program should be carefully assessed prior to implementation for characteristics that might impede its acceptance, and steps should be taken to alter those characteristics; and (3) strategies for change should be designed to reflect the organizational and social environments into which the new program is to be incorporated.

MOTIVATING AND SUSTAINING BEHAVIORAL CHANGE

Once the attention of a targeted audience has been captured through appropriate messages, there remains the task of getting people to act. Social and behavioral science research offers some guidance:

- To begin behavioral change, people must be motivated; they must also believe that the changes being proposed will do some good, and they must believe that they have a reasonable chance of successfully accomplishing those changes. Moreover, the proposed changes should be consistent with the individual's existing beliefs and values.
- People often need assistance and support to change unhealthy behaviors, and many will not be completely successful in adhering to new behavior patterns.
- It is often easier to get people to modify a behavior than to eliminate it.
- Incremental changes and modifications, rather than global life-style changes, are more realistic goals for most people.

- Offering choices among alternative behaviors for change is often more effective than rigidly prescribing a single behavior.

People at risk for AIDS are less likely to attempt a complete alteration of their behavior than they are to adopt protective measures that allow them to pursue their long-standing goals and interests in life. Thus, for many, condoms will be more acceptable than abstinence; for some IV drug users, the sterilization of injection equipment may be more acceptable than detoxification or methadone treatment. Although "heroic" efforts to achieve radical changes in behavior are appealing and provide dramatic stories, the reality is that, for most people, attempts to achieve major life-style or global changes will probably fail.

Thus, for many individuals, strategies that seek to modify behavior rather than to achieve global behavioral change are more likely to succeed. Examples abound to support this point; to take just two: gout sufferers will more readily take a daily pill of allopurinol than adopt draconian diets, and some IV drug users will modify their injection behavior rather than attempt to give up drugs entirely. Furthermore, successful modification of behavior will not be achieved through one treatment or by one exposure to an intervention program. Significant long-term behavioral change will require continuous support as new behaviors evolve over time. Thus, **the committee recommends that programs to facilitate behavioral change be approached as long-term efforts, with multiple and repeated strategies to initiate and sustain behavioral change over time.**

In the sections that follow, the committee reviews some of the factors that motivate behavioral change to reduce the risk of HIV infection, including perceived self-efficacy, altruistic motives, and knowledge of antibody status. Because HIV infection is a fatal threat for which there is no biomedical "magic bullet," it will be necessary to maintain behavioral changes for an indefinite period, perhaps for a lifetime. Therefore, the committee also considers the problems associated with sustaining behavioral change and assesses the adequacy of the change that has occurred to date.

Self-Efficacy

People who consciously change their behavior and maintain such change must believe that (1) a particular behavior will result in a desired outcome (i.e., outcome expectations), and (2) they are capable of executing that behavior (i.e., efficacy expectations) (Bandura, 1977; Strecher et al., 1986). Perceived ability is not necessarily congruent with actual past performance. Rather, it is the perception of one's abilities or self-efficacy that is important in an individual's assessment of whether or not she or he can execute specific behaviors in specific situations. This means that expectations of one's capability or self-efficacy are variable and can be molded. The concept of self-efficacy has been used in programs to stimulate new health behaviors (e.g., initiate contraceptive use), inhibit existing behaviors (e.g., stop cigarette smoking), and disinhibit behaviors (e.g., resume sex after a heart attack) (Strecher et al., 1986). Programs that focus on self-efficacy help individuals change their behavior by building their sense of competency and by teaching them the necessary skills.

Strategies based on self-efficacy were originally designed to prevent the use of tobacco and have been adapted to drug-use prevention; they are now being applied to AIDS education efforts. Effective smoking prevention programs have been designed around the principles of a social influence model that identifies messages and arguments in favor of smoking from peers, adults, and the media, and teaches teenagers how to counter those messages (Polich et al., 1984). The intent of these programs is twofold: (1) to raise the level of general social skills (including expression, conversation, and assertiveness) and specific social skills related to the target behaviors, and (2) to promote self-efficacy. Teaching skills to resist both subtle and explicit pressures to smoke from peers and the media has been shown to delay the onset of smoking among junior high school students and thus reduce the number of smokers by 30 to 60 percent (Durell and Bukoski, 1984; Polich et al., 1984). Program activities have been led by classroom teachers and trained peers; the curricula presented by peers appear to have more impact on smoking behavior (Battjes, 1985). There is differential success reported among younger adolescents who have not yet begun to smoke or who are only experimenting with tobacco (Battjes, 1985). More research is needed to understand the program's effects on different groups, especially minority adolescents.

The use of condoms will also depend on an individual's sense of empowerment—whether that person perceives himself or herself as capable of making the necessary behavioral changes to reduce risk. Notions of capability affect whether people will consider changing behaviors, what actions they choose, how much effort they apply to a situation, how long they persevere, how well change is maintained, and the amount of discomfort associated with making a behavioral change. Expectations of self-efficacy vary with three aspects of an individual's self-perception: magnitude, strength, and generality. Magnitude refers to how capable a person believes himself or herself to be: if expectations are low, he or she will attempt only simple tasks. Strength refers to an individual's perception of the probability of successfully completing a task. Generality refers to taking a sense of efficacy from one task to others (Strecher et al., 1986). The repetition of difficult behaviors that are found to be protective enhances perceptions of self-efficacy and reduces defensive behavior. If perceptions of self-efficacy are deficient, situations may not be managed in accordance with what the individual *knows* to be effective.

Empirical studies of homosexual men and IV drug users have found that higher levels of self-efficacy contributed to reducing high-risk behavior and increasing activity associated with lower levels of risk (Catania et al., 1988). In a study of homosexual men, self-efficacy was found to be the variable most powerfully associated with level of risk activity (McKusick et al., 1987). Other studies support the importance of self-efficacy in the adoption of safer sex behaviors (Joseph et al., 1987b). Among IV drug users recruited through detoxification treatment centers, self-efficacy was also associated with increased condom use (Catania et al., 1988).

Altruism

Not all behavior reflects self-interest: altruism prevails in more situations than is generally recognized. People have a strong tendency to identify with "their" group and to behave for its benefit; thus, the altruism displayed by those who reduce or eliminate high-risk behaviors is quite understandable. Studies of diverse groups of gay men (Coates et al., 1988a) have shown that those who are seropositive take *more* precautions against spreading the virus than those who are seronegative (who presumably are protecting themselves). Similar altruism has been demonstrated among IV drug users: some of the behavioral changes among IV drug users have been made to protect sexual partners and trusted needle-sharing partners (Des Jarlais, 1987).

HIV Antibody Testing

There are important individual and societal benefits to be derived from making voluntary HIV testing and counseling available on demand to all who wish to know their antibody status. For example, people who know their serologic status have been able to change some risk-associated behaviors; in addition, the knowledge of seropositivity can lead to early recognition and treatment of life-threatening infections. Before the availability of any treatment for HIV infection, individuals concerned about the stigma and discrimination associated with antibody testing argued that the risks associated with testing outweighed the benefits. Now, however, with the possibility that AZT (zidovudine) may be used for the treatment of early stages of HIV infection, testing, in conjunction with counseling and treatment for both HIV and opportunistic infections, can provide real benefits to infected individuals. Moreover, if voluntary antibody testing is not provided through alternative test sites to all who seek it, some individuals may feel compelled to use the blood-banking system as a testing venue, thus increasing the risk of contaminating the blood supply.

HIV antibody testing has been found to be valuable in changing some risk-associated behaviors in specific populations. More is known about the effects of testing among homosexual and bisexual men than about its effects among IV drug users, adolescents, or women at high risk of HIV infection. In general, studies have found positive behavioral effects associated with antibody testing among homosexual men in the United States, Canada, and Europe (Farthing et al., 1987; Fox et al., 1987b; Godfried et al., 1987; Willoughby et al., 1987; Coates et al., 1988a; McCusker et al., 1988). Yet there are other studies that have not found an association between knowing a positive test result and reducing risk-associated behavior (Doll et al., 1987; Pesce et al., 1987; Soucy, 1987). In two studies, homosexual men who learned that they were seropositive were more likely to eliminate or decrease unprotected insertive anal intercourse than either seronegative men or seropositive men who did not know their antibody status (Fox et al., 1987b; McCusker et al., 1988); however, in one study (McCusker et al., 1988), an awareness of test results was not associated with a decrease in unprotected receptive anal intercourse. Studies of the effects of testing on the behavior of homosexual men (Fox et al., 1987a; McCusker et al., 1988) have been confounded by the fact that seropositive men reported higher initial levels of most risk-associated behaviors at the outset of the study than did seronegative men, thus leaving more room for change.

Of the limited number of studies in this country that have looked at the effects of HIV antibody testing on the behavior of IV drug users, all have shown consistent findings of reduced risk-taking behavior following testing and counseling (Casadonte et al., 1986, 1988;

Cox et al., 1986). IV drug users who were found to be seropositive reported more risk reduction than those who were seronegative. In addition, more change was seen in relation to the reduction or elimination of injection or to the sharing of injection equipment than was seen in sexual behavior. Some of the moves to more responsible behavior came at considerable cost, including the dissolution of previously stable intimate relationships (Des Jarlais, 1987).

Psychiatric morbidity associated with HIV testing has been a continuing issue of concern. Unfortunately, the limited studies that have been conducted report divergent findings. In one small study of 15 seropositive IV drug users recruited from methadone clinics in New York City, learning of a positive antibody status was not associated with serious psychological sequellae (Casadonte et al., 1988). A separate study of 66 pregnant women from the New York City area (Cancellieri et al., 1988) compared 25 seropositive drug users with 41 seronegative drug users. The study found increased feelings of guilt regarding the health of the unborn child in the seropositive women, together with anxiety when drug-related symptoms were confused with HIV-related symptoms. Notification of test results was associated with the increased use of crack in both seropositive and seronegative women, which in turn led to paranoid psychotic episodes along with suicidal or homicidal behavior.

Other studies illuminate additional problems associated with antibody testing. In one large survey of homosexual men (Lyter et al., 1987), the anticipation of psychological difficulties in dealing with a positive test result was the most common reason for refusing to learn about test results among those who had volunteered for HIV screening and had undergone extensive pretest counseling. Those who declined to be informed of their results were more likely to be young, nonwhite, and less educated then those who agreed to know their results. In another study, seropositive men were more likely than seronegative men to report a break-up of their primary relationships (Coates et al., 1987). Finally, a study of suicides in New York found alarmingly high rates among men with AIDS.[7] Marzuk and colleagues (1988) found that men aged 20–59 with AIDS were 36 times more likely to commit suicide than men in the same age group who were not diagnosed with AIDS.

Despite the fact that public health officials recommend testing to encourage and support behavioral change, both this committee and the IOM/NAS AIDS committee find that further studies are

---

[7]Because the suicides documented among these men were obvious and for the most part violent, these rates are thought to underestimate the true level.

necessary to assess the impact of testing on behavioral change and psychiatric morbidity, including suicide. Research is needed to determine why change occurs and how it is sustained in some individuals but not in others. Moreover, more knowledge is needed about how individuals in various at-risk groups decide whether to be tested. Part of the process surely includes weighing the risks of discrimination (including the loss of housing and insurance benefits) and the psychological distress associated with testing against its benefits. It is to be hoped that data from the CDC community demonstration and AIDS prevention projects noted earlier in this chapter will help fill these and other gaps in knowledge.

New studies of the impact of serologic testing on risk-associated behavior will have to take into account the potential effects of differential participation in testing programs. On the one hand, individuals who are more concerned about their health may be more likely to seek testing and counseling for HIV infection or to undergo diagnostic evaluations more frequently than those who are less concerned about their health. On the other hand, individuals who know or suspect they are infected may be less likely to seek testing. Data from a serologic testing program (conducted in an STD clinic) showed that seropositive individuals were more likely than seronegative persons to decline testing (Hull et al., 1988). Clearly, it will be important to ascertain the extent and direction of self-selection bias in future studies.

In no case, however, will testing be a panacea to prevent the spread of HIV infection, and it should not be the centerpiece of a health education program. Motivating, directing, and sustaining behavioral change should involve multiple strategies, with antibody testing as but one of the available means to achieve these goals. In addition, the problems that attend the whole issue of antibody testing must be addressed. Institutional support, including the provision of counseling and the guarantee of confidentiality, is needed to maximize the effectiveness of testing. Legal protection against discrimination and guarantees of humane treatment will also need to be put in place at the federal level. At present, however, from a public health perspective, it is indefensible not to have testing available for those individuals who believe it will benefit their capacity to alter risk-associated behaviors. **The committee recommends that anonymous HIV antibody testing with appropriate pre- and posttest counseling be made available on a voluntary basis for anyone desiring it.** This recommendation concurs with that of the IOM/NAS AIDS committee (IOM/NAS, 1988).

Sustaining Behavioral Change

Even when desired change has occurred, there remains the problem of sustaining the changed behaviors over time. Considerable variation occurs in the length of time behavioral change will persist. High relapse rates have been reported in studies of a variety of health behaviors, although a critical review of experimental studies and their methodologies indicates that the problem of relapse has sometimes been overstated (Green et al., 1986). For chronic health threats (e.g., HIV infection), a lifelong adherence to health-promoting behaviors (in this case, safer sex and safer injection behaviors) is necessary. It is therefore important to understand the factors associated with relapse and its prevention.

"Temptation"—that is, availability in the environment—is commonly believed to be the cause of relapse. Yet careful studies have shown that negative emotions—such as stress, depression, and anxiety—are the most common precursors of relapse. In addition, alcohol or drugs may contribute to relapse; the combination of alcohol or drugs with sex has been associated with high-risk activities among homosexual and bisexual men (Stall et al., 1986). Although it is not known with any certainty whether the probability of lapsing is constant over time (Brownell et al., 1986), there are clearly psychological, environmental, and social factors that affect it. Learned coping responses, including skills training and relapse rehearsal, can lead to increased perceptions of self-efficacy and decrease the probability of relapse (Marlatt, 1982).[8]

Relapse prevention involves a self-management technique to help individuals either to refrain from a specific set of behaviors or to limit the occurrence of those behaviors. It includes a number of components: a conscious rethinking of the skills needed to resist risk-associated activity, relapse action and planning, behavioral contracting and rehearsal, and the mastery of new skills (Mantell, no date). The technique is based on principles of social learning theory and combines skills training and cognitive intervention (Marlatt, 1982). Originally developed to manage addictive behaviors, relapse prevention is suitable for impulse control and the control of indulgent behaviors that require immediate gratification and are followed by delayed negative consequences. Many different strategies are used in relapse prevention; current HIV intervention programs, for example, are evaluating the efficacy of diaries for gay and bisexual

[8]For addictive behaviors, such as heroin use, there are also physiological issues that must be addressed to prevent relapse.

men to help them monitor the cognitive, social, and emotional antecedents of their high-risk behaviors (Coxon, 1986). Other interventions that protect against relapse may also help begin desired behavioral change.

The length of an intervention program can affect the stability of behavioral change. In evaluating programs, it is important to distinguish between short-term and long-term prevention strategies. Sometimes there may be a tradeoff between expedient intervention strategies that result in short-term changes in behavior and the slower, more difficult programs that target long-term education and life-style changes to achieve congruence between behavior and the values, beliefs, and other attributes of the individual. Long-term drug treatment provided through therapeutic communities and short-term detoxification for IV drug use illustrate the two poles of this continuum of intervention length. (Unfortunately, the available data are not adequate to make definitive statements about the relative efficacy of long-term versus short-term drug treatment programs.)

Drug treatment programs are obvious points for reaching IV drug users at risk of HIV infection and are effective in decreasing the frequency of infection, thus decreasing the likelihood of spreading AIDS. It is obvious, however, that an IV drug user must first have access to treatment if treatment is to have an effect. Currently, there are waiting lists for IV drug treatment programs in every major urban area in the country (IOM/NAS, 1988). In Chapter 3, the committee recommends expanding drug treatment programs to accommodate anyone wanting treatment. Individuals who are motivated to take action need assistance to do so; they should be provided with programs to change risk-associated behavior and to sustain those changes. As stated in the previous chapter, serving the diverse needs of disparate populations is apt to require multiple strategies. Moreover, sustained treatment contact is needed: a single experience with an intervention program is usually insufficient to effect lasting change.

The common belief that one slip necessarily leads to complete relapse is not substantiated by research in relapse prevention. The incorrect picture that has been fostered by this notion may have come from focusing only on those who have relapsed while not taking into account those who have not. It is particularly important to overcome the idea of "one fatal slip" among IV drug users. As Des Jarlais has noted:

> Given the exigencies of daily life for an IV drug user, it is unlikely that the new risk reduction behavior can always be maintained.

> Thus there must also be an additional belief that the occasional slip in risk reduction behavior does not negate the need for continuing risk reduction. (1987:12)

It is unreasonable to expect that changes in risk-associated behavior will be constant over an individual's lifetime. Both the individual and the environment in which he or she lives are dynamic. The grave consequences of HIV infection require continued efforts to facilitate change in those behaviors associated with risk and to support change that has already occurred. Therefore, **the committee recommends that programs consider the psychological, social, biological, and environmental factors that may affect relapse; learned coping responses, including skills training and relapse rehearsal, should be taught to increase perceptions of self-efficacy.**

It is not yet clear how to influence the behavior of those individuals who persist in high-risk activities despite intervention efforts. The lessons that have been learned from smoking cessation programs indicate that even long-term educational efforts are sometimes ineffective with persistently noncompliant groups. As discussed earlier in this chapter, more education does not inevitably lead to more change. Nevertheless, some approaches have been seen to offer the potential for influencing persistent behavior. Increasing a person's level of self-efficacy appears to be helpful. Programs to heighten individuals' awareness of the capacity of drugs and alcohol to impair judgment, especially in sexual situations, may also facilitate risk reduction. Combining approaches offers additional possibilities. In a randomized trial of a multifaceted face-to-face program for homosexual men with long histories of high-risk activities, significant risk reduction was seen after 12 weeks of education, cognitive self-management training, and the development of strong social support systems (Kelly et al., 1987a). In addition, there are forces greater than the individual (e.g., peer support and supportive social conditions) that need to be mobilized in oder to evoke and sustain appropriate behaviors; some of these forces are discussed later in this chapter.

Assessing Change

There is a notion that change is only significant or "real" if it has occurred in all targeted individuals and is permanent. Those who insist on so absolute a definition of change are unrealistic, and they will be eternally disappointed in the actual achievements of risk-takers (and in the social scientists who design the intervention programs to facilitate those achievements). It is highly unlikely that such a standard for behavioral change can be met sufficiently widely to make it a satisfactory program goal. As stated earlier, the modification of behavior and incremental change are usually easier to achieve than global change; in addition, any change that has occurred may be difficult to maintain. A more reasonable and appropriate standard of judgment can be formulated as the question: Is the change that has already occurred sufficient to reduce the spread of HIV infection within a community, thereby decreasing the likelihood that a risk-taking person will encounter an infected individual?

Unfortunately, there is limited information available on the distribution of sexual and drug-use behaviors (see Chapters 2 and 3) against which behavioral change can be measured. (Without such information, it is also difficult to target resources and programs; it is impossible to monitor program effects.) For some parts of the United States, appropriate current data simply do not exist. The available self-reported data on behavioral change show irregular patterns over time and across groups. For example, data from a longitudinal study of homosexual and bisexual men from San Francisco (Ekstrand and Coates, 1988) indicated that 33.9 percent of the respondents reported unprotected receptive anal intercourse in 1985; only 8.3 percent continued to report this practice in 1987 (T. J. Coates, University of California at San Francisco, personal communication, August 1988). Yet there is strong concern that the behavioral modifications demonstrated in homosexual men from urban epicenters of the epidemic may not have occurred among gay men from rural areas or from urban areas that are thought to have low infection rates (Coates et al., 1988b). Data from a number of studies give support to the belief that safer sex practices have not been adopted equally throughout the country.

- Between May and December 1986, 65 percent of men participating in a large prospective, longitudinal study of homosexual men in Pittsburgh reported at least one episode of unprotected anal intercourse (Valdiserri et al., 1987).
- Homosexual men surveyed in Mississippi in 1987 reported an average of 19.7 partners in the past year with whom they had experienced unprotected receptive anal intercourse (Kelly et al., 1987a).
- Of men recruited through a gay support organization in New Mexico in 1985, 67 percent reported that they

practiced unprotected anal intercourse (C. C. Jones et al., 1987).

- In 1986, 21 percent of men interviewed in Boston reported anal intercourse without the use of condoms (McCusker et al., 1988).
- Even in New York City, an epicenter of the epidemic, homosexual men surveyed in 1985 reported using condoms only 20 percent of the time they engaged in anal intercourse (Martin, 1987).

As noted in Chapter 2, the incidence of STDs has been used as a surrogate marker for sexual behaviors associated with HIV infection. The uneven declines shown in gonorrhea and syphilis incidence data confirm the abovementioned self-reports of persisting high-risk sexual behavior. Although STD incidence has declined in San Francisco, Atlanta, New Orleans, San Diego, and Denver, increases in syphilis have been seen in Miami, Newark, Houston, Dallas, and Boston (Coates et al., 1988b). Chancroid is a sexually transmitted disease that has been implicated as a cofactor for HIV infection in Africa. Since 1981 numerous outbreaks of chancroid have been reported in the United States, and it has become endemic in several areas including urban areas in Florida, California, and New York. Between 1971 and 1980, a mean of 878 cases of chancroid was reported annually in the United States; in 1986, 3,418 cases were reported (Schmid et al., 1987).

There are some data to indicate that behavioral change has also occurred among IV drug users, albeit with variation across locations. A sample of IV drug users recruited through methadone maintenance programs in New York City in 1984 reported behavioral change to reduce the risk of contracting AIDS: approximately 30 percent reported the increased use of clean or new injection equipment and reduced needle-sharing (Friedman et al., 1986). In addition, although no change in needle-sharing behavior was seen between 1985 and 1987 in a sample of IV drug users recruited from a drug treatment center in San Francisco (Becker and Joseph, 1988), the proportion that reported it usually or always sterilized with bleach increased from 6 percent to 47 percent over this period (Chaisson et al., 1987).

Much less is known about the behavior of IV drug users who live in areas that have no active research programs. Even in areas in which intervention programs have been established, complete risk-reducing change is unlikely to have occurred throughout the at-risk population. Moreover, little is known about how existing change is maintained over time.

Impediments to Individual Action: The Example of Condom Use

The principles of behavioral change discussed above may be difficult to implement. These principles presume an empowered, active individual rather than a passive one, as well as realistically achievable paths of action. The following example may be helpful in clarifying some of the obstacles people may encounter when they attempt to change their behavior. (A broader discussion of barriers to action is presented in Part III of this report.)

A male high school student has heard that AIDS is a deadly sexually transmitted disease and that condoms may be helpful in preventing it. Being sexually active, he is reluctant to abandon a behavior that has been pleasurable. However, being quite sensible besides, he is not prepared to continue to take life-threatening risks. There are several questions he might well be expected to ask himself: Where do I get condoms? How do I negotiate the purchase with the local pharmacist? How do I figure out when and how to put a condom on? What do I do if my partner doesn't want me to use them? Answering these questions is apt to require information, skills, practice, and a sense that one is capable of doing these things.

The answers to these and other questions apparently elude many adolescents. A survey of black male adolescents in grades 7 through 12 from an urban area found that more than half thought they needed parental permission to purchase condoms (S. D. Clark et al., 1984; Grieco, 1986). Almost half (43 percent) said the embarrassment involved in purchasing condoms inhibited their use. Of those students who reported using condoms, there were more who had obtained them from another person than from a store. Twelve percent reported stealing their first condom.

Homosexual men have also reported cultural and practical barriers to condom use. In a study of gay men from the Pittsburgh area, the following perceptions of condoms were noted: they spoil sex (22 percent); they are embarrassing to buy (18 percent); they are found objectionable by sexual partners (16 percent); they are not readily available (22 percent); and they are used only by heterosexuals for contraceptive purposes (26 percent) (Valdiserri et al., 1987). When men who "always" used condoms for insertive anal intercourse were compared with men who "never" used them, nonusers tended to be younger, less educated, less concerned about risk, less convinced of condom efficacy in preventing the spread of HIV, and more likely to have used alcohol or other drugs during sex (Valdiserri et al., 1988). Indeed, the health education literature is replete with examples of motivated individuals who nevertheless do not undertake recommended behavioral changes because they perceive numerous barriers to be associated with these actions (Janz and Becker, 1984).

The use of condoms to prevent sexually transmitted HIV infection requires both the belief that condoms will prevent the spread of infection and the social and practical skills to acquire and use them. The question of condom efficacy in the prevention of STDs—in particular, infection from HIV—has fueled the debate about whether condoms are a reasonable method of AIDS prevention. It is obviously desirable and wise to caution potential users about the possible failure of condoms and the associated risks of such failure; it is also important, however, to consider the manner in which such a warning is given and the possible negative impact of exaggerated risk and of being led astray by perceived authorities. The following quotation comes from *Parade* magazine ("Special Intelligence Report," April 24, 1988:6), which is distributed in Sunday newspapers to households throughout the country.

> **Warning!** People who use condoms to prevent the spread of sexually transmitted diseases, such as AIDS, gonorrhea and syphilis, should know that they do not provide 100% protection. In recent tests, 12% of the condoms made in the U.S. and 21% of those made abroad failed. The Food and Drug Administration tests condoms by submitting them to federal water-leakage standards in the lab. If more than four condoms out of 1000 are found defective, the FDA rejects the entire batch from which the samples have been drawn. Imported condoms consistently show a higher failure rate than domestic brands.
>
> Unfortunately, there is virtually no scientific data on the failure rate of condoms as used by humans. Last April, the FDA wrote condom manufacturers explaining that, as a result of HIV infection, "it has become very important that users be fully aware that latex condoms provide protection, but do not guarantee it, and that protection is lost if condoms are not used properly." Properly used or not, a defective condom is, of course, worthless.

This information is only partly correct and very misleading. The article claimed that 12 percent of domestic condoms fail; in fact, 12 percent of *batches* fail (CDC, 1988a). A batch is rejected (i.e., fails) if 4 of 1,000 (0.4 percent) of condoms do not pass a water leakage test, a test that may or may not mimic the stresses and strains of in vivo use. Moreover, foreign manufacturers with two or more batches that fail to meet FDA standards are placed on an automatic detention list; their products are detained at the port of entry and are not distributed throughout the country (CDC, 1988a). Without doubt, there is some risk of breakage (and therefore infection) associated with condom use, although such risk is difficult to estimate. Nevertheless, it is clear that intercourse (vaginal or anal) using a condom is much safer than intercourse without one. Consequently, in the case of the *Parade* article, the "warning" may well do more harm than good in reducing the spread of HIV infection.

In its brochure, "AIDS and the Education of Our Children," the U.S. Department of Education stressed three phrases in its one-page section on condoms and AIDS: (1) the use of condoms can reduce but by no means eliminate the risk of contracting AIDS; (2) condoms can and do fail; and (3) maintaining strict moral standards is the most appropriate way to avoid AIDS (U.S. Department of Education, 1987:16). Focusing on the risk of condom failure in this way can lead to feelings of hopelessness and frustration, which in turn can lead to unprotected intercourse. Indeed, messages that stress the failure of condoms rather than their capacity to protect have been shown to dissuade young adults from believing that condoms are an effective means of preventing HIV infection.[9] It is clear, however, that protected intercourse, although not perfectly safe, is still safer than unprotected intercourse.

SOCIAL SUPPORT FOR BEHAVIORAL CHANGE

Individuals do not act in a vacuum: rather, action occurs in a social environment. Thus, if AIDS prevention programs are to be successful, they must take into account several important facts about the social factors that affect individual change. First, people are less likely to behave in ways that will incur the disapproval of others in their social group; people tend to conform to the "shoulds" and "oughts" of behavior specified in the norms of their community. (For example, behavioral change reported by homosexual men has been influenced by changes in the accepted standards and expectations for sexual behavior [i.e., normative shifts] in this group.) Second, some social and community structures foster healthy behaviors and behavioral change; others inhibit them. (It is sensible to expect that anonymous testing, in contrast to other formats of testing, will yield more credible information and may also lead to desirable changes in behavior.) The identification and mobilization of social factors that support behavioral change are thus extremely important components of AIDS prevention programs. Programs that seek to

---

[9] Approximately 100 Yale University students were assigned to one of two groups receiving logically equivalent but differently worded messages on condom failure. They were asked: "Should the government allow this condom to be advertised and sold as an effective method for preventing the spread of AIDS?" Almost 90 percent of the students who were told that condoms were 95 percent effective answered yes; only 42 percent of the students who were told that condoms had a 5 percent failure rate concurred with the statement (Dawes, 1988).

change behavior must inevitably confront the diverse and complex social forces that motivate and shape the behaviors at issue.

Family, Group, and Community Beliefs

There is increasing evidence that social support has an effect on the health status of individuals. Such support appears to be especially important in the management of chronic disease or in situations in which long-term behavioral change is required to prevent or ameliorate disease (Becker, 1985). For example, family support has been shown to be important in cuing and reinforcing appropriate behaviors for obesity, hypertension, arthritis, and coronary heart disease (Becker, 1985; Morisky et al., 1985). Families and other groups can affect an individual's adherence to prescribed behaviors by providing material, cognitive, and psychological support. The greater the compatibility of family roles and beliefs, the greater the support for health behaviors and the greater the likelihood that the individual will initiate and sustain them.

Social support comes in many forms, and it can affect individual action in many ways. In the early days of the AIDS epidemic, for instance, gay men turned to their communities for information about the disease and for an interpretation of relevant information. Yet social support for health behavior goes beyond the provision and interpretation of information, and this broader definition implies the need for additional resources and the possibility of other problems. For example, the services needed to prevent and treat drug use require federal, state, and local resources, the appropriation and coordination of which may be problematic. The current shortage of treatment slots and the establishment of fees to enter treatment constitute socially erected barriers to prevention. An additional barrier may be a community's resistance to locating programs in the local neighborhood.

A number of the factors that have contributed to the spread of infection among Hispanics (or Latinos) provide poignant examples of the failure of societal and community structures to support individual action to prevent AIDS. Grass-roots Latino political organizations did not make AIDS a high-priority issue early in the epidemic, nor did they claim to represent homosexual Latino men. Indeed, the high level of stigma associated with homosexuality in the Hispanic family and community is thought to have led to the denial of same-sex orientation and susceptibility to AIDS that has been seen among Latino men. The risk of abandonment by family and friends appears real to Hispanic men who may have had sex with other men.[10] In addition, support from larger societal structures has been limited. Minority populations in the United States have received fewer health resources and endured greater morbidity and mortality from a range of health problems. AIDS is yet another health threat that will differentially affect Latino and other minority communities (Fullilove, 1988; Peterson and Bakeman, 1988).

Subgroups of women also suffer from the lack of social support to prevent AIDS. Cultural constraints can inhibit women from taking a more active role in bringing condoms to a sexual relationship (Mantell et al., in press). For example, Latino gender roles make it difficult for some women even to broach the subject of sex or condoms. Moreover, condoms interfere with reproduction and are therefore at odds with cultural ideals of virility and womanhood (Mantell et al., in press). Even within a long-standing intimate relationship, a woman may not have sufficient power to effect change. Messages and programs that place the burden of condom use on women without parallel education efforts for men are not reasonable when the culture equates such behavior among women with prostitution or moral laxness. Programs that focus exclusively on women give them the responsibility for protecting themselves and their offspring from AIDS, but many women do not have sufficient power to prevent sexual transmission of this disease.[11]

Social forces can also modify perceptions and expectations, however, which in turn can motivate and sustain behavioral change. Friends may report confidentially a very pleasurable sexual experience that involved the use of a condom; they may also reinforce the notion that others expect protected intercourse. Moreover, as Catania and coworkers note: "Belief in our abilities to accomplish change may be influenced by observing that people similar to us can successfully accomplish change" (1988:14).

The responses of others are particularly important in the case of IV drug use. Peer approval is a significant component in the initial use of IV drugs and is also a factor in the sharing of injection equipment. It is logical, therefore, to consider peer approval as a potential strategy to reinforce risk-reducing behaviors. Indeed, data from one study in New York City indicated that the participation of friends in risk-reducing activities was the strongest predictor of behavioral change among IV drug users (Friedman et al., 1987). In addition, a study of methadone patients from the New York City area (Des

[10]See C. McGraw, "Lack of Effort to Combat AIDS in Latino Community Criticized," *Los Angeles Times*, February 26, 1988:II1.

[11]See S. G. Boodman, "Hispanic Culture Redefines AIDS Fight: Communication Problems, Moral Traditions Hinder Efforts," *The Washington Post*, December 28, 1987:A1.

Jarlais, 1987) showed that change was occurring along the lines of friendship groups and not among isolated individuals, indicating the important role of peer support in initiating and sustaining behavioral change. A sense of group identity and social community among homosexual men has also supported measures to prevent the spread of AIDS. Perceptions that one's peers were reducing risk-associated behavior have been shown to be correlated with individuals' reports of change in their own behavior (Joseph et al., 1987a). Common life-styles, attitudes, and beliefs form a strong basis for group identity, and field observations of communities of gay men (Coates and Greenblatt, in press) have shown that the sense of group identity and social community is very important in leading people to take protective measures against the spread of HIV infection.

Normative beliefs also affect what an individual will do to prevent infection. The theory of reasoned action (Ajzen and Fishbein, 1980) proposes that the intention to act depends in part on subjective normative beliefs about what others think one should or should not do. Behaviors that are considered the norm or that convey social approval provide a reward, a sense of benefit, to the individual who behaves in such a fashion. Similarly, unacceptable behavior can be inhibited by the predicted social disapproval of such action. The response of individuals to the perceived normative climate will affect their behavior: people develop notions about what others think of their behavior, and their subsequent actions reflect some sense of how important this is to them. Thus, for example, if the use of sterile injection equipment becomes normative within the IV drug-using population, individual users will feel pressured to sterilize their works.

Community-Level Intervention Programs

Community-level approaches to prevent HIV infection provide information, skills training, and a social environment that supports and sustains individual behavioral changes. In their efforts to change health-related behaviors, community-level programs bring together a number of diverse program components. They can also direct intervention strategies and the flow of information through existing structures and groups, thus influencing a broader audience than would be reached by more individual efforts.

Community-level programs are designed to produce enough change in enough people to prevent the spread of infection and to alter norms that are relevant to the behaviors associated with risk. They create a social environment that reminds the individual that safer behavior is viewed as preferable to risky behavior. There are two important points of impact. First, community-level interventions can reach a critical mass of individuals, providing information, motivation, and skills training. Second, by working through a variety of local agencies, changes in norms can be achieved. If normative behavior has changed, it increases the likelihood that, for example, sex partners will expect to engage in low-risk behavior. If a critical mass has been reached, motivated, and changed, and if community norms have shifted, it is less likely that any given individual will indulge in high-risk behavior. "The objective is to create a sum greater than the parts through synergistic action around community-wide AIDS prevention events and activities" (Coates et al., 1988b:22).

Communities can be defined by various criteria: they may consist of individuals who share behavioral patterns (e.g., IV drug users or homosexual men); they may have a common racial, ethnic, or sexual identity; they may share a common geographic area or organization (e.g., a school or prison). Regardless of the definition, intervention strategies should take into account the leaders and organizations of the community in the design of intervention programs. Authority figures and trusted opinion leaders can be important allies in achieving health goals. Although the initial stimulus for action may come from outside (for example, from the public health department or a university-based research program), it must still be accepted by and incorporated into community structures. The committee agrees with Coates and Greenblatt's (in press) statement that "[c]hange may require ideas and technology from the outside, but adoption, maintenance, and adaptation require the explicit collaboration of individuals and agencies from within the community." **The committee recommends that, to the extent possible, community-level interventions to prevent the spread of HIV infection address simultaneously information, motivational factors, skills, prevailing norms, and methods for diffusing innovation.**

Community-level intervention methods have been successfully applied to the prevention of a range of diseases, including cardiovascular disease and cancer. Annual evaluation data from the well-designed Stanford Three-Community Study (Farquhar et al., 1977) indicated that communities exposed to a media-based campaign reduced hypertension, blood cholesterol, and cigarette use by approximately 25 percent; individuals who were given additional skills training and social support reduced their risk by approximately 30 percent. Most of those reporting change had maintained it for three years. In another instance, a community-based program to reduce teenage pregnancy (modeled on the Stanford program) was able to delay the age of initial intercourse and increase the consistent use of contraceptives among teenagers who were sexually active (Vincent et al., 1987). It is hoped that evaluation data from CDC-supported community demonstration projects currently under way in Dallas, Denver, Albany, New York City, Seattle, Chicago, and Long Beach will help to identify the primary factors associated with facilitating and maintaining behavioral change to prevent HIV infection.

Community-level attempts to prevent drug use take into account the environment in which that behavior occurs. Such approaches have relied on information campaigns to communicate the adverse effects of drug use and to motivate people to refrain from using drugs; they have also involved the formation of collaborative and cooperative relationships among parents, schools, and community agencies to heighten concern about the problems associated with drug use and to take steps to alter organizations (e.g., "head shops") and situations that facilitate drug use (Durell and Bukoski, 1984). A program in California called Parents Who Care provides support to adolescents by giving drug-free parties and cooperatively setting guidelines for curfews and social activities (Polich et al., 1984).

The San Francisco area offers an excellent model of community-level intervention. Very early in the epidemic, the San Francisco AIDS Foundation began a community-based HIV risk reduction program. A nonprofit corporation, the Stop AIDS Project, was formed to work with grass-roots gay organizations. Because many gay men had already reported knowledge of AIDS and change in relevant behaviors, the focus of the Stop AIDS program activities moved beyond individual change to social and cultural change that included raising individual awareness of peer support for safer sex practices and promoting further normative change in the local community. Changes that had already occurred among gays were emphasized to show the larger group that a shift in norms was occurring. The cooperation and participation of leaders in the gay community facilitated education efforts and lent credibility to the project's activities.

The Stop AIDS project has now broadened its approach to the problem by reaching out to other risk groups and by enlisting other organizations in efforts to prevent further spread of infection. The University of California at San Francisco, through its AIDS Health Project, and Pacific Mental Health Services, through Operation Concern, joined this endeavor to provide health consultation and support groups for those at risk. The Instituto Familiar de la Raza and the Bayview Hunter's Point Foundation assisted with outreach activities to minority communities and education efforts. The Women's AIDS Network and the California Prostitutes Education Project are addressing the needs of women at high risk of HIV infection. Another part of the San Francisco community-level program provided AIDS prevention education to IV drug users and relied on a number of organizations and outreach workers to contact substance abusers on the street and in outpatient and inpatient treatment facilities (Doll and Bye, 1987).

Independent research projects in the San Francisco area have found substantial decreases in the number of men engaging in high-risk sexual behavior. Because many AIDS-related activities have occurred simultaneously in San Francisco, it is difficult to discover a causal relationship between particular elements of the community-based program and specific outcomes. However, there are indications that change occurring in San Francisco during the program's operation is apt to be related to community-based efforts. Almost 7,000 homosexual and bisexual men attended at least one small group meeting on safer sex practices; this number is thought to represent approximately 10 percent of the local gay population. A 1986 telephone survey found that 86 percent of homosexual and bisexual men interviewed were aware of the media campaign. More men remembered specific messages about sex than about drugs. Twelve percent had attended at least one educational activity (Doll and Bye, 1987).

The San Francisco experience highlights the following seven elements of a successful community-based program:

1. strong leadership from within the targeted community;
2. market research to identify appropriate messages and communication channels to reach the target audience;
3. programs to inform and motivate the target audience;
4. activities to facilitate social and cultural change;
5. use of multiple channels of communication;
6. grass-roots participation; and
7. research documenting baseline levels of high-risk behavior and behavioral change, noting, where possible, the factors related to a failure to change (Communication Technologies, 1987).

In the case of AIDS, fostering community norms that allow those at risk to avail themselves of help is critical in controlling the spread of HIV infection. To empower the individual, it is necessary to empower the community, which in turn may require changes in institutions and structures. Institutional factors, such as legal and religious sanctions, can foster community norms and structures that either facilitate or impede individual action, and those institutions that operate in and have credibility with the community must be used in efforts to change human behavior. Schools, churches, health care providers, the media, and workplaces are important venues for affecting health behavior. Analyses of local resources can identify potential links to the local population and may provide clues to the best ways to reach specific groups. Ideally, the objectives and priorities for community-based programs should be established through a process that includes input from the groups that make up that community (Green and McAlister, 1984).

Impediments to Effecting Behavioral Change

As noted earlier in this chapter, there are sometimes substantial barriers to implementing the strategies that have been designed to change human health-related behavior. For example, people often hold incorrect stereotypical notions about the problem and about those at risk. These problematic perceptions slow progress in preventing further infection because they frequently lead to operationalization of poor ideas and tend to retard reasoned action.

Prejudice and stigma (see Chapter 7) have caused some people to believe that certain groups are incapable of changing their behavior, but data from surveys of IV drug users, prostitutes, and homosexual men do not support this notion. In general, it is important to point out that the groups at highest risk of infection in this epidemic also respond most favorably to the conditions under which all people respond best—that is, supportive economic, political, and social conditions. Clearly, there are variations in health and other behaviors across ethnic and racial groups; yet there are also common threads linking all people that should not be overlooked.

In-Groups Versus Out-Groups: Creating Distance From Risk

Many people believe that individuals who engage in high-risk behavior are quite different from everyone else, and they therefore conclude that risk-taking individuals will not respond to intervention strategies designed to halt the spread of HIV infection. This exaggerated sense of difference between oneself or one's group (in-group) and others (out-group) has limited effective interventions in the AIDS epidemic. Four important phenomena may operate when the perceptions of in-groups are compared with those of out-groups: (1) people tend to see in-groups as superior (ethnocentrism); (2) they tend to perceive in-groups as more complex and heterogeneous than out-groups (out-group homogeneity); (3) they tend to exaggerate the differences between their own group and other groups (contrast and accentuation effects); and (4) they tend to perceive events in a manner that is consistent with the expectations and goals of their group (assimilation) (Dawes et al., 1972; Rothbart et al., 1984). These phenomena have an impact on how problems are defined and solved and on how people are perceived and treated.

The operation of these phenomena can result in distorted perceptions of minorities and their risk of HIV infection, as illustrated in the following example. Minority communities in the United States have suffered a disproportionate burden of infection (Sabatier, 1988). In a 1987 *Washington Post* editorial, "AIDS: The Real Danger . . ." (June 7:B7), social critic George F. Will did not find it surprising that blacks and Hispanics account for disproportionate numbers of cases of AIDS: "After all, many people are caught in the culture of urban poverty precisely because they have never been given the basic skills of social competence: they do not regulate their behavior well, least of all in conformity with public-health bulletins." The distinction that Mr. Will makes between poor, urban ethnic minorities and what he calls "the general heterosexual population" heightens the reader's perceptions of the differences between groups.

The committee believes it is counterproductive to focus on differences that are not related to behavioral change. To prevent further infection, people have to change risk-associated behavior; to begin to make appropriate behavioral changes, people must recognize that AIDS is a potential problem for them personally. Therefore, to lay blame, to label those at risk as socially, economically, or behaviorally inferior, is to alienate people who are seeking to understand their personal susceptibility and to discourage them from assessing their risk. In addition, to portray the problem as one that primarily affects minority populations deflects attention away from the need for nonminorities to take preventive action.

It is vital to dispel the belief that individuals who engage in high-risk behaviors are so different from most of the population or live with so high a level of psychopathology that they cannot be motivated by the same concerns or goals as others in the population and are therefore not likely to be influenced by any of the intervention strategies that the behavioral sciences have to offer. Although there are certainly important differences between out-groups and in-groups, these differences can be identified and taken into account when planning interventions. Moreover, too strong a focus on such differences may negate those similarities that are bound to exist. There is no doubt that many factors affect the differential responses people have to one strategy or another. Still, exaggerating the differences between in-groups and out-groups will prevent an appropriate assessment of personal susceptibility and can generate a sense of hopelessness.

IV Drug Users

An example of this hopelessness is the public's perception that IV drug users are unable to alter their drug and sexual behaviors to prevent either the acquisition or spread of the disease. There is a pervasive sense that drug users are self-destructive and uninterested in their own health and that they therefore cannot be expected to be concerned about the health of others. Although social organizational constraints and the physiology of addiction make changes in behavior difficult for this at-risk population, data show that some IV drug users have already taken action to protect their own health and that of others.

Skeptics might question the reliability of self-reported data collected from IV drug users, but there are other, perhaps more objective, indicators of behavioral change. In New York City, as more and more addicts have become aware of the risk posed by used injection equipment, the market for sterile illicit needles and syringes has been growing. For those who cannot give up their drug habit, rising numbers are trying to inject drugs in a safer fashion. Of 22 illicit needle sellers surveyed in New York City, 18 reported an increase in sales over the past year; 4 specifically mentioned AIDS as the cause for increased demand (Des Jarlais and Friedman, 1987). Sadly, as discussed in the previous chapter, some of this demand is being met on the black market with counterfeit sterile injection equipment. Almost one-half of those selling needles reported occasionally repackaging used equipment for resale as new. Other drug dealers have been using new works as a marketing device for bags of heroin (Des Jarlais, 1987). These data highlight both the strength of the demand for clean injection equipment and the dangers of relying on illicit markets for distribution. It is clear, however, that many IV drug users want to and can change some of their behavior, and the social barriers to such change should be removed.

Female Prostitutes

Considerable concern has also been expressed about the role that female prostitutes may play in spreading HIV infection. The link between multiple sexual partners and increased risk for AIDS was established in the homosexual population. Many people fear that prostitutes (who by definition have multiple sex partners) will not adopt safer sex practices with their clients and will therefore be the conduit through which HIV infection will spread to the heterosexual population. Yet the existing data on prostitutes do not support this concern (see Chapter 2). The threat that prostitutes pose to any given heterosexual contact appears to be greater in personal relationships than in paying ones. The cultural values that surround intimate relationships, including notions of love and trust, do not foster condom use. Unsafe sex may be a part of the definition of a personal relationship for women who work in the sex industry.

The term *women in the sex industry* has been coined to describe the diverse group of women who exchange sex for money, goods, or services (see discussion of prostitution in Chapter 2). A survey of these women (Cohen, 1987) found that important prerequisites to AIDS intervention efforts included program designs that reflected the needs and perceptions of the target population and outreach to those in need through relationships based on caring, respect, and honesty. The design phase of this survey permitted input from the target population; respondents asked that they not be treated impersonally (as patients are often treated) or as objects of intellectual or ethical curiosity. Researchers who have made an impartial, informed effort to understand the needs of this population feel that, in return, they have benefited from their subjects' increased participation and frankness (Cohen, 1987).

As is the case with needle sterilization among IV drug users, women in the sex industry who are at risk for AIDS are more likely to modify their behavior than to make global changes in their life-styles. Clearly, the threat of further HIV transmission posed by prostitutes could be removed by eliminating prostitution. However, this is unlikely to occur as long as there is a demand for the services offered by women in the sex industry and as long as women perceive that such employment is the best or only kind available to them. Therefore, effective prevention programs must understand and make appeals to the real goals of the targeted population, and the social barriers to implementing such programs should be removed. It should not be assumed that the goals held by those proposing change are necessarily those of the individuals to be reached. Rather, there is a need to interact with the group to determine what these goals are.

Innovative and Controversial Approaches to Behavioral Change

In its recent report, the IOM/NAS AIDS committee concluded that "the HIV epidemic should prompt a reexamination of the fiscal and institutional barriers that impede effective public health efforts in all program areas related to the control of HIV infection" (IOM/NAS, 1988:62). The threat posed by HIV infection does not permit the luxury of proceeding as with other diseases; this is not business as usual. Therefore, for some behaviors and in some populations, dramatic, innovative steps will be needed to prevent the spread of infection.

Two such innovative approaches to facilitating behavioral change—both of which are sources of controversy—are the provision of sterile needles for individuals who persist in IV drug use and intensive school sex education programs. The committee finds both of these approaches to be promising; nevertheless, it concludes that systematic, well-designed program evaluations (and planned program variations) are needed to determine the effectiveness of these strategies in preventing disease.

Sterile Needle Programs

There is no controversy about whether sterile needles help to prevent the spread of AIDS among IV drug users. Rather, debate centers on whether sterile needles would be used if they were made available and whether programs to make them available would have harmful side effects (e.g., prolonging drug use or increasing its rate) that would outweigh their benefits. The committee finds no convincing evidence that current legal restrictions decrease drug use and no evidence (from other countries) that easing access to injection equipment increases the number of new drug users or the levels of drug use among existing IV drug users. To date, needle distribution programs in this country are currently in the planning stage; therefore, no data are currently available on the effect of this approach among IV drug users in the United States.

The belief that IV drug users would not protect themselves by using sterile needles is best expressed by a 1988 editorial written by Tottie Ellis for *USA Today.* The editorial, entitled "Clean Needles Idea Is Menace to Society," states: "To assume that anyone who is so irresponsible as to get on heroin would then become sensible enough to use clean needles or sterilize them is as contradictory as a cat with wings" (February 9:10A). The belief expressed in this statement is that a single behavior (IV drug use) is diagnostic of a global personality characteristic (irresponsibility) that implies with certitude an entire set of other behaviors.[12] Yet almost all research on the subject challenges the existence of global personality characteristics. The inconsistent arguments that a sterile needle program would be ineffective because irresponsible people who do not care about their health would not use it and because it would encourage drug use appear to be based more on in-group/out-group prejudice than on logic.

In countries in which sterile needle programs have been implemented, IV drug users have taken advantage of their offerings (Des

[12] For a review of the concept of global personality, see Shweder (1979).

Jarlais and Hunt, 1988). An estimated 50 percent of IV drug users in Amsterdam have used its "needle exchange program" (Buning et al., 1988). As discussed in the previous chapter, data from Amsterdam (Buning, 1987), where needle exchange programs have been in place for several years and the sale of injection equipment is legal, indicated no increase in the number of IV drug users; they did indicate an increase in the demand for treatment. There is also evidence that the program led to a decrease (from almost 90 percent to less than 50 percent) in the percentage of IV drug users who injected more than once a day (Des Jarlais, 1987). It is important to note, however, that the provision of sterile needles has been insufficient to prevent the spread of HIV and hepatitis among IV drug users in Amsterdam.

Controlled experiments are required to assess the impact of sterile needle programs in this country. Careful evaluation will be needed to provide evidence of the effect of such programs on the initiation of new IV drug users and on the drug-use patterns of those who are already injecting drugs. The committee recognizes that instituting sterile needle programs will not be easy; it will take money, expertise, scientific review, and care in execution as well as public and political support. Moreover, it will take time. It is highly unlikely that any one study of needle exchange programs will be definitive; multiple efforts, using planned variations of approaches in different populations with appropriate evaluation, will be needed to build a sound base of knowledge about this innovative strategy. Thus, **the committee recommends that well-designed, staged trials of sterile needle programs, such as those requested in the 1986 Institute of Medicine/National Academy of Sciences report *Confronting AIDS*, be implemented.**

Education Programs for Teenagers

The committee focuses on teenage sexual behavior because a substantial number of adolescents are sexually active and have dismal rates of consistent contraceptive use and alarmingly high rates of STDs. The relevant data that are summarized below are presented in detail in Chapter 2. Sexual experimentation without the benefit of barrier contraceptives (i.e., condoms) and a history of STDs indicate that adolescents are also at risk for HIV infection. The fact that there have been few documented cases of AIDS among adolescents is in part a function of the lengthy time between acquisition of the infection and the diagnosis of AIDS.

Data from the 1983 National Longitudinal Survey of Youth (Moore et al., 1987:Appendix Table 1.4) found that, by the end of adolescence (age 19), 83 percent of all young men and 74 percent of all young women have engaged in sexual intercourse. Many people believe that very early onset of sexual intercourse is a problem seen only among disadvantaged youths—that middle-class and nonminority adolescents do not engage in intercourse. Although it is true that minority youth are more likely than nonminority youth to have had intercourse as teenagers, the difference between black and white never-married girls reporting intercourse has decreased since 1971 (Moore et al., 1987:Appendix Table 1.2).

American teenagers, in contrast to their peers in other industrialized countries, are notoriously poor contraceptive users (J. B. Jones et al., 1985). Approximately half of all teenagers do not use contraceptives the first time they have sexual relations, and there is often irregular or no use after the first intercourse (Zelnik and Shah, 1983; Moore et al., 1987:Appendix Table 2.1). This lack of contraceptive use results in substantial rates of pregnancy among young women. In a sample of sexually active female adolescents who reported never using contraception, 48 percent of whites and 52 percent of blacks reported a premarital first pregnancy within 24 months of experiencing first intercourse (Moore et al., 1987:Appendix Table 3.5). Even among those who reported that they always used a contraceptive method, premarital pregnancies occurred in approximately 10 percent of young women in the sample within two years of the onset of intercourse.

Excluding homosexual men and prostitutes, sexually active teenage girls have the highest rates of gonorrhea, cytomegalovirus, chlamydia, and pelvic inflammatory disease of any age/sex group (Bell and Hein, 1984; Cates and Raugh, 1985; Mosher, 1985). The risk factors for STDs in adolescence include early onset of intercourse and no or irregular contraceptive use.

There are several ways to alter the high rates of STDs and unintended pregnancies among adolescents and the behaviors that can transmit HIV. The IOM/NAS AIDS committee found that "school-based educational programs are an essential part of efforts to increase awareness of the risk of HIV and to combat the spread of infection" (IOM/NAS, 1988:66). The Presidential Commission on the Human Immunodeficiency Virus Epidemic (1988) concurred. This committee has considered two important strategies for preventing infection in the adolescent population: school-based sex education programs and school-based clinics.

An often-cited concern about providing sex education is the intuitive and generally untested notion that sex education leads to sexual activity (Hayes, 1987). If teenagers have not learned about sex, the argument goes, then they will not engage in it. Does sex education precipitate or encourage sexual behavior? There is little evidence to support this notion. Large-scale evaluations of school-based programs in the United States suggest that sex education does not promote early sexuality (Zelnik and Kim, 1982; Furstenberg et al., 1986). However, these programs do appear to increase knowledge about reproduction, especially in younger adolescents, and they may even promote contraceptive use among sexually active teens (although variations in program design and implementation and few large-scale evaluations make the interpretation of these data more difficult) (Kirby, 1984). In Western Europe, where youths receive much more extensive sexual education, rates of sexual activity are no higher than those reported in the United States, but rates of contraceptive use are higher and rates of teenage pregnancy are lower (J. B. Jones et al., 1985).

Another concern about school-based sex education programs surrounds the belief that parents will not accept sex education outside the home for their children. Parents report being very concerned that their offspring become sexually responsible adults; many also report that they are very uncomfortable talking about reproductive and sexual issues with their children (Brooks-Gunn, 1987). In addition, although sex education was once believed to be solely the province of the family, the responsibility for sex education has in fact shifted in part to the school system. In the early 1980s, three quarters of all school districts provided some sex education (Kirby and Scales, 1981). The specter of HIV infection may increase the already high proportion of parents wishing to have sex education in the schools. In a recent national survey by Harris, virtually all parents (94 percent) wanted AIDS education in schools.[13]

Given the virtual unanimity among parents to include AIDS education in school curricula, why does the controversy surrounding such programs persist? The crux of the problem seems to be whether frank, explicit instruction will be allowed. Existing sex education programs are neither intensive nor extensive. Guttmacher's (1981) survey of school districts revealed that three quarters of the school districts surveyed provided reproductive information, but only one quarter of them included the reduction of sexual activity and teenage childbearing in their goals. In addition, most sex education programs are short (10 hours or less); fewer than 10 percent of all students have taken comprehensive programs of 40 hours or more (Kirby, 1984).

---

[13]A 1988 *Children's Magazine* article ("When AIDS Comes to School," a special report from Rodale Press) reported that 94 percent of parents responded that schools should take special steps when Harris pollsters asked them the following question: "In schools where NO child is suspected of having AIDS or carrying the AIDS antibodies, should the school take special steps to educate teachers and students about the disease, or are no special steps necessary?"

It is likely that sex education curricula will be expanded in coming years, given the concerns about AIDS (Boyer et al., 1988). Large urban school districts in this country have already initiated AIDS education programs, although current programs tend to be short and nonspecific. To successfully prevent risk-associated behavior, AIDS education programs must begin before the behavior is initiated. Therefore, AIDS education should begin in elementary school, and programs should take into account the cognitive differences of various age groups, differences that affect their ability to understand HIV transmission. Similarly, community concerns about the "appropriateness" of information need to be considered. AIDS education programs can begin in elementary school; the focus of such programs should be to allay excessive anxiety. In junior high school, the topic of sexual transmission would be included in the curriculum. In high school, more information would be added, including HIV transmission by homosexual and heterosexual behaviors, skills training and decision making, and the effective use of contraceptive methods (DiClemente et al., 1987).

The committee supports school-based AIDS education efforts for adolescents that encompass planned program variations and evaluation to provide information on educating youths more effectively about the risks posed by HIV infection. These programs need to inform both male and female, and both homosexual and heterosexual, adolescents.[14]

Most intervention programs that try to prevent adolescent drug use and pregnancy operate in the schools. An obvious and serious limitation to school-based programs is their inability to reach those adolescents who are not in school. For example, many drug users drop out of school before they make the decision to inject drugs (Des Jarlais and Friedman, 1987). It is important that prevention efforts located in the schools begin at a sufficiently early age to reach those at high risk for drug use, early sexual experimentation, and dropping out of school. Other programs are needed to reach beyond the schools to make contact with dropouts, runaways, and unemployed adolescents on the street and in the various institutions that serve adolescent populations.

School-based clinics, a hotly debated major programmatic effort that has been implemented in some communities, are another approach to dealing with a range of health-related problems in the adolescent population, including unintended pregnancy, contraceptive use, and the prevention of HIV and other sexually transmit-

[14]The IOM/NAS (1988) AIDS committee recommended the development of programs to reach youth who were just becoming homosexually active.

ted infections (Brooks-Gunn and Furstenberg, in press). Typically, other services are also provided, including physical examinations, treatment for illness and injury, immunization, and drug and alcohol programs. Most programs require parental consent, with blanket permission for all health services offered. Test results and consultations are confidential. Evaluations of school-based clinics are currently being conducted, with promising results reported for some programs (Edwards et al., 1980; Zabin et al., 1986). Given the resistance evidenced in some communities, however, it remains to be seen how many school-based clinics will be opened in the coming decade. The committee believes that such clinics require the systematic evaluation of planned variations to understand in what settings and for which individuals these programs can promote contraceptive use and HIV prevention.

The committee recommends that sex education be available to both male and female students and that such education include explicit information relevant to the prevention of HIV infection. Comprehensive services for adolescents, both those offered in the community and in the school context, should include components that focus directly on the high-risk behaviors—unprotected sex and IV drug use—that are associated with the spread of HIV infection.

In focusing its attention on the problems associated with preventing HIV infection among adolescents, the committee was not able to address AIDS prevention outside the context of sex education and school-based clinics. Nevertheless, the committee recognizes that the majority of school-based AIDS education takes place outside these venues and that joint efforts involving the schools and communities may hold the greatest promise for preventing HIV infection, other STDs, and unintended pregnancies (Vincent et al., 1987). The CDC Guidelines for Effective School Health Education to Prevent the Spread of AIDS (CDC, 1988b), as well as the Presidential AIDS Commission, the Institute of Medicine, and other national health and education organizations, have recommended that AIDS education be integrated within a planned and comprehensive school health education program. Age-appropriate curricula that address HIV prevention, sex education, and drug prevention education have been proposed for children in kindergarten through grade twelve. A comprehensive school program that is integrated into community efforts is needed to prevent the unnecessary problems that result when categorical efforts are developed in isolation and without broader public and administrative support. The committee finds health education for children of all ages, especially as it relates to HIV prevention, to be a very important issue and one that it hopes to address in detail in future activities.

THE ROLE OF PLANNED VARIATIONS AND EVALUATION

It was the committee's hope that those factors clearly associated with altering sexual and drug-use behaviors could be identified by examining the evaluation data of well-designed programs. Unfortunately, such data do not exist. There are self-reported data on relevant behavioral change: some IV drug users report changes in needle-sharing practices and increased sterilization of injection equipment, while some homosexual men report less unprotected anal intercourse. Yet little attention has been paid to understanding how and why these changes have occurred or the extent to which they have been instituted by different groups in different places.

Altering the course of the AIDS epidemic will depend on an iterative process in which intervention programs are implemented, their effects assessed, and a new and better set of intervention programs designed and implemented. Any intervention program is likely to involve many aspects, each of which would require choosing from a set of possible alternatives (there may be several choices available among target groups and approaches to them, media, program materials, delivery modes, timing, and so forth). The "best" choice is not always clear for at least some of these aspects. This fact poses a strategic opportunity that should not be lost: *progress in program improvement can be much accelerated by deliberately using two or more alternatives for some of the key choices.* This strategy has been referred to in this chapter as *planned variation.* **The committee recommends that planned variations of key program elements be systematically and actively incorporated into the design of intervention programs at an early stage.**

There are great advantages to conditions in which several admissible variants can be tried out in parallel. First, some successful combination is more likely to emerge if several promising variants are used. Second, ideas that are actually inferior can be more promptly identified and dropped. Third, ideas that are actually superior can be more quickly recognized. Fourth, a broader understanding of what works and why it works can build up a systematic base of knowledge. The principles of behavior discussed in this chapter form the basis for selecting the most promising program variations. **The committee recommends that the Public Health Service**

and others conducting or supporting intervention programs ensure the implementation of planned variations in AIDS messages, programs, and campaigns.

Careful evaluation is crucial to improving the nation's ability to contain the spread of HIV infection. If the United States is to build its capacity to intervene effectively to retard the spread of HIV, it must learn from ongoing prevention programs. To learn from such programs, they must be evaluated. The current situation does not appear to reflect a misperception of the need for evaluation or a lack of desire to conduct it. Rather, there are insufficient resources to conduct such work at the program implementation level. It may be most helpful to begin marshaling and allocating evaluation resources at the federal level. The next chapter discusses these and other issues related to the evaluation of AIDS interventions.

In sum, learning new behaviors and breaking established patterns of behavior that are known to be associated with risk will not be simple, nor will complete change be achieved. What is important to remember, though, is that people can change. It is also important to note that many stereotypical notions about the behavior of those at highest risk are not only incorrect but may slow the process of preventing further infection. Multiple strategies that repeat a coherent message are necessary to initiate and support behavioral change. Creating and sustaining behavioral changes in people have many aspects: producing an awareness of threat and the motivation to change while providing people with alternative ways of behaving; involving the relevant community or communities in such efforts; and creating economic, political, and social environments that support the new behaviors. Strategies that focus only on the individual must be supplemented with strategies that address those macro-level conditions that cause or reinforce high-risk behavior.

REFERENCES

Ajax, L. (1974) How to market a nonmedical contraceptive: A case study from Sweden. In M. H. Redford, G. W. Duncan, and D. J. Prager, eds., *The Condom: Increasing Utilization in the United States.* San Francisco: San Francisco Press, Inc.

Ajzen, I., and Fishbein, M. (1980) *Understanding Attitudes and Predicting Social Behavior.* Englewood Cliffs, N.J.: Prentice-Hall.

Bandura, A. (1977) Self-efficacy: Toward a unifying theory of behavioral change. *Psychological Review* 34:191–215.

Battjes, R. J. (1985) Preventing adolescent drug abuse. *International Journal of the Addictions* 20:1113–1134.

Becker, M. H. (1970) Sociometric location and innovativeness: Reformulation and extension of the diffusion model. *American Sociological Review* 35:267–282.

Becker, M. H. (1985) Patient adherence to prescribed therapies. *Medical Care* 23:539–555.

Becker, M. H., and Joseph, J. G. (1988) AIDS and behavioral change to reduce risk: A review. *American Journal of Public Health* 78:394–410.

Bell, T., and Hein, K. (1984) The adolescent and sexually transmitted diseases. In K. K. Holmes, P. A. Mardh, P. S. Sparling, and P. J. Wiesner, eds., *Sexually Transmitted Diseases*. New York: McGraw-Hill.

Brandt, A. M. (1987) *No Magic Bullet*. New York: Oxford University Press.

Brooks-Gunn, J. (1987) Pubertal processes and girls' psychological adaptation. In R. Lerner and T. T. Foch, eds., *Biological-Psychosocial Interactions in Early Adolescence*. Hillsdale, N.J.: Lawrence Earlbaum Associates.

Brooks-Gunn, J., and Furstenberg, F. F. (In press) Adolescent sexual behavior. *American Psychologist*.

Boyer, C. B., Brooks-Gunn, J., and Hein, K. (1988) Preventing HIV infection and AIDS in children and adolescents: Behavioral research and intervention strategies. *American Psychologist* 43:958–964.

Brownell, K. D., Marlatt, G. A., Lichtenstein, E., and Wilson, G. T. (1986) Understanding and preventing relapse. *American Psychologist* 41:765–782.

Buning, E. C. (1987) Prevention Policy on AIDS Among Drug Addicts in Amsterdam. Presented at the Third International AIDS Conference, Washington, D.C., June 1–5.

Buning, E. C., Hartgers, C., Verster, A. D., et al. (1988) The Evaluation of the Needle/Syringe Exchange in Amsterdam. Presented at the Fourth International AIDS Conference, Stockholm, June 12–16.

Cancellieri, F. R., Holman, S., Sunderland, A., Fine, J., Bihari, B., and Landesman, S. (1988) Psychiatric and Behavioral Impact of HIV Testing in Pregnant Drug Users. Presented at the Fourth International AIDS Conference, Stockholm, June 12–16.

Casadonte, P. P., Des Jarlais, D. C., Smith, T., et al. (1986) Psychological and Behavioral Impact of Learning HTLV-III/LAV Antibody Test Results. Presented at the Second International AIDS Conference, Paris, June 23–25.

Casadonte, P. P., Des Jarlais, D. C., Friedman, S., and Rotrosen, J. (1988) Psychological and Behavioral Impact of Learning HIV Test Results in IV Drug Users. Presented at the Fourth International AIDS Conference, Stockholm, June 12–16.

Catania, J. A., Kegeles, S. M., and Coates, T. J. (1988) Towards an Understanding of Risk Behavior: The CAPS' AIDS Risk Reduction Model. University of California at San Francisco.

Cates, W., Jr., and Raugh, J. L. (1985) Adolescents and sexually transmitted diseases: An expanding problem. *Journal of Adolescent Health Care* 6:1–5.

Centers for Disease Control (CDC). (1988a) Condoms for prevention of sexually transmitted diseases. *Morbidity and Mortality Weekly Report* 37:133–137.

Centers for Disease Control (CDC). (1988b) Guidelines for effective school health education to prevent the spread of AIDS. *Morbidity and Mortality Weekly Report* 37(Suppl. S-2).

Chaisson, R. E., Osmond, D., Moss, A. R., Feldman, H. W., and Bernacki, P. (1987) HIV, bleach, and needle sharing (letter). *Lancet* 1:1430.

Check, W. A. (1987) Beyond the political model of reporting: Nonspecific symptoms in media communications about AIDS. *Reviews of Infectious Diseases* 9:987–1000.

Clark, N. M. (1987) Social learning theory in current health education practice. In W. B. Ward, S. K. Simonds, P. D. Mullen, and M. H. Becker, eds., *Advances in Health Education and Promotion,* vol. 2. Greenwich, Conn.: JAI Press, Inc.

Clark, S. D., Zabin, L. S., and Hardy, J. B. (1984) Sex, contraception, and parenthood: Experience and attitudes among urban black young men. *Family Planning Perspectives* 16:77–82.

Coates, T. J., and Greenblatt, R. M. (In press) Behavioral change using interventions at the community level (draft). In K. K. Holmes, P A. Mardh, P. S. Sparling, and P. J. Wiesner, eds., *Sexually Transmitted Diseases.* New York: McGraw-Hill.

Coates, T. J., McKusick, L., Morin, S. F., Charles, K. A., Wiley, J. A., Stall, R. D., and Conant, M. D. (1985) Differences Among Gay Men in Desire for HTLV-III/LAV Antibody Testing and Beliefs About Exposure to the Probable AIDS Virus: The Behavioral AIDS Project. Presented at the Annual Meeting of the American Psychological Association, Los Angeles, August.

Coates, T. J., Morin, S. F., and McKusick, L. (1987) Behavioral consequences of AIDS antibody testing among gay men. *Journal of the American Medical Association* 258:1889.

Coates, T. J., Stall, R. D., Kegeles, S. M., Lo, B., Morin, S. F., and McKusick, L. (1988a) AIDS antibody testing: Will it stop the AIDS epidemic? Will it help people infected with HIV? *American Psychologist* 43:859–864.

Coates, T. J., Stall, R. D., and Hoff, C. C. (1988b) Changes in Sexual Behavior Among Gay and Bisexual Men Since the Beginning of the AIDS Epidemic. Background paper prepared for the Health Program, Office of Technology Assessment, U.S. Congress, Washington, D.C.

Cohen, J. B. (1987) Three Years' Experience Promoting AIDS Prevention Among 800 Sexually Active High Risk Women in San Francisco. Presented at the National Institute of Mental Health/National Institute on Drug Abuse Research Workshop on Women and AIDS, Bethesda, Md., September 27–29.

Cohen, J. B. (No date) Condom Promotion Among Prostitutes. University of California at San Francisco.

Communication Technologies. (1987) *A Report on Designing an Effective AIDS Prevention Campaign Strategy for San Francisco.* San Francisco: Communication Technologies.

Cox, C. P., Selwyn, P. A., Schoenbaum, E. E., et al. (1986) Psychological and Behavioral Consequences of HTLV-III/LAV Antibody Testing and Notification Among Intravenous Drug Abusers in a Methadone Program in New York City. Presented at the Second International AIDS Conference, Paris, June 23–25.

Coxon, A. P. M. (1986) Report of a Pilot Study: Project on Sexual Lifestyles of Non-heterosexual Males. Social Research Unit, University College, Cardiff, U.K.

Darrow, W. W. (1987) Condom Use and Use-Effectiveness in High-Risk Populations. Presented at the CDC Conference on Condoms in the Prevention of Sexually Transmitted Diseases, Atlanta, Ga., February 20.

Dawes, R. M. (1988) Measurement Models for Rating and Comparing Risks: The Context of AIDS. Presented at the conference, Health Services Research Methods: A Focus on AIDS, sponsored by the Health Services Research and Demonstration Grants Review Committee of the National Center for Health Services Research and Health Care Technology Assessment and the University of Arizona, Department of Psychology, Tucson, June 2–4.

Dawes, R. M., Singer, D., and Lemons, F. (1972) An experimental analysis of the contrast effect and its implications for intergroup communication and the indirect assessment of attitude. *Journal of Personal and Social Psychology* 21:281–295.

Dawson, D. A., Cynamon, M., and Fitti, J. E. (1988) AIDS knowledge and attitudes for September 1987: Provisional data from the National Health Interview Survey. In *Advance Data from Vital and Health Statistics,* No. 148. DHHS Publ. No. (PHS) 88-1250. Hyattsville, Md.: Public Health Service, National Center for Health Statistics.

Des Jarlais, D. C. (1987) Effectiveness of AIDS Educational Programs for Intravenous Drug Users. Background paper prepared for the Health Program, Office of Technology Assessment, U.S. Congress, Washington, D.C.

Des Jarlais, D. C. (1988) HIV Infection Among Persons Who Inject Illicit Drugs: Problems and Progress. Presented at the Fourth International AIDS Conference, Stockholm, June 12–16.

Des Jarlais, D. C., and Friedman, S. (1987) HIV infection among intravenous drug users: Epidemiology and risk reduction (editorial review). *AIDS* 1:67–76.

Des Jarlais, D. C., and Hunt, D. E. (1988) AIDS and intravenous drug use. AIDS Bulletin, National Institute of Justice, U.S. Department of Justice.

DiClemente, R. J., Zorn, J., and Temoshok, L. (1986) Adolescents and AIDS: A survey of knowledge, attitudes, and beliefs about AIDS. *American Journal of Public Health* 76:1443–1445.

DiClemente, R. J., Boyer, C. B., and Mills, S. J. (1987) Prevention of AIDS among adolescents: Strategies for the development of comprehensive risk-reduction health education programs. *Health Education Research* 2:287–291.

DiClemente, R. J., Boyer, C. B., and Morales, E. S. (1988) Minorities and AIDS: Knowledge, attitudes, and misconceptions among black and Latino adolescents. *American Journal of Public Health* 78:55–57.

Doll, L. S., and Bye, L. L. (1987) AIDS: Where reason prevails. *World Health Forum* 8:484–488.

Doll, L. S., Darrow, W., O'Malley, P., Bodecker, T., and Jaffe, H. (1987) Self-Reported Behavioral Change in Homosexual Men in the San Francisco City Clinic Cohort. Presented at the Third International AIDS Conference, Washington, D.C., June 1–5.

Durell, J., and Bukoski, W. (1984) Preventing substance abuse: The state of the art. *Public Health Reports* 99:23–31.

Edwards, L., Steinman, M., Arnold, K., and Hakanson, E. (1980) Adolescent pregnancy prevention services in high school clinics. *Family Planning Perspectives* 12:6–14.

Ekstrand, M., and Coates, T. J. (1988) Prevalence and Change in High Risk Behavior Among Gay and Bisexual Men. Presented at the Fourth International AIDS Conference, Stockholm, June 12–16.

Emmons, C. A., Joseph, J. G., Kessler, R. C., et al. (1986) Psychosocial predictors of reported behavior change in homosexual men at risk for AIDS. *Health Education Quarterly* 13:331–345.

Farquhar, J. W., Wood, P. D., and Breitrose, I. T. (1977) Community education for cardiovascular health. *Lancet* 1:1191–1195.

Farthing, C. F., Jessen, W., Taylor, H. L., Lawrence, A. G., and Gazzard, B. G. (1987) The HIV Antibody Test: Influence on Sexual Behavior of Homosexual Men. Presented at the Third International AIDS Conference, Washington, D.C., June 1–5.

Flay, B. R. (1987) Mass media and smoking cessation: A critical review. *American Journal of Public Health* 77:153–160.

Fox, R., Ostrow, D., Valdiserri, R., VanRaden, B., and Polk, B. F. (1987a) Changes in Sexual Activities Among Participants in the Multicenter AIDS Cohort Study. Presented at the Third International AIDS Conference, Washington, D.C., June 1–5.

Fox, R., Odaka, N. J., Brookmeyer, R., and Polk, B. F. (1987b) Effect of HIV antibody disclosure on subsequent sexual activity in homosexual men. *AIDS* 1:241–246.

Friedman, S. R., Des Jarlais, D. C., and Sotheran, J. L. (1986) AIDS health education for intravenous drug users. *Health Education Quarterly* 13:383–393.

Friedman, S. R., Des Jarlais, D. C., Sotheran, J. L., Garber, J., Cohen, H., and Smith, D. (1987) AIDS and self-organization among intravenous drug users. *International Journal of the Addictions* 22:201–219.

Friedman, S. R., Sotheran, J. L., Abdul-Quader, A., Primm, B. J., Des Jarlais, D. C., Kleinman, P., Mauge, C., Goldsmith, D. S., El-Sadr, W., and Maslansky, R. (1988) The AIDS epidemic among blacks and Hispanics. *Milbank Quarterly* 65(Suppl. 2):455-499.

Fullilove, R. E. (1988) Minorities and AIDS: A review of recent publications. *Multicultural Inquiry and Research on AIDS* 2:3–5.

Furstenberg, F. F., Moore, K. A., and Peterson, J. L. (1986) Sex education and sexual experience among adolescents. *American Journal of Public Health* 75:1331–1332.

Godfried, J. P., VanGriensven, G., Tielman, R. A. P., Goudsmit, J., VanDerNoordaa, J., DeWolf, F., and Coutinho, R. A. (1987) Effect of HIVab Serodiagnosis on Sexual Behavior of Homosexual Men in the Netherlands. Presented at the Third International AIDS Conference, Washington, D.C., June 1–5.

Green, L. W., and McAlister, A. L. (1984) Macro intervention to support health behavior: Some theoretical perspectives and practical reflections. *Health Education Quarterly* 11:322–339.

Green, L. W., Wilson, A. L., and Lovato, C. Y. (1986) What changes can health promotion achieve and how long do these changes last? The trade-offs between expediency and durability. *Preventive Medicine* 15:508–521.

Greer, A. L. (1977) Advances in the study of diffusion of innovation in health care organizations. *Milbank Memorial Fund Quarterly: Health and Society* 55:505–532.

Grieco, A. (1986) Cutting the Risks for STDs. Winter Park, Fla.

Guttmacher, A. (1981) *Teenage Pregnancy: The Problem Hasn't Gone Away.* New York: Alan Guttmacher Institute.

Hayes, C. D., ed. (1987) *Risking the Future: Adolescent Sexuality, Pregnancy, and Childbearing,* vol. 1. Washington, D.C.: National Academy Press.

Hochhauser, M. (1987) Readability of AIDS Educational Materials. Presented at the Annual Meeting of the American Psychological Association, New York, August.

Hull, H. F., Bettinger, C. J., Gallaher, M. M., Keller, N. M., Wilson, J., and Mertz, G. J. (1988) Comparison of HIV-antibody prevalence in patients consenting to and declining HIV-antibody testing in an STD clinic. *Journal of the American Medical Association* 260:935–938.

Institute of Medicine/National Academy of Sciences (IOM/NAS). (1988) *Confronting AIDS: Update 1988.* Washington, D.C.: National Academy Press.

Janz, N. K., and Becker, M. H. (1984) The health belief model: A decade later. *Health Education Quarterly* 11:1–47.

Job, R. F. S. (1988) Effective and ineffective use of fear in health promotion campaigns. *American Journal of Public Health* 78:163–167.

Jones, C. C., Waskin, H., Gerety, B., et al. (1987) Persistence of high-risk sexual activity among homosexual men in an area of low incidence of the acquired immunodeficiency syndrome. *Sexually Transmitted Diseases* 14:79–82.

Jones, J. B., Forrest, J., Goldman, N., Henshaw, S., Lincoln, R., Rosoff, J., Westoff, C., and Wulf, D. (1985) Teenage pregnancy in developed countries: Determinants and policy implications. *Family Planning Perspectives* 17:53–63.

Joseph, J. G., Montgomery, S. B., Kessler, R. C., et al. (1987a) Behavioral Risk Reduction in a Cohort of Homosexual Men: Two Year Follow-up. Presented at the Third International AIDS Conference, Washington, D.C., June 1–5.

Joseph, J. G., Montgomery, S. B., Emmons, C. A., Kessler, R. C., Ostrow, D. B., Wortman, C. B., O'Brien, K., Eller, M., and Eshleman, S. (1987b) Magnitude and determinants of behavioral risk reduction: Longitudinal analysis of a cohort at risk for AIDS. *Psychological Health* 1:73–96.

Kelly, J. A., St. Lawrence, J. S., Hood, H. V., et al. (1987a) Behavioral Interventions to Reduce AIDS Risk Activities. University of Mississippi Medical Center.

Kelly, J. A., St. Lawrence, J. S., Brasfield, T. L., and Hood, H. V. (1987b) Relationship Between Knowledge About AIDS and Actual Risk Behavior in a Sample of Homosexual Men: Some Implications for Prevention. Presented at the Third International AIDS Conference, Washington, D.C., June 1–5.

Kirby, D. (1984) *Sexuality Education: An Evaluation of Programs and Their Effects.* Santa Cruz, Calif.: Network Publications.

Kirby, D., and Scales, P. (1981) An analysis of state guidelines for sex education instruction in public schools. *Family Relations* 31:229–237.

Kotler, P., and Zaltman, G. (1971) Social marketing: An approach to planned social change. *Journal of Marketing* 35:3–12.

Lashley, K. S., and Watson, J. B. (1922) *A Psychological Study of Motion Pictures in Relation to Venereal Disease Campaigns.* Washington, D.C.: U.S. Interdepartmental Social Hygiene Board.

Lave, L. B. (1987) Health and safety risk analyses: Information for better decisions. *Science* 236:291–295.

Lyter, D. W., Valdiserri, R. O., Kingsley, L. A., Amoroso, W. P., and Rinaldo, C. R. (1987) The HIV antibody test: Why gay and bisexual men want or do not want to know their result. *Public Health Reports* 102:468–474.

Mantell, J. E. (No date) Prevention of HIV Infection Among Women: Issues and Recommended Initiatives. Gay Men's Health Crisis, New York City.

Mantell, J. E., Schinke, S. P., and Akabas, S. H. (In press) Women and AIDS prevention. *Journal of Primary Prevention.*

Marlatt, G. A. (1982) Relapse prevention: A self-control program for the treatment of addictive behaviors. In R. B. Stuart, ed., *Adherence, Compliance and Generalization in Behavioral Medicine.* New York: Brunner/Mazel.

Martin, J. L. (1987) The impact of AIDS on gay male sexual behavior patterns in New York City. *American Journal of Public Health* 77:578–581.

Marzuk, P. M., Tierney, H., Tardiff, K., Gross, E. M., Morgan, E. B., Hsu, M. A., and Mann, J. J. (1988) Increased risk of suicide in persons with AIDS. *Journal of the American Medical Association* 259:1333–1337.

McCusker, J., Stoddard, A. M., Mayer, K. H., Zapka, J., Morrison, C., and Saltzman, S. P. (1988) Effects of HIV antibody test knowledge on subsequent sexual behaviors in a cohort of homosexually active men. *American Journal of Public Health* 78:462–467.

McKusick, L., Horstman, W., and Coates, T. J. (1985) AIDS and sexual behavior reported by gay men in San Francisco. *American Journal of Public Health* 75:493–496.

McKusick, L., Coates, T. J., Wiley, J. A., Morin, S. F., and Stall, R. (1987) Prevention of HIV Infection Among Gay and Bisexual Men: Two Longitudinal Studies. Presented at the Third International AIDS Conference, Washington, D.C., June 1–5.

Moore, K. A., Wenk, D., Hofferth, S. L. (ed.), and Hayes, C. D. (ed.) (1987) Statistical appendix: Trends in adolescent sexual and fertility behavior. In S. L. Hofferth and C. D. Hayes, eds., *Risking the Future: Adolescent Sexuality, Pregnancy, and Childbearing.* Vol. 2, *Working Papers and Statistical Appendixes.* Washington, D.C.: National Academy Press.

Morisky, D. E., DeMuth, N. M., Field-Fass, M., Green, L. W., and Levine, D. M. (1985) Evaluation of family health education to build social support for long-term control of high blood pressure. *Health Education Quarterly* 12:35–50.

Mosher, W. D. (1985) Reproductive impairments in the United States, 1965–1982. *Demography* 22:415–430.

Office of Technology Assessment (OTA). (1988) How Effective Is AIDS Education? A staff paper in OTA's Series on AIDS-Related Issues, Health Program. Office of Technology Assessment, Washington, D.C.

Pappas, L. S. (1987) Promoting Condoms for Gay Men. Presented at the CDC Conference on Condoms in the Prevention of Sexually Transmitted Diseases, Atlanta, Ga., February 20.

Pesce, A., Negre, M., and Cassuto, J. P. (1987) Knowledge of HIV Contamination Modalities and Its Consequence on Seropositive Patients' Behavior. Presented at the Third International AIDS Conference, Washington, D.C., June 1–5.

Peterson, J., and Bakeman, R. (1988) The epidemiology of adult minority AIDS. *Multicultural Inquiry and Research on AIDS* 2:1–2.

Polich, J. M., Ellickson, P. L., Reuter, P., and Kahan, J. P. (1984) *Strategies for Controlling Adolescent Drug Use.* Santa Monica, Calif.: Rand Corporation.

Potts, M. (No date) Using Controversy to Promote Condoms. Family Health International, Research Triangle Park, N.C.

Pratt, W. F., and Hendershot, G. E. (1984) The use of family planning services by sexually active teenagers. *Population Index* 50:412–413.

Presidential Commission on the Human Immunodeficiency Virus Epidemic. (1988) *Report of the Presidential Commission on the Human Immunodeficiency Virus Epidemic.* Washington, D.C.: Government Printing Office.

Reuben, N., Hein, K., Drucker, E., Bauman, L., and Lanby, J. (1988) Relationship of High-Risk Behaviors to AIDS Knowledge in Adolescent High School Students. Presented at the Annual Research Meeting, Society for Adolescent Medicine, New York City, March 24–27.

Rogers, E. M. (1962) *Diffusion of Innovations.* New York: Free Press.

Rogers, E. M., and Adhikarya, R. (1980) Diffusion of innovations: An up-to-date review and commentary. In D. Nimmo, ed., *Communication Yearbook 3.* New Brunswick, N.J.: Transaction Books.

Rosenstock, I. M. (1960) What research in motivation suggests for public health. *American Journal of Public Health* 50:295–302.

Rothbart, M., Dawes, R., and Park, B. (1984) Stereotyping and sampling biases in intergroup perception. Pp. 109–134 in J. R. Eiser, ed., *Attitudinal Judgment.* New York: Springer-Verlag.

Sabatier, R. (1988) *Blaming Others: Prejudice, Race, and Worldwide AIDS.* Washington, D.C.: The Panos Institute.

Schmid, G. P., Sanders, L. L., Blount, J. H., and Alexander, E. R. (1987) Chancroid in the United States. *Journal of the American Medical Association* 258:3265-3268.

Shweder, R. A. (1979) Rethinking culture and personality theory: A critical examination of two classical postulates. *Ethos* (Fall):255–278.

Soucy, J. (1987) Human Immunodeficiency Virus Antibody Disclosure and Behavior Change. Presented at the Annual Meeting of the American Psychiatric Association, Chicago, Ill., May 9–14.

Stall, R., Wiley, J., McKusick, L., et al. (1986) Alcohol and drug use during sexual activity and compliance with safe sex guidelines for AIDS: The AIDS behavioral research project. *Health Education Quarterly* 13:359–371.

Strecher, V. J., DeVellis, B. M., Becker, M. H., and Rosenstock, I. M. (1986) The role of self-efficacy in achieving health behavior change. *Health Education Quarterly* 13:73–91.

Sutton, S. R. (1982) Fear-arousing communications: A critical examination of theory and research. In J. R. Eiser, ed., *Social Psychology and Behavioral Medicine.* New York: John Wiley & Sons.

Turner, C. F., Miller, H. G., and Barker, L. (In press) AIDS research and the behavioral and social sciences. In R. Kulstad, ed., *AIDS 1988: A Symposium.* Washington, D.C.: American Association for the Advancement of Science.

U.S. Department of Education. (1987) *AIDS and the Education of Our Children: A Guide for Parents and Teachers.* Washington, D.C.: U.S. Department of Education.

Valdiserri, R. O., Lyter, D., Callahan, C., et al. (1987) Condom Use in a Cohort of Gay and Bisexual Men. Presented at the Third International AIDS Conference, Washington, D.C., June 1–5.

Valdiserri, R. O., Lyter, D., Leviton, L. C., Callahan, C. M., et al. (1988) Variables influencing condom use in a cohort of gay and bisexual men. *American Journal of Public Health* 78:801–805.

Vincent, M., Clearie, A. F., and Schluchter, M. D. (1987) Reducing adolescent pregnancy through school and community-based education. *Journal of the American Medical Association* 257:3382–3386.

Watters, J. K. (1987) Preventing Human Immunodeficiency Virus Contagion Among Intravenous Drug Users: The Impact of Street-Based Education on Risk Behavior. Presented at the Third International AIDS Conference, Washington, D.C., June 1–5.

Weinstein, N. D. (1987) Unrealistic optimism about susceptibility to health problems: Conclusions from a community-wide sample. *Journal of Behavioral Medicine* 10:481–500.

Willoughby, B. M., Schechter, T., Boyko, W. J., Craib, K. J. P., Weaver, M. S., and Douglas, B. (1987) Sexual Practices and Condom Use in a Cohort of Homosexual Men: Evidence of Differential Modification Between Seropositive and Seronegative Men. Presented at the Third International AIDS Conference, Washington, D.C., June 1–5.

Winkelstein, W., Samuel, M., Padian, N. S., et al. (1987) The San Francisco Men's Health Study. III. Reduction in human immunodeficiency virus transmission among homosexual/bisexual men, 1982–1986. *American Journal of Public Health* 77:685-689.

Zabin, L. S., Hirsch, M. B., Smith, E. A., Strett, R., and Hardy, J. B. (1986) Evaluation of a pregnancy prevention program for urban teenagers. *Family Planning Perspectives* 18:119–126.

Zelnik, M., and Kim, Y. J. (1982) Sex education and its association with teenage sexual activity, pregnancy, and contraceptive use. *Family Planning Perspectives* 14:117–126.

Zelnik, M., and Shah, F. K. (1983) First intercourse among young Americans. *Family Planning Perspectives* 15:64–70.

5

Evaluating the Effects of AIDS Interventions

Previous chapters of this report have dealt with understanding the behaviors that transmit HIV, monitoring the spread of infection, and designing and implementing intervention programs to oppose the further spread of the disease. The committee has called for the implementation of planned variations of programs to determine how best to facilitate change in those behaviors associated with risk. Making those determinations requires sound evaluations of the different program variations. Yet evaluation is rarely part of a program's activities.

In its review of existing intervention programs, the committee was distressed to find a dearth of associated evaluation activity. Committee members were also disappointed to see a lack of data on behavioral variables for those evaluations that had been conducted. The committee believes that the time has come to make a commitment to the rational design of intervention strategies and to careful evaluation of the effectiveness of those strategies through controlled experiments that use carefully defined populations. Knowledge must be gained from current intervention programs to improve future efforts. Evaluation is the process that will enable us to learn from experience. **The committee recommends that the Office of the Assistant Secretary for Health take responsibility for an evaluation strategy that will provide timely information on the relative effectiveness of different AIDS intervention programs.**

The political realities of evaluation point to both positive and negative aspects of the process. On the one hand, good evaluations can generate support for effective programs. Well-publicized findings of evaluation activities can legitimately defend successful programs that may be viewed as politically sensitive or controversial, while gestures that were merely symbolic can be shown to be ineffective. On the other hand, evaluation efforts are likely to show that programs are less effective than might be hoped. Perfect studies and absolute, permanent change in behavior are standards that are rarely, if ever, met. Every effort should be made to ensure that evidence of imperfect improvement is not used to overturn programs that may be viewed as politically undesirable.

There is every reason to believe that the nation can and will do better in determining which interventions change behavior and which do not. Discussions with many people who have been on the front lines of AIDS prevention activities since the early days of the epidemic reveal their desire for evaluation of their work. To date, however, most of these individuals have not conducted evaluations—not because they were unwilling but because they lacked the capability. The links between those who provide services and manage programs, on the one hand, and those who conduct research and evaluation, on the other hand, have not been strong in the past.

This chapter discusses basic approaches to and problems inherent in conducting controlled experiments and evaluations. The committee recognizes that it will not meet the needs of all readers: for some, it will be too basic. For those who are not yet familiar with the techniques of experimental design and evaluation, however, we hope it will be a useful introduction. Yet it must be noted that any document such as this cannot take the place of individual, program-specific consultation. It is therefore imperative to establish supportive, productive linkages among program and evaluation professionals so that future prevention efforts can result in sound, useful information.

DIMENSIONS OF EVALUATION

It is not always easy to learn from experience, but it is certainly possible. To increase the likelihood of such learning requires the advance planning of evaluations as well as the precise, controlled execution of programs. Good evaluation does not just happen; it must be planned for and arranged. Evaluation is a systematic process that produces a trustworthy account of what was attempted and why; through the examination of results—the outcomes of intervention programs—it answers the questions, "What was done?" "To whom, and how?" and "What outcomes were observed?" Well-designed evaluation permits us to draw inferences from the data and addresses the difficult question: "What do the outcomes mean?" Well-executed evaluations provide credible information about program effectiveness. Such information is critical to developing rational policies, allocating limited resources, and serving needs in a targeted, productive, and economical fashion.

Ensuring complete, high-quality evaluation requires advance specification of the program. Thus, in preparing for an evaluation, the design of a program can sometimes be improved by increasing its specificity and establishing standards of performance at the outset. At its best, a process in which program innovations are informed by feedback from careful, prompt evaluations can lead to the timely elimination of ineffective concepts and designs and the selection and adoption of effective ones.

A successful evaluation of an intervention program must provide answers to several key questions:

1. What were the objectives of the intervention?
2. How was the intervention designed to be conducted?
3. How was the intervention actually conducted?
   - Who participated?
   - Were there any unexpected problems?
   - What parts of the program were easier to conduct than was anticipated?
   - What parts were harder?
4. What outcomes were observed, and how were they measured?
5. What were the results of the intervention?

These questions are presented in a logical order of progression; they are also ranked according to the ease with which they can be answered—those at the end are harder to answer than those at the beginning. It is not uncommon to find reports of programs that use the term *evaluation* to refer to activities that would answer only the first three questions. The committee does not follow that usage. Evaluation refers to the whole set of questions, with particular emphasis on the last two.

It is important to distinguish between the outcomes of the program and the results of the intervention: an outcome denotes what occurred; an evaluation seeks to determine whether the outcome resulted from the intervention or from some other external factor.

Program Objectives

An intervention program may start with a protocol—a document that includes a description of the intervention, the activities to be undertaken, the groups targeted to receive the intervention, and the roles and responsibilities of the individuals or groups undertaking the tasks. (Frequently, funding agencies require such a document from organizations or individuals who are applying for a grant or seeking a contract to support the program.) This protocol is an integral part of an intervention: it should spell out unambiguously the objectives of the program and how they will be measured, as well as the operational content of the work to be performed. The program objectives are the desired outcomes. They do not, for example, specify an intent to spend a certain sum on an activity or to deliver a certain number of advertisements or pamphlets; rather, they relate to the reasons that motivate the program. Objectives state the outcomes the program seeks to achieve.

Program Design

Two key elements in program design are defining the measures of the outcome or effect of the program and selecting the treatment unit. A variety of outcome measures can be chosen for study. It may help to conceptualize them along two dimensions: (1) their relevance as indicators of program achievement and (2) the feasibility of actually measuring them. For example, both the behavior and knowledge of subjects may be affected by a program; yet the former, although harder to measure, may be more relevant to the program's objectives. Many AIDS prevention programs have chosen knowledge as the outcome measure; it is easier to gauge than behavior but less relevant to the process of preventing the spread of HIV infection. It is not unusual for programs to include multiple outcome measures that vary in importance.

The treatment unit refers to the body to which the intervention will be applied. Variations in this construct and in outcome measures are illustrated in the following four examples of intervention programs.

- Two different pamphlets on the same subject are prepared. They are sent to individuals calling an AIDS hot line and are distributed in an alternating sequence. The outcome to be measured is whether recipients return a card asking for more information.

- Two discussion/instruction curricula about AIDS and HIV infection are prepared for use in high school health education classes. The outcome to be measured is the score on a test of knowledge.
- A subset of all STD clinics in a large standard metropolitan statistical area is randomly chosen to introduce a change in fee schedules. The outcome to be measured is the change in patient load.
- A community-level prevention program establishes a coordinated set of interventions involving community leadership, social service agencies, the media, community associations, and other groups. The two outcomes to be measured are knowledge (as assessed by testing) and condom sales in the community's retail outlets.

These fictitious interventions are applied to very different treatment units. In the first example, the treatment unit is an individual person who receives either pamphlet A or pamphlet B. If either "treatment" were to be applied again, it would be applied to a person. In the second example, the high school health education class is the treatment unit; everyone in a specific class is given either curriculum A or curriculum B. If either treatment were to be applied again, it would be applied to a class. The treatment unit in the third example is the clinic. In the fourth example, the treatment unit is the whole community.

To make inferences from the results of an evaluation, the treatment units that are analyzed must correspond to those that are sampled. For example, when organizations or groups are randomly chosen to receive a given intervention, the sample size is the number of organizations or groups. Because individuals within each broader unit do not yield independent observations, they cannot be used as statistical units.

The consistency of the outcome measures or effects of a particular intervention during repetitions of it is critical in appraising the intervention. It is important to remember that repetitions of a treatment or intervention are counted as the number of treatment units to which the intervention is applied.

Planning the intervention program and planning its evaluation should go hand in hand. The evaluation plan is an appropriate part of the protocol, which should state how the measurement and analysis of intended outcomes will be conducted. The comparisons to be used to assess the program's results are also part of an evaluation plan.

Program Implementation

Whatever results are judged to have occurred because of an intervention, they must relate to the program as it was actually carried out rather than to the program as it was planned or intended. Thus, it is necessary to determine what services were in fact delivered, to whom, and how.

Evaluations that address the actual execution of the program are usually called process evaluations or implementation analyses—that is, if the evaluator's role is passive. When the evaluator takes a more active role, these efforts are referred to as trouble shooting or formative evaluations. Process evaluation has three important purposes: (1) to verify that planned services are actually offered and received, (2) to determine how the quality or extent of a service varied, and (3) to develop ideas about how to improve the organization or delivery of services.

The best of such evaluations recognize that no policy is ever fully implemented and no service ever delivered exactly as planned. Evaluation that discovers, for instance, that a fraction of the condoms received by individuals remained unused, that many free needles were stolen or not received by the target group, or that "counseling" in some cases was based on inaccurate and naive information is important. There are many good examples of formative evaluations. For example, in a study of whether a special community-based program for the severely and persistently mentally ill worked better than conventional approaches, Brekke and Test (1987) undertook an approach that monitored a sample of clients regularly over three years to determine where treatment took place, the amount and nature of treatment, who received it, and how continuity of care was achieved. Similarly, in a multisite study of which of three regimens worked best to ameliorate the problems of patients afflicted with mental depression, Waskow (1984) and Elkin and colleagues (in press) ensured that therapists used the treatment variation that they had agreed to use and determined how they did so. Their work included the development of manuals that stipulated guidelines, the preparation of training regimens for therapists, and studies of interactions between clients and therapists; their evaluation data also included more conventional measures of the number, frequency, and length of therapy sessions.

Process evaluations can be designed in different ways to focus more squarely on the treatment target. Recent work conducted by the Center for AIDS Prevention Studies in San Francisco investigated three stages in the prevention process: (1) ensuring that individuals who engage in high-risk behavior know they are doing so; (2) understanding how, why, and when commitments are made to reduce such behavior; and (3) understanding the factors that influence the way people seek out and act on alternative approaches to risk behavior reduction (Catania et al., 1988). The best of such process evaluations also direct attention to the families and partners of individuals at high risk in an attempt to understand the frequency and character of support from those sources and how that support may discourage or foster high-risk behavior.

Well-executed process evaluations also make plain the standards or criteria against which an organization's performance will be judged. Standardized criteria for assessing programs have been established in some substantive areas by different groups and organizations. The American Public Health Association has developed criteria for health education programs that have been used in the design of a university-based AIDS program that seeks to reduce risk-associated behavior (Valdiserri et al., 1987).

Defining and Measuring Outcomes

As noted earlier, there are two dimensions to outcome measures: relevance and feasibility. Often, there are many possible outcome measures inherent in the design of an intervention, and their relevance is obvious. For example, consider an instructional program aimed at persuading people to use condoms. Each of the following questions corresponds to at least one outcome measure:

- Did the subjects attend the program?
- Did they pay attention?
- Did they understand the message correctly?
- Did they believe and accept it?
- Did they thereafter use condoms?
- Did they benefit from that behavior?

The questions become progressively harder to answer; in addition, the answer to each succeeding question is more important than the one before it. The choice of an outcome measure or measures is largely a matter of balancing importance against feasibility. In the case of AIDS, the issue of time must also be considered. The extent and character of current condom use are important pieces of information, but the need to use condoms goes beyond the present. Moreover, the lengthy incubation period of HIV may mean that answers to the later questions on the list may only be acquired some years in the future, when the effect of condom use on HIV prevalence can be seen.

Obstacles to the feasibility of outcome measurement, the second of the two dimensions, span a wide range of difficulty. An outcome may simply be impossible to measure. For example, the incidence of HIV infection in the general population is not known because such knowledge would require repeated serologic testing of a very large probability sample of the population, which is currently impossible. For an outcome like sexual behavior, which is effectively impossible to observe, one can use surrogates or verbal reports about the behavior. Other obstacles to measurement are illustrated in the following examples:

- the failure of a respondent to understand what is asked—in some STD clinics, there are concerns that clients may not understand the term vaginal intercourse;
- nonresponse, perhaps by withholding cooperation—Hull and colleagues (1988) reported that the 18 percent of their sample of patients from an STD clinic who refused antibody testing contained more seropositives than the 82 percent who were tested;
- the sheer difficulty of collating information from many sources for each subject—this has been a problem in measuring the costs associated with health care utilization;
- fearful and inaccurate responses from people who are worried about their vulnerable status or from those who are concerned about legal strictures that may threaten them;
- perplexity about how to measure complex concepts, such as perceived self-efficacy; and
- cultural and linguistic barriers that may lead to noncooperation and misunderstanding on the part of respondents, investigator, or both.

The extent and severity of such obstacles will necessarily influence which outcome measures are chosen for study. Although they may not be widely known, there are many instruments to measure such constructs as the quality of life, depression, perceived self-efficacy, and satisfaction with care, as well as instruments for measuring knowledge and comprehension (Mitchell, 1985).

Once the outcome measure or measures have been chosen (perhaps following a pilot test, a procedure the committee endorses), there remains the task of actually doing the measuring. Often, a difficult measurement problem can be solved by using a surrogate. For example, the incidence of STDs can serve as a prompt, sensitive indicator of behavioral change to prevent sexually acquired HIV infection because STDs and HIV can be spread by the same behaviors. If a particular outcome is simply too difficult to measure accurately, a major component of that outcome may serve as a reasonable alternative. Thus, ascertaining the total costs of medical care for each of many AIDS patients can be daunting, but accurate figures for the number of days spent in the hospital, in the intensive care unit, and in nursing facilities may be readily available. Although these estimates ignore unit costs and omit the cost of such items as drugs and respiratory therapy, they may be better outcome measures than the conceptually complete but inaccurately measured total cost.

Finding a good surrogate for outcomes that are difficult to measure and devising ways to cross-check those measures call for ingenuity and imagination.

Inferring Results: The Value of Controlled Experiments

Good evaluations can provide accurate descriptions of the intervention process and measure the outcomes. Yet there remains the problem of inferring the effects of the intervention. Describing the process and stating the results are not sufficient. A good evaluation should say something about the relationship between the intervention and the outcome. A patient who receives a worthless treatment for the common cold is still likely to get better within a week because that is what usually happens with a cold, with or without the benefit of treatment. To infer that a given intervention has produced a particular effect involves comparing what did happen with the intervention to what would have happened without it. Because it is not possible to make this comparison directly, inference strategies rely on proxies for what would have happened. Such proxies include the patient's past history and comparison groups of various sorts.

In some circumstances, extrapolating a trend from a patient's pretreatment history as a proxy for what would have happened is the best that can be done. Yet extrapolation is always problematic: past records may be incomplete, and it is impossible to control for all intervening factors. This type of approach should probably be used as a near-to-last resort.

Under certain conditions, comparison groups can be quite useful for inferring results, although defining and recruiting a suitably similar control group can be difficult. For example, after selecting ethnically similar control and treatment groups, an investigator may find that one group is, on average, older, sicker, or more educated. There are evaluation strategies that attempt to adjust for the differences between the two groups, but making those adjustments is seldom easy. Three types of information or knowledge are required: (1) knowledge of intervening variables that also affect the outcome of the intervention and that consequently need adjustment to make the groups comparable; (2) measurements on all intervening variables for all subjects; and (3) knowledge of how to make the adjustments properly, which in turn requires an understanding of the functional relationship between the intervening variables and the outcome variables. Satisfying each of these information requirements is likely to be more difficult than attaining the primary goal of the activity, which, simply stated, answers the question, "Does this intervention produce beneficial effects?"

With differently constituted groups, inferences about results are hostage to uncertainty about the extent to which the observed outcome actually results from the intervention and is not an artifact of intergroup differences. Fortunately, there is a remedy: establish one, singly constituted group in which to assess treatment effects. To be included in the group, individuals must satisfy the inclusion and exclusion criteria for the study. A subset of this group is then randomly chosen to receive the intervention, thus forming two comparable groups. They are not identical, but because they are two random samples drawn from the same population, they are as similar as is possible. Moreover, they are not systematically different in any respect, which is important for all variables—those known and those as yet unidentified—that can influence the outcome. Dividing a singly constituted group into random and therefore comparable subgroups cuts through the tangle of causation and establishes a basis for the valid comparison of treated and untreated subjects.

After establishing two or more comparable subgroups, a good evaluation must ensure that outcome measurement is performed symmetrically for all subjects. For example, if treated subjects are examined and tested at hospital A and untreated subjects are examined and tested at hospital B, it is impossible to determine whether observed differences are due to treatment or are merely artifacts of noncomparable outcome measurement. The foregoing ideas are central to randomized clinical trials and randomized field experiments, which are discussed in the next section. Although highly desirable, partitioning strategies of this type are not practical for every question. The nonparticipation of some individuals or high attrition rates among participants may cause an investigator to use methods that are less satisfactory for inferring results. This, unfortunately, has been the case with randomized trials of some drug treatment strategies: for example, many IV drug users prefer methadone maintenance over detoxification, making it difficult to recruit subjects for random assignment treatment studies.

Constraints on Evaluation

The above sections have described the basic characteristics of evaluation. Three additional considerations are discussed here. First, the size of the study, or the number of treatment units, is a function of several factors. Budget constraints may influence the size of the study, in all likelihood, by setting the upper limits. Moreover, time limits may affect the capacity to coordinate a study and thus set limits on the number of units.

In addition to pragmatic considerations, there are important statistical issues. The major one is determining how large a sample must be to reliably detect the impact of an intervention strategy with a stated (albeit hypothetical) degree of effectiveness. Analyses of statistical power help to avoid study designs that are not sufficiently sensitive to detect an intervention's effects. Analyses of power can dictate an increase in the size of the study to achieve the necessary sensitivity, or, occasionally, suggest a reduction in size, thus saving time and other resources.

Finally, in planning programs and evaluations, consideration should be given to pilot tests. The committee strongly believes that every intervention program and every evaluation program should be tested in advance, on a small scale and in a realistic way, to identify problems before more substantial resources are expended. It is possible to avoid using funds or other resources on programs or evaluations that, with a small pilot test, can easily be seen to be infeasible. A large number of AIDS intervention programs are currently being implemented. Good evaluations of these programs may be difficult to perform; they will almost certainly be expensive. To improve the likelihood that high-quality evidence of program effectiveness will be obtained, it would be justified to focus what are necessarily finite resources on the best-designed, best-implemented intervention programs.

RANDOMIZED FIELD EXPERIMENTS

An important component of a well-designed and well-executed study is the random assignment of individuals (or groups) to alternative treatment protocols. In this section, we propose and examine the use of the randomized field experiment in the behavioral sciences. A randomized field experiment is a particular kind of controlled experiment; it requires that individuals, organizations, or other treatment units be randomly assigned to one of two or more treatments or program variations. Random assignment ensures that the estimated differences between the groups so constituted are statistically unbiased; that is, that any differences in effects measured between them are a result of treatment. The absence of statistical bias in groups constituted in this fashion stems from the fact that random assignment prevents systematic differences among them, differences that can and usually do affect groups composed in ways that are not random. In other words, randomization ensures that hidden systematic group differences will not be erroneously identified as real differences that can be attributed to the effects of a program. (Of course, this guarantee about random outcome must be probabilistically hedged, and that is what the significance test does: it points to differences that are too large to reasonably attribute to group disparities induced by the randomization.)

Over the past decade, the number and quality of randomized field tests for planning and evaluation have increased dramatically. This methodological approach has proved to be as important for behavioral field trials of AIDS intervention strategies as it has been shown to be for clinical trials of chemotherapeutic agents. **The committee recommends the expanded use of randomized field experiments for evaluating new intervention programs on both individual and community levels.**

Examples

Designing and conducting randomized field experiments are demanding tasks; the examples in this section may be helpful in understanding the feasibility of using this type of experiment under various conditions.

Coates and coworkers (1987) tested a new stress management training intervention with men who were infected with HIV. The program sought to understand the effects of stress management on risk-associated behaviors and immune functions. Individuals were randomly assigned to the treatment or to a waiting list, which constituted the control group. The results showed a decrease in the number of sexual partners for the experimental group, but there was no discernible effect on immune functions.

Valdiserri and colleagues (1986) and Leviton and coworkers (1988) mounted field tests comparing two risk intervention strategies targeted at homosexual and bisexual men. The participants were randomly assigned to one of two small groups; each group received either a treatment that stressed information or a treatment that stressed information and the development of social and coping skills. Follow-up studies at 6 and 12 months suggested that information and skills training brought considerably more benefits than information alone, a finding that accords generally with the evaluation of similar programs for other health problems.

The feasibility of formal randomized tests in some clinical settings has been shown in programs that are designed to increase knowledge about and compliance with regimens to treat and prevent venereal disease. For example, Solomon and DeJong (1986a) randomly assigned clinic patients with gonorrhea to videotape instructions or to a control condition (no videotape). The results showed that tape viewers understood more about the disease than patients who did not view the videotape and also exhibited increased willingness to return to the clinic for follow-up care (to test for cure). However, viewing the videotape produced no detectable effect on whether patients informed their sex partners of exposure to infection.

In another research effort, videotapes to increase condom use among STD patients were tested at Boston City Hospital. The study, which used randomly constituted viewing and nonviewing groups in two experiments, found that viewing had a remarkable impact on patients' redemptions of coupons for free condoms. The researchers presumed that the redemption of coupons meant the increased use of condoms (Solomon and DeJong, 1986c).

Specially developed venereal disease videotapes and redesigned packaging for antibiotic treatments (in this case, tetracycline) are other interventions that have been tested in randomized field experiments (Solomon et al., 1986). Clinic patients who were assigned randomly to the tape and specially packaged antibiotics exhibited a 10-fold increase in their adherence to the prescribed regimen in comparison with those assigned singly to a group receiving only conventional therapeutic instructions. The videotape also had a measurable effect on delaying patients' reported resumption of sexual behavior.

Formal randomized field experiments of programs directed at IV drug users are not common, but they could be an important tool for learning more about reducing risk-associated behavior in this group. For example, a program conducted in Baltimore (McAuliffe et al., 1987) provided IV drug users with information about AIDS and the sterilization of injection equipment. The outreach workers who disseminated the information were ex-addicts who were randomly assigned to work in half of the targeted urban areas. The analyses of the program compared knowledge levels and risk reduction in the areas serviced by outreach workers with knowledge and risk reduction in areas in which they did not work. The outcome measures showed remarkable changes in knowledge for the group receiving the treatment (information), but in contrast to other studies (see Chapter 3), there was no detectable program effect on the reduction of risk-associated behavior.

In evaluations of programs that have been designed to reduce risky behavior among adolescents, the treatment units have been institutions (e.g., schools), classrooms, and individuals. In testing "soft" or so-called gateway drug education programs for seventh- and eighth-grade students, for example, Moskowitz and colleagues (1984) randomly assigned school classrooms either to participate in an innovative program or to be part of a control (no program) group. The two groups of classrooms were approximately equivalent; there were no evident systematic differences that could be thought to influence estimates of the outcomes. The results, based on tracking the two groups over time, revealed few long-term effects. Similarly, in other studies, schools have been matched and randomly assigned to promising "cooperative learning strategies" for classroom instruction related to substance abuse (Moskowitz et al., 1983). Blythe and coworkers (1981) and Schinke and colleagues (1981) tested intensive interpersonal skills training in a pregnancy prevention program for female adolescents that used singly constituted groups to which girls were randomly assigned. These experiments and others (e.g., Schinke et al., 1981) were undertaken to estimate the relative effects of various programs on adolescents' abilities to identify problems and to resist and handle pressure that put them at risk. Participants in the experimental group reviewed by Schinke and colleagues (1981) were better informed, more committed to postponing pregnancy and using contraceptive devices, and more able to resist peer pressure than individuals in the control group.

Benefits and Costs of Well-Designed Experiments

The scientific and social benefits of randomized field experiments such as the ones described above are many. Most importantly, such experiments permit a fair, unbiased comparison among treatments (or interventions), and they provide a statistically legitimate statement of one's confidence in the comparison. If AIDS prevention strategies are implemented as well-designed, well-evaluated experiments to reduce the risks associated with HIV, they can provide solid evidence about the efficacy of specific approaches.

The institutional and policy benefits of using a randomized experimental approach include (1) the recognition that hard-to-do research can in fact be done and (2) the recognition that better evidence is obtainable to inform decisions about allocating resources in the prevention and treatment of HIV infection. It is clear that the superior quality of the evidence from randomized experiments is recognized by agencies that are responsible for informing policy makers; see, for example, Chelimsky (1988) on AIDS; the U.S. General Accounting Office (1986) on pregnancy prevention programs; the Institute of Medicine (1985) on medical devices; and Haynes and colleagues (1979) on compliance with therapeutic regimens.

Randomized field experiments also encourage those who manage such projects to pay more attention to details that contribute to the proper execution and evaluation of the program. A well-planned program enables managers to anticipate the relative size of program effects and when effects will appear and to improve the search for, recruitment into, and retention of subjects in treatment protocols (Riecken et al., 1974).

The main barrier to such rigorous experiments is that they are difficult to design and execute. In addition to the skills, money, and integrity that are demanded, there are ethical and legal problems, and, often, formidable institutional resistance. Some of these problems can be resolved, as discussed in the next section.

Threshold Conditions for Randomized Experiments

Regardless of the feasibility and benefits of randomized tests of AIDS prevention programs, such tests are not always appropriate. Ethical propriety is an important aspect of whether a randomized test is an appropriate approach.

The Federal Judicial Center (1981), the research arm of the U.S. Supreme Court, recently examined this topic, outlining four threshold conditions that must be present if randomized experiments are to be considered for use in the judicial system. These conditions are also applicable, within limits, to tests of new programs or to program variations that are designed to reduce the risk of HIV infection:

1. Does present practice or policy need improvement?
2. Is there significant uncertainty about the effectiveness of the proposed treatment?
3. Are there acceptable alternatives to randomized experiments?
4. Will the results of the experiment be used to improve practice or policy?

Affirmative answers to these questions justify serious consideration of the use of randomized experiments. A fifth consideration concerns the role of coercion in recruiting subjects, a condition that must be considered for AIDS interventions, especially among such vulnerable populations as institutionalized men and women.

Does Present Practice or Policy Need Improvement?

In reviewing AIDS intervention programs, there appear to be very few areas that do not need improvement. As this report has shown, far more knowledge is needed about (1) locating individuals who are at risk for HIV infection; (2) making programs more acceptable to those at highest risk, including adolescents; (3) making programs more effective; and (4) eliciting more accurate information from those who are reluctant or who fear to reveal themselves. Each of these needs is important.

Is There Significant Uncertainty About the Effectiveness of the Proposed Treatment?

Whether there is "significant uncertainty" about a proposed innovation is often a matter of debate. For AZT (i.e., zidovudine), a treatment proposed for early HIV infection, its severely toxic effects as well as potentially beneficial effects engendered one kind of uncertainty that led to early, controlled tests of the drug. Additional uncertainties about appropriate dose levels for AZT and other newer drugs, the appropriate conditions for their use, and interactions with other treatments also help to justify randomized experiments that are designed to reduce doubts about a proposed treatment.

In the case of AIDS, an understandable inclination toward wishful thinking and competing interests often complicate the normal uncertainty inherent in evaluating a new treatment. The developers of a new drug regimen or therapeutic approach, or of a prevention program, for example, may be convinced that their innovation is effective, a conviction that is based on their evidence. Yet competitors may hold a contrary view based on other evidence. The strength of these convictions (which may stem in part from vested interests) makes the independent evaluation of the effectiveness of new treatments extremely important. It also underscores the need for randomized experiments, which preclude unconscious or deliberate attempts to bias results by using blind (and random) allocation of individuals to alternative treatments and, when possible, blind measurement.[1]

Are There Acceptable Alternatives to Randomized Experiments?

In one sense, the question of whether there are good alternatives to randomized experiments is easy to answer. Random assignment produces equivalent groups that make subsequent comparisons as unambiguous as possible. The approach allows evaluators to disentangle the effects that result from differently constituted groups from the effects of the intervention, a distinction that in turn can prevent a good intervention from appearing worthless and a harmful one from appearing productive. For example, based on nonrandomized tests, oxygen-enriched environments for premature infants were initially thought to be beneficial. Subsequent randomized experiments showed that the treatment actually put infants at risk for vision loss. Similarly, the results of experiments on the Salk vaccine and anticoagulant drug therapy for acute myocardial infarction, as well as on other medical interventions, were different depending on whether randomized or other program approaches were used. (See Bunker et al. [1977] for case histories of these and other interventions.)

Two methodological research technologies, quasi-experimentation (Cook and Campbell, 1979) and econometric modeling, have been developed to assess the quality of outcome data from experiments in which random assignment has not been used. These methods depend heavily on existing data and strong theory, however, both of which are usually absent or fragmentary and inchoate for new target groups and programs. Individuals who are at risk of HIV infection, for example, are properly classifiable as a new target group because there are limited data and theory on their behavior

[1] Blinding refers to the processes that prevent the people who measure outcomes from knowing whether the respondent was in the treatment or control group.

and responsiveness to specific intervention strategies. This lack of information reinforces the need for randomized field tests of proposed HIV intervention programs.

In another sense, the question of whether there is a sound alternative to randomized experimentation is difficult to answer. The appropriateness of alternative methods must be judged in relation to the setting in which they will be applied. There may be justification, for example, in running a simple before-and-after evaluation if the only plausible explanation for a change is the intervention. Alternatively, a statistical model may be used to predict what would have happened to individuals in the absence of the program—that is, provided the model has been shown to work well in other situations and the conditions that affect the model's performance have not changed. Unfortunately, using these alternative methods requires great technical skill, and the user must still accept some threat to the validity of inferences.

Will the Results of the Experiment Be Used to Improve Practice or Policy?

No one can guarantee that good evidence will be used in any public forum or, for that matter, in any scientific one. Indeed, bad evidence or a lack of evidence has been used on more than one occasion, in both democratic and totalitarian societies. One has only to recall, for example, Lysenko's genetics or the use of laetrile, orgone boxes, and other useless "medications" to realize that decisions are made and programs established regardless of the state of the data that exist to support them.

Yet the fact that some policy makers (and patients) have depended on unreliable evidence does not mean that high-quality data, once collected, will not be used or that sound data should not be collected. In fact, as noted earlier in this chapter, evidence from randomized experiments in the social sciences has become increasingly important to decision making over the last decade.

Voluntary Participation

In considering the use of experiments in institutional contexts, the Federal Judicial Center (1981) noted that special attention must be paid to the mandatory character of the criminal justice system, in contrast to the "voluntary" character of social and sociomedical systems. Regardless of the institutionalized status of program participants, however, researchers must be extremely wary of introducing or allowing coercive program elements. One way to do so involves the informed consent of subjects. Other devices to ensure that coercion is eliminated include the use of institutional review boards to oversee the design and execution of programs, although institutional review boards have the responsibility to oversee only research; other program and administrative actions fall outside their purview. Efforts to ensure that all appropriate legal and ethical proprieties are observed in tests of HIV prevention programs—that there is no explicit or implicit pressure to participate—must go well beyond simple efforts to ensure informed consent on the part of participants and the confidentiality of study results.

Organizations as the Treatment Unit in Field Experiments

In the first section of this chapter, the committee discussed the treatment unit, which is either a person or another entity to which the treatment is applied. This section considers in more detail the use of organizations as the units of treatment for randomized field experiments.

Chapters 2, 3, and 4 of this document note the role of the social environment in molding individual behavior. In fact, the principles of behavior that are spelled out in Chapter 4 recognize that any behavior undertaken by an individual will be inhibited or facilitated by community structures and conditions. Consequently, community structures or organizations are appropriate and important targets for intervention programs. The term *community organization* is used to denote a variety of formal and informal units; thus, towns, neighborhoods, youth gangs, and pharmacies, diverse though they may be, are all appropriate units for controlled randomized tests of AIDS intervention programs.

The primary motive in considering the use of communities as treatment units in randomized field experiments is that of practicality. Research findings on health promotion and disease prevention indicate that community-level approaches can be very effective (Farquhar et al., 1977; Vincent et al., 1987). It has been difficult, however, to evaluate programs that involve only one or two communities. For example, programs that have used cities as the treatment unit—one city as the experiment and another as the control—have found differences in the composition of the cities and the manner in which different groups gain access to the program (Betsey et al., 1985). Furthermore, the ways in which cities have measured outcomes of programs have differed. Even when cities appear to be similar, it is impossible to guarantee that they have been matched on all the variables that may affect the outcome measures. To learn more about the efficacy of variants of community-level programs, we need studies that randomly assign multiple communities to treatment or control regimens.

There is some research that offers guidance in this kind of experimental design. Programs to prevent smoking have matched cities and then randomly assigned one city of each matched pair to an intensive antismoking program. These community-level interventions have used the mass media, as well as face-to-face interactions at work sites and public locations and in other areas. In other studies, schools and classrooms have been randomly assigned to programs to prevent the use of alcohol, cigarettes, and marijuana (Schaps et al., 1982; Moskowitz et al., 1984). Villages in India, Korea, and Puerto Rico have been randomly assigned to alternative fertility control programs to ascertain the best methods of decreasing birth rates and the health risks associated with pregnancy (Hill et al., 1959; R. Freedman et al., 1969). There are also other examples of programs that have used random assignments of neighborhoods, stores, and community-based organizations for a variety of health promotion programs.

Although there are no examples among AIDS prevention programs of the randomized assignment of organizations to treatment or control groups, strategies that have been employed for non-AIDS programs can provide useful information. The staff performance studies now being undertaken in franchise stores (R. F. Boruch, Northwestern University, personal communication, October 12, 1988) may shed some methodological light on programs to increase access to condoms through pharmacies. This research seeks to understand the effects of the vendor's demeanor and his or her degree of familiarity on customer's patterns of buying. Other research has used households that have been randomly chosen to receive alternative direct mailing strategies to identify methods to increase awareness of commercial products (Magidson, 1988a,b). The information derived from such tests would be far better than that derived from, for example, focus group approaches to determine the effect of media campaigns on people's knowledge and attitudes about AIDS.

Yet there are certain special issues that arise in the use of organizations as the treatment unit in large-scale field experiments. These issues have not received thorough attention in the past, largely because such experiments have been few in number. But if the strategy of using organizations as the treatment unit can be helpful in learning how to resolve problems in the settings in which they occur, then careful consideration must also be given to the methodological and practical constraints of this approach.

The consequences of using organizations or communities as the treatment unit include expense and a reduction of purported statistical power (true power is a function of the number of units that are actually sampled and not the number of individuals). If, for example, there is an average of m individuals evaluated in each of n units, then the sample size is n. To achieve a comparable study based on randomly chosen individuals, the number of observations that are collected and analyzed must be increased by a multiplicative factor of m. Consequently, effort and expense are expanded by this same factor, which must be taken into account or subsequent evaluation will be inadequate.

An obvious preliminary issue to be resolved concerns the use of official records to measure outcomes. Record-keeping practices differ significantly among cities and other relevant units such as schools, hospitals, police departments, and the like. Developing core methods to measure knowledge—about condoms, for example, or the use of condoms—is essential. These methods will also help to stabilize differences that may occur in measurement quality if the units receiving the treatment improve their record-keeping methods over the course of the program while the control units do not. For instance, cities that have been randomly assigned to a needle exchange program may become more attentive to mortality among IV drug users. As a result, mortality attributed to AIDS may increase in those cities relative to control cities simply because the measures used to gauge mortality have become more accurate. This problem is not different, in principle, from those that occur in programs that randomly assign individuals to alternative treatments. When official records are found to be disparate and vulnerable to artifactual change, formal surveys can be used to improve the quality of and the capability to interpret outcome measurement data.

Another concern about community-level experiments involves the ability to adapt a treatment protocol to local conditions; this adaptation can be achieved by keeping the core elements of the treatment constant while varying other elements as needed. Such an approach requires measurements that allow evaluators to know the degree to which a treatment has been varied. Local demands are not unique to randomized field experiments, however; demonstration projects have also been required to be responsive to local conditions.

A problem that is unique to randomized field experiments is the random allocation of organizations to alternative treatments. For example, recruiting cities to participate in a program will require political leadership and bureaucratic skill. Fortunately, there are precedents for this work. Major collaborative studies in medicine have generated a body of knowledge about the administration of large clinical trials. Although these programs involve individuals as the treatment unit, the administrative and managerial lessons to be learned from such studies are pertinent in the case of larger units. Similarly, the large-scale social experiments that have been conducted over the past 15 years on economic welfare, insurance, and the like also provide valuable information.

SPECIAL CONCERNS OF EVALUATION IN THE CONTEXT OF HIV INFECTION AND AIDS

Research on HIV infection and AIDS presents many methodological challenges. Although some of them have been met, at least in part, by research programs on other sensitive, controversial, or illegal behaviors, there are methodological impediments inherent in this epidemic that can be overcome only by first investing in methodological research. Such research is necessary to provide the tools to understand complex behaviors that are enacted in diverse social situations. This section outlines several of those challenges.

Target Groups

AIDS prevention must necessarily focus on groups for whom risk-associated behavior is common. This criterion means that intervention programs will be directed toward groups that may be unfamiliar and inaccessible to the research community. For example, as Chapter 3 noted, IV drug users have good reasons to remain invisible; if and when they can be located, researchers may find themselves stymied by communication barriers. Linguistic and cultural minorities present analogous demands and challenges. The fact that 25 percent of patient admissions to STD clinics are teenagers means that there is also an urgent need to better understand the beliefs, attitudes, motivations, and social networks of people in that age group.

These circumstances raise two problems that demand the serious attention of those conducting HIV- and AIDS-related research. First, special efforts must be made to increase access to hard-to-reach individuals and to elicit valid, reliable information from them. Second, in evaluating the effects of new intervention programs, hard-to-locate individuals must not only be found but must also be recruited for and engaged in the program.

The problems of identifying, engaging, and retaining participants in experiments that are designed to learn which of several strategies works better have been severe enough in the medical arena to receive sophisticated lay attention.[2] Evidence on the problem has also emerged from randomized field experiments on training programs for vulnerable groups such as youths (Betsey et al., 1985) and minority women who are single parents (Boruch et al., 1988); from tests of criminal justice projects (Boruch et al., 1988); and from other sources.

There are many reasons why it is difficult to recruit sufficiently large samples for research programs. First, "guesstimates" of the number of individuals in need of a new service or alternative service may be wrong. (Recent examples of major disagreements about numbers include the claims about the number of homeless people in Chicago [Rossi, 1987, 1988] and the number of individuals who were expected to contract swine flu [Silverstein, 1981].) One of the more subtle reasons for recruitment problems lies partly in the need to design the evaluation so that it is sensitive to the variations in outcome that can occur with different kinds of people. Such a design requires not only a sufficiently large sample but also homogeneous groups (with respect to age, sexual preference, or other characteristics). Focusing on homogeneous groups means developing clear eligibility requirements for participation in a program. Meeting these requirements leads to the exclusion of a sizable fraction of a larger, more heterogeneous potential target population. The tension between ensuring both sensitivity and adequate sample size has been examined in such texts as Friedman and colleagues (1985) and Riecken and coworkers (1974).

Developing the ability to locate and identify individuals who are at risk for AIDS and then engage them in field tests requires new information and perhaps new methods. At least four approaches that have been applied to resolving such problems in other settings are worth considering. First, preevaluation studies by ethnographers can help to identify and provide some understanding of the groups in which risk-associated behavior is prevalent. This kind of study involves careful observation and controlled interaction with

[2]See, for example, the history of diabetes control and its complications in F. Allen's *Wall Street Journal* article, "Diabetes Study Aimed at Gauging the Benefit of Strict Regimen Finds Recruiting Hard," March 31, 1987:33.

individuals from groups of interest. Such work can be helpful in developing better ways to identify and recruit people for projects; to understand their mobility, thus permitting investigators to follow a group over time; and to determine measures that will increase their willingness and capacity to participate. Other essential, early approaches include preevaluation surveys and the exploitation of existing local data systems. At best, these surveys or systems improve a researcher's ability to estimate the size of the target groups and the extent to which they are more or less eligible. Local data systems on the incidence of relevant behaviors, such as adolescent pregnancy, drug-related delinquency, and criminal activity, may provide a better statistical characterization of the groups. However, these data should be supplemented with surveys or ethnographic studies for the level of detailed understanding required for good program planning. Moreover, a researcher must consider whether existing data are trustworthy.

A second approach that could be taken is a pilot study of a planned experiment. The pilot study serves as a miniature experiment, incorporating the important elements of the larger effort, such as participant location, recruitment, engagement, and random assignment. Pilot studies have been helpful in improving the quality of programs in various situations, including judicial settings and corrections contexts.

A third approach to recruiting and retaining individuals for participation in research focuses on outreach specialists who can communicate well with potential subjects and community groups, generate interest, and help ensure the continued participation of the sample. Outreach specialists have been used in manpower training experiments involving economically vulnerable women and other hard-to-reach groups. In turn, outreach worker training can be informed by local ethnographic work and those with experience in longitudinal surveys of other hard-to-reach groups (e.g., homeless people or IV drug users). Knowledge of local networks, community-based organizations, and the local media is extremely helpful. Engaging the interest and cooperation of potential respondents, using culturally appropriate incentives, and minimizing such disincentives as transportation problems or threats of social sanctions will improve both the rate of participation in the experiment and the quality of the evaluation.

Finally, formal methodological research is needed to understand how and why individuals cooperate in AIDS research and to enhance their cooperation. Clausen and colleagues (1954) conducted early work on cooperation: they surveyed parents to understand why they chose to cooperate with field experiments of the Salk polio vaccine, which was administered to their children. More recently, others have conducted methodological research on additional medical questions (Waskow, 1984; L. M. Friedman et al., 1985).

Information Base

Evaluators can draw on a large panoply of measurement devices (e.g., questionnaires and other instruments), interview techniques, and various research designs that have been developed and applied in diverse behavioral and social science contexts. For many areas, however, measurement is more the product of a craft than of scientific development. Few instruments have been systematically tested for reliability and validity. For some of the groups at greatest risk for HIV infection—namely, IV drug users, men who have sex with other men but who do not define themselves as homosexuals, and linguistically and culturally isolated groups—there is very little information. These deficits in knowledge pose special problems for planning interventions to prevent the spread of HIV infection and for the evaluations of those programs.

Objectives of AIDS Intervention Programs

The main objective of an AIDS intervention program in the United States is to retard the spread of HIV infection. Yet HIV infection is a difficult outcome to measure. At present, there is only one reliable population-based measure: the prevalence of infection in newborn infants in 30 metropolitan areas (see Chapter 1). This ongoing survey provides accurate information about the level of infection among childbearing women and thus offers an important vantage point from which to view the future spread of infection. The survey provides data on the geographical location of infection, but it does not include much other descriptive information. It will gather trustworthy information on a segment of the population, but it will probably be insufficiently specific to measure the effectiveness of interventions targeted at specific groups. The lack of more detailed information (e.g., the mother's address, her membership in treatment programs, her educational level, and other identifiers) to accompany the seroprevalence data collected by the survey is a necessary consequence of the need to protect those individuals who bear the social and physical burdens of infection. Protecting the privacy of research subjects is an important issue, which is discussed in the next section of this chapter.

In addition to the newborn serologic survey, information about certain sentinel[3] populations will be collected during CDC's family of surveys. These samples include individuals recruited from certain hospitals, STD clinics, drug treatment clinics, and the like. (For more detail, see Chapter 1.) It is unclear how useful these data may be in evaluating intervention programs, but the possibility of using at least some of the information should be carefully yet vigorously explored.

HIV has spread quickly within some groups. Changes in attitudes and risk-associated behavior also appear to have occurred rapidly in some subsets of the groups at highest risk to acquire AIDS. Some researchers have argued that there are few remarkable differences to be seen in their studies of knowledge and attitudes about AIDS because of the vast, rapid changes that have been occurring at the national level. Such changes leave little room for measuring improvements that might otherwise have been induced by a new intervention. The rapidity and pervasiveness of change indicate that efforts to understand the effects of intervention programs pose challenges that have not previously been encountered. There may be ceilings on the size of the effect that any intervention may produce; to try to identify further small changes may not be warranted. The value of measuring relatively small increments of change will depend in part on the risk that is associated with the behaviors that are being altered.

In measuring behavioral change, it is important to remember that change is dynamic and its measurement, at times, quite fallible. The quality of measurement of certain behaviors may not allow researchers to discern whether in fact change has really occurred. Improved surveys of IV drug users, for instance, may show an increase in drug use when no increase has actually happened; such differences simply reflect the use of more accurate measures. Changes of this sort in the quality of measurement are entirely plausible and complicate even the best evaluation designs (Campbell and Stanley, 1966).

Some of the chronic problems associated with HIV transmission in U.S. society have origins that preceded the onset of the AIDS epidemic. Determining the best tactics to reduce such practices as IV drug use and the health risks associated with prostitution will

---

[3]In epidemiology, sentinel groups are the harbingers of potential infection for the larger population.

require the design and delivery of better intervention programs with good evaluations.

Ethical Issues

Questions of individual privacy and the confidentiality of a person's research record often loom large in AIDS program evaluations. Positive serologic status constitutes sensitive information, as does self-reported drug use, prostitution, or anal intercourse; these latter behaviors can also make the individual who engages in them vulnerable to a variety of social and legal sanctions. The ethical propriety of a randomized experiment that is designed to establish whether a particular program intervention works is also a major issue.

Considerable progress has been made in understanding how to reduce or eliminate privacy problems at both the individual and experimental levels (National Research Council, 1975). This experience stems largely from research on sensitive topics other than AIDS (e.g., illicit drug use).

Three approaches have been useful in protecting privacy and attempting to meet individual interests in ways that do not compromise the quality of the data or the evaluation. Procedural approaches have used nontechnical devices, such as eliciting information from individuals who remained anonymous; this approach has been used frequently in AIDS prevention programs. Its limitations are not inconsequential: it is impossible to ascertain the reliability of self-reported data if the individual cannot be located or identified. Allowing a respondent to use an alias can obviate this difficulty. This approach was used in a seroprevalence study of prostitutes (Darrow, 1988).

Statistical approaches permit the collection of data that can provide specific information on behavior and selected demographic characteristics without permitting the identification of any individual. However, these procedures are cumbersome and therefore of limited usefulness in some settings. They have been used to good effect in studying illicit drug use among adolescents and other populations (Boruch and Cecil, 1979).

Legal approaches, such as the Public Health Services Act (P.L. 91-513), provide protection against the use of research records for any nonresearch purpose. PHS protection is afforded in two ways. First, it provides explicit protection for research records on identifiable individuals that are generated by the National Center for Health

Statistics and its contractors; it also protects individual records generated by the National Center for Health Services Research. Second, the act permits the secretary of the Department of Health and Human Services (DHHS) to award special confidentiality certificates to researchers who undertake work on mental health topics that fall within the PHS purview. However, the protection provided by this second mechanism is limited in several respects: for example, the confidentiality certificate is discretionary, and certain kinds of judicial access to records are excluded from protection. Details on the benefits, limitations, and opportunities to be gained from improving legal approaches are discussed in Gray and Melton (1985) and in Boruch and Cecil (1979).

Approaches to resolving ethical problems engendered by randomized experiments have been a topic of serious interest since the early 1970s. Thoughtful treatments of constitutional law and the court's views of randomized tests are given in Breger (1983), Teitlebaum (1983), and Rivlin and Timpane (1971).

Threshold conditions for deciding whether certain fundamental ethical standards have been met have been developed for research in other sensitive areas. The monograph of the Federal Judicial Center (1981) that was discussed earlier provides a helpful enumeration of the criteria for making such decisions. Contemporary ethical problems in biomedical research have been considered in a range of publications, workshops, and training programs offered under the aegis of the DHHS Office of Protection of Human Subjects in Research.

Other technical approaches to the design of more ethical experiments are also important (Cook and Campbell, 1979). For example, it may be ethical to randomly allocate some individuals to a new treatment and others to a no-treatment control group when resources for the intervention are very scarce and its effectiveness has not been established. As resources become more plentiful and alternative options are devised, however, the comparison of different treatments acquires a more ethical hue. Statistical technology permits researchers to vary the ratio of those receiving one treatment or another, thus maximizing the number of people who might be helped by what is believed to be an effective strategy. The proper use of such methods increases the likelihood of providing valuable services while maintaining the sensitivity of the evaluation.

Attrition and Noncompliance

Individuals or organizations may agree to take part in a controlled experiment and then later refuse to participate. Important methodological and inference problems result from the attrition or failure of subjects to comply with the treatment to which they have been assigned. Even under controlled conditions, attrition and noncompliance rates can induce biases in estimates of program effects; in poorly controlled experiments, such estimates become indefensible. Problems of this sort are not new. Lashley and Watson's (1922) studies of the effects of motion pictures on condom use among U.S. servicemen are an early illustration: because fewer than 800 of 1,200 viewers responded to their surveys, there had to be concern about the validity of their findings.

A more recent example of a randomized experiment estimated the effect of a behavior modification program on delinquent behavior (Ostrom et al., 1971). Some members of the groups assigned to therapy failed to attend sessions regularly; some failed to attend sessions at all. In other words, some were noncompliers in the sense of failing to adhere to the treatment. In comparing the full randomized groups (i.e., ignoring noncompliers), the researchers could detect no effect of treatment on delinquent activity. They then compared the results for compliers only with the whole control group, under the presumption that such an analysis produces easily interpretable results. In fact, however, they could not know which members of the control group would have participated in the modification program consistently had they been assigned to it. (It is arguable, for example, that those who would have participated are those most likely to shed a delinquent life-style.) By comparing a selected subgroup of those randomly assigned to treatment with the entire control group, the authors confounded their finding: they created a situation in which the estimate of the program's effect is tangled inextricably with unknowable differences between the treatment group and the control group.

Attrition and noncompliance problems occur in experiments on various topics, including studies of drug trials (L. M. Friedman et al., 1985: Chapter 13); income maintenance programs (Hausman and Wise, 1979; Boeckmann, 1981); manpower training programs (Betsey et al., 1985; Boruch and Dennis, 1986); and criminal justice research (Boruch et al., 1988). To the extent that there is a high rate of attrition, the data become less defensible and analyses become much more complicated. Different attrition processes may cause estimates of program effects to be inflated, deflated, or left unchanged relative to the true effect. To the extent that the noncompliance rate is high, the temptation to compare subgroups is great; giving in to this temptation may seriously compromise the validity of the study.

Survey research conducted over the past 20 years has provided a great deal of information about controlling attrition. Reports on this topic regularly appear in such periodicals as the *Annual Proceedings of the American Statistical Association*, *Evaluation Review*, *Proceedings of the Annual Census Conference*, and *International Statistical Review*. Bibliographies have been issued by the National Center for Health Services Research, the National Center for Health Statistics, and the U.S. Department of Education. Field tests have been conducted to determine better ways to locate respondents, provide incentives, reduce disincentives, and track and remind respondents to participate. Attention has been paid to applying these findings in a variety of research settings, including face-to-face interviews and telephone surveys.

Despite the richness of research in this area, however, it is insufficient to address all of the questions that arise in the design of AIDS intervention programs. More is known about tracking adolescents over long periods of time than about the other groups of interest. It is especially important to learn more about retaining contact with particularly vulnerable groups such as IV drug users, who are not reached by the treatment system or by other organizations that serve this population. The gaps in knowledge about attrition and noncompliance invite the serious consideration of methodological research to understand how to reach the hard to reach, how to locate and maintain close contact with them, and how to improve the capacity and willingness of such individuals to participate in research and evaluation.

Measurement and Observation

Eliciting accurate information from vulnerable individuals is not easy. For example, self-reports by IV drug users of their needle-sharing habits may be systematically distorted. The distortion may be deliberate as a result of threats, real or imagined, of legal or social sanctions. Such distortion is not uncommon in studies in related areas—substance abuse, sexual activity, and the like. Distortion may also be systematic and not deliberate—that is, attributable to simple memory lapse. For example, research (e.g., Mathiowetz, 1987) shows that reporting on spells of unemployment is remarkably imperfect. It would be surprising if memory-related causes of distortion were any less influential in the recalling of drug-use or sexual activity. Finally, self-reported data may be subject to nonsystematic variation that can be regarded as random. Interviewers, for instance, may vary subtly in the way they elicit information from drug dealers; the dealers in turn may vary in the accuracy of their reports on the sale of clean needles.

The research literature on the accuracy of self-reported data on sensitive behavior is sparse because such research is extremely difficult. It is especially important to understand the relationship between self-reports and actual behavior, but it is rare to see research projects that can correlate self-reported data with direct, independent observation or with observations that are arguably more accurate than retrospective self-reports. This pattern argues for methodological research that:

- correlates self-reported data with direct observations of IV drug use and the shared use of needles;
- correlates retrospective self-reports of sexual behavior among prostitutes, IV drug users, and others at risk for HIV infection with monitoring (e.g., more frequent interviews or the use of diaries) that is more proximate to the time of condom use or the use of other protections against infection; and
- investigates the cognitive processes that individuals use to answer sensitive questions (e.g., memory flaws and distortion that is not deliberate).

Although to date such research has not been extensive, the organizational mechanisms to support it are in place. The National Laboratory for Collaborative Research in Cognition and Survey Measurement at the National Center for Health Statistics, and the grant mechanisms of the National Center for Health Services Research and the National Institute of Mental Health, are important resources for such activities, which are likely to take considerable time and consume other resources. Yet the problems engendered by inadequate knowledge of the quality of self-reported behavior will persist unless the matter is given serious attention. For example, self-reported data collected in surveys on drug use are generally thought to be reliable; that is, the reports remain constant for an individual from one time to the next. However, less is known about the validity of these data—the extent to which self-reports reflect actual behavior. Clearly, memory decay can occur, but the impact of the passage of time on reported data depends on the salience of the events and the manner in which questions are asked, among other factors.

The litany of difficulties presented in this chapter is not intended to discourage evaluation activity. On the contrary: it is hoped that, by discussing the various methodological, legal, and ethical hurdles, each can, in some degree, be dealt with and made more tractable as experience is acquired. Indeed, each difficulty stands to benefit from the systematic approach and cumulation of knowledge that typify good programs of evaluation.

IMPLEMENTING GOOD EVALUATIONS

Evaluation tends to evoke sentiments on the part of those being evaluated that are similar to the responses inspired by a visit from an auditor or by interaction with a customs inspector. The feelings and fears are not surprising; nevertheless, they have impeded productive collaborative arrangements and severely diminished the returns that are otherwise attainable from good evaluation. Some of the impediments arise from program practitioners' lack of access to individuals with expertise in the area of evaluation. **The committee recommends that evaluation support be provided to ensure collaboration between practitioners and evaluation researchers.**

The challenge to leadership and management is to remove impediments to evaluation. An effective strategy should, inasmuch as possible, remove all basis for the fear and trepidation that has existed in the past. In essence, this means that no person or unit should be punished as a result of an evaluation. In making this strong statement, the committee recognizes that occasionally justified punishment will be withheld. Yet that may be a small cost to pay for fostering program evaluation, which is a valuable part of an organization's process of self-criticism.

Oversights and problems are inevitable. The occurrence of some mistakes, some errors, some imperfections is not generally cause for punitive action; properly viewed, they present opportunities. If something goes wrong, evaluation may allow an understanding of how and why the problem occurred. This understanding in turn can enable a change or adjustment that may forestall similar error in the future. An organization that adopts this ethos and is recognized by staff to have done so, can learn much more effectively from its own experience.

People can learn from both successes and failures. Unfortunately, however, descriptions of failed interventions are less likely to be published than reports of successful ones, and they accrue little prestige for those who conduct them. Yet the publication of negative research results can forestall further unfruitful efforts. Because available resources are limited, it is important to try to repeat successful interventions and not to repeat the clear failures. In reviewing AIDS intervention programs, the committee found that the descriptive information typically published about an actual intervention does not provide sufficient detail to permit its replication. Therefore, **the committee recommends to the research community that the results of well-conducted evaluations be published, regardless of the intervention's effectiveness. The committee further recommends that all evaluations publish detailed descriptive information on the nature and methods of intervention programs, along with evaluation data to support claims of relative effectiveness.**

The resources required to perform evaluations include money, personnel with relevant expertise, and the time and attention of managers. All are essential components of the process, and some are not always readily available. It is evident that choices of emphasis and allocation must be made. Indeed, not every program should receive a full-blown evaluation, although every intervention should probably receive at least some minimal assessment, if only to know what was done and what actually occurred over the course of the program. Setting priorities for the use of evaluation resources appears to rest on several factors: the importance of the intervention, the extent of existing knowledge concerning it, the perceived value of additional information, and the estimated feasibility of the assessment. In order to use available evaluation resources most efficiently, **the committee recommends that only the best-designed and best-implemented intervention programs be selected to receive those special resources that will be needed to conduct scientific evaluations.**

In this chapter and those that precede it, we urge that interventions to prevent the spread of HIV be conducted in accordance with two principles: (1) planned variants of new interventions should be systematically used and should replace the "one-best-shot" approach; and (2) evaluations of new initiatives should be planned in advance and carefully executed. The committee believes that following these two principles will result in more effective programs of education and behavioral change in a shorter time frame. This belief rests on the following propositions:

1. More information is developed and conserved when the evaluation of planned variants is carried out.
2. Good program ideas are more promptly recognized and accepted.
3. Less effective ideas are more promptly recognized and eliminated.
4. Agreement on the relative merits of alternatives is easier to reach and can be effected with more confidence when there are systematically acquired data concerning plausible alternatives.

When possible, for at least each major type of intervention and each major target population, a minimum of two intervention programs should be subjected to rigorous evaluations that are designed to produce research evidence of the highest possible quality. Variants of intervention programs should be developed for and tested in different populations and in different geographic areas using random assignment strategy accompanied by careful evlauation. When ethically possible, one of the variants should be a nontreatment control.

The committee recognizes that difficulties will attend the effort to adopt this strategy, difficulties that include not only the challenges of unfamiliarity and the extra work required to prepare several variants of a brochure, curriculum, radio message, or other intervention tool, but also the problems of actually performing evaluations. All such endeavors call for skills and additional resources that may be in short supply for the agencies that are already heavily committed to coping with AIDS. Despite the difficulties, we believe the achievable benefits are too important to pass by. The first steps to implement the ideas discussed above should be taken promptly. **The committee recommends that CDC substantially increase efforts, with links to extramural scientific resources, to assist health departments and others in mounting evaluations.** State and local health departments as well as education departments will likely require additional resources as they mount evaluation efforts.

The committee sees two steps as sufficient to initiate this process. First, CDC (and any other agency that undertakes AIDS prevention programs) should assign to some administrative unit the responsibility for ensuring the use of planned variants of intervention programs and for overseeing a system of evaluating such programs. Second, there should be easy access to extramural resources to help with the task of evaluation. These resources might be consultants, commercial research organizations, committees of outside experts, or some combination of these individuals and bodies.

BIBLIOGRAPHY

The entries below include references cited in the chapter and other publications of interest. Citations with an asterisk are material relevant to guidelines and standards of evidence for evaluation.

Ackerman, A. M., Froman, D., and Becker, D. (1987) The multiple risk factor intervention trial: Implications for nurses. *Progress in Cardiovascular Nursing* 2:92–99.

Alexander, J. F., and Parsons, B. V. (1973) Short-term behavioral intervention with delinquent families: Impact on family practices and recidivism. *Journal of Abnormal Psychology* 81:219–225.

American Psychological Association, Committee for the Protection of Human Participants in Research (1982). *Ethical Principles in the Conduct of Research with Human Participants.* Washington, D.C.: American Psychological Association.

Barcikowski, R. S. (1981) Statistical power with group mean as the unit of analysis. *Journal of Educational Statistics* 6:267–285.

Barnes, B. A. (1977) Discarded operations: Surgical innovation in trial and error. In J. P. Bunker, B. A. Barnes, and F. Mosteller, eds., *Costs, Risks, and Benefits of Surgery.* New York: Oxford University Press.

Becker, M. H. (1985) Patient adherence to prescribed therapies. *Medical Care* 25:539–555.

Berk, R. A. (1986) Anticipating the Social Consequences of a Catastrophic AIDS Epidemic. Department of Sociology, University of California at Santa Barbara.

Berk, R. A., and Rauma, D. (1983) Capitalizing on nonrandom assignment to treatments: A regression discontinuity evaluation of a crime control program. *Journal of the American Statistical Association* 78:21–27.

Berk, R. A., et al. (1985) Social policy experimentation: A position paper. *Evaluation Review* 9:387–429.

*Bernstein, I. N., and Freeman, H. E. (1975) *Academic and Entrepreneurial Research.* New York: Russell Sage Foundation.

Betsey, C. L., Hollister, R. G., and Papageorgiou, M. R., eds. (1985) *Youth Employment and Training Programs: The YEDPA Years.* Washington, D.C.: National Academy Press.

Blythe, B. J., Gilchrist, L. D., and Schinke, S. (1981) Pregnancy prevention groups for adolescents. *Social Work* 26:503–504.

Boeckmann, M. (1981) Rethinking the results of a negative income tax experiment. In R. F. Boruch, P. M. Wortman, and D. S. Dordray, eds., *Reanalyzing Program Evaluations.* San Francisco: Jossey-Bass.

Boruch, R. F., and Cecil, J. S. (1979) *Assuring Confidentiality of Social Research Data.* Philadelphia: University of Pennsylvania Press.

Boruch, R. F., and Dennis, M. (1986) Understanding respondent cooperation: Field experiments versus surveys. Pp. 296–318 in *Proceedings: Second Annual Research Conference.* Washington, D.C.: U.S. Department of Commerce.

Boruch, R. F., Dennis, M., and Carter-Greer, K. (1988) Lessons from the Rockefeller Foundation's Experiments on the Minority Female Single Parent Program. *Evaluation Review* 12:396–426.

Boruch, R. F., McSweeny, A. J., and Soderstrom, J. (1978) Bibliography: Illustrative randomized experiments for program planning, development, and evaluation. *Evaluation Quarterly* 4:655–696.

*Boruch, R. F., and Pearson, R. (1988) Comparative evaluation of longitudinal surveys. *Evaluation Review* 12:3–58.

Boruch, R. F., Reiss, A., Larntz, K., Andrews, A., and Friedman, L. (1988) Report of the Program Review Team: Spouse Assault Replication Project. National Institute of Justice, Washington, D.C.

Breger, M. J. (1983) Randomized social experiments and the law. Pp. 97–144 in R. F. Boruch and J. S. Cecil, eds., *Solutions to Ethical and Legal Problems in Social Research.* New York: Academic Press.

Brekke, J. S., and Test, M. A. (1987) An empirical analysis of services delivered in a model community treatment program. *Psychosocial Rehabilitation Journal* 10:51–61.

Brownell, K. D., Marlatt, G. A., Lichtenstein, E., and Wilson, G. T. (1986) Understanding and preventing relapse. *American Psychologist* 41:762–782.

Bunker, J. P., Barnes, B. A., and Mosteller, F. (1977) *Costs, Risks, and Benefits of Surgery.* New York: Oxford University Press.

Campbell, D. T., and Stanley, J. S. (1966) *Experimental and Quasi-Experimental Designs for Research.* Chicago: Rand-McNally.

Catania, J. A., Kegeles, S. M., and Coates, T. J. (1988) Towards an Understanding of Risk Behavior: The CAPS' AIDS Risk Reduction Model (ARRM). Center for AIDS Prevention Studies, Department of Psychiatry and Department of Medicine, University of California at San Francisco. January.

*Chalmers, T. C. (1981) A method for assessing quality of a randomized control trial. *Controlled Clinical Trials* 2:31–49.

Chelimsky, E. (1988) Educating People at Risk of AIDS. Testimony before the U.S. Congress, Committee on Governmental Affairs. U.S. General Accounting Office, Program Evaluation and Methodology Division, Washington, D.C. June 8.

Clausen, J. A., Seidentefeld, M. A., and Deasy, L. C. (1954) Parent attitudes toward participation of their children in polio vaccine trials. *American Journal of Public Health* 44:1526–1536.

Coates, T. J., McKusick, L., Kuno, R., and Sites, D. P. (1987) Stress Management Training Reduces Number of Sexual Partners but Does Not Enhance Immune Function in Men Infected with Human Immunodeficiency Virus (HIV). University of California at San Francisco.

Condiotte, M. M., and Lichtenstein, E. (1981) Self-efficacy and relapse in smoking cessation programs. *Journal of Consulting and Clinical Psychology* 49:648–658.

Conner, R. F. (1982) Random assignment of clients in social experimentation. In J. E. Sieber, ed., *The Ethics of Social Research: Surveys and Experiments.* New York: Springer-Verlag.

Cook, T., and Campbell, D. T. (1979) *Quasi-Experimentation.* Boston: Houghton-Mifflin.

*Cordray, D. S. (1982) An assessment of the utility of the ERS standards. *New Directions for Program Evaluation* 15:67–82.

Darrow, W. W. (1988) Behavioral research and AIDS prevention. *Science* 239:1477.

*Davis, H. R., Windle, C., and Sharfstein, S. S. (1977) Developing guidelines for program evaluation capability in community mental health centers. *Evaluation* 4:25–34.

Deniston, O. L., and Rosenstock, I. M. (1972) The Validity of Designs for Evaluating Health Services. School of Public Health, University of Michigan.

Dennis, M. (1988) Implementing Randomized Field Experiments: An Analysis of Civil and Criminal Justice Research. Ph.D. dissertation, Department of Psychology, Northwestern University.

Des Jarlais, D. C. (1987) Effectiveness of AIDS Educational Programs for Intravenous Drug Users. Background paper prepared for the Health Program, Office of Technology Assessment, U.S. Congress, Washington, D.C.

Dondero, T. J., Pappaioanou, M., and Curran, J. W. (1988) Monitoring the levels and trends of HIV infection: The Public Health Service's HIV surveillance program. *Public Health Reports* 103:213–220.

Elkin, I., Pilkonis, P. A., Docherty, J. P., and Sotsky, S. (In press) Conceptual and methodological issues in comparative studies of psychotherapy and pharmacotherapy. *American Journal of Psychiatry.*

Farquhar, J. W., Maccoby, N., and Wood, P. D. (1985) Education and community studies. Chapter 12 in W. W. Holland, R. Detels, and G. Knox, eds., *Oxford Textbook of Public Health.* London: Oxford University Press.

Farquhar, J. W., Wood, P. D., and Breitose, I. T. (1977) Community education for cardiovascular health. *Lancet* 1:1191–1195.

Federal Judicial Center. (1981) *Social Experimentation and the Law.* Washington, D.C.: Federal Judicial Center.

Ferber, R., Sheatsley, P., Turner, A., and Waksberg, J. (1980) *What Is a Survey?* Washington, D.C.: American Statistical Association.

Fienberg, S. E., Martin, M. E., and Straf, M. L., eds. (1985) *Sharing Research Data.* Washington, D.C.: National Academy Press.

Flay, B. R. (1986) Efficacy and effectiveness trials and other phases of research in the development of health promotion programs. *Preventive Medicine* 15:451–474.

Fraker, T., and Maynard, R. (1985) *The Use of Comparison Group Designs in Evaluations of Employment Related Programs.* Princeton, N.J.: Mathematics Policy Research.

Fraker, T., and Maynard, R. (1987) Evaluating comparison group designs with employment related programs. *Journal of Human Resources* 22:195–227.

Freedman, D., Pisani, R., and Purves, R. (1978) *Statistics.* New York: W. W. Norton.

Freedman, R., Takeshita, J. Y., et al. (1969) *Family Planning in Taiwan: An Experiment in Social Change.* Princeton, N.J.: Princeton University Press.

Freeman, H. E., and Rossi, P. H. (1981) Social experiments. *Milbank Memorial Fund Quarterly—Health and Society* 59:340–374.

Friedman, L. M., Furberg, C. D., and DeMets, D. L. (1981) *Fundamentals of Clinical Trials.* Boston: John Wright.

Friedman, L. M., Furberg, C. D., and DeMets, D. L. (1985) *Fundamentals of Clinical Trials,* 2d ed. Littleton, Mass.: PSG Publishing, Inc.

Friedman, S. R., De Jong, W. M., and Des Jarlais, D. C. (1988) Problems and dynamics of organizing intravenous drug users for AIDS prevention. *Health Education Research: Theory and Practice* 3:49–58.

Glaser, E. M., Coffey, H. S., et al. (1967) *Utilization of Applicable Research and Demonstration Results.* Los Angeles: Human Interaction Research Institute.

*Gordon, G., and Morse, E. V. (1975) Evaluation research. In A. Inkeles, ed., *Annual Review of Sociology,* vol. 10. Palo Alto, Calif.: Annual Reviews, Inc.

Gray, J. N., and Melton, G. B. (1985) The law and ethics of psychosocial research on AIDS. *University of Nebraska Law Review* 64:637–688.

Harkin, A. M., and Hurley, M. (1988) National survey on public knowledge of AIDS in Ireland. *Health Education Research* 3:25–29.

Hausman, J. A., and Wise, D. A. (1979) Attrition bias in experimental and panel data: The Gary (Indiana) income maintenancy experiment. *Econometrica* 47:455–473.

Haynes, R. B., Taylor, D. W., Snow, J. C., Sackett, D. L., et al. (1979) Appendix 1: Annotated and indexed bibliography on compliance with therapeutic and preventive regimens. In R. B. Haynes, D. W. Taylor, and D. L. Sackett, eds., *Compliance in Health Care.* Baltimore, Md.: Johns Hopkins University Press.

Hill, R., Stycos, J. M., and Back, K. W. (1959) *The Family and Population Control: A Puerto Rican Experiment in Social Change.* Chapel Hill: University of North Carolina Press.

Holland, P. W., and Rubin, D. B. (1986) Research designs and causal inferences: On Lord's paradox. In R. Pearson and R. Boruch, eds., *Survey Research Designs.* Lecture Notes in Statistics No. 38. New York: Springer-Verlag.

Hull, H. F., Bettinger, C. J., Gallaher, M. M., Keller, N. M., Wilson, J., and Mertz, G. J. (1988) Comparison of HIV-antibody prevalence in patients consenting to and declining HIV-antibody testing in an STD clinic. *Journal of the American Medical Assocation* 260:935–938.

Institute of Medicine. (1985) *Assessing Medical Technologies.* Washington, D.C.: National Academy Press.

Jaffe, H. W., Rice, D. T., Voight, R., Fowler, J., and St. John, R. (1979) Selective mass treatment in a venereal disease control program. *American Journal of Public Health* 69:1181–1182.

Janz, N. K., and Becker, M. H. (1984) The health belief model: A decade later. *Health Education Quarterly* 11:1–47.

Job, R. F. (1988) Effective and ineffective use of fear in health promotion campaigns. *American Journal of Public Health* 78:163–167.

*Joint Committee on Standards. (1981) *Standards for Evaluations of Programs, Projects and Materials.* New York: McGraw-Hill.

Kadane, J. (1986) Progress toward a more ethical method for clinical trials. *Journal of Medicine and Philosophy* 11:285–404.

Klein, N. C., Alexander, J. F., and Parsons, B. V. (1977) Impact of family systems intervention on recidivism and sibling delinquency. *Journal of Consulting and Clinical Psychology* 45:469–474.

LaLonde, R. J. (1986) Evaluating the econometric evaluations of training programs with experimental data. *American Economic Review* 76:604–619.

Lashley, K. S., and Watson, J. B. (1922) *A Psychological Study of Motion Pictures in Relation to Venereal Disease Campaigns.* Washington, D.C.: U.S. Interdepartmental Social Science Board.

Leamer, E. E. (1978) *Specification Searches: Ad Hoc Inference with Nonexperimental Data.* New York: John Wiley & Sons.

Levine, R. (1987) Community Consulting. Presented at the annual meetings of the American Psychological Association, Symposium on Clinical Trials in AIDS, New York, August 30.

Leviton, L., Valdiserri, R. O., Lyter, D. W., Callahan, C. M., Kingsley, L. A., and Rinaldo, C. R. (1988) AIDS Prevention in Gay and Bisexual Men: Experimental Evaluation of Attitude Change from Two Risk Reduction Interventions. Presented at the annual meeting of the American Evaluation Assocation, New Orleans, La., October 19.

Light, R., and Pillemer, D. (1984) *Summing Up: The Science of Reviewing Research.* Cambridge, Mass.: Harvard University Press.

Magidson, J. (1988a) CHAID, LOGIT and log linear modeling. In *Marketing Information Systems.* New York: McGraw-Hill and Data Pro Research.

Magidson, J. (1988b) Progression beyond regression. *DMA (Direct Marketing Association) Research Council Newsletter* 4:6–7.

Mathiowetz, N. (1987) Response error: Correlation between estimation and episodic recall tasks. Pp. 430–435 in *Proceedings of the Survey Research Methods Section: American Statistical Association.* Washington, D.C.: American Statistical Association.

Mathiowetz, N., and Duncan, G. J. (1984) Temporal patterns of response errors on retrospective reports of unemployment and occupation. Pp. 652–657 in *Proceedings of the Survey Research Methods Section: American Statistical Association.* Washington, D.C.: American Statistical Association.

McAuliffe, W. E., Doering, S., Breer, P., Silverman, H., Branson, B., and Williams, K. (1987) An Evaluation of Using Ex-Addict Outreach Workers to Educate Intravenous Drug Users About AIDS Prevention. Presented at the Third International AIDS Conference, Washington, D.C., June 1–5.

*McTavish, D. G., Cleary, J. D., Brent, E. C., Perman, L., and Knudsen, K. R. (1977) Assessing research methodology: The structure of professional assessments of methodology. *Sociological Methods and Research* 6:3–44.

Meier, P. (1972) The biggest public health experiment ever: The 1954 field trial of the Salk poliomyelitis vaccine. In J. M. Tanur, F. Mosteller, W. Kruskal, R. F. Link, R. S. Peters, and G. Rising, eds., *Statistics: A Guide to the Unknown.* San Francisco: Holden-Day.

Miller, W. R. (1986) Inpatient alcoholism treatment. *American Psychologist* 41:794–805.

Mitchell, J. V., Jr., ed. (1985) *The Ninth Mental Measurements Yearbook*, 2 vols. Lincoln: Buros Institute of Mental Measurements, University of Nebraska.

Morisky, D. E., DeMuth, N. M., Field-Fass, M., Green, L. W., and Levine, D. M. (1985) Evaluation of family health education to build social support for long term control of high blood pressure. *Health Education Quarterly* 12:35–50.

Moskowitz, J., Malvin, J. H., Schaeffer, G. A., and Schaps, E. (1983) Evaluation of a cooperative learning strategy. *American Educational Research Journal* 20:687–696.

Moskowitz, J., Malvin, J. H., Schaeffer, G., and Schaps, E. (1984) An experimental evaluation of a drug education course. *Journal of Drug Education* 14:9–22.

Moskowitz, J., Schaps, E., Malvin, J., Schaeffer, G., and Condon, J. (1981) An Evaluation of an Innovative Drug Education Program: Follow-Up Results. Report to the National Institute on Drug Abuse. Pacific Institute for Research and Evaluation, Napa, Calif.

Moskowitz, J. M., Schaps, E., Malvin, J. H., and Schaeffer, G. A. (1984) The effects of drug education at follow-up. *Journal of Alcohol and Drug Education* 30:45–49.

*Mosteller, F. M., Gilbert, S. P., and McPeek, B. (1980) Reporting standards and research strategies: Agenda for an editor. *Controlled Clinical Trials* 1:37–58.

National Cancer Institute. (1988) *Summary: Community Intervention Trial for Smoking Cessation.* Bethesda, Md.: National Institutes of Health.

National Research Council. (1975) *Protecting Individual Privacy in Evaluation Research.* Report of the Committee on Federal Agency Evaluation Research. Washington, D.C.: National Academy Press.

National Research Council. (1982) *An Analysis of Marijuana Policy.* Report of the Committee on Substance Abuse and Habitual Behavior. Washington, D.C.: National Academy Press.

Ostrom, T. M., Steel, C. M., Rosenblood, L. K., and Mirels, H. L. (1971) Modification of delinquent behavior. *Journal of Applied Social Psychology* 1:118–136.

*Pear, R. (1984) Taking the measure, or mismeasure of it all. *New York Times,* August 28.

Public Health Service. (1988) *Understanding AIDS: A Message from the Surgeon General.* Rockville, Md.: Public Health Service.

Reisner, L., David, J., and Turnbull, B. (1988) *Evaluation of the Chapter I Technical Assistance Centers (TAC).* Report to the U.S. Department of Education. Washington, D.C.: Policy Studies Associates.

Riecken, H. W., Boruch, R. F., Campbell, D. T., Caplan, N., Glennau, T. K., Pratt, J. W., Rees, A., and Williams, W. W. (1974) *Social Experimentation: A Method for Planning and Evaluating Social Programs.* New York: Academic Press.

Rivlin, A. M., and Timpane, M., eds. (1971) *Ethical and Legal Issues of Social Experimentation.* Washington, D.C.: Brookings Institution.

Robertson, L. S., Kelley, A. B., O'Neill, B., Wixom, L. W., Eiswirth, R. S., and Haddon, W. (1974) A controlled study of the effect of television messages on safety belt use. *American Journal of Public Health* 64:1071–1080.

Rosenbaum, P. (1987) A nontechnical introduction to statistical power and control of bias. Pp. 174–185 in J. Steinberg and M. Silverman, eds., *Preventing Mental Disorders.* Rockville, Md.: National Institute of Mental Health.

Rossi, P. (1987) Estimating the number of homeless in Chicago. Pp. 1–7 in *Proceedings of the Section on Survey Research Methods: American Statistical Association.* Washington, D.C.: American Statistical Association.

Rossi, P. (1988) *Homelessness in America: Social Research and Policy.* New York: Twentieth Century Fund.

Rubin, D. (1974) Estimating causal effects of treatments in randomized and nonrandomized studies. *Journal of Educational Psychology* 66:688–701.

Rubin, D. (1977) Assignment to treatment group on the basis of a covariate. *Journal of Educational Statistics* 2:1–26.

Ruffin, J. N., Grizzle, J. E., Hightower, N. C., McHardy, G., Shull, H., and Krisher, J. B. (1969) A cooperative double blind evaluation of gastric freezing in the treatment of duodenal ulcer. *New England Journal of Medicine* 281:16–19.

Rutstein, D. C. (1969) The ethical design of human experiments. *Daedalus* 98:523–541.

Schaps, E., et al. (1981) A review of 127 drug education prevention evaluations. *Journal of Drug Issues* 11:17–43.

Schaps, E., Moskowitz, J., Condon, J., and Malvin, J. (1982) A process and outcome evaluation of a drug education course. *Journal of Drug Education* 12:353–364.

Schinke, S., Blythe, B. J., and Gilchrist, L. (1981) Cognitive-behavioral prevention of adolescent pregnancy. *Journal of Counseling Psychology* 28:451–454.

Schneider, A. L. (1980) Effects of status offender deinstitutionalization in Clark County, Washington. Presented at the annual convention of the American Society of Criminology, San Francisco, Calif., November 5–8.

Severy, L. J., and Whitaker, J. M. (1982) Juvenile diversion: An experimental analysis of effectiveness. *Evaluation Review* 6:753–774.

Silverstein, A. M. (1981) *Pure Politics and Impure Science: The Swine Flu Affair.* Baltimore, Md.: Johns Hopkins University Press.

Smith, T. W. (1983) The hidden 25 percent: An analysis of nonresponse on the 1980 General Social Survey. *Public Opinion Quarterly* 47:386–404.

Solomon, M. Z., and DeJong, W. (1986a) The impact of clinic based educational videotapes on male gonorrhea patients' knowledge and treatment behavior. Appendix A in Final Report to the Center for Prevention Services, Centers for Disease Control: October 1, 1983–September 30, 1986. Educational Development Center, Newton, Mass.

Solomon, M. Z., and DeJong, W. (1986b) Recent sexually transmitted disease prevention efforts and their implications for AIDS health education. *Health Education Quarterly* 13:301–316.

Solomon, M. Z., and DeJong, W. (1986c) STD prevention through condom use: Changing patients' knowledge, attitudes, and behavior. Appendix A in Final Report to the Center for Prevention Services, Centers for Disease Control: October 1, 1983–September 30, 1986. Educational Development Center, Newton, Mass.

Solomon, M. Z., DeJong, W., and Jodrie, T. A. (1986) Improving drug-regimen adherence among patients with sexually transmitted disease. Appendix A in Final Report to the Center for Prevention Services, Centers for Disease Control: October 1, 1983–September 30, 1986. Educational Development Center, Newton, Mass.

Strecher, V. J., DeVellis, B., Becker, M., Rosenstock, I. M. (1986) The role of self efficacy in achieving health behavior change. *Health Education Quarterly* 13:73–91.

Teitlebaum, L. E. (1983) Spurious, tractible, and intractible legal problems: A positivist approach to law and social science. Pp. 11–48 in R. F. Boruch and J. S. Cecil, eds., *Solutions to Ethical and Legal Problems in Social Research.* New York: Academic Press.

Thistlethwaite, D. L., and Campbell, D. T. (1969) Regression-discontinuity analysis: An alternative to the ex-post facto experiment. *Journal of Experimental Psychology* 51:309–317.

Tobler, N. (1986) Meta-analysis of 143 adolescent drug prevention programs: Quantitative outcome results of program participants compared to a control or comparison group. *Journal of Drug Issues* 16:537–567.

Trochim, W. (1984) *Research Design for Program Evaluation: The Regression Discontinuity Approach.* Beverly Hills, Calif.: Sage.

*U.S. Department of Education, National Institute of Education. (1977) *The Joint Dissemination Review Panel Ideabook.* Washington, D.C.: National Institute of Education.

*U.S. General Accounting Office. (1975) *Evaluation and Analysis to Support Decision-making.* Washington, D.C.: U.S. General Accounting Office.

*U.S. General Accounting Office. (1978) *Assessing Social Program Impact Evaluations: A Checklist Approach.* Washington, D.C.: U.S. General Accounting Office.

U.S. General Accounting Office. (1986) *Teenage Pregnancy: 500,000 Births but Few Tested Programs.* PEMD-86-16 BR. Washington, D.C.: U.S. General Accounting Office.

Valdiserri, R. O., Leviton, L., et al. (1986) A Randomized Trial Evaluating Two Interventions Promoting AIDS Risk Reduction (proposal submitted to CDC). University of Pittsburgh.

Valdiserri, R. O., Lyter, D. W., Leviton, L. C., Stoner, K., and Silvestre, A. (1987) Applying the criteria for the development of health promotion and education to AIDS risk reduction programs for gay men. *Journal of Community Health* 12:199–212.

Vincent, M., Clearie, A. F., and Schlucter, M. D. (1987) Reducing adolescent pregnancy through school and community-based education. *Journal of the American Medical Association* 257:3382–3386.

Waskow, J. E. (1984) Specification of the treatment variable in the NIMH treatment of depression collaborative research program. In J. Williams and R. L. Spitzer, eds., *Psychotherapy Research.* New York: Guilford Press.

Weinstein, N. D. (1987) Unrealistic optimism about susceptibility to health problems: Conclusions from a community-wide sample. *Journal of Behavioral Medicine* 10:481–500.

Part III

Impediments to Research and Intervention

In Parts I and II of this report, we discussed the two primary modes of transmission of HIV infection: sexual activity and IV drug use. We also documented the incomplete state of scientific knowledge about those behaviors and the behavioral interventions that might retard HIV's future spread. Understanding the behaviors and intervening to modify them are necessary to control the spread of HIV infection. Yet sexual behavior and drug use occur in a social context of strong and often conflicting beliefs that can create barriers to both understanding and intervention. In this part of the volume, we consider some of those barriers. Chapter 6 describes some of the obstacles to adequate support of relevant behavioral and social research and presents recommendations to overcome them. Chapter 7 describes the barriers to potentially effective interventions to control the AIDS epidemic. Our purpose is to suggest that the understanding and prevention of AIDS must ultimately be seen in a broader context of cultural, political, and social realities.

6

Barriers to Research

The twentieth century has witnessed unprecedented advances in the ability to diagnose and treat infectious diseases. Yet the discovery of effective chemotherapies and vaccines has not guaranteed success in controlling sexually transmitted infection. For example, although penicillin has been an important and effective part of the campaign against syphilis and gonorrhea for more than 40 years, these sexually transmitted diseases have persisted, and their incidence has risen with the changes that have occurred in sexual mores. Brandt (1987) has argued that these diseases pose a complex problem in which the biology of the parasite and of its host interact with a variety of social and environmental factors that codetermine the pattern of the spread of the disease. Thus, the efficacy of therapies and vaccines can be overwhelmed by social changes—for example, the weakening of the link between sex and marriage, changes in patterns of nonmarital sexual behavior, or declines in the use of particular contraceptive methods.

Disease prevention, then, calls for more than biomedical technologies. It also requires a sophisticated comprehension of individual and social behavior patterns and the ability to design interventions in accord with that comprehension. This is particularly true for STDs and, as the previous chapters of this report have made clear, for halting the spread of HIV infection. Awareness of the role that the social and behavioral sciences can play in designing and implementing preventive strategies in health promotion and disease control has increased significantly during the past two decades. In 1979, for example, a committee of the Institute of Medicine that was charged to review principles for health research concluded that there was a need for a concept of the health sciences "that is much broader than was the view as recently as ten years ago" (IOM/NAS, 1979:25). It recommended that approaches that equated health research with biomedical research be expanded to recognize the importance of the behavioral and social sciences—as well as statistics and epidemiology—for research on disease prevention and health maintenance: "The committee regards this broadened concept as a desirable advance in policy formation, and supports efforts to translate this perspective into tangible and adequate support for the full complement of the health sciences" (1979:25).

Writing three years later, the IOM/NAS Steering Committee on Health and Behavior (Hamburg et al., 1982:Chapter 19) echoed these conclusions and urged increased funding, multidisciplinary collaborative research programs, and a number of other specific actions: increasing the number of behavioral scientists appointed to medical school faculties, expansion of M.D.–Ph.D. programs to include psychology and sociology, and increased use of behavioral and social scientists on review panels for the National Institutes of Health (NIH). The committee also argued that funding levels for behavioral research on health were not commensurate with the available research opportunities:

> Many substantial opportunities for research do in fact exist. They offer promise of clarifying linkages of health and behavior and the potential of suggesting more effective therapeutic and preventive interventions in the future. This being the case, the present low level of funding of research deserves serious re-examination. It would be tragic to allow a prolonged decline in support at a time of expanding scientific opportunity. (Hamburg et al., 1982:319)

In its concluding remarks on the situation that existed in 1982, the committee recognized one significant set of barriers to broader views of health-related research:

> Prejudices and inherent complexities have presented formidable obstacles to efforts to link biological and behavioral phenomena . . . [but the] practical problems of clinical medicine and public health demand novel conjunctions and open-minded, cooperative explorations. . . . (1982:321–322)

Since 1982 some progress has been made in enhancing the role of the social and behavioral sciences in medical research and practice. There has been, for example, an increase in the number of social and behavioral scientists on the faculties of schools of medicine and

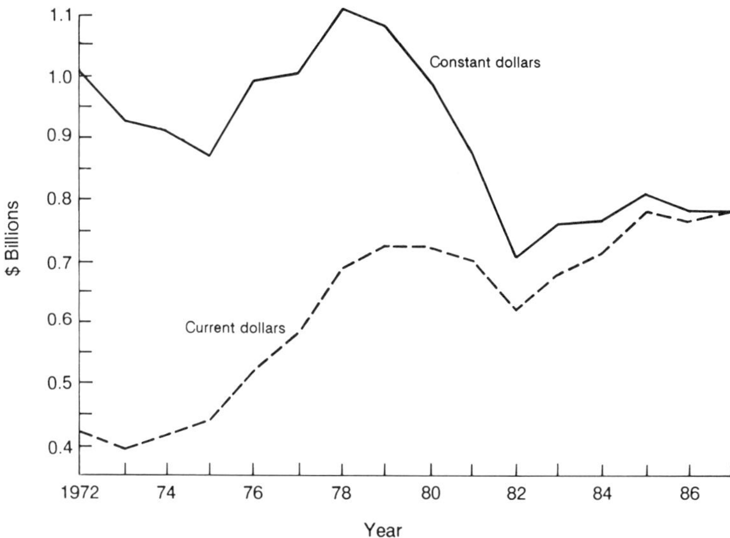

FIGURE 6-1a Trends in federal support for behavioral and social science research (in current and constant 1987 dollars). Source data are from the National Science Foundation's *Federal Funds for Research and Development,* cited in Gerstein and colleagues (1988:252).

public health.[1] Federal funding for research in the behavioral and social sciences, however, has declined. As Figure 6-1a illustrates, the funding available for behavioral and social science research (of all types) in 1987 was 25 percent less than in 1972 in constant dollar terms (i.e., adjusting for inflation). This decline in federal support was not due to an across-the-board cut in federal support for scientific research: federal support for other research increased by 36 percent during this same period (Figure 6-1b). It should also be noted (as indicated by the dotted line in Figure 6-1b) that funding of behavioral and social research of all types has been a barely visible fraction of the federal research budget in every year between 1972 and 1987.

The key role of prevention in the control of the AIDS epidemic has led to a renewed appreciation of the need for behavioral and social research. As early as 1985, the Office of Technology Assessment

[1]Tabulations from the biennial Survey of Doctorate Recipients conducted by the National Research Council's Office of Scientific and Engineering Personnel indicate that the estimated number of behavioral and social sciences Ph.D.s employed in medical schools increased steadily from 2,229 in 1977 to 4,730 in 1985 and remained at this level (4,694) in 1987. It is the committee's impression that a parallel increase occurred in schools of public health, although the available data do not permit estimates to be made of the number of doctoral recipients employed in these schools.

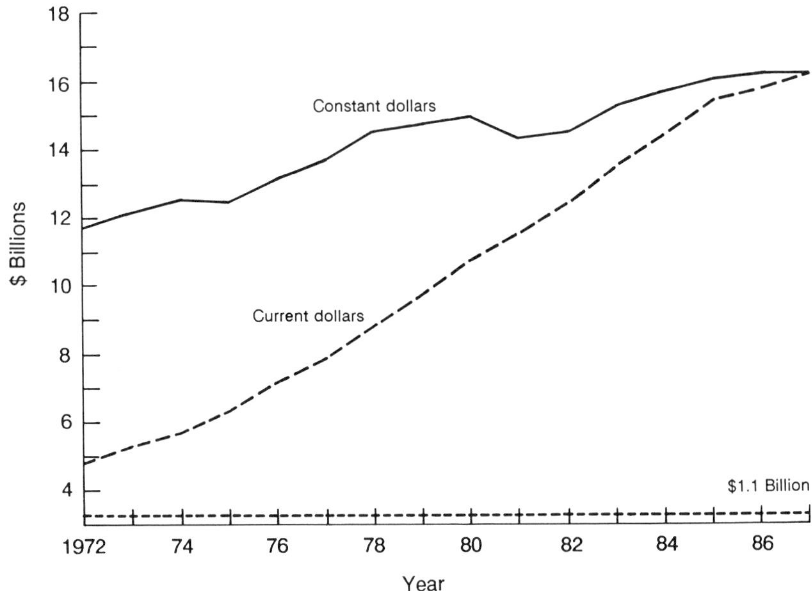

FIGURE 6-1b Trends in federal support for other research (in current and constant 1987 dollars). Source data are from the National Science Foundation's *Federal Funds for Research and Development,* cited in Gerstein and colleagues (1988:252).

questioned whether adequate funds were being devoted to behavioral research on AIDS prevention strategies:

> By directive [of the Department of Health and Human Services], the response to AIDS has concentrated on research into the biology of AIDS. Psychological and social factors related to AIDS, the service needs of AIDS patients, and public education and prevention have not been considered funding priorities. . . . The distribution of resources to activities not directly involving the etiologic agent remains an issue. Of particular importance is the question of whether sufficient resources are being devoted to the investigation of factors affecting the transmissibility of AIDS, treatment, public education, and prevention. (1985:31)

One year later, the IOM/NAS Committee on a National Strategy for AIDS also noted the crucial role to be played by behavioral interventions in controlling the AIDS epidemic, and it discussed the consequences of inadequate funding for social and behavioral research:

> . . . the knowledge base in the behavioral and social sciences needed to design approaches to encourage behavioral change is more rudimentary because of chronic inadequate funding. This lack of behavioral and social science research generates some of

> the most important and immediate questions surrounding the epidemic. (IOM/NAS, 1986:230–231)

Our own committee, which is composed largely of behavioral and social scientists, agrees with the conclusion previously reached by our biomedical colleagues. We have not, however, taken it as our task to assess the relative funding allocated to biomedical versus behavioral research. The committee observes, however, that a large number of serious and pressing needs for behavioral and social research have not been met because of a lack of funding or (in cases such as sex research) because of the hesitancy of federal health officials to support research that might provoke congressional criticism.[2] This history of unfunded research needs has hobbled attempts to understand the AIDS epidemic. The preceding chapters have described some of these needs; two examples deserve reiteration:

- The AIDS epidemic has created a great demand for data on the prevalence and patterns of IV drug use in the United States. Lack of funding, however, has forced the closing of the data archive that was established to catalog and store data from past research studies.
- In 1987, statisticians began to develop and apply methods that use counts of AIDS cases to infer the spread of HIV infection. These methods require reliable information about the distribution of incubation periods from HIV infection to the diagnosis of AIDS (see Chapter 1). Yet as a result of funding limitations and the cost of tracing participants, it has not been possible to follow all men with long-term HIV infection in the cohort study that has enrolled the largest number of men infected during the first stage of the epidemic.

In the preceding chapters of this report, the committee has recommended the funding of specific research efforts to better understand the behaviors that transmit HIV infection.

In addition to removing the barriers imposed by a history of underfunding of basic social and behavioral research, the committee believes that current AIDS research efforts are often hindered by clearance procedures imposed by the Office of Management and Budget (OMB) on the collection of survey data. These clearance procedures (mandated by the Paperwork Reduction Act of 1980)

---

[2]The National Institute of Mental Health, for example, was awarded a "Golden Fleece Award" in April 1978 by Senator William Proxmire for funding a study of behavioral and social relationships in a Peruvian brothel.

can impose delays of several months between the time a researcher prepares a research design and the time the content and wording of the survey form are approved by OMB. This procedure not only retards research but may discourage careful pilot testing because each new version of a survey questionnaire requires clearance if it is to be administered to more than nine persons. Given the urgent unmet research needs related to AIDS, ways to speed up research must be found. **The committee recommends that serious consideration be given to exempting research on HIV infection and AIDS from the requirements of the Paperwork Reduction Act.**

COLLABORATION IN RESEARCH

Equally as important as the removal of barriers to social and behavioral research on AIDS is the facilitation of contact between all of the relevant researchers in the field. Interdisciplinary collaboration is crucial to an understanding of the complex set of biological, psychological, and social problems that affect the AIDS epidemic. Research on the dynamics of HIV transmission, for example, has come to involve not only experts in virology and infectious disease but experts in survey measurement and sample design.

Just as it has been essential for AIDS researchers to collaborate across the boundaries of unfamiliar disciplines, so, too, has it been vital to develop collaborations between scientists and the communities with which they work. Indeed, it would appear that much of the best behavioral and statistical research on AIDS has resulted from the joint efforts of university scientists, government agencies (at all levels), and organizations rooted in the communities that have borne the brunt of the AIDS epidemic. Although these collaborations have not always been easy to arrange or free from conflict, the practical and scientific payoffs have been substantial. Research aimed at the design, implementation, and evaluation of AIDS interventions depends in many important ways on the organizations that can represent and reach the communities that are the targets for those interventions. Beyond providing entry into these communities, collaboration with organizations and individuals in the community can enrich the research process and improve the chances that the interventions will be effective. To help foster this crucial collaboration, the committee believes that, to the maximum extent possible, talented, well-trained, and dedicated workers should be recruited from within the communities in which interventions will be conducted. These workers should be involved in decision making at all levels, from central coordination and funding to local outreach and education.

Attempts to break down social barriers may sometimes be more difficult than arranging collaborations across the boundaries of academic specialities. Differences in social origins, economic status, or life-style may sometimes lead to misunderstandings on both sides. Yet despite such misunderstandings, the differences that can at times make these collaborations difficult also make them indispensable. Efforts to design and implement effective AIDS education without the collaboration of local communities will only multiply these misunderstandings. **The committee recommends that intervention programs at all levels increase the involvement of minority researchers and minority health care workers to assist in reaching and involving the black, Hispanic, and gay communities.**

Collaboration can take many forms, and unfortunately, some of those forms may amount to little more than "window dressing." Communities may be "involved," for example, by appointing community representatives to consult with medical and behavioral scientists who are designing interventions for these communities. When convened in good faith, such groups may help to improve the interventions. Their potential influence is limited, however, by the time group members are able to donate to this activity, their understanding of the research process, and the receptivity of the scientists involved. Obviously, when such groups are convened to placate community activists or to satisfy the requirements of a federal contract, the prospects are bleak that the group will contribute to improving the intervention.

The history of collaboration between communities and researchers has been quite mixed. It is claimed, for example, that poor communication between public health officials and the gay community impeded early prevention efforts (Shilts, 1987). As "outsiders," public health officials were sometimes unaware of the behavioral patterns, social habits, and political sensitivities that required consideration in planning intervention strategies. On the positive side, the committee notes that a number of creative arrangements have been developed to foster collaboration through the multidisciplinary AIDS research centers established by the National Institute of Mental Health (NIMH). For example, in San Francisco, academic research groups have established strong linkages with institutions in the black, Hispanic, and gay communities. These institutional connections have been strengthened in turn by the recruitment from those communities of physicians and behavioral scientists who were working in service delivery positions. These individuals have been invited to work on research projects in collaboration with the AIDS center at the University of California at San Francisco (UCSF). Besides providing the UCSF research teams with colleagues familiar with and familiar to the community, these arrangements will ultimately increase the cadre of minority scientists skilled in AIDS research.

A key ingredient in UCSF's ability to forge these links has been the university's flexibility regarding appointment policies and its willingness to appoint minority scientists with service delivery backgrounds in the community to staff positions equivalent to those of research scientists recruited from academia. So, for example, UCSF was able to appoint a talented black female physician without a research background in AIDS to the junior faculty to work on AIDS prevention research. Besides helping to blur the distinctions between community service and academic research, faculty appointments for talented service providers may be the sine qua non for their participation in research. Many of these practitioners have family and other financial obligations that preclude their acceptance of positions carrying typical postdoctoral stipends. UCSF's ability to make such appointments has been assisted by encouragement from responsible NIMH staff and by the funding NIMH provides for the university's AIDS activities. The committee believes that continued attention needs to be paid to fostering such innovative institutional arrangements.

In addition, the collaborative efforts begun with federal support should be sustained. Much of the required behavioral and social research on AIDS prevention requires large multidisciplinary teams of scientists with close working relationships with many of the different communities in which interventions must be conducted. Recent initiatives, particularly those of NIMH, have been instrumental in forming such multidisciplinary teams in cities that are current foci of the AIDS epidemic.

The special funding mechanisms used to support the AIDS centers are an important complement to more traditional grant-making procedures, and they have stimulated interesting and innovative collaborative research. Moreover, such arrangements have the potential for rapidly enlarging the pool of talented senior AIDS investigators by bringing established scientists into this research area. The committee believes that it would be a serious mistake to curtail funding for these new initiatives in favor of more traditional means of research.

Funding strategies that rely entirely on unsolicited grant mechanisms supporting individual or small groups of researchers at work on narrowly focused topics are unlikely to stimulate the wide range of needed AIDS research in a reasonable period of time. **The committee recommends that support of multidisciplinary centers for research on AIDS prevention be viewed as a long-term commitment to allow sustained collaborative efforts, including valuable prospective studies.**

FEDERAL RESEARCH PERSONNEL

In addition to the need for research funding and increased collaboration, there is a crucial need to enlarge the behavioral and social science staff of the federal agencies charged with formulating and coordinating the national response to the epidemic. As the lead agency for AIDS prevention and surveillance activities, CDC has struggled mightily to respond to this important charge; yet organizational and staffing constraints have compromised its ability to do so.

At the heart of CDC's traditional mode of infectious disease control is the rapid location of disease, followed by treatment, vaccination, or isolation to prevent its spread. With AIDS, however, there is neither a treatment nor a vaccine, and isolation or quarantine of HIV-infected individuals is inappropriate, given that the spread of the disease does not occur through chance or casual interactions. Thus, CDC's traditional mode of disease control does not fit the needs of the AIDS epidemic, and the agency has had to evolve rapidly to mount a prevention strategy based on behavioral change and education.

When the AIDS epidemic began, CDC employed fewer than 40 Ph.D.-level behavioral scientists, and the agency had limited connections with the behavioral science community. CDC thus lacked the organizational and research infrastructure to appreciate the role of the behavioral sciences in disease prevention and has had to build bridges to the behavioral research community in order to formulate reasonable approaches in its response to the epidemic. Creating an appropriate behavioral and social science infrastructure will take time; it will also require the continuing attention of CDC's senior management to ensure that there is an appropriate increase in staff trained in the relevant social and behavioral sciences.

In this regard, the committee notes that it would be desirable to broaden the pattern of recruitment for CDC's Epidemiologic Intelligence Service (EIS) to include a greater number of behavioral

TABLE 6-1 Persons Trained Between 1951 and 1987 by CDC's Epidemiologic Intelligence Service, by Profession

Scientific Field	Number Trained
Selected categories of biomedical scientists	
Physicians	1,318
Veterinarians	103
Epidemiologists	40
Microbiologists	11
Dentists	5
All statisticians and social scientists	
Statisticians	44
Anthropologists	5
Demographers	4
Sociologists	2
Total	1,570

SOURCE: CDC (1987).

and social scientists. The EIS provides broad training in epidemic surveillance and control and is an important source of trained personnel for surveillance and public health activities. Since 1951 the EIS has trained over 1,500 individuals, including 1,300 physicians, but it has trained only 11 social scientists (Table 6-1). The involvement of more such scientists might bring to the agency social and behavioral research skills that are needed to complement the biomedical skills of physicians and other biological scientists in disease prevention. It could also broaden the scope of the training experience. Finally, it might foster the development of collegial relationships among individuals from different research backgrounds that could serve as a catalyst for future collaborative efforts or as an entry into an informational network in another discipline.

In this regard, the committee would emphasize that the staffing of the EIS is but a minor (and rather specialized) example of CDC's needs. The committee notes that CDC is presently managing a portfolio of more than $150 million in behavioral research and intervention programs with a small, severely overextended cadre of persons trained in relevant disciplines. Of approximately 4,500 employees at CDC, fewer than 40 are Ph.D.-level behavioral and social scientists (and only a fraction of these are working in areas related to AIDS). From the beginning of the AIDS epidemic until the spring of 1988, only one behavioral scientist was added to CDC's staff to work full-time on AIDS.

Immediate Needs

The committee believes there is a pressing need to expand substantially the cadre of behavioral, social, and statistical scientists working in the area of AIDS research within agencies of the federal government. The committee offers three recommendations concerning specific staff needs and one suggestion as to how these needs could be met in a timely and flexible fashion.

First, the committee recommends that the number of trained behavioral and social scientists employed in AIDS-related activities at federal agencies responsible for preventing the spread of HIV infection be substantially increased. Next, the committee encourages a consideration of further expertise in the areas of survey sampling and design. As detailed in Chapter 1, survey data will result in a better product if the surveys are planned and conducted with more timely and greater input from individuals with expertise in relevant fields. At present, the CDC AIDS program does not employ a sampling statistician; as of May 24, 1988, it employed only four Ph.D.-level statisticians in its Statistics and Data Management Branch. The recent organizational move of the National Center for Health Statistics (NCHS) to CDC could provide some of the needed expertise. The role played by NCHS staff has been constrained, however, by the agency's incomplete integration into CDC's AIDS activities. **The committee recommends that the CDC AIDS program increase its staff of persons knowledgeable about survey sampling and survey design, and that it exploit the methodological expertise of the National Center for Health Statistics.**

Finally, the committee notes that, often, educational activities undertaken or supported by CDC and other federal agencies have not undergone rigorous evaluation; in some cases in which evaluations have been done, uninformative criteria were used to measure the effects of the program. Examples of such criteria include measuring the impact of educational efforts in terms of the numbers of brochures distributed or assessing changes in knowledge in what is presumed to be the target audience with little or no information being collected on risk-associated behavior. In many instances, these oversights or omissions reflect the inexperience of those conducting the evaluation. **The committee recommends that, in addition**

to experienced survey scientists, CDC obtain technical assistance to evaluate intervention programs it is currently funding.

In making these recommendations, the committee is painfully aware of two impediments that may thwart administrators who seek to implement them. One impediment arises from the delays imposed by the federal personnel system; the second arises from overcrowding at CDC's Atlanta facility. On the latter need, the committee would note that the Presidential Commission on the HIV Epidemic recommended that long-delayed plans to expand and modernize CDC's Atlanta facility be implemented. It is to be hoped that plans to enlarge the facility will take into account the need to accommodate the new staff recommended in this report.

A more difficult logistical problem may be encountered in recruiting appropriate staff. In addition to the delays caused by the federal personnel system, senior scientists may be reluctant to relocate on a permanent basis. The committee notes, however, that one- or (preferably) two-year appointments of "visiting scientists" might provide quick access to needed personnel. These positions (and other junior positions, perhaps of longer duration) might be filled through Intergovernmental Personnel Agreements (IPAs) or through the PHS fellowship program. Use of these mechanisms would provide PHS management with flexibility in meeting changing staffing needs. Therefore, **the committee recommends the use of PHS fellowship programs and IPAs as an interim means for rapidly enlarging the cadre of senior behavioral and social scientists working on AIDS programs at CDC and other PHS agencies.**

Future Needs

In the longer term, planning must begin to train the next generation of researchers. The present cadre of AIDS researchers has been recruited from a wide range of specialities in the behavioral, social, and statistical sciences. This range suggests that an adequately broad and rigorous training in these areas may provide reasonable preparation for work in this field. Nonetheless, much is being learned by AIDS researchers that is not now included in graduate training within these disciplines. For example, even well-trained graduate students are unlikely to be familiar with such topics as the use of back-extrapolation methods to generate estimates of HIV infection from AIDS case data; procedures for reducing bias when obtaining self-reports of intimate sexual behaviors; or methods for developing comprehensive instruments with carefully worded questions to maximize the likelihood of enumerating and understanding factors that encourage or inhibit behavioral change. These skills, which are now being acquired by the current generation of researchers, must find their way into the training programs that will produce the next generation of AIDS scientists. Although it may be too early to prescribe the format of such programs, it is not too early for those concerned with graduate training to begin planning to integrate this material into graduate and postgraduate curricula. Similarly, federal agencies (including the National Institutes of Health; the Alcohol, Drug Abuse, and Mental Health Administration; the Centers for Disease Control; and the Health Resources and Services Administration) must begin to consider how their programs can be used to ensure that appropriately trained researchers will be available for future work to halt the spread of AIDS.

REFERENCES

Brandt, A. M. (1987) *No Magic Bullet: A Social History of Venereal Disease in the United States Since 1880,* expanded ed. New York: Oxford University Press.

Centers for Disease Control (CDC). (1987) *1987–1988 EIS Directory.* Atlanta, Ga.: Epidemiology Intelligence Service and Epidemiology Program Office, Centers for Disease Control.

Gerstein, D., Luce, R. D., Smelser, N. J., and Sperlich, S., eds. (1988) *The Behavioral and Social Sciences: Achievements and Opportunities.* Washington, D.C.: National Academy Press.

Hamburg, D. A., Elliot, G. R., and Parron, D. L., eds. (1982) *Health and Behavior: Frontiers of Research in the Biobehavioral Sciences.* Washington, D.C.: National Academy Press.

Institute of Medicine/National Academy of Sciences (IOM/NAS). (1979) *DHEW Research Planning Principles: A Review.* Washington, D.C.: National Academy of Sciences.

Institute of Medicine/National Academy of Sciences (IOM/NAS). (1986) *Confronting AIDS: Directions for Public Health, Health Care, and Research.* Washington, D.C.: National Academy Press.

Office of Technology Assessment (OTA). (1985) *Review of Public Health Service's Response to AIDS.* Washington, D.C.: Office of Technology Assessment.

Shilts, R. (1987) *And the Band Played On: Politics, People, and the AIDS Epidemic.* New York: St. Martin's Press.

7

Social Barriers to AIDS Prevention

The previous chapters have discussed in detail the two primary modes of transmission of HIV infection: sexual activity and IV drug use. At present, controlling the spread of HIV infection requires both a scientific understanding of these behaviors and a societal commitment to behavioral intervention sufficient to reduce the transmission of HIV infection. Yet fulfilling these requirements will be difficult: cultural and social beliefs and feelings about these behaviors can generate conflict that impedes efforts to understand them and interventions to modify them.

Initially, this chapter describes some of the societal conflicts that have characterized America's response to the AIDS epidemic. Subsequently, from a more conjectural perspective, it considers ways in which an understanding of these conflicts may be informed by a historical view of stigmatization as it has characterized other epidemics.

SOCIAL RESPONSE TO EPIDEMICS

It is important to clarify our use of the word *epidemic*, which is now commonly associated with the presence of HIV infection in the U.S. population. (For example, the recent presidential commission was named the Presidential Commission on the Human Immunodeficiency Virus *Epidemic*.) In fact, as Shilts (1987) reports, gaining official recognition of AIDS as an epidemic in the United States was not easy, although *epidemic* is loosely used in everyday discourse. For most people, it means a disease that affects a large number of people; thus, debates can arise over how large the affected population must be for a health problem to be called an epidemic. Recently, for example, columnist James J. Kilpatrick noted that many more persons are afflicted with heart conditions and cancer than with AIDS, which prompted him to write, "What's the big deal about AIDS?"[1]

In the scientific sense, epidemic disease refers not so much to the number of people affected but to the unexpected increase of a disease in a community. Thus, epidemic disease is defined as "the occurrence in a community or region of cases of an illness, specific health-related behavior, or other health-related events, clearly in excess of normal expectancy" (Kelsey et al., 1986:212). Most commonly, an epidemic disease appears unexpectedly, and the number of affected people increases rapidly within the population. Given the record of the last seven years, HIV infection clearly fulfills the definition of an epidemic.

The scientific definition, however, must be supplemented by the historical meaning of *epidemic*. That meaning is vividly captured by the etymology of the word, which in ancient Greek means "upon the people." Historically, many epidemics have fallen on the community as great calamities, affecting not only the individuals in the community but the structure of the community itself. A debilitating or lethal disease, striking many persons suddenly and often inexplicably, throws the community into disorder. An epidemic in this sense is quite literally a social, cultural, and political disease (McNeil, 1976).

The devastating effect of an epidemic on a community can evoke strong political and social responses. During the plagues of medieval Italy, civil authorities exerted a strong, even draconian influence (Cipolla, 1973). Similarly, during the cholera and yellow fever epidemics of nineteenth-century America, business and commercial interests moved to control the disaster (Rosenberg, 1962). In almost all major epidemics, community life has been seriously disrupted by the presence of a mass of seriously ill and dying people. At the same time, an epidemic necessitates the rapid mobilization of the community to counter the spread of illness and death.

Such mobilization is never easy. Social, cultural, political, and economic institutions are built for the day-to-day activities of communal living; they are not quickly or easily modified to deal with catastrophe. Indeed, because catastrophe is so threatening to the familiar, these institutions may resist being reshaped to meet the needs of a crisis. A "business-as-usual" attitude may obscure the harsh truth that the community is seriously threatened, and familiar ways of dealing with familiar problems may be applied to what is

[1]James J. Kilpatrick, "Aren't We Overreacting to AIDS?," *Washington Post*, June 9, 1988:A19.

really novel or out of the ordinary. Thus, in most major epidemics of which there are accurate histories, medicine was slow to realize that it was confronting an unfamiliar problem; disease was diagnosed incorrectly, and the prevention or therapy measures used to contain it were consequently inadequate (Winslow, 1943).

The AIDS epidemic has also evoked a traditional response: it has been defined as primarily a medical problem, to be solved primarily by medical science. As this report has stressed, however, AIDS is also a social problem. The virus is transmitted through human behaviors; as such, the problem needs to be solved by social means that facilitate change in risk-associated behaviors. Yet the social response to the AIDS epidemic in America has produced a number of conflicts and paradoxes that may result from social processes similar to those that have characterized the history of societal responses to other epidemics.

As noted above, an epidemic is properly understood as the cases of a disease that occur in unexpectedly high numbers in a community. Epidemics spread from place to place, and the term *pandemic* is used to describe excess disease in many countries. Many epidemics rage for a time—days, months, years—and then subside. Sometimes cases disappear altogether or become increasingly rare as smallpox and diphtheria have done in the United States. Other epidemic diseases "settle in" and become an expected part of the illness burden that a society bears. In this situation, the number of cases does not show the rapid increase that originally called attention to the epidemic; instead, the disease persists at a relatively constant level, becoming, in scientific terms, "endemic"—literally, "dwelling with the people."

Some people believe that the nation can relax, once it is announced that "the epidemic is over." Yet such an announcement can be dangerously ambiguous. If a disease disappears or is conquered by medical science, then relaxation is appropriate: for example, yellow fever, which devastated the United States in the nineteenth century, is no longer a threat. If the disease becomes endemic, however, it continues to dwell in the community, doing its damage less dramatically but just as surely. The mutation of a disease from epidemic proportions to endemic status is thus cold comfort. It is likely that HIV infection will be endemic in the United States for a long time and will also continue to be epidemic in certain groups.

The following section offers examples that illustrate some of the ways in which social barriers have already impeded effective responses to the AIDS epidemic and ways in which such barriers will hinder attention to the disease in the future if AIDS becomes endemic.

COMMUNICATING ABOUT SEX

Reticence about discussing sexual issues is common among Americans. Because HIV infection is spread by sexual activities, frank discussions of AIDS have suffered from that reticence, a factor that has limited the public debate necessary for political action. Even more serious, however, is the broadly accepted notion, shared by "liberals" and "conservatives" alike, that government simply has no business dealing with sexuality. Liberals maintain that sexuality is a private matter between consenting adults and that police power has no place in the bedroom. Conservatives hold that sexuality is a matter of values and is best dealt with in the setting of a family's moral and religious beliefs; the schools, or any other public agency, have no right to usurp the family's educational role. In addition, some major religious bodies claim the sexual education of adherents as their exclusive domain; sometimes these bodies even object to educational efforts that are not directed specifically at their adherents but that might, in their view, "taint" them or lower moral standards within society in general. This view makes discussions of sexuality religiously sensitive as well. Thus, from both ends of the political spectrum, government action related to sexuality is problematic. In addition, the United States has a long history of institutional barriers to communication about (as well as treatment of) sexually transmitted diseases. The examples that follow are from Brandt (1987).

- In 1822 the Massachusetts General Hospital excluded all venereal disease patients from admission. During the period 1851 to 1881, syphilitics were admitted upon special approval of the board of trustees, but they were required to pay double rates. Revised rules in 1881 again forbade their admission (p. 43).
- In 1912 the U.S. Post Office confiscated Margaret Sanger's pamphlet *What Every Girl Should Know* because it considered the references to syphilis and gonorrhea "obscene" under prevailing laws (p. 24).
- The film "Fit to Fight," the centerpiece of anti-venereal disease propaganda during World War I, was declared obscene by the New York State Board of Censors—a ruling that was upheld by the circuit court. New York License Commissioner John F. Gilchrist told the court: "The fact that a small body of specialized medical opinion supports the picture . . . does not free a given picture from the vice of violating the standards of morality" (p. 124).

- In November 1934 the Columbia Broadcasting System scheduled a radio appearance by New York State Health Commissioner Thomas Parran, Jr. Parran planned to review the major problems confronting public health officers. That talk was never delivered. Moments before air time, CBS informed Parron that he could not mention syphilis or gonorrhea by name during the broadcast (p. 122).
- During the 1960s the American Medical Association instituted a publicity campaign for the control of syphilis and gonorrhea, but it deleted the names of the diseases from its advertisements (p. 176).
- In 1964 NBC canceled plans for a two-part drama on two popular series ("Dr. Kildare" and "Mr. Novak") because the story involved a high school student who contracted a sexually transmitted disease. The NBC network spokesman claimed: "If the drama were to be valid, it would have to contain passages and dialogue, including a discussion of sexual intercourse, that the network considers inappropriate for television" (p. 176).
- In 1982 the Texas State Commission of Education recommended deletion of all references to venereal disease in its textbooks. The deputy commissioner stated: "The bottom-line issue, is when you're talking about sexually transmitted diseases you're relating it to 'How do you get it' " (p. 176).

In the past several years, a number of examples reveal how potentially effective AIDS education activities were prohibited or delayed because of similar social barriers. The following section considers three: (1) the refusal to accept condom advertising on network television; (2) requirements that federal AIDS education materials be phrased in ways that are inoffensive to most educated adults; and (3) attempts to use federal AIDS campaigns that present factual information about HIV transmission to deliver a message about desirable moral behavior. The final section of the chapter considers some of the lessons learned from past epidemics and how they can be applied to AIDS/HIV.

BARRIERS TO ACTION: RECENT EXAMPLES

Condom Advertising on Network Television

Television is a major source of information in U.S. society. Yet television coverage of AIDS is currently limited to dramatic presentations, news broadcasts, and public service announcements—often with the very limited message that viewers should "find out" about AIDS. The role of sexuality is seldom discussed explicitly, and TV networks refuse to accept commercial advertisements for condoms.

Cultural reticence about sexuality strongly influences the mass media. Until recently, direct references to sexual acts were sedulously banned from newspapers; motion pictures were carefully censored by the "Hayes Office" to ensure that visual and verbal sexuality were drastically muted. Television was equally restrictive. In the last two decades, there has been less reticence in TV dramatic presentations and in advertising, but network executives continue to insist that their audiences are not ready to accept certain sorts of ads.

During 1987, representatives of the broadcast media testified before the House Subcommittee on Health and the Environment regarding their policies toward paid advertisements for condoms.[2] The broadcast representatives stated that, historically and currently, the television networks had endeavored to accommodate the changing views of their audience; nevertheless, they concluded that the AIDS epidemic had not yet sufficiently changed their audiences' sensitivities about condom advertising and that they could not support it. Thus, one network representative, Alfred R. Schneider of ABC, stated:

> [A] significant portion of our viewers feel contraceptive commercials are inappropriate or offensive, because they appear within or adjacent to programs that they may be viewing with their families, and these commercials appear without warning and out of context. These concerns have been the basis for our long standing policy against carrying such advertising on the ABC Television Network. (U.S. House of Representatives, 1987:48)

Yet despite this advertising policy for a sexual prophylaxis, television soap operas and dramatic presentations sometimes involve sexual material that might be judged inappropriate or offensive by some viewers. Television soap operas, for example, frequently depict erotic and adulterous encounters; yet several of these shows have become prime-time success stories with large audiences. Indeed, television series like "Dallas" and "Dynasty," which feature characters who acquire several sexual partners during a single season, might prove an ideal context for advertisements that promote responsible contra-

[2]Testimony was provided by Ralph Daniels, Vice-President, Broadcast Standards, National Broadcasting Co., Inc.; George Dessart, Vice-President, Program Practices, CBS Broadcast Group; and Alfred R. Schneider, Vice-President, Policy and Standards, Capital Cities/ABC, Inc. For the text of their testimony, see U.S. House of Representatives (1987).

ceptive behavior and preventive action against sexually transmitted diseases. Careful scheduling of condom advertisements might go a long way toward reaching audiences who would be comfortable with discussions of sexuality. Furthermore, since audiences may be more influenced by the thematic content of programs than by advertising, television shows—particularly those whose characters engage in behaviors that risk the transmission of HIV infection—could perform a public service by dealing frankly with the issue of condom use.

Although the major television networks will not accept commercial advertising for condoms,[3] data from a number of public opinion polls indicate that a substantial majority of American adults would not be offended by condom advertisements (Table 7-1). A 1987 Associated Press survey, for example, found a 2-to-1 majority in favor of condom ads on television; numerous other national surveys support these findings. In fact, the proportion of American adults who indicate that they *would* object to condom advertisements on television (17 to 32 percent) is no greater than the proportion (32 percent) who object to ads for products that are now widely advertised on network television (e.g., tampons).[4]

Communicating with Inoffensive Language

Because HIV is transmitted by sexual behavior, education about transmission must refer to that behavior in a manner that can be understood and retained by the audience. In 1986 the IOM/NAS report *Confronting AIDS* recommended the removal of impediments to the use of frank and explicit language in AIDS education. These impediments, however, have proved quite resistant.

Historically, there has been a strong social reluctance in the

---

[3]Recently, the three major television networks agreed to broadcast a public service advertising campaign that promotes the use of condoms to prevent the spread of HIV (see R. Rothenberg, "3 Networks Agree to Run Condom Ads in AIDS Fight," *New York Times,* October 1, 1988:35). This change of policy is commendable. There is more that can be done, however, including permitting condom manufacturers to advertise their products.

[4]Of the 1,348 adults interviewed in a national survey conducted by the Associated Press between June 1 and June 10, 1987, 32 percent found television commercials for products other than condoms to be objectionable; most frequently cited were "feminine hygiene products" (tampons, sanitary napkins, and the like). Questions were worded as follows: "Are there any commercials other than condom advertisements now on TV that you find objectionable?" and "What other commercials are objectionable to you?" (The second question was asked only of those who said "yes" to the previous question.)

United States to speak or write about sexuality in explicit terms. Despite recent indications of greatly increased tolerance for sexual explicitness in the media and literature, that reluctance remains strong in much of the population; it is particularly strong in instances that involve the education of children and adolescents. Thus, public discussion of the modes of transmission of, and methods of protection against, HIV infection is marked by omissions and circumlocutions: the omissions include a lack of reference to homosexuals in some messages; the circumlocutions include use of the phrase "exchange of bodily fluids" in early discussions as a euphemism for sexual intercourse with ejaculation, among other things (Check, 1987).

The problem of explicit language is undeniably complex. To begin with, the term *explicit* is itself unclear. It may mean any direct reference to sex, sex organs, or sexual activity. It may refer to the use of colloquial or common words rather than technical or medical terms. It may mean the use of slang or "crude" terms. In addition, the choice of words in a message may be dictated by diverse communication goals. Clarity of expression may require the use of a certain vocabulary; credibility with certain audiences may require use of a different vocabulary. Sustaining interest and attention or making points forcefully and unforgettably would, again, require a certain vocabulary and style. Thus, educationally effective language must be measured by several criteria. Unfortunately, the only measurement criterion urged by opponents of explicit language seems to be politeness. The committee believes that, during an epidemic, politeness is a social virtue that must take second place to the protection of life.

The use of frank language in AIDS education has been hampered by federal guidelines adopted in response to congressional pressure that restrict all language used in AIDS education in the United States. The federal language guidelines that are used by organizations receiving funds from CDC to produce AIDS education materials include the following directive:

> a. Language . . . to describe dangerous behaviors and explain less risky practices concerning AIDS should use terms or descriptors necessary for the target audience to understand the messages.
>
> b. Such terms or descriptions should be those which a reasonable person would conclude should be understood by a broad cross-section of educated adults in society, or which when used to communicate with a specific group, such as homosexual men, about high risk sexual practices, would be judged by a reasonable person to be inoffensive to most educated adults beyond that group (CDC, 1988b).

TABLE 7-1 Public Opinion on Television Condom Advertising

Question	Survey and Date	Opinion (percentage)		
		Favor Ads	Oppose Ads	Unsure[a]
Some TV stations have been asked to show commercials that advertise condoms. Do you think TV stations should show commercials for condoms or not?	Associated Press, June 1–10, 1987 (N = 1,348)	63	28	9
Some TV stations now show commercials for condoms because they may help prevent the spread of AIDS. Do you think commercials for condoms should be on TV or not?	ABC/*Washington Post*, March 5–9, 1987 (N = 511)	75	23	2
The Surgeon General and the National Academy of Sciences have called for a campaign to reduce the spread of AIDS with, among other things, much greater use of condoms. Would you favor or oppose the use of advertisements on TV to promote the use of condoms to prevent the spread of AIDS?	Louis Harris, Jan. 28–Feb. 1, 1987 (N = 1,250)	74	23	3

Do you approve or disapprove of advertisements on the use of condoms as a way to help prevent the spread of AIDS?	NBC/*Wall Street Journal*, Jan. 4, 1987 (N = 800)	79	17	4
As you know, there has been considerable discussion lately about ways to prevent sexually transmitted diseases. In this regard, do you favor or oppose commercials for condoms, that is, male contraceptives, being shown on television in your area?	Gallup Organization, March 2–11, 1987 (N = 502)	69	24	7
Do you agree or disagree with the statement: advertisements for condoms should be on TV and radio.	Mark Clements Research, June 4–21, 1987 (N = 1,003)	67[b]	32[c]	1

NOTE: All data are from a compilation prepared by the Roper Center of various telephone surveys of the adult population of the United States. (Alaska and Hawaii, which comprise 0.5 percent of the national population, were not included in the sampling frame of all surveys.)

[a]Includes "don't know" responses and "no answers."
[b]Combines 42 percent who "strongly" agree and 25 percent who "slightly" agree.
[c]Combines 12 percent who "slightly" disagree and 20 percent who "strongly" disagree.

As the last sentence notes, the language to be used in AIDS prevention messages for gay men must be inoffensive to the educated heterosexual population. This least-common-denominator formula for providing information on the prevention of a fatal disease would keep CDC-funded projects from following the committee's recommendations to make "information available in clear, explicit language in the idiom of the target audience" (see Chapter 4). The committee firmly believes that the grave consequences of HIV infection require that education messages leave no room for misunderstanding about risk-associated behaviors. In the face of a deadly threat, conventions about polite or "inoffensive" language should not be allowed to impede effective communication about the sexual and drug-using behaviors that risk transmission of HIV. In this regard, it is instructive to note the responses of governments outside the United States to the epidemic. The politically conservative government of Great Britain, for example, launched a massive, sexually explicit educational campaign in early 1987. At the time, Britain had fewer than one tenth the number of AIDS cases as had occurred in the United States. Similarly, during the last three years, countries around the world have provided their populations with an assortment of explicit messages on ways to reduce the risk of HIV infection (World Health Organization Special Programme on AIDS, 1988). For instance, a Brazilian poster follows many of the recommendations offered by the committee in Chapter 4. It laudably combines a positive message with specific information—using the idiom of the people—on how to protect oneself. The slogan "Love doesn't kill" is supplemented with the following advice: "You can have sexual relations with security using a latex condom, a rubber. The condom can keep AIDS away from you, but doesn't keep you away from the one you love." The following informative announcement comes from the Republic of Ghana:

> You need to know the facts in order to demystify the disease.
>
> AIDS is not a gay disease.
>
> You can be infected just by one contact—teach your children so that their first sexual experience will not be a death sentence.
>
> You cannot detect who is a carrier just by looking at them—they look just as normal and healthy as you. (World Health Organization Special Programme on AIDS, 1988)

In contrast to the messages promoted by these governments, the United States has made what some observers have called slow and halting movements toward the dissemination of explicit educational materials (Feinberg, 1988). Conflict over public discussion of sexual behaviors has certainly contributed to this delay.

Federal AIDS Education Efforts

Communicating Facts Versus Moral Suasion

On October 14, 1987, the U.S. Senate voted 94 to 2 in support of an amendment to the 1988 Department of Health and Human Services appropriations bill that required the following: "All AIDS educational, informational, and preventive materials and activities for school-aged children and young adults shall emphasize—(1) abstinence from sexual activity outside of a monogamous marriage; and (2) abstinence from the use of illegal intravenous drugs."[5] This amendment crystallized in public law one side of a continuing public debate over the content of federally sponsored AIDS education.

For several years, federal AIDS education efforts have stumbled over disputes about the need to offer "realistic" advice about the protective value of condoms (and bleach) versus counterclaims that the AIDS epidemic requires moral education to promote abstinence from sex prior to marriage, fidelity within marriage, and avoidance of drugs. Evidence of this conflict can be found by comparing the statements issued in 1986 by the surgeon general (U.S. Department of Health and Human Services, 1986) with those distributed to every school district by the U.S. Department of Education in 1987. The surgeon general's brochure recognized the protective value of sexual abstinence and monogamous relationships with uninfected partners, but it also advised the following:

> If your partner has a positive blood test showing that he or she has been infected with the AIDS virus or you suspect that he or she has been exposed by previous heterosexual or homosexual behavior or use of intravenous drugs with shared needles or syringes, a rubber (condom) should always be used during (start to finish) sexual intercourse (vagina or rectum). (1986:17)

The surgeon general's report subsequently encouraged teenagers to "say NO to sex" (p. 18), but it did so after instructions about condoms had been provided. In contrast, the U.S. Department of Education publication emphasized "moral education":

> What is to be done? The surest way to prevent the spread of AIDS in the teenage and young adult population is for schools and

[5] *Congressional Record,* October 14, 1987, S-14217.

> parents to convey the reasons why adolescents should be taught restraint in sexual activity and why illegal drug use is wrong and harmful. Although messages urging responsibility and restraint have been given before, the emergence of the AIDS threat has given them even greater importance. (1987:9)

The Department of Education brochure also paid considerable attention to the risk of condom failure, which was highlighted in a sidebar explaining that "condoms can and do fail."

Similar conflicts within the federal government have produced extensive delays in the approval of several high-visibility products of AIDS education efforts. For example, during the summer of 1987 the federal government announced it would mail an AIDS information brochure to every American household. First, however, the text of this 1987 brochure went through a lengthy round of drafting and revision that involved staff from the Public Health Service, the Office of the Assistant Secretary for Health and Human Services, the Domestic Policy Council, and the Office of Management and Budget (Booth, 1987). Finally, after 45 million copies of the brochure were printed in 1987, the mailing was canceled.

Although that draft of the brochure was never mailed, its content reveals much about the barriers within U.S. society regarding communication about sex.[6] The document (Public Health Service, 1987) mentioned the use of condoms to prevent the transmission of HIV in only one place: "If you are sexually active: Enter into a mutually faithful, single-partner relationship with an uninfected person, or at least be sure to reduce your risk by using condoms." It contained several references to abstinence, monogamy, and family values ("family" or "families" appeared 12 times), but the word "gay" appeared only once—in a quotation from a front-line AIDS worker (Booth, 1987).

For adolescents, the brochure advised in large, highlighted type that "Teenagers Should Avoid Drugs and Sex." The text noted: "If you are a young person: Discuss and understand and live by your family's values. Say 'no' to drugs. And say 'no' to sex until you are ready to enter into a mutually faithful, single-partner relationship with an uninfected person."

This advice does not recognize the realities of teenage sexual behavior. As the data presented in Chapter 2 indicate, the majority of young Americans begins having sex during their teens, and the majority of those who have had sex reports having more than one

---

[6]See J. Estill, "45 Million Brochures on AIDS Printed," *Washington Post*, October 25, 1987:A22.

partner.[7] Besides requiring a revolution in adolescent sexual behavior, advice that young people say "no" to sex until they are ready to enter into a single-partner relationship with an *uninfected* partner is problematic from a practical standpoint. It presumes widespread availability of information about the HIV status of potential sexual partners, which is not a realistic assumption.[8] By confounding moral advice with information, the brochure would have provided little practical information for sexually active adolescents—homosexual or heterosexual—who were not prepared to enter into mutually faithful, single-partner relationships.

Subsequently, another brochure, *Understanding AIDS* (Public Health Service, 1988), was mailed to American households in June 1988; it does, in fact, communicate in a value-free manner with simple and explicit language that avoids moralizing. The committee commends this Public Health Service effort, and it hopes that future AIDS education efforts will follow the example set in this document and in the original 1986 surgeon general's report on AIDS (U.S. Department of Health and Human Services, 1986).

Efforts to educate IV drug users have suffered from similar problems. For example, the National Institute on Drug Abuse prepared a pamphlet to inform drug users about AIDS and the risks posed by needle-sharing; the pamphlet stressed the importance of sterilizing injection equipment before use (if the drug user was unable to discontinue the use of drugs). When the institute submitted this document for approval prior to release and distribution, however, approval was refused, and a White House aide was quoted as saying that this information would be released by the government "over our collective dead bodies" (Aiken, 1987:97).

The committee believes that, even if current sexual or drug-use practices meet with public disapproval, the reality of these practices

---

[7]Data from the 1983 National Longitudinal Survey of Youth (Moore et al., 1987:Appendix Table 1.4) found that 83 percent of boys and 74 percent of girls reported being sexually active by the end of their teens. Moreover, Zelnik (1983), in a 1979 probability sample of teenagers residing in metropolitan areas of the United States, found that 51 percent of sexually active 15- to 19-year-old girls reported having two or more sexual partners; 16 percent reported four or more partners.

[8]Indeed, it is important to remember that current tests for antibodies to HIV may not reveal infection during a "window" of time (2 to 14 months) after the infection occurs. Thus, the advice to wait until one can establish a monogamous relationship with an uninfected partner assumes a willingness on the part of the advisee to: (1) accept some level of risk (from undetected new infection), (2) delay intercourse until the window of undetectable infection is past, or (3) use other methods, such as condoms, to reduce risk during this period.

must be taken into account when making public health recommendations. Moreover, even for those who find these practices and the discussion of them morally repugnant, the value of saving human lives and preserving the health of the public should weigh as an equally important consideration.

Reflecting Values Versus Imposing Them

Government decisions to emphasize moral education for AIDS prevention have been enacted against a background of public opinion that has become, in general, more tolerant of nonmarital heterosexual intercourse. Indeed, as discussed in Chapter 2, the twentieth century has seen a progressive uncoupling of sexual behavior from marriage. As a result, the nonmarital heterosexual experiences of young women now parallel those of young men more closely (see, for example, Figure 2-3a in Chapter 2). Again, as already discussed in Chapter 2, this trend may have begun as early as the turn of the century.

The climate of increasing social tolerance for nonmarital sex can be observed most reliably during 1972–1988, for which there are a reliable set of standardized national indicators of public attitudes. For example, Figure 7–1 shows that increasingly large proportions of the public reported an acceptance of premarital (hetero)sexual intercourse: the proportion saying that sex before marriage is "not wrong at all" rose from 28 percent in 1972 to 41 percent in 1988. In addition, more than 80 percent of respondents said that birth control information should be made available to teenagers. (This percentage rose from 81 percent in 1974 to 86 percent in 1983.[9])

Some of the federal guidelines regarding AIDS education in schools require that programs be consistent with the moral values of parents and the community; others require that the values presented in the programs correspond to those stated in the previous section

---

[9]Results are taken from five national survey measurements made in the General Social Survey during 1974–1983. (Measurements were not made after 1983 using this question.) The survey asked the question: "Do you think birth control information should be available to teenagers who want it, or not?" (The question immediately preceding this one noted that some states had laws prohibiting distribution of birth control information to everyone.) Despite the results on the question of birth control information, however, the overwhelming majority of respondents thought that sexual relations between young teens were wrong. When asked, "What if they are in their early teens, say 14 to 16 years old. In that case, do you think sex relations before marriage are always wrong, almost always wrong, wrong only sometimes, or not wrong at all?," respondents in 1988 answered as follows: always wrong, 69 percent; almost always wrong, 16 percent; wrong only sometimes, 12 percent; not at all wrong, 4 percent.

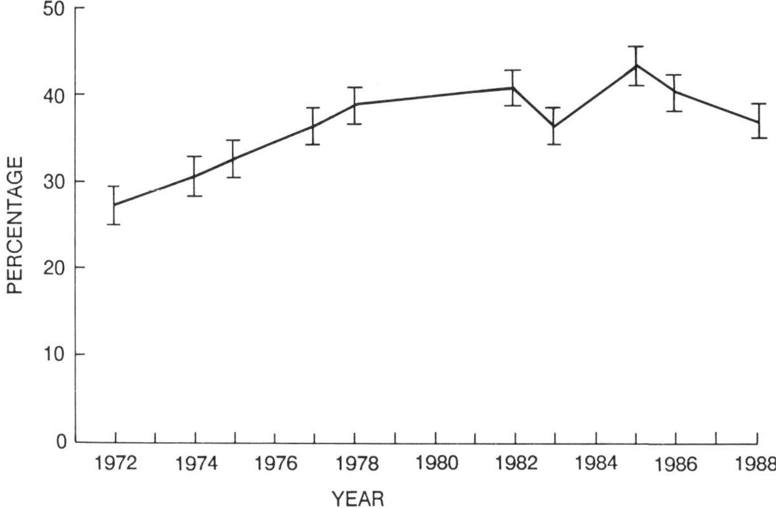

FIGURE 7-1 Percentage of American adults who report that they believe it is "not wrong at all" for a man and woman to have sexual relations before marriage, 1972–1988. Estimates are derived from surveys of probability samples of the noninstitutional adult population of the continental United States, conducted by the General Social Survey program of the National Opinion Research Center (University of Chicago; see J. A. Davis and Smith, 1988). Sample sizes each year were approximately 1,500; samples were restricted to persons 18 years of age and older. Error bars denote approximately ±1 standard error around the estimates. The estimates have been weighted to reflect the varying probabilities of selection for persons in households with different numbers of eligible adults. The question presented to respondents was: "There's been a lot of discussion about the way morals and attitudes about sex are changing in this country. If a man and woman have sex relations before marriage, do you think it is always wrong, almost always wrong, wrong only sometimes, or not wrong at all?"

(i.e., sexual relations should occur only in the context of monogamous marriage) (CDC, 1988c). Such guidelines flatly ignore the pluralistic nature of the country. Anxious to avoid offending some minorities by the presentation of fact, government guidelines of this kind attempt to *impose* values on others. It is not surprising that the resulting contradictions lead to poor communication. One simple way to avoid these contradictions—and to strengthen communication—is to leave out the moral dimension of such messages and allow individuals and families to supply value judgments. This approach embodies a respect for private beliefs that is consistent with the philosophy of government programs in other areas.

HISTORICAL LESSONS

The Effects of Epidemics on Poor People and Minorities

The preceding examples suggest that there may be similarities between America's response to the AIDS epidemic and the social history of other epidemics discussed at the outset of this chapter. One may note, for example, a "business-as-usual" attitude in the refusal of television executives to relax the ban on condom advertising despite the threat posed by the AIDS epidemic. Another unstated similarity between past epidemics and the current AIDS epidemic is their disproportionate impact on the poor. Past epidemics of infectious diseases decimated poor people in the great cities and had less serious effects on more well-to-do people (Rosenberg, 1962:Chapter 3). The AIDS epidemic is beginning to repeat this theme. Epidemiological surveillance data suggest that there is a disproportionately high incidence of AIDS among the poorer segments of American society (regardless of sexual orientation or drug use). Data from New York City, for instance, indicate that there are geographic concentrations of AIDS cases and HIV infection in the city's poorest neighborhoods (New York State Department of Health, 1988).

Although CDC surveillance data do not permit a breakdown of AIDS cases by socioeconomic status, the reported distribution of AIDS cases across racial and ethnic groups suggests a similar phenomenon (CDC, 1988a). Blacks and Hispanics, for example, represent 11 percent and 8 percent, respectively, of the U.S. population; yet 26 percent of all AIDS cases have been diagnosed in blacks, and 15 percent of all cases have been diagnosed in Hispanics. Among women and children with AIDS, blacks and Hispanics dominate: more than 70 percent of the women and 75 percent of the children with AIDS are either black or Hispanic (Guinan and Hardy, 1987; CDC, 1988a). AIDS cases have occurred 14 times more frequently among black women and 9 times more frequently among Hispanic women than among white women; cumulative AIDS incidence rates for black and Hispanic children are 12 and 7 times higher, respectively, than the rate for white children (Curran et al., 1988).

The disproportionate percentage of AIDS cases among blacks and Hispanics is thought to reflect higher rates of HIV infection among black and Hispanic IV drug users, their sex partners, and their infants (Allen and Curran, 1988; Curran et al., 1988).[10] It has

---

[10]Of 12,721 cases of AIDS reported among IV drug users (as of July 18, 1988), 6,454 were diagnosed among blacks, and 3,721 were diagnosed among Hispanics. Of 906

been predicted that AIDS morbidity and mortality rates may remain particularly high among young and middle-age poor men because large numbers of IV drug users in some cities are already infected with HIV (Curran et al., 1988).

In epidemics during times long past, the poor were sometimes locked into their houses or into their districts and left to die, abandoned by doctors and clergy alike. In this epidemic, the ability to reach across class boundaries to educate and modify behavior is vital to controlling the spread of disease. Yet this capability is not easily acquired. Educators, researchers, and providers of care are almost inevitably from the middle or upper classes. Frequently, they may have little knowledge of the culture or conditions of poorer people, which may make their efforts to assist and engage them blundering and clumsy. A few may have scant sympathy for the plight of the poor, understanding little about their health or other needs. Moreover, even when knowledge, sympathy, and understanding are present, differences of language, values, and life-style can make effective collaboration and communication difficult. Crafting messages and programs that reach the affected population may consequently be fraught with problems.

As the AIDS epidemic becomes endemic, new problems will afflict poor and minority people. Once the dramatic impact of epidemic growth recedes, seriously affected groups may be effectively abandoned. Some of these groups are already underserved in terms of health care resources (K. Davis et al., 1987; Manton et al., 1987; Jaynes and Williams, in press); they may be even more at risk of delayed diagnosis and treatment (K. Davis et al., 1987; Manton et al., 1987).

The endemic presence of HIV in the IV drug-using population may have similar effects. Drug prevention and drug treatment programs have generally had low priority in federal, state, and city budgets. In addition, although the health needs of drug-using individuals are significant, drug users receive little sympathy from the general population and frequently find it difficult to gain access to the health care system because of poverty and a lack of health insurance. IV drug users often have mixed feelings about entering the health care system, feelings that may be fed, in part, by a fear of detection of criminal activity. Those IV drug users that do gain access to health

---

cases among children under five years of age, 728 were diagnosed in black and Hispanic children. Of 2,815 cases thought to be due to heterosexual transmission, 2,273 were among blacks and Hispanics (CDC, 1988a:Tables B and I).

care frequently find that the system is poorly equipped to deal with their needs.

Stigma

One social phenomenon that has been characteristic of past epidemics is the stigmatization of persons who contract a dread disease. This process affects not only the treatment of infected persons but the ways in which uninfected individuals and the society as a whole respond to an epidemic. Some people, including various political and social leaders, have already stigmatized the victims of AIDS, seeking to exclude them from society as lepers were once driven out (e.g., Sabatier, 1988). Others have complained that, because gays, minorities, and drug users were already stigmatized groups in our society, their needs as the groups at highest risk have been ignored and their already limited opportunities in society have been threatened and further restricted. Understanding how stigmatization works is crucial to reducing its impact.

Defining Stigma

Stigma, in ancient Greek, meant a tattoo mark or a brand, and *stigmatias* was a branded culprit or a runaway slave. In contemporary terms, *The Concise Oxford Dictionary* defines stigma as a negative "imputation attaching to a person's reputation; a stain on one's good name."

The ancient and modern meanings differ notably. In the ancient meaning, the stigma is a visible mark on the body; in the modern, it is an opinion in the mind of one person about the moral status of another. Yet both meanings convey a similar message: the person, whether physically or morally marked, is not fully human and ought to be excluded from human society in some way.

In recent years, the concept of stigmatization has been studied by social scientists who have observed that, in all societies, certain persons and groups are selected for different and usually deprecating treatment. Goffman (1963:3) defined stigma as "an attribute that is deeply discrediting." In many instances, people do bear some observable sign that distinguishes them—such as skin color or language or life-style—but the sign, in itself, is not the stigma. Rather, in its sociological meaning, the stigma is the set of ideas, beliefs, and judgments that the majority or dominant group holds about some other group.

These beliefs are not merely negative; they often characterize members of the stigmatized group as dangerous or as deserving of punishment for some vague offense or moral improbity. Group members may be considered dangerous because their very existence threatens the dominant group's sense of primacy, power, or safety. By simply being different, they may cast doubt on the rightness or perfection of the dominant group's way of life. The characteristics imputed to the stigmatized group—for example, inclination to crime, laziness, inferior intelligence, and the like—result from biased, limited observation and are supported by illogical, tortuous arguments. The stigma becomes a predominant description of members of the group, effectively hiding most of their real features. Stigma thus becomes not merely a cliché but a menacing, mean cliché.

Effects of Stigmatization

Throughout history, stigmatization, in the modern sense of designating a group or social class as blameworthy and dangerous, has frequently appeared in times of epidemic disease. Leprosy offers the classic example of a stigmatizing disease. Individuals who were marked with its lesions were forced to live "outside the camp" (Gussow and Tracy, 1970). During the great plagues of the fourteenth century, Jews were blamed for poisoning the wells, and terrible retribution followed. (One pope of the era attempted, with little success, to refute the charges [Tuchman, 1978].) During the cholera and yellow fever epidemics of the nineteenth century in the United States, the poor were blamed because of their "uncleanliness" and immigrants were blamed because of their "immorality" (Rosenberg, 1962). During smallpox epidemics in San Francisco in the latter years of the nineteenth century, blame fell on the city's Chinese inhabitants (Trauner, 1978). Even as late as the 1940s, Norwegian immigrants were accused of being the vectors of polio (Benison, 1974). The panic and uncertainty that accompany epidemic disease may lead to a desperate search for explanations—often, personalized ones. Many people must have theological and moral reasons for their plight—as Albert Camus demonstrated so brilliantly in *The Plague*. Stigmatization seems to provide a partial (although spurious) answer to essentially unanswerable questions. The convenience of having an already despised or suspect group in the vicinity allows for quick attribution of causality and blame.

There are many other effects of stigmatization. A problem that primarily affects a stigmatized group is of little concern to the dominant society; thus, scientific interest, funding priorities, social support, and legal protections, all of which come from the dominant society, may not appear until the threat touches the dominant society itself. When these elements do appear, they are often overtly and covertly punitive, in keeping with the dominant society's general attitude toward the group. The stimulus of compassion, usually so important in rousing a society to help the afflicted, is absent. In consequence, important public health measures may be undermined, for the affected persons hide themselves, refraining from action that might identify them as belonging to the guilty, dangerous group. Finally, the burden of solving the problem is placed on the stigmatized themselves; they must change their abode or their habits, or give up their freedom.

Stigmatization can also distort the stigmatized group's view of itself (Ainlay et al., 1986). Group members may suffer from a sense of inadequacy, powerlessness, and unworthiness because these messages are constantly directed at them by the dominant society. Even when they are able to acknowledge their risks, they may feel incapable of defending themselves; consequently, vigorous, brave efforts from within the group are needed for members to break free of these imputations. Yet while these views prevail, they can deeply affect the group's ability to stimulate itself to action. In addition, the genuine fears that punitive actions will be taken in the name of public health may limit the group's willingness to cooperate with even reasonable measures. The phenomenon of stigmatization may inhibit a clear understanding of an epidemic and rational management of prevention and treatment programs. In fixing blame on individuals, it obscures the social and institutional dimensions so necessary to sound public health measures. To blame the victim is to absolve social institutions of their responsibilities.

Stigmatization has other effects as well. Convictions about the moral inferiority of the stigmatized may undermine confidence in educational interventions and make the dominant groups reluctant to provide resources for such efforts. Paradoxically, while "voluntary behaviors" are condemned, those who exercise them are often said to be "unable to change." Moreover, the branding involved in stigmatization can inhibit people from seeking treatment, from being tested, and from availing themselves of educational and support programs. Empirical data needed to track the course of the epidemic can be difficult to obtain because the stigmatized hide themselves from investigators who, in the view of the stigmatized, represent the dominant society. Members of the dominant society who themselves become infected and who can contribute to the spread of disease may react by psychological denial or secrecy—to avoid being stigmatized. In all these ways, the planning and execution of sound public health measures are hindered. *The committee believes it is imperative that such stigmatization not affect government programs.* Whatever effect stigmatization may have had in the past is not of concern here, but any present effects it is having must be remedied as soon as they are discovered.

Stigma and the AIDS Epidemic

The AIDS epidemic has engendered stigmatization since its inception. The fact that infection has been largely confined to male homosexuals and IV drug users has made stigmatization almost inevitable, for these groups were already the objects, to a greater or lesser degree, of the deprecating judgments that constitute stigmatization. The AIDS epidemic has added to opinions already held about these groups the new belief that they are dangerous to the whole society, not only because they exist, are different, or are outlaws but because they can infect people outside their group with a lethal disease. Thus, the stigmatization to which these groups have previously been subject has been reinforced, and one of its primary effects, the imputation of blame—both for being the cause of the epidemic and for "bringing it on themselves"—has become a menacing cliché.

In this epidemic, the rationale for such stigmatization rests on the fact that AIDS is transmitted by seemingly voluntary behaviors that are widely disapproved of in the broader society. In the vocabulary of some religions, these behaviors are called "sinful." Accusers can say to victims, "If you hadn't behaved in this or that shameful or sinful way, this wouldn't have happened to you." This direct attribution of responsibility feeds one of the essential features of stigmatization: blameworthiness. It allows the society to feel justified in excluding victims from concern or in banishing them from the community. One group that is especially prone to stigmatization is gay men. Figure 7-2 shows the survey responses of national samples of the American adult population to questions asking whether homosexual sex was "always wrong," whether homosexuals should be allowed to give speeches or teach in colleges, and whether books advocating homosexuality should be permitted in public libraries.

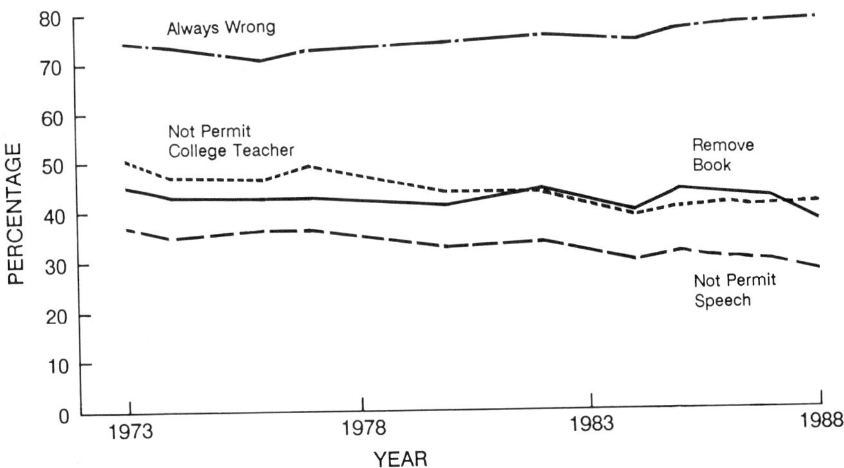

FIGURE 7-2 Public opinions about homosexual sex and the civil rights of homosexuals, 1972–1988. Questions included the following:

> "1. What about sexual relations between two adults of the same sex—do you think it is always wrong, almost always wrong, wrong only sometimes, or not wrong at all?
>
> 2. What about a man who admits that he is a homosexual—
>   a. Suppose this admitted homosexual wanted to make a speech in your community. Should he be allowed to speak or not?
>   b. Should such a person be allowed to teach in a college or university, or not?
>   c. If some people in your community suggested that a book he wrote in favor of homosexuality should be taken out of your public library, would you favor removing this book, or not?"

SOURCE: Tabulated from the General Social Surveys conducted by the National Opinion Research Center (University of Chicago) (J.A. Davis and Smith, 1988). See the caption to Figure 7-1 for details of the survey and tabulation procedures.

The survey data indicated that, throughout 1973–1988, the vast majority of Americans (70–77 percent) said that homosexual sex was "always wrong"; in addition, substantial proportions also said they would forbid speeches (27–37 percent) and college teaching (39–50 percent) by homosexuals and would remove books favoring homosexuality from public libraries (37–45 percent). These data suggest a source of the conflict that has hampered efforts to combat AIDS, and they illustrate the particular vulnerability of gay Americans to stigmatization.

Legal Status of Homosexual Behaviors

The uneven tolerance found in surveys of public opinion regarding different types of human sexuality is mirrored in the law. Private heterosexual behaviors between two consenting adults appear to be constitutionally protected, even if the man and woman are not married. However, as recently as 1986, the Supreme Court ruled that states could enforce criminal sanctions against consensual homosexual behaviors, even when practiced by adults in the privacy of their own home (*Bowers* v. *Hardwick,* No. 85-140, June 30, 1986). Although the statute[11] at issue was not limited to homosexuals, the Court's majority held that "the only claim properly before the court [was the] challenge to the statute as applied to consensual homosexual sodomy." Furthermore, in a 5-to-4 decision, it ruled that

> (a) The Constitution does not confer a fundamental right upon homosexuals to engage in sodomy.
> (b) Against a background in which many States have criminalized sodomy and still do, to claim that a right to engage in such conduct is "deeply rooted in this Nation's history and tradition" or "implicit in the concept of ordered liberty" is, at best, facetious.
> (c) There should be great resistance to expand the reach of the Due Process Clauses to cover new fundamental rights.
> (d) The fact that homosexual conduct occurs in the privacy of the home does not affect the result.
> (e) Sodomy laws should not be invalidated on the asserted basis that the majority belief that sodomy is immoral is an inadequate rationale to support the laws. (478 U.S. at 186)

The four dissenting justices advanced as their first argument in rebuttal that

> the court's almost obsessive focus on homosexual activity is particularly hard to justify in light of the broad language Georgia has used. Unlike the Court, the Georgia Legislature has not proceeded on the assumption that homosexuals are so different from other citizens that their lives may be controlled in a way that would not be tolerated if it limited the choices of those other citizens. (478 U.S. at 200)

In the opinions of the nine U.S. Supreme Court justices, as in the opinion of the public, there is a cleavage in attitudes toward private sexual behaviors that depends on the sexual orientation of the participants. The Court's decision—as recognized in both the minority

---

[11]The statute (Georgia Code Annotated at 16-6-2, 1984) held that "(a) A person commits the offense of sodomy when he performs or submits to any sexual act involving the sex organs of one person and the mouth or anus of another. . . . (b) A person convicted of the offense of sodomy shall be punished by imprisonment for not less than one nor more than 20 years. . . ."

and majority statements—outlaws behaviors between homosexuals that would be constitutionally protected if practiced by two heterosexuals.[12]

Such animosity toward the sexual behavior of gay men, which is evident in public opinions and laws, has complicated public discussions of the AIDS epidemic and hindered the development of public policies to curb its spread. Although IV drug users were infected early in the epidemic and in some locations outnumber gay men with AIDS, AIDS was initially perceived in the United States as a "gay disease." This perception has conditioned much of the American reaction to the disease and has called forth the ambivalences and conflicts that surround American attitudes toward sexuality in general and homosexuality in particular.

Gays and racial minorities are also threatened from another quarter. They may fear that the social acceptance and civil rights they have only recently won and tenuously hold may be eroded. They have had to fight hard to demonstrate that, because they were different, they were not dangers to the society at large; now, they may be seen as dangers because they may be viewed as "sources" of a lethal disease. Finally, in this epidemic, not one but several stigmatized groups are affected. They may share little sympathy for one another and will often be at pains to distinguish among themselves. Efforts at education, prevention, and the formation of policy may be fragmented as a result.

If the AIDS epidemic taxes the health care system as heavily in the future as is now predicted, the public, already lacking in

---

[12]A heterosexual couple joined in the original case, stating that they wished to engage in the proscribed sexual behaviors but were "chilled and deterred" by the statute and the arrest of the homosexual plaintiff. A federal district court dismissed their claim, ruling that "because they had neither sustained nor were in immediate danger of sustaining any direct injury from the enforcement of the statute," they did not have proper standing to maintain the action. The federal Court of Appeals affirmed that judgment, and the heterosexual couple did not challenge the ruling in the Supreme Court. The inability to apply the Georgia sodomy statute to heterosexuals also caused three of the four dissenters on the Court to conclude that the "State must assume the burden of justifying a selected application of its law. Either the persons to whom Georgia seeks to apply its statute do not have the same interest in 'liberty' that others have, or there must be a reason why the State may be permitted to apply a generally applicable law to certain persons that it does not apply to others" (478 U.S. at 218). Elsewhere in this case, the dissenters noted that "indeed, the Georgia Attorney General concedes that Georgia's statute would be unconstitutional if applied to a married couple. See Transcript of Oral Argument, 8, stating that the application of the statute to a married couple 'would be unconstitutional' because of the 'right of marital privacy as identified by the Court in Griswold.'" The dissenters go on to state that "[p]aradoxical as it may seem, our prior cases thus establish that a state may not prohibit sodomy within the sacred precincts of marital bedrooms, Griswold, 381 U.S. at 485, or, indeed, between unmarried heterosexual adults" (478 U.S. at 218).

sympathy for these groups, may resent that they are drawing upon resources that could be used for "better" purposes—just as many resent programs meant to help the "unworthy" (as opposed to the "worthy") poor. Should AIDS become endemic within a group, it may even appear rational to some people to deny care to its victims so that they "die out" and no longer make claims on society's scarce resources.

An immediate concern involves the provision of the one approved drug (AZT, or zidovudine) that has been shown to be effective in delaying the progression of disease in individuals who have been diagnosed as having AIDS. The use of AZT could claim substantial financial resources: a year of treatment can cost from $10,000 to $20,000 per person. Data on the efficacy of AZT in preventing the progression of disease among asymptomatic infected individuals are not yet available. However, a senior federal scientist, in response to questions concerning the use of AZT for early stages of the disease, was quoted as saying: "When that happens, we are in for a very bad day. We don't have enough AZT for a million people, and this country could not afford to pay for it if we did."[13]

Toward Dispelling Stigma

The deeply rooted social pathology of stigmatization is not easy to dispel. Even when revealed for what it is, the psychological and social mechanisms that support stigmatization may resist eradication. Rational appeals to understanding are necessary and sometimes useful, but they are often frustrated by forces deeper than reason. It may be that the dominant group in society must begin to recognize that the maintenance of stigma has deleterious effects on itself as well as on those who are stigmatized. In addition to widely shared humanitarian reasons for helping those at risk of disease, utilitarian purposes and self-interests are also served by establishing a suitable social climate for preventive action. In the AIDS epidemic, fears that the disease would spread from high-risk groups into the general population stimulated concern and, eventually, the mobilization of resources, as Shilts described so forcefully in his 1987 book *And the Band Played On.*

The public has thus far repudiated the worst forms of stigmatizing punishment. Although calls for quarantining all of the infected—even for branding infected persons—have been heard, they have been

---

[13]See M. Specter, "450,000 AIDS Cases Seen by '93; Experts Say Costs Could Bankrupt Public Hospitals," *Washington Post,* June 5, 1988:A7.

rejected by voters and policy makers. Protections for confidentiality have been erected. However, stigmatization works in subtle and insidious ways that must be continuously countered. Health professionals have a particular responsibility in this regard. They can counter the growth of stigmatization by the ways in which they define the disease, label those who are affected by it, serve their needs, and become their advocates. It has been noted that such professional behavior has helped in destigmatizing several conditions (e.g., leprosy and epilepsy); similarly, mental retardation and psychiatric disease may be on the way to destigmatization as a result of professional definition and advocacy (Volinn, 1983).

The media also bear a particular responsibility because the stories they choose to portray and the language and images they choose to use may reinforce or counteract stigma. Churches, whose involvement in stigma has historically been great—both as objects and agents—can preach an enlightened view and demand of their adherents sympathy and justice. Educators can devise forms of education that not only avoid the clichés of stigma but also communicate facts in frank and fair language. Politicians can shun the temptation to exploit the epidemic for their own interests.

In general, the American political system, while ostensibly designed to protect the weak and disadvantaged, is often stymied by the task of protecting the stigmatized. As noted earlier in this chapter, stigma often imputes dangerousness to a population and attempts, in effect if not in name, to outlaw that population. Thus, a politician who undertakes to advocate for the stigmatized takes on a most unpopular task: to protect by law the outlaw. Politicians in an elected system may be hesitant to adopt the unpopular cause; consequently, the stigmatized often live with diminished legal protection.

The law may influence the social process of stigmatization by prohibiting certain behaviors that are inspired by it. However, this influence will usually be indirect because the law does not reach the attitudes that underlie stigmatization (except by educating and motivating). Stigmatization must be distinguished from discrimination: the former is the valuation of the stigmatized class as dangerous or undesirable; the latter is the actual behavior and social practices that place the stigmatized person at a disadvantage in society. Antidiscrimination laws can restrain the behaviors that disdavantage a social group, but they influence the valuation of that group by the rest of society only slowly and partially.

The law performs many functions in society. It can constrain and punish some behaviors and enable or encourage others. Although the primary purpose of law is not education, educational messages can be communicated to the public by statutes and their enforcement. In the AIDS epidemic, the law has functioned in all of these ways. In the United States, laws have been framed to protect the public against infection and to protect the rights and confidentiality of infected persons. Efforts to enact the most extreme forms of constraint, such as quarantine or isolation, have failed; at the same time, the usual principles of criminal and civil law have been invoked to restrain harmful behavior by infected persons. Efforts to ensure the privacy of infected persons have usually succeeded because it is apparent to legislators and judges that educational programs and care are inhibited by the unwanted exposure of a person's infected state. Measures to ensure nondiscrimination in jobs, housing, and health insurance have taken various forms (Gostin and Curran, 1987; Gostin and Ziegler, 1987; Dickens, 1988).

The educational messages conveyed by the law would seem to be significant influences on behavior. Thus, confidentiality, which is widely assumed to be necessary to the efficacy of educational programs leading to behavioral changes, must be upheld and maintained. Otherwise, the obvious threat of discrimination that attends public disclosure of infection status would deter individuals from undergoing testing or seeking assistance. Although the precise effects of any form of legislation are difficult to ascertain, the law must protect HIV-positive individuals from discrimination. Failure to do so would not only conflict with the ethical foundation of American society but would also make the epidemic unmanageable.

REFERENCES

Aiken, J. H. (1987) Education as prevention. Pp. 90–105 in H. L. Dalton, S. Burris, and the Yale AIDS Law Project, eds., *AIDS and the Law.* New Haven, Conn.: Yale University Press.

Ainlay, S. C., Becker, G., and Coleman, L. M., eds. (1986) *The Dilemma of Difference.* New York: Plenum Press.

Allen, J. R., and Curran, J. W. (1988) Prevention of AIDS and HIV infection: Needs and priorities for epidemiologic research. *American Journal of Public Health* 78:381–386.

Benison, S. (1974) Poliomyelitis and the Rockefeller Institute: Social effects and institutional response. *Journal of the History of Medicine* 29:74–92.

Booth, W. (1987) The odyssey of a brochure on AIDS. *Science* 237:1410.

Brandt, A. M. (1987) *No Magic Bullet: A Social History of Venereal Disease in the United States Since 1880,* expanded ed. New York: Oxford University Press.

Centers for Disease Control (CDC). (1988a) *AIDS Surveillance Weekly Report, November 14, 1988.* Atlanta, Ga.: Centers for Disease Control.

Centers for Disease Control (CDC). (1988b) Content of AIDS-related written materials, pictorials, audiovisuals, questionnaires, survey instruments and educational sessions in Centers for Disease Control assistance programs. *Federal Register* 53:6034–6036.

Centers for Disease Control (CDC). (1988c) Guidelines for effective school health education. *Morbidity and Mortality Weekly Report* 37(Suppl S-2):1–14.

Check, W. A. (1987) Beyond the political model of reporting: Nonspecific symptoms in media communications about AIDS. *Reviews of Infectious Diseases* 9:987–1000.

Cipolla, C. M. (1973) *Cristofano and the Plague.* London: Collins.

Curran, J. W., Jaffe, H. W., Hardy, A. M., Morgan, W. M., Selik, R. M., and Dondero, T. J. (1988) Epidemiology of HIV infection and AIDS in the United States. *Science* 239:610–616.

Davis, J. A., and Smith, T. W. (1988) *General Social Surveys, 1972–1988: Cumulative Codebook.* Chicago: National Opinion Research Center, University of Chicago.

Davis, K., Lillie-Blanton, M., Lyons, B., Mullan, F., Powe, N., and Rowland, D. (1987) Health care for black Americans: The public sector role. *Milbank Quarterly* 65(Suppl. 1):213–247.

Dickens, B. M. (1988) Legal rights and duties in the AIDS epidemic. *Science* 239:580–586.

Feinberg, H. V. (1988) Education to prevent AIDS: Prospects and obstacles. *Science* 239:592–596.

Goffman, E. (1963) *Stigma: Notes on the Management of Spoiled Identity.* Englewood Cliffs, N.J.: Prentice-Hall.

Gostin, L., and Curran, W. J. (1987) Legal control measures for AIDS: Reporting requirements, surveillance, quarantine, and regulation of public meeting places. *American Journal of Public Health* 77:214–218.

Gostin, L., and Ziegler, A. (1987) A review of AIDS-related legislative and regulatory policy in the United States. *Law, Medicine and Health Care* 15:5–16.

Guinan, M. E., and Hardy, A. (1987) Epidemiology of AIDS in women in the United States. *Journal of the American Medical Association* 257:2039–2042.

Gussow, Z., and Tracy, G. S. (1970) Stigma and the leprosy phenomenon: The social history of a disease in the nineteenth and twentieth centuries. *Bulletin of the History of Medicine* 45:425–449.

Institute of Medicine/National Academy of Sciences (IOM/NAS). (1986) *Confronting AIDS: Directions for Public Health, Health Care, and Research.* Washington, D.C.: National Academy Press.

Jaynes, J. P., and Williams, R. M., Jr., eds. (In press) *A Common Destiny: Blacks and American Society.* Report of the Committee on the Status of Black Americans. Washington, D.C.: National Academy Press.

Kelsey, J. L., Thompson, W. D., and Evans, A. S. (1986) *Methods in Observational Epidemiology.* New York: Oxford University Press.

Manton, K. G., Patrick, C. H., and Johnson, K. W. (1987) Health differentials between blacks and whites: Recent trends in mortality and morbidity. *Milbank Quarterly* 65(Suppl. 1):129–199.

McNeil, W. H. (1976) *Plagues and Peoples.* New York: Doubleday.

Moore, K. A., Wenk, D., Hofferth, S. L. (ed)., and Hayes, C. D. (ed.) (1987) Statistical appendix: Trends in adolescent sexual and fertility behaviors. In S. L. Hofferth and C. D. Hayes, eds., *Risking the Future: Adolescent Sexuality, Pregnancy, and Childbearing.* Vol. 2, *Working Papers and Statistical Appendixes.* Washington, D.C.: National Academy Press.

New York State Department of Health. (1988) *AIDS in New York State: Through 1987.* Albany: New York State Department of Health.

Presidential Commission on the Human Immunodeficiency Virus Epidemic. (1988) *Final Report of the Presidential Commission on the Human Immunodeficiency Virus Epidemic.* Washington, D.C.: Government Printing Office.

Public Health Service. (1987) *What You Should Know about AIDS* (brochure). Washington, D.C.: Public Health Service.

Public Health Service. (1988) *Understanding AIDS* (brochure). Washington, D.C.: Public Health Service.

Rosenberg, C. E. (1962) *The Cholera Years.* Chicago: University of Chicago Press.

Sabatier, R. (1988) *Blaming Others: Prejudice, Race, and Worldwide AIDS.* Washington, D.C.: The Panos Institute.

Shilts, R. (1987) *And the Band Played On: Politics, People, and the AIDS Epidemic.* New York: St. Martin's Press.

Trauner, J. J. (1978) The Chinese as medical scapegoats. *California History* 57:70–84.

Tuchmann, B. W. (1978) *A Distant Mirror: The Calamitous 14th Century.* New York: Knopf.

U.S. Department of Education. (1987) *AIDS and the Education of Our Children: A Guide for Parents and Teachers.* Washington, D.C.: U.S. Department of Education.

U.S. Department of Health and Human Services. (1986) *Surgeon General's Report on Acquired Immune Deficiency Syndrome.* Washington, D.C.: U.S. Department of Health and Human Services.

U.S. House of Representatives. (1987) *Condom Advertising and AIDS.* Hearing Before the Subcommittee on Health and the Environment of the Committee on Energy and Commerce, House of Representatives. Serial No. 100-1. 100th Cong., 1st sess. February 10.

U.S. Supreme Court. (1986) *Bowers* v. *Hardwick,* No. 85-140, Argued March 31, 1986, Decided June 30, 1986. *United States Reports* 478:186–220.

Volinn, T. I. (1983) Health professionals as stigmatizers and destigmatizers of diseases. *Social Science Medicine* 17:385–393.

Winslow, C. E. (1943) *The Conquest of Epidemic Disease.* Princeton, N.J.: Princeton University Press.

World Health Organization Special Progamme on AIDS. (1988) *Folio, A Collection of AIDS Health Promotion Materials.* Geneva: World Health Organization.

Zelnik, M. (1983) Sexual activity among adolescents: Perspective of a decade. Pp. 21–33 in E. R. McAnarney, ed., *Premature Adolescent Pregnancy and Parenthood.* New York: Grune & Stratton.

Appendixes

APPENDIX

A

The Committee's Recommendations

MONITORING THE EPIDEMIC'S COURSE

The committee recommends that an appropriate federal agency mount a continuing program to monitor HIV testing at all laboratories doing such testing.

The committee recommends that CDC and other agencies with HIV/AIDS data gathering and reporting functions review their data disclosure practices, searching for rules and setting policies that continue to safeguard confidentiality but do so at the least practical cost in information.

The committee recommends that efforts be made to reformulate the CDC family of seroprevalence surveys as probability samples.

The committee recommends instituting a continuing anonymous probability survey of the HIV serostatus of women who are clients of clinics that provide abortion services.

The committee recommends that the newborn infant seroprevalence survey be extended to include all children born in the United States.

HUMAN SEXUAL BEHAVIOR AND AIDS

The committee recommends that the Public Health Service support vigorous programs of basic social and behavioral research on human sexual behavior, particularly through such agencies as the National

Institutes of Health; the Alcohol, Drug Abuse, and Mental Health Administration; and the Centers for Disease Control.

The committee recommends that data be collected to estimate the prevalence of the sexual risk-taking behaviors associated with the acquisition and spread of HIV infection in various populations, including those at higher and lower risk.

The committee recommends that funding be provided (and continued over time) to support prospective longitudinal studies of sexual behavior, and that high priority be given to studies of the social and societal contexts of sexual behaviors.

The committee recommends that the Public Health Service support research in those subsets of the population that are at increased risk of HIV infection.

The committee recommends immediate steps to close the vast gaps in our knowledge of the relationship of sexual behavior and drug and alcohol use.

The committee recommends that resources be invested in methodological research to develop better procedures to obtain information from hard-to-reach groups.

The committee recommends that an independent review of STD data collection systems be undertaken and sufficient resources provided to undertake any improvements that may be required.

The committee recommends that the Public Health Service immediately begin a research program to determine the extent to which the use of condoms and spermicides reduces the risk of HIV transmission. This program should include investigations of the current use of these products, how that use might be modified, and—equally important—how these products themselves may be modified to encourage uses compatible with human skills and dispositions.

The committee recommends a concerted effort to upgrade and standardize (when possible and desirable) the procedures used to gather behavioral data in clinical and biomedical research settings.

The committee recommends that funding agencies, both public and private, encourage the sharing of data relevant to HIV infection and AIDS that have been gathered by federal and extramural researchers, within the limits set by scientific priority and confidentiality. To facilitate such sharing, the committee recommends that a data archive be established to support secondary analyses of these data.

The committee recommends that local public health authorities ensure that treatment for all sexually transmitted diseases is readily available to all persons who may seek such treatment.

The committee recommends that local public health authorities ensure that condoms are readily available to all sexually active persons.

AIDS AND IV DRUG USE

The committee recommends that well-designed, staged trials of sterile needle programs, such as those requested in the 1986 Institute of Medicine/National Academy of Sciences report *Confronting AIDS*, be implemented.[1]

The committee recommends that high priority be given to studies of the social and societal contexts of IV drug use and IV drug-use prevention efforts.

The committee recommends that high priority be given to research on the natural history of IV drug use, with an emphasis on prospective longitudinal studies of the factors associated with initiation into and cessation of IV drug use.

The committee recommends that high priority be given to studies of the sexual and procreative behavior of IV drug users, including methods to reduce sexual and perinatal (mother–infant) transmission of HIV.

The committee recommends that the appropriate government authorities take immediate action to (1) provide drug treatment upon request for IV drug users throughout the country; (2) sustain and expand current programs that provide for "safer injection" to reach all current IV drug users in the nation on a continuing basis and with appropriate research evaluation; and (3) establish data collection systems for monitoring present AIDS prevention efforts for IV drug users.

---

[1]In the text of the report, this recommendation appears in Chapter 4.

The committee recommends that high priority be given to research that will lead to improved drug-use treatment, including studies of relapse prevention and of treatment for cocaine dependence. Applied research should include planned variation and evaluation of experimental programs.

The committee recommends that high priority be given to studies of IV drug users who are not in contact with health care, drug-use treatment, or criminal justice systems.

The committee recommends that high priority be given to methodological studies to determine ways of improving the quality of self-reports of sexual and drug-use behavior.

The committee recommends that high priority be given to research on the estimation of the current number of IV drug users in the United States and of seroprevalence rates among different groups of IV drug users.

FACILITATING CHANGE IN HEALTH BEHAVIORS

The committee recommends making information available in clear, explicit language in the idiom of the target audience.

The committee recommends that AIDS prevention messages strike a balance in the level of threat that is conveyed.

The committee recommends that television networks present more public service messages on those behaviors associated with HIV transmission and practical measures for interrupting the spread of infection.

The committee recommends that television networks accept condom advertisements.

The committee recommends that programs to initiate and sustain changes in risk-associated behavior take into account how the targeted population perceives and understands risk.

The committee recommends that innovative approaches to AIDS prevention programs be introduced in a planned manner that reflects well-established principles about the adoption and diffusion of new ideas.

The committee recommends that programs to facilitate behavioral change be approached as long-term efforts, with multiple and repeated strategies to initiate and sustain behavioral change over time.

The committee recommends that anonymous HIV antibody testing with appropriate pre- and posttest counseling be made available on a voluntary basis for anyone desiring it.

The committee recommends that programs consider the psychological, social, biological, and environmental factors that may affect relapse; learned coping responses, including skills training and relapse rehearsal, should be taught to increase perceptions of self-efficacy.

The committee recommends that, to the extent possible, community-level interventions to prevent the spread of HIV infection address simultaneously information, motivational factors, skills, prevailing norms, and methods for diffusing innovation.

The committee recommends that sex education be available to both male and female students and that such education include explicit information relevant to the prevention of HIV infection.

The committee recommends that planned variations of key program elements be systematically and actively incorporated into the design of intervention programs at an early stage.

The committee recommends that the Public Health Service and others conducting or supporting intervention programs ensure the implementation of planned variations in AIDS messages, programs, and campaigns.

EVALUATING THE EFFECTS OF AIDS INTERVENTIONS

The committee recommends that the Office of the Assistant Secretary for Health take responsibility for an evaluation strategy that will provide timely information on the relative effectiveness of different AIDS intervention programs.

The committee recommends the expanded use of randomized field experiments for evaluating new intervention programs on both individual and community levels.

The committee recommends that evaluation support be provided to ensure collaboration between practitioners and evaluation researchers.

The committee recommends to the research community that the results of well-conducted evaluations be published, regardless of the intervention's effectiveness.

The committee recommends that all evaluations publish detailed descriptive information on the nature and methods of intervention programs, along with evaluation data to support claims of relative effectiveness.

The committee recommends that only the best-designed and best-implemented intervention programs be selected to receive those special resources that will be needed to conduct scientific evaluations.

The committee recommends that CDC substantially increase efforts, with links to extramural scientific resources, to assist health departments and others in mounting evaluations.

BARRIERS TO RESEARCH

The committee recommends that serious consideration be given to exempting research on HIV infection and AIDS from the requirements of the Paperwork Reduction Act.

The committee recommends that intervention programs at all levels increase the involvement of minority researchers and minority health care workers to assist in reaching and involving the black, Hispanic, and gay communities.

The committee recommends that support of multidisciplinary centers for research on AIDS prevention be viewed as a long-term commitment to allow sustained collaborative efforts, including valuable prospective studies.

The committee recommends that the number of trained behavioral and social scientists employed in AIDS-related activities at federal agencies responsible for preventing the spread of HIV infection be substantially increased.

The committee recommends that the CDC AIDS program increase its staff of persons knowledgeable about survey sampling and survey design, and that it exploit the methodological expertise of the National Center for Health Statistics.

The committee recommends that, in addition to experienced survey scientists, CDC obtain technical assistance to evaluate intervention programs it is currently funding.

The committee recommends the use of PHS fellowship programs and Intergovernmental Personnel Appointments (IPAs) as an interim means for rapidly enlarging the cadre of senior behavioral and social scientists working on AIDS programs at CDC and other PHS agencies.

APPENDIX

B

Supplemental Data

This appendix[1] presents a variety of data to supplement the discussion of sexual behavior in Chapter 2. Table B-1 summarizes data from several studies of the proportions of young men and young women reporting first sexual intercourse at (or before) various ages. These data span the period 1958–1973; it should be noted that most of these studies used convenience samples drawn from particular high schools or colleges. Table B-2 presents parallel data (broken down by birth cohort) from a national probability sample of young women conducted in 1982 (the National Survey of Family Growth, or NSFG), and Table B-3 presents similar data collected by Zelnik and Kantner (1985) from probability samples of young women residing in metropolitan areas of the United States in 1971, 1976, and 1979. Table B-4 (adapted from work reported by Klassen and colleagues in this volume) provides a parallel tabulation from the 1970 Kinsey Institute survey broken down by birth cohort. Figures B-1 and B-2 plot the data from these tables.[2]

Table B-5 presents a tabulation of the number of sexual partners reported by never-married young women in the 1979 Zelnik and Kantner survey. Table B-6 compares measurements of heterosexual activity for the 1944–1949 birth cohort that were made in the 1982 NSFG and in the 1970 Kinsey Institute survey. Although a definitive

[1]References cited in this appendix can be found in the Chapter 2 bibliography.

[2]To make the plots "readable," only the 1979 survey data from Zelnik and Kantner have been plotted. For the 1944–1949 cohort from a national probability sample, we have plotted only the 1970 Kinsey Institute survey data; a tabulation of data for women in this birth cohort in the NSFG can be found in Table B-6. The reader should note that the 1970 Kinsey Institute survey data reflect sexual contact to orgasm and not necessarily intercourse.

interpretation cannot be made, the higher rates of sexual activity reported in the 1970 Kinsey Institute survey may plausibly reflect the fact that the "activity" measured in that study was sexual contact to orgasm, whereas the NSFG measured reported intercourse.

Tables B-7 and B-8 elaborate data reported by Fay and colleagues (in press). Table B-7 cross-tabulates the homosexual experience of ever-married men (including number of male partners) by their premarital heterosexual experience. As noted in the commentary by Fay and coworkers (in press), although these data show substantial heterogeneity of same-gender and across-gender sexual contacts, the data are quite sparse, and the missing data problems are severe. Table B-8 provides a parallel tabulation for never-married men; however, owing to the paucity of available data ($N = 135$ never-married men), the table does not break down the men's same-gender sexual experience by number of same-gender partners.

TABLE B-1 Percentage of Sexually Active Males and Females by Age (or grade in school) Reported in Selected Studies Conducted Between 1958 and 1973

Study	Date of Survey	Sample	Age or Grade	Sexually Active: Percentage (N) of Males		Sexually Active: Percentage (N) of Females	
Christensen and Gregg (1970)	1958	Midwestern college	18–22[a]	51	(213)	21	(142)
	1968	Midwestern college	18–22[a]	50	(245)	34	(238)
Simon et al. (1972)	1967	Probability sample of college students	17 or less	25		7	
			18	36		19	
			19	63		30	
Vener and Stewart (1974)	1969	Western shore communities, Michigan[b]	14	21	(208)	10	(197)
			15	26	(193)	13	(195)
			16	31	(217)	23	(200)
			17–18	38	(179)	27	(142)
	1973	Western shore communities, Michigan[b]	14	32	(220)	17	(218)
			15	38	(191)	24	(220)
			16	38	(176)	31	(190)
			17–18	34	(173)	35	(185)
Jessor and Jessor (1975)	1972	High school students, Rocky Mountain region	Grade 10	21	(75)	26	(96)
			Grade 11	28	(60)	40	(82)
			Grade 12	33	(51)	55	(64)
DeLamater and MacCorquodale (1979)	1973	Students, University of Wisconsin[c]	13	2.1[d]		0.2[d]	
			14	2.8		0.9	
			15	6.3		3.3	
			16	17.8		8.6	
			17	37.0		21.2	
			18	57.2		40.1	
			19	66.2		52.3	
			20	72.0		57.6	
			21	74.3		59.5	

1973	Nonstudents, Madison, Wisconsin[e]	13	2.3[f]	0.0[f]
		14	5.4	0.3
		15	13.6	2.0
		16	25.9	10.6
		17	44.5	24.2
		18	64.5	43.3
		19	69.9	55.3
		20	74.4	62.8
		21	77.6	68.9
		22	79.0	70.6

NOTE: In this table, years of age mean during the respondents' *N*th year, not before their *N*th birthday. Small samples studied (1968 and 1972) by Bauman and Wilson (1974) have not been included because *N*s for each sex were between 68 and 107 and published tabulations are not broken down by age.

[a]Age range of 18–22 is estimated for respondents since they were all college undergraduates at the time of the surveys (1958 and 1968).

[b]Described as follows (Vener and Stewart, 1974:729): "This community has a school district which serves 25,000 residents—Seventy per cent of the respondents' fathers have a high school diploma and approximately 25 per cent have completed four years of college. The community contains one public junior and senior high school and is located less than 5 miles from the nearest SMSA . . . of approximately 150,000 and approximately 20 miles from another SMSA of 360,000."

[c]A 6 percent random sample of undergraduates at the University of Wisconsin at Madison. There were 1,141 potential respondents identified in the sample, and interviews were ultimately conducted with 985 respondents, representing a completion rate of about 82 percent of the total sample.

[d]For tabulations from student samples, the authors had samples of 432 for males and 431 for females. These *N*s should apply to all retrospective reports for precollege ages. For older ages, the sample decreases as follows: for males, 19.5 percent aged 18 or under; 41.1 percent under 19; 62.9 percent under 20; and 84.0 percent under 21; and for females, 18.7 percent aged 18 or under; 46.9 percent under 19; 71.3 percent under 20; and 88.4 percent under 21.

[e]Sample selected from people aged 18 to 23 who resided in Madison, Wisconsin, but who were not students at the university. Sample was drawn from residences listed in the Madison telephone directory. Authors (pp. 44–45) indicate that 96 percent of residences in the area had telephones, but no indication is given of the proportion of residences that had unlisted telephone numbers. For this nonstudent sample, 1,134 individuals were identified in screening calls. (Data are not presented on the proportion of residential households that could not be screened.) Of these persons, 79 moved before an interview could be scheduled. Interviews were completed with 663 (62.8 percent) of those contacted.

[f]For tabulations from nonstudent samples, authors had samples of 220 for males and 293 for females. These *N*s should apply to all retrospective reports for ages 13–17. For older ages, the total sample decreases as follows: for males, 23.6 percent of sample age 18; 38.6 percent under 19; 54.5 percent under 20; 65.9 percent under 21; and 82.7 percent under 22; and for females, 20.8 percent of sample age 18; 40.9 percent under 19; 53.9 percent under 20; and 70.3 percent under 21.

TABLE B-2 Cumulative Percentage of U.S. Teenage Women in the 1982 National Survey of Family Growth (NSFG) Who Reported Premarital Sexual Intercourse, by Age and According to Race and Birth Cohort

Race	Birth Cohort									
and Age	1938–1940	1941–1943	1944–1946	1947–1949	1950–1952	1953–1955	1956–1958	1959–1961	1962–1964	1965–1967
Total	(*N* = 383)	(*N* = 444)	(*N* = 479)	(*N* = 664)	(*N* = 745)	(*N* = 805)	(*N* = 786)	(*N* = 707)	(*N* = 897)	(*N* = 848)
13	0.9	0.3	0.3	0.9	0.4	0.5	1.3	2.0	0.9	1.9
14	2.1	0.8	1.1	2.8	0.8	3.0	3.6	4.0	4.0	5.9
15	3.0	2.5	2.2	4.6	3.1	6.3	8.7	9.2	9.8	12.6
16	7.4	7.4	7.1	10.1	6.6	14.5	17.9	18.9	23.1	[a]
17	14.0	14.3	13.2	19.0	13.8	26.4	28.3	33.0	37.8	[a]
18	23.0	22.7	22.6	29.3	26.9	43.1	45.5	46.4	54.0	[a]
19	32.2	33.3	31.7	40.2	42.6	58.8	58.8	61.5	[a]	[a]
20	38.9	39.1	40.8	48.9	55.9	68.4	68.2	68.3	[a]	[a]

White	(N = 235)	(N = 273)	(N = 296)	(N = 393)	(N = 422)	(N = 449)	(N = 405)	(N = 385)	(N = 599)	(N = 538)
13	0.5	0.2	0.0	0.9	0.0	0.3	1.0	1.7	0.3	1.7
14	1.3	0.6	0.3	2.4	0.3	2.8	3.0	3.0	3.4	5.0
15	1.3	2.0	1.0	3.7	2.2	5.6	7.6	7.9	8.3	11.0
16	4.5	6.3	5.1	8.6	4.6	12.9	16.1	16.8	20.8	[a]
17	10.2	10.9	10.7	17.0	11.2	24.0	25.6	29.9	34.8	[a]
18	18.4	18.5	19.1	27.2	23.4	39.6	42.5	43.0	50.9	[a]
19	27.2	28.3	27.6	37.2	38.7	55.5	55.2	58.4	[a]	[a]
20	33.3	34.2	37.0	45.6	52.5	65.5	64.9	65.3	[a]	[a]
Black	(N = 148)	(N = 171)	(N = 183)	(N = 271)	(N = 323)	(N = 356)	(N = 381)	(N = 322)	(N = 298)	(N = 310)
13	4.3	1.4	2.7	0.5	3.5	1.5	3.0	4.0	4.6	3.2
14	8.5	2.3	8.0	5.5	5.5	4.5	7.6	10.0	7.9	10.5
15	15.7	6.9	13.2	12.1	10.5	11.0	15.3	18.0	19.4	20.4
16	28.9	16.3	23.5	21.6	22.0	27.0	29.3	32.1	37.0	[a]
17	42.7	41.8	33.9	34.1	33.0	44.8	44.5	52.8	57.3	[a]
18	57.8	56.3	51.9	45.1	54.5	69.2	64.0	68.6	73.1	[a]
19	70.6	73.0	66.3	62.2	73.6	83.1	81.0	81.4	[a]	[a]
20	81.7	77.9	73.9	74.2	83.1	90.4	88.8	87.7	[a]	[a]

SOURCE: Hofferth et al. (1987:49, Table 3), calculated from the 1982 NSFG. Reprinted with permission.

[a]Data censored by the survey date.

TABLE B-3 Percentage of Women 15–19 Years of Age Who Had Premarital Intercourse, by Age, Marital Status, and Race, in the 1971, 1976, and 1979 Surveys Conducted by Kantner and Zelnik

Age and Marital Status	1971			1976			1979		
	Total	White	Black	Total	White	Black	Total	White	Black
15	14.8	11.8	31.2	18.9	14.2	38.9	22.8	18.5	41.7
16	21.8	17.8	46.4	30.0	25.2	55.1	39.5	37.4	50.9
17	28.2	23.2	58.4	46.0	40.0	71.9	50.1	45.8	74.6
18	42.6	38.8	62.4	56.7	52.1	78.4	63.0	60.3	77.0
19	48.2	43.8	76.2	64.1	59.2	85.3	71.4	68.0	88.7
(*N*)	(2,739)	(1,758)	(981)	(1,452)	(881)	(571)	(1,717)	(1,034)	(683)

NOTE: Sample restricted to women in metropolitan areas. Unweighted sample size is shown in parentheses; $N \geq 107$ for each age-race cell.

SOURCE: Zelnik (1983).

TABLE B-4 Cumulative Proportion of Respondents in the 1970 Kinsey Institute Survey Reporting Premarital Sexual Contact to the Point of Orgasm Before Given Birthdays by Gender and Year of Birth

Age and Gender	Year of Birth 1944–1949	1938–1943	1931–1937	1921–1930	1911–1920	Pre-1911
Before 14						
Male	15.5%	12.4%	12.7%	12.5%	3.4%	6.9%
Female	4.1	1.9	1.1	1.5	2.7	0.8
Before 15						
Male	23.0	20.6	26.5	18.5	8.8	10.1
Female	7.3	5.1	2.7	2.6	3.6	1.3
Before 16						
Male	36.6	33.0	38.1	30.2	14.7	16.4
Female	15.4	9.8	6.4	4.8	4.9	1.7
Before 17						
Male	52.8	49.0	48.6	44.0	29.9	25.9
Female	26.4	19.6	11.2	7.0	8.4	4.2
Before 18						
Male	67.7	62.9	60.2	53.9	43.1	32.8
Female	37.8	32.7	17.0	10.7	11.6	5.0

Continued

TABLE B-4 *Continued*

Age and Gender	Year of Birth 1944–1949	1938–1943	1931–1937	1921–1930	1911–1920	Pre-1911
Before 19						
Male	78.9	76.3	70.7	65.9	55.4	42.6
Female	50.0	38.8	23.4	16.6	13.8	5.4
Before 20						
Male	83.9	79.4	75.1	72.4	62.3	48.3
Female	56.1	46.7	27.1	20.7	16.0	7.1
Before 21						
Male	87.6	80.9	80.1	74.1	66.2	52.1
Female	58.1	51.4	28.7	23.6	18.2	8.4
Before 22						
Male	89.4	83.0	82.9	75.9	69.1	55.2
Female	60.6	53.7	30.9	27.3	20.9	8.8
Before 23						
Male	90.1	84.5	83.4	77.6	71.1	57.7
Female	61.8	55.6	31.4	28.8	23.6	9.2
Total	100%	100%	100%	100%	100%	100%
N (Male)	161	194	181	232	204	317
N (Female)	246	214	188	271	225	239

SOURCE: Secondary analysis of data from the 1970 Kinsey Institute survey.

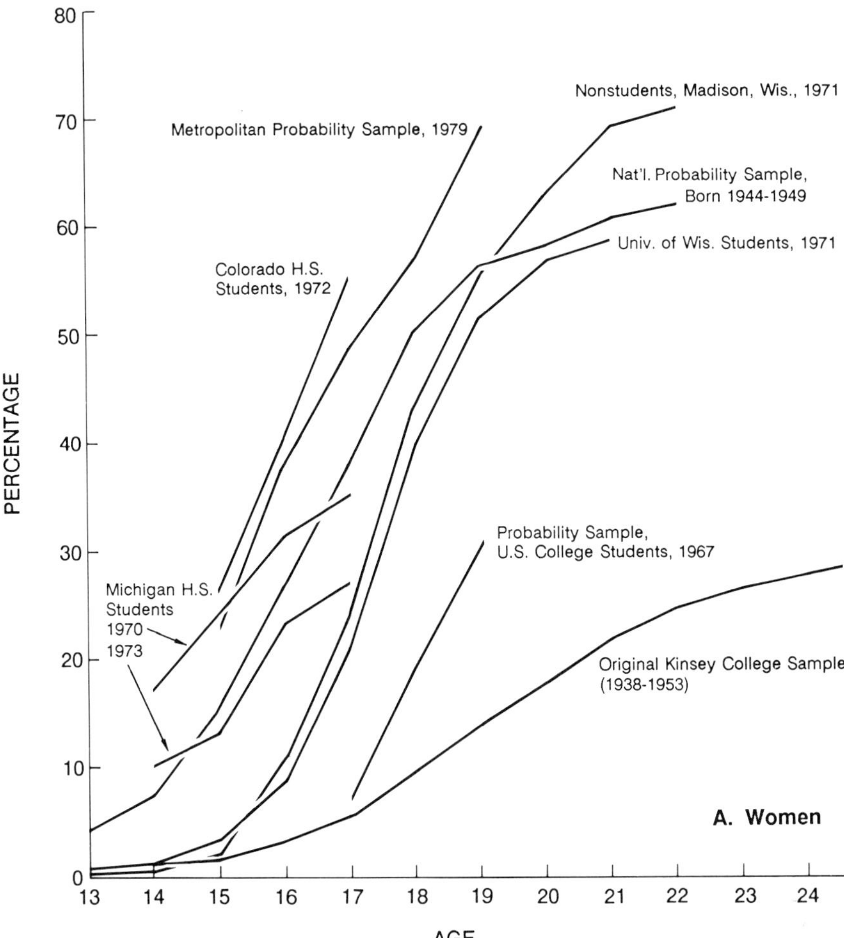

FIGURE B-1 Proportion of females reporting premarital sexual intercourse (by age) in selected studies. NOTE: In the 1970 Kinsey Institute survey, respondents reported sexual contact to orgasm of either partner (not intercourse). SOURCE: Tables B-1 to B-4.

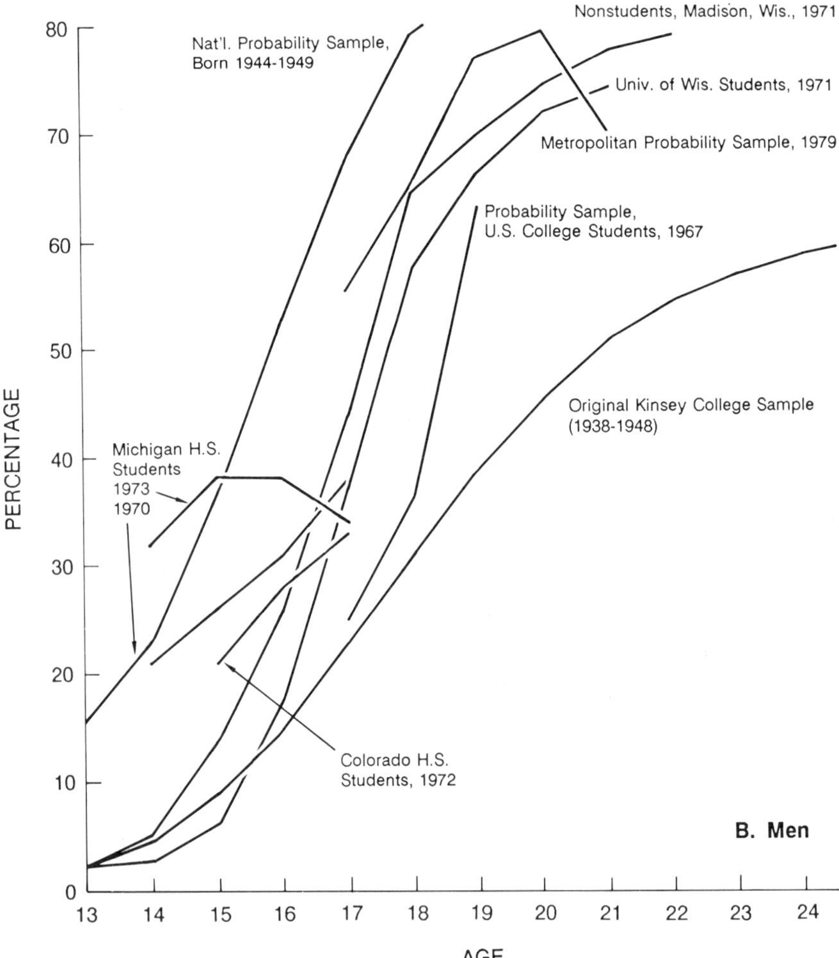

FIGURE B-2 Proportion of males reporting premarital sexual intercourse (by age) in selected studies. NOTE: In the 1970 Kinsey Institute survey, respondents reported sexual contact to orgasm of either partner (not intercourse). SOURCE: Tables B-1 to B-4.

TABLE B-5 Total Number of Heterosexual Partners Reported in the 1979 Kantner and Zelnik Survey by Never-Married Young Women Residing in Metropolitan Areas[a]

Number of Sexual Partners	Age 15	16	17	18	19
None	77.5%	62.3%	51.5%	43.3%	31.2%
1	15.0	18.0	25.0	23.4	27.1
2	3.4	11.2	7.4	10.7	12.5
3	2.5	6.1	6.8	8.6	14.0
4	0.9	0.6	1.5	5.1	4.5
5	0.0	0.5	1.9	2.4	2.4
6	0.4	0.3	0.9	1.0	2.5
7–9	0.3	0.4	2.1	1.3	2.8
10 +	0.0	0.6	2.7	4.1	2.9
Total	100%	100%	100%	100%	100%
N	313	364	314	300	275

NOTE: Secondary analysis of data provided by the Data Archive on Adolescent Pregnancy and Pregnancy Prevention from the data set collected in 1979 by Zelnik and Kantner (1985). Percentages were tabulated using sampling weights encoded in the data set; *N*s shown in last row of table are unweighted. Five cases were excluded from this analysis due to missing data.

[a]The survey sample was restricted to young women residing within the standard metropolitan statistical areas of the United States.

TABLE B-6 Cumulative Percentage of Female Respondents Born Between 1944 and 1949 Reporting Premarital Sexual Contact to the Point of Orgasm in 1970 Kinsey Institute Survey and Cumulative Percentage Reporting Sexual Intercourse in 1982 National Survey of Family Growth (NSFG)

	Survey and Cohort	
Age	Kinsey 1944–1949	NSFG 1944–1949
Before 14	4.1%	2.1%
Before 15	7.3	3.6
Before 16	15.4	8.8
Before 17	26.4	16.6
Before 18	37.8	26.5
Before 19	50.0	36.6
Before 20	56.1	45.5

NOTE: Estimates from 1982 NSFG are weighted means of estimates for two birth cohorts (1944–1946 and 1947–1949) reported in Hofferth et al. (1987:49, Table 2). The sample *N*s (479 and 664) for the cohorts were used as weights in estimating the percentages for the combined group (1944–1949). Almost identical results are obtained if the size of these cohorts in the 1980 census are used as the weights.

SOURCE: Secondary analysis of 1970 Kinsey Institute Survey data and Hofferth et al. (1987).

TABLE B-7 Observed Counts from the 1970 Kinsey Institute Survey of Currently or Previously Married Men by Number of Reported Heterosexual Partners Before Marriage and Number of Lifetime Homosexual Partners by Age at Last Homosexual Contact

Number of Male Partners	Number of Female Partners Before Marriage						
	None or Future Spouse Only	1–4	5–9	10–19	20 +	NA/REF	Total
No male partners	264	216	130	113	79	80	882
Last contact before age 20							
1 male partner	11	19	2	6	5	4	47
2–4	6	12	5	12	10	4	49
5–9	0	1	2	0	1	1	5
10 +	1	0	0	1	2	0	4
NA/REF	1	1	3	2	2	3	12
Last contact at age 20 +							
1 male partner	5	1	1	0	0	1	8
2–4	0	4	3	4	1	1	13
5–9	0	0	3	1	1	0	5
10 +	0	1	0	3	2	0	6
NA/REF	10	8	1	0	0	4	23
Nonrespondents, age at last contact[a]	8	7	12	6	5	12	50
Nonrespondents, homosexual experience[b]	53	36	25	27	11	59	211
Total	359	306	187	175	119	169	1,315

NOTE: NA/REF = no answer/refused.

[a]Respondents with reported homosexual experience but for whom it could not be established whether the age at last contact was before or after age 20.

[b]Nonrespondents to all of the questions on homosexual experience.

SOURCE: Secondary analysis of 1970 Kinsey Institute survey data.

TABLE B-8 Observed Counts from the 1970 Kinsey Institute Survey of Never-Married Men by Number of Reported Lifetime Heterosexual Partners by Age at Last Homosexual Contact

Number of Male Partners	Number of Female Partners: None or Future Spouse Only	1–4	5–9	10–19	20 +	NA/REF	Total
Homosexual contact							
None	12	10	11	19	16	21	89
Last contact before age 20	0	3	2	2	0	3	10
Last contact at age 20 +	1	3	3	1	1	3	12
Nonrespondents, age at last contact[a]	3	3	0	0	0	6	12
Nonrespondents, homosexual experience[b]	1	0	3	0	0	8	12
Total	17	19	19	22	17	41	135

NOTE: NA/REF = no answer/refused.

[a]Respondents with reported homosexual experience but for whom it could not be established whether the age at last contact was before or after age 20.

[b]Nonrespondents to all of the questions on homosexual experience.

SOURCE: Secondary analysis of 1970 Kinsey Institute survey data.

Background Papers

On the Accuracy of Estimates of Numbers of Intravenous Drug Users

Bruce D. Spencer

The purpose of this paper is to assess the accuracy of estimates of the numbers of intravenous drug users (IVDUs) that were published in the November 30, 1987 report "A Review of Current Knowledge and Plans for Expansion of HIV Surveillance Activities" (hereafter, the "Review"), submitted by the Centers for Disease Control (CDC) to the Domestic Policy Council.[1] The purpose is not to develop alternative estimates but rather to see whether the published estimates are accurate enough to be relied upon for estimating and forecasting the extent of human immunodeficiency virus (HIV) infection. As will be made clear, the published estimates are fraught with problems. The accuracy of the estimates is not ascertainable by objective means because the estimates are based largely on guesses. In the author's judgment, the estimates could well be off by a factor of 2, in either direction.

Although this paper will appear to be highly critical of the ways that various researchers and agency personnel have estimated numbers of IVDUs, appreciation and respect are owed to researchers for producing the estimates that we have of numbers of IVDUs. Considerable ingenuity has been used by a number of researchers

The author is from the Department of Statistics, Northwestern University, and the Methodology Research Center, NORC. He is grateful for helpful comments from Lincoln Moses, John Newmeyer, I. Richard Savage, and James Schmeidler.

[1]The report later appeared as the supplement to the December 18, 1987 *Morbidity and Mortality Weekly Report,* 36, No. S-6.

in attacking this difficult estimation problem. This paper does not say that the estimates should have been produced by alternative procedures; indeed, few constructive suggestions are made. Rather, it concludes that the estimates are simply highly inaccurate and form a weak basis for any policy or program decisions.

Before proceeding to discuss the estimates themselves, the reader should understand the statistical concept of accuracy. The following discussion is intended to elucidate, rather than confuse; the reader who wishes to skip it should proceed to the next section.

Let X refer to the published estimate of the number of IVDUs and let θ refer to the true number of IVDUs, that is, the number to be estimated. One may think of X as fixed and known, since it is published, and of θ as fixed but unknown. The error in X, namely ε, is the difference between X and θ; $\varepsilon = X - \theta$. When the accuracy of X is referred to, a statement is being made about beliefs concerning the magnitude of ε. Except on rare occasions when θ is known with a much smaller error than ε, the value of ε is uncertain. This uncertainty will be represented by a probability distribution for ε. The key features of the distribution are its mean, which measures the bias or systematic error in X, and its variance, which measures the unreliability of X. The bias may be decomposed into the sum of two component biases, one arising because X is designed to measure the wrong concept (i.e., the wrong definition of IVDU underlies X) and the other arising from systematic error in the measurement process. Summary measures of accuracy may be developed in various ways, but the most common is root-mean-square error (RMSE), the square root of the sum of the variance and the squared bias.

Two alternative interpretations of probability will now be discussed. Under one interpretation, the "relative frequency" (RF) interpretation, the estimate X is viewed as a realization of a stochastic process; for example, if X is based on the results of randomly selected samples, then the randomization inherent in the sampling gives rise to a probability distribution for X (i.e., different samples would give rise to different estimates of X). Other, nonsampling bases for error in X can also be endowed with a randomization distribution; for example, response errors in surveys can be viewed as occurring at random (perhaps with bias as well as variance). For another example (see "Newmeyer's Ratio Estimate"), consider ratio-estimators X of the form $X = \hat{A}Y$, where Y is the number of reports of drug-related emergency room episodes reported in the Drug Abuse Warning Network (DAWN) and $\hat{A}$ is an estimate of A, with A defined as the ratio of θ to the expected value of Y. Here Y is random and $\hat{A}$ has error when viewed as an estimate of A, and the latter error and Y may be correlated.

Not all estimates X are conducive to the RF interpretation; for example, some estimates of X are called "informed guesstimates" (never *un*informed guesstimates, though) and are not produced by a repeatable process. In such cases, a relevant notion of probability is based on the view that a person's beliefs about θ may be represented by a probability distribution; this interpretation will be referred to as a "personalistic Bayesian" (PB) perspective. The PB viewpoint explicitly incorporates subjective opinion, whereas the RF viewpoint does not. However, application of the RF model inevitably uses subjective opinion in the specification of the randomization model to be used to assess the mean and variance of the distribution. In either case, RF or PB, the problem of *whose opinion* arises. In this paper, the author's opinion is represented. Coming from a nonexpert in the area of drug abuse, these opinions represent those of experts whose views have been encountered as well as a sufficient degree of skepticism acquired from experience in assessing the accuracy of demographic statistics and from watching experts be overconfident about their expertise (see also Mosteller, 1977, in this regard).

WHAT IS THE DEFINITION OF INTRAVENOUS DRUG USER?

The first problem with estimates of the number of intravenous drug users is the definition of IVDU. Many IVDUs shoot opioids, principally heroin, and many do not. W. R. Lange (personal communication, 1988) believes that, at least in some communities such as Baltimore, "approximately 20% of IVDUs are primary cocaine and amphetamine users who do not on a regular basis abuse opioids intravenously." Many varieties of patterns of needle use exist. Some persons inject drugs subcutaneously ("skin poppers") and do not even use needles; although they are not IVDUs if they do not use needles, they are at risk of HIV infection to the extent that they share injection equipment with drug users who are infected with HIV. Some IVDUs are hard-core addicts who inject drugs multiple times each day; other IVDUs are successful upper middle class users, who inject less frequently. Other IVDUs inject multiple times daily for a few months and then stop; still others inject only a few times per year. Some IVDUs have been shooting for a long time; others, only recently. Whether an IVDU did most injecting prior to 1975 or in a later year will greatly affect the risk of HIV infection.

Gerstein (1976) distinguished four types of heroin-using IVDUs. The first two types are hard-core users who are "strung out"; the third type consists of "people with dual identities . . . who may be strung out, but often at low levels. . . . These are people whose status as members of the heroin community is often secret, hidden from a whole set of close associations: family and friends. These may or may not be identified on the street as addicts, depending on their mode of scoring and the stage of their careers." The fourth type is IVDUs who are not usually strung out on heroin. "These may be 'chippies', 'weekenders', or 'sandbox users' as opposed to 'boot-and-shoe addicts', 'stone junkies', 'dope fiends', and 'real hypes'. They may or may not score directly on the street. . . . Sometimes these peoples are situational heroin users—the current lover of a strung-out user, for example." Gerstein believes, based on field experience and study of the epidemiological literature on heroin that there are about two or three type 4 IVDUs for every type 1–3 IVDU (Gerstein, 1976).

What is the right choice of definition? For estimating the number of seropositive persons in the United States, the precise definition is largely irrelevant as long as it is consistent with other definitions being employed.

For example, Table 14 in the "Review" estimates the total number of infected people in eight (presumably nonoverlapping) population subgroups:

1. exclusively homosexual,
2. other homosexual,
3. regular IVDU,
4. occasional IVDU,
5. hemophiliac A,
6. hemophiliac B,
7. heterosexuals without specific identified risks, and
8. others.

The estimates of total infected persons in each group are derived by multiplying the number of persons in the group by the seropositivity rate and summing. Thus, if R_j is the seropositivity rate for group j and if N_j is the size of group j, the total number of infected persons in the population is

$$R_1N_1 + R_2N_2 + R_3N_3 + R_4N_4 + \cdots + R_8N_8.$$

If group 4 were split into two groups, say $4a$ and $4b$, with rates R_{4a} and R_{4b} and sizes N_{4a} and N_{4b}, then the total number of infected persons in the population may be expressed as:

$$R_1N_1 + R_2N_2 + R_3N_3 + R_{4a}N_{4a} + R_{4b}N_{4b} + \cdots + R_8N_8,$$

which equals the previous total because $R_4 = (R_{4a}N_{4a} + R_{4b}N_{4b})/N_4$ and $N_4 = N_{4a}+N_{4b}$. Thus, changing the definitions or compositions of the groups does not affect the estimate of the total number infected as long as the group sizes N_j and seropositivity rates R_j are appropriate to the group as defined. (Of course the groups should comprise the whole population and be nonoverlapping.)

This is not to say that for other purposes the definition is irrelevant. For example, for studying transmission of the infection, one would wish to estimate seroprevalence for IVDUs classified by frequency of injection, how long they had been shooting, whether they shared needles and with whom, if and how long they had been infected, the stage of the infection, and so on. In this case, the definition should be focused so that the groups of IVDUs are homogeneous. Thus, the definition of IVDU might well exclude or otherwise distinguish chippies from other users. The definition implicitly used by Newmeyer (1988) in his method (described later) has this feature.

WHAT DEFINITIONS ARE USED IN THE "REVIEW"?

The "Review" distinguishes two types of IVDUs: *regular* users who inject at least weekly and *less frequent or occasional* users who inject less often than regular users but have used drugs more than once or twice. Two sets of national estimates were produced for each type of IVDU, the original Public Health Service estimates for 1986 ("Review," Table 13) and the revised estimates ("Review," Table 14) for 1987. These are listed in Table 1.

TABLE 1 Public Health Service (1986, 1987) Estimates of HIV Prevalence Among IV Drug Users

Type of IV Drug User	Estimated Number	Approximate Seroprevalence (%)	Total Number Infected
Original estimate (1986)			
Regular	750,000	30	225,000
Occasional	750,000	10	75,000
Total	1,500,000		300,000
Revised estimate (1987)			
Regular	900,000	25	225,000
Occasional	200,000	5	10,000
Total	1,100,000		235,000

In assessing these estimates, critical questions concern what population definitions were actually used in estimating the total number of each type of IVDU and in estimating the seroprevalence rates. How different are the operational definitions? How accurate are the estimates for the populations as operationally defined?

WHAT POPULATION DEFINITION WAS USED FOR ESTIMATING SEROPREVALENCE?

Seroprevalence rates were estimated by a weighted average of seroprevalence rates for each state, with the weights proportional to the estimated number of IVDUs in the state (discussed later). Seroprevalence estimates for a state were based on rates observed in specific locations, primarily from data obtained from intraveneous (IV) drug abuse treatment facilities in major cities (Dougherty, 1987); presumably these rates were not simply averaged across the entire state. The data were mostly gathered in 1986 and 1987, but some were gathered in 1984 and 1985. Because seroprevalence rates may change rapidly upward in only a year (as seems to have occurred in New York and Edinburgh), even the 1986 data are out of date for estimating seroprevalence in 1987, let alone 1988. The effect of outdated data on local seroprevalence rates may be to bias the estimates downward to an unknown but possibly appreciable extent.

John Dougherty has suggested that the rates, which "are from the few drug abuse treatment facilities in which planned studies have been conducted," may be underestimates. He noted that many "drug treatment professionals report that IV drug users more likely to be infected with HIV (i.e., engage in more risky behaviors) tend not to seek treatment at drug centers where HIV testing is known to occur but prefer programs in which there is not testing." However, the extent of the avoidance of such treatment programs depends on how much *real* choice a user has of treatment program and whether testing is optional. Dougherty (1987) also notes that "several other lines of evidence indicate that seroprevalence rates are higher for drug users not receiving treatment than for those in treatment programs" (although this author has not seen such evidence). Furthermore, the drug treatment programs include many persons who no longer use needles to inject drugs. At first blush, these considerations would seem to indicate that the estimated seroprevalence rates would be low estimates (for the cities in which they were based). However (even if the judgment of drug treatment professionals is accepted for the moment), merely because the IV drug users more likely to be infected *tend* not to seek treatment at the centers in the studies does not mean that the rates are underestimated since the chippies and other occasional users—who may have very low rates of infection—might be even more underrepresented in the studies. Whether the rates are underestimated due to underrepresentation of the whole IV drug-using population or not depends on who should be included in the denominator of the rate, and that, as noted earlier, depends on the inclusiveness of the definition of IVDU. The suggestion of Newmeyer (1988) that the definition of IVDU exclude chippies has merit; it is important, however, that they be excluded both from the defined population of IVDUs and from the tested groups used to estimate seroprevalence of IVDUs.

The kinds of settings in which the seroprevalence estimates for IVDUs were made include methadone maintenance programs, drug-free treatment programs, detoxification programs, the "street" (seroprevalence testing performed in addicts not currently in treatment programs), and other kinds of drug treatment programs. The clinics and treatment programs were not selected at random, nor were members in the programs selected at random. How well do the populations "sampled" match the population definitions used for developing numbers of regular and occasional IVDUs? This is not known, but there is no reason why they should be close; it has been impossible to pin down any expert with an opinion on this question. As shown in the following section, the population definitions used for estimates of numbers of IVDUs are exceedingly vague regarding frequency of injection. How exactly were the seroprevalence estimates developed for each state and how were the differences between seroprevalence rates for regular and occasional users estimated? Again, we do not know.

HOW WERE NUMBERS OF IVDUs ESTIMATED?

Overview

The revised estimate of 1.1 million IVDUs was chosen by the CDC from among several alternative estimates available at the time. The alternative methods of estimation underlying the numbers in the "Review" are described in the next three sections. These methods are based on aggregation of state agencies' estimates, on national-level estimates for different kinds of drug abusers, and on the assumption (Lange's approach) that the proportions of the adult population in large cities who are IVDUs are constant within classes of cities. The

Newmeyer ratio estimate represents an alternative method that was not considered by the CDC in choosing its estimate.

Three general kinds of techniques are used for estimating the numbers of IVDUs. Terminology varies somewhat, but the practice of the National Association of State Alcohol and Drug Abuse Directors (NASADAD) will be used (Butynski et al., 1987:41–42) to classify them as "direct," "indirect," or "informed guesstimates." *Direct estimates* may be based on the National Household Survey on Drug Abuse (NHS) run by the National Institute on Drug Abuse (NIDA), on dual-systems estimates, or on backward extrapolation. *Indirect estimates* are based on a fitted regression model that attempts to relate indicator data such as number of burglaries or heroin-related deaths to prevalence of IVDUs. Estimates of numbers of IVDUs are obtained by substituting observed (or predicted) values of the indicators into the regression model. Note that the estimation of the regression coefficients depends on the availability of direct estimates. Finally, so-called *informed guesstimates* are produced by one or more people looking at any available indicators or other correlates of IVDU prevalence and making a loose guess about the number of IVDUs. Both the indirect estimation and the informed guesstimation are dependent on direct estimates somewhere along the line. Thus, the accuracy of any estimates of the number of IVDUs can be no greater than the accuracy of the direct estimates. A brief description of the three direct estimation methods is now provided.

The NHS attempts to measure drug use and prevalence in the general household population aged 12 and over. The survey excludes by design persons living in transient households or in institutions (including university dormitories and prisons), persons in the military, and persons with no fixed residence. Many heroin users will, therefore, not be covered by the survey. Also, even within the population not excluded, the survey suffers from biases due to nonresponse and underreporting of drug use. Thus, cocaine and amphetamine users may be covered by the survey but may decline to report themselves as drug abusers. The extent of bias in the survey results is unknown but potentially enormous.[2]

Back-extrapolation methods use data on AIDS deaths and HIV

[2]For example, the decennial census is believed to miss as many as 15 percent of all black males aged 20–44; the percentage of IVDUs missed by the census is surely much higher. If 30 percent of the drug abusers are not covered by the census, and if only one in two drug abusers surveyed would admit being a drug abuser, then the number of drug abusers reported by the survey will tend to be only 35 percent of the actual number.

prevalence to estimate the number of IVDUs. Based on seroprevalence studies and on models of disease progression, estimates of the probability that an IVDU will have had AIDS are represented, for example, by P. Then estimates of the number of AIDS cases among IVDUs are developed, N. The number of IVDUs is then estimated by the ratio N/P. Such a technique was used by Newmeyer (1988) to estimate the number of IVDUs in New York City; his method is discussed at the end of this section.[3]

Difficulties with the method are attributable to errors in the estimates P and N. The estimate P is based on nonrandom samples subject to severe but unknown selection biases, as well as errors in the model of disease progression. The estimate N must successfully correct for underreporting of AIDS deaths. In- or out-migration of IVDUs from the geographic area of interest is also a problem, but probably of lesser magnitude. An advantage of this technique is the consistency in the definition of IVDU, as discussed earlier.

Dual-systems estimates, also known as tag-recapture estimates, are perhaps the most widely used direct estimates. One begins with two lists of IVDUs, for example, a list of persons in heroin treatment programs and a list of persons treated in emergency rooms for adverse reactions to heroin abuse. If there are a people on both lists, b people on the first list but not the second, and c people on the second list but not the first, then one may estimate the probability P that an IVDU is on the first list by the fraction of people on the second list who are also on the first list, $P = a/(a+c)$. The number of IVDUs who are on the first list is $N = a+b$. Then the total number of IVDUs is estimated by N/P, or $(a+b)(a+c)/a$. A number of problems with dual-systems estimates have been recognized, both in the drug abuse literature and in the statistical literature (Wolter, 1986). Problems include errors in classifying individuals as to membership on one list

---

[3]Newmeyer also describes a variation on this method in his unpublished note "Four Readily Applicable Methods to Estimate Drug Abuse Prevalence" (personal communication, 1988):

> The method is to ascertain from the medical examiner's [coroner's] toxicology data the relative proportion of decedents with methadone metabolites to decedents with heroin metabolites (metabolite is simply a chemical produced by the body's metabolism of a drug.) If this ratio is, say, 1 to 5, and if it is known that there are 2,000 persons receiving methadone maintenance in the city, it can be hazarded that there are about 10,000 persons attempting to maintain themselves on heroin.

Note that the validity of this method rests on an assumption of equal death rates for methadone and heroin users. For other discussions of the back-extrapolation method, see Brookmeyer and Gail (1986, 1988) and Medley et al. (1987).

or two, possible multiple appearances of an IVDU on a list, variabilities in the selection probabilities for different types of individuals (some IVDUs are more likely to appear on the list than others), migration of IVDUs in and out of the geographic area between the times that the two lists are created, and causal effects of being on one list—enrollment in a treatment program may lessen the chance of a drug-related emergency room incident. The errors arising from variability in selection probabilities and causal effects are sometimes jointly referred to as "correlation bias." Triple-systems estimates are sometimes advocated (Woodward et al., 1984), but the same basic problems remain.

Aggregation of State Agencies' Estimates

State drug abuse authorities submit plans for treating drug abuse to the Alcohol, Drug Abuse, and Mental Health Administration (ADAMHA). These plans contain estimates of numbers of IVDUs in each state. The numbers are developed by the states from a variety of sources, including surveys, treatment data, and drug indicator data. It is worth noting that the state agencies compile the numbers for political purposes, including obtaining block grant funds from ADAMHA (which would put upward pressure on the numbers) and informing state legislators (which could put upward or downward pressure on the numbers, depending on the state). NIDA staff reviewed the states' plans and interviewed the agency directors in California, Illinois, Michigan, New Jersey, New York, and Pennsylvania to confirm the numbers reported in the plans. Those reviews merely verified that the numbers were reported correctly and not that the numbers reported were accurate. In this way, the total number of IVDUs was estimated at 1.28 million.

Also, according to Butynski et al. (1987:41–42), NASADAD asked each state alcohol and drug agency to:

> provide estimates relating to IV drug abuse for Fiscal Year (FY) 1986 for the total number of client admissions to treatment and total number of IV drug abusers in the State. . . . Seventeen (17) states provided data on the total number of IV drug abusers in the State.[4] The highest estimates of IV drug abusers were provided by New York, California, and Texas, in that order. . . . States were also asked to report the basis for their estimates of

[4]The following states were excluded: Alabama, Alaska, Arizona, Arkansas, Colorado, Delaware, District of Columbia, Florida, Georgia, Hawaii, Idaho, Indiana, Kansas, Kentucky, Louisiana, Maine, Montana, Nebraska, Nevada, New Mexico, North Carolina, North Dakota, Ohio, Oklahoma, Oregon, Puerto Rico, South Carolina, South Dakota, Tennessee, Utah, Vermont, Virginia, Virgin Islands, Washington, West Virginia, and Wyoming.

> the total drug abuser population. The largest number of responding States [10] reported that their estimates were based upon indirect measures or indicators. Three States reported that only "guesstimates" were used, and four States indicated that a combination of methods [i.e., a combination of a "guesstimate" and another method] was used.

The total number of IVDUs reported for the 17 states was 1.067 million. If the state plan estimates for the other 33 states, Puerto Rico, the District of Columbia, and the Virgin Islands are included, the total increases to 1.447 million.

The national estimates described above can be no better than the state estimates they are based on. Individual states use quite different methods to estimate the number of IVDUs. Estimation methods for three states (Illinois, California, and New York) and three cities (Chicago, Los Angeles, and New York) are now described.

Illinois and Chicago

The estimate for Illinois is based on data from the Client Oriented Data Acquisition Process (CODAP) and the National Household Survey on Drug Abuse. CODAP collects limited demographic and drug-use information about clients in participating federally or state-funded drug abuse programs. Illinois uses the CODAP and the NHS data to estimate several components. First, the Illinois Department of Alcoholism and Substance Abuse uses the CODAP data for all participating programs to estimate the fraction F_1 of narcotics abusers in Illinois who inject drugs. Second, the proportion F_2 of the U.S. population who are narcotics abusers is estimated from data collected by the NHS. Finally, the estimate of the number of IVDUs in Illinois is derived as $PF_2 \times F_1$, with P equal to the total population of Illinois. The method for estimating the number of IVDUs in Chicago is analogous, with Chicago figures used instead of Illinois figures (Jerome Gross, personal communication, May 20, 1988). The downward bias in the NHS-based estimate of F_2 makes the estimates very untrustworthy.

California and Los Angeles

The estimates of the number of IVDUs in California are formed as the sum of the estimates of numbers of IVDUs shooting amphetamine and cocaine and those shooting opiates. Apparently, persons who inject more than one of these drugs are counted more than once. First, let us consider estimation of amphetamine- and cocaine-shooting IV-DUs. NHS 1983 data from the western region of the country were used to estimate a prevalence rate for the use of amphetamine and cocaine. The estimated prevalence rate was multiplied by the size of the at-risk population to estimate the number of amphetamine and cocaine users. Data from DAWN and the California Drug Abuse Data System (CALDADS) as well as "street data" were used to estimate the fraction of drug abusers who administered the drugs intravenously; the estimates were subjectively adjusted downward slightly to account for selection bias. Then the latter figures were multiplied by the estimated number of amphetamine and cocaine users to estimate the number of amphetamine and cocaine shooters in 1985. Those figures were assumed constant at 97,000 for the years following 1985. As with Illinois, the downward bias of the NHS prevalence rate subjects the California estimate of number of amphetamine and cocaine shooters to great downward bias.

The number of persons shooting opiates is based on extrapolation from a nonlinear regression model fitted to data more than 10 years old. Specifically, a regression was fitted to predict estimated prevalence rates for fiscal years 1974–1975, 1975–1976, 1976–1977, and 1977–1978 from indicators including number of drug-induced deaths, burglaries, new admissions to treatment programs, and number of hepatitis B cases. The prevalence estimates were based on work by John Newmeyer.[5] A quadratic trend was fitted, which leads one to believe that the model was overfitted (only four data points were used to estimate at least three parameters). Rates of prevalence for future years were predicted from values of the indicator data from those years. The model was last run on fiscal year 1982–1983 data, for which the estimate was 102,500. The estimate was subjectively adjusted to 125,000 for fiscal year 1986–1987; numbers are assumed constant since then. The extent of extrapolation, overfitting, and possible weakness in the direct estimates used to calibrate the regression model makes these estimates untrustworthy. The total estimate of IVDUs in California is thus 220,000. The number is taken to refer to hard-core users (Susan Nisenbaum, personal communication, 1988).

The estimate of the number of IVDUs in Los Angeles County is based on multiplication of the number of IVDUs in treatment by a factor. The factor is about 4 or 5 and is based on examination of drug indicator data, but explicit models were not used. The

[5]The manner in which Newmeyer's estimates were prepared is not known, but it is believed that they were based on dual-systems estimation (Susan Nisenbaum, personal communication, 1988).

estimate (about 70,000) includes regular users and occasional users; including users in remission might push the estimate up to 120,000 or more (Donald McAllister, personal communication, 1988). As the accuracy of the factor is unknown, so too is the accuracy of the estimate. However, there is no reason to assume that the accuracy is any higher than that for Chicago.

New York State and New York City

The estimate of the number of IVDUs in New York State is derived as the ratio of the New York City estimate to the fraction F of narcotic abusers in the state who are estimated to reside in New York City; F is estimated from the NHS (Schmeidler and Frank, n.d.). The current estimate for New York City is 240,000. The accuracy of F may be reasonably good to the extent that biases in the NHS cancel out, since F is the ratio of two NHS estimates of narcotic abusers.

The estimate of the number of IVDUs in New York City is based on extrapolation of past estimates of prevalence. In brief, the past estimates were based on regression estimation using drug indicators as predictors, and the regression models were estimated by using a combination of Narcotics Registry and dual-systems estimates. The method is complicated because some of the predictor variables became unavailable and had to be predicted on the basis of other, available indicators. The models are designed to estimate the number of heroin addicts, and those estimates are used without modification to estimate numbers of IVDUs in New York City.

A somewhat more detailed summary of the estimation of the number of IVDUs in New York City follows (Schmeidler et al., 1978). The discussion is longer than that for the other cities because the method is more complicated, more information was available on how New York City's estimates were prepared, and the estimates of the number of IVDUs in New York City are especially critical (see the discussion of Newmeyer's estimate, below).

- The first principal component of 12 indicators of heroin use was computed and used as a predictor variable for regression estimates of numbers of heroin addicts.
- Values of the "dependent variable" (numbers of heroin addicts) for 1970–1974 were provided by the numbers of heroin addicts reported in the New York Narcotics Register, adjusted for duplication, reporting of drugs other than heroin, incarceration, relocation, death, non-addiction, and false inclusion. These adjustments were

largely guesses (particularly the adjustments for death, relocation, and incarceration) and are problematic. The numbers were also adjusted[6] by dual-systems estimates of the numbers of heroin addicts not reported in the Register. Absence of data on the extent of drug abuse or demographic characteristics for persons in the Register meant that no poststratification could be employed and correlation bias could be high, leading to downward pressure on the estimates. Matching errors (false nonmatches) probably occurred, leading to upward pressure (see Woodward et al., 1984). Further upward pressure is present because the population is not closed and the adjustments for out-migration from the population were imperfect. Sampling error is also present. In this way, estimates of the number of heroin addicts in 1970–1974 were prepared.

- Then regression models were fitted to predict smoothed successive differences of logs of 1970–1974 numbers of heroin addicts from the first principal component.
- Estimates for 1975 through 1979 were based directly on the regression model.
- The estimates for 1980 and onward are described as "guesstimates." For example, the estimate for 1980 was taken to be the same as for 1976 because the DAWN reports of heroin-related emergency room admissions were similar for the two years, and the DAWN indicator was believed to be a strong correlate of the number of heroin addicts. The estimate for 1981 was based on quadratic extrapolation from the estimates for 1977–1980.

Despite the commendable ingenuity shown in the methodology for developing the estimates of the number of IVDUs in New York City, the estimates must be regarded as highly suspect. Of most concern are the "guesstimates" used to adjust the Registry data and the fact that the current estimates of the numbers of IVDUs

[6]The adjustments for false positives—people newly reported who had not been previously reported to the Register—were applied to the number denoted as c in the "Overview." An adjustment for "inactivation"—to correct for the fact that not all previously identified persons will persist in their status (due to death, incarceration, cessation of addiction)—was applied to the number denoted as b in the "Overview." Both adjustments are described as "guesstimates," especially the second.

are largely "guesstimates." Although New York City's application of the dual-systems method may be better than most (due to high coverage of the Register), the combination of errors in the dual-systems estimates used to fit the regression is also of concern, as is the change in the viability of the regression model over time. Of course, the regression estimates were not used directly for making estimates for the 1980s, but they do enter into the development of the "guesstimates."

The estimates for New York State are even less accurate, due to error in the factor F described above.

National Estimates

NIDA also explored some arithmetic with national estimates to derive an estimate of 1.1 million IVDUs.[7]

500,000	estimated heroin addicts in 1982
+250,000	heroin IV users, not addicts (NIDA estimate)
+475,000	cocaine heavy users
−150,000	overlap in cocaine/heroin use
+25,000	nonheroin, noncocaine IV users (NIDA estimate)
1,100,000	total.

The author is unaware of the descriptions of the methodology underlying these estimates.

Lange's Approach

Lange utilized several assumptions to develop an estimate of the total number of IVDUs (and their seroprevalence, which is interesting but will not be discussed here). His estimate of the total number of IVDUs is 1.6 million. His first assumption is that the proportion of IVDUs in the general (adult?) population is fairly stable among cities of comparable sizes, and he assumes ratios of 1/25 for cities larger than one-half million and 1/30 for those between 300,000 and 500,000. (These ratios may be interpreted as number of IVDUs in cities in a given size range divided by total population in those

[7]The source for this is an unauthored, undated document "Estimated Number of IV Drug Abusers in U.S." The estimated number of heroin addicts in 1982 is taken from Shreckengost (1983); estimates for the number of heroin IV users who are not addicts and the number of users of IV drugs other than heroin and cocaine are supplied by NIDA; the estimate of the number of cocaine heavy users was reported in the 1985 National Household Survey on Drug Abuse.

cities.) The first assumption is based on "the opinion of many that one-half of IVDU's live in New York City ... and that between 70–75% of them reside in 24 of the largest metropolitan areas. . . ." His second assumption is that 95 percent of the IVDUs in the United States reside in the 50 largest cities. The estimate of 1.6 million follows (W. Robert Lange, personal communication, 1988). There is probably more heterogeneity in the proportions of IVDUs in the cities than Lange's figures imply, although that flaw need not be critical for estimating the total number of IVDUs across the cities. The accuracy of Lange's estimate is unknown.

Newmeyer's Ratio Estimate

John Newmeyer recently developed a method for estimating the number of IVDUs in Standard Metropolitan Statistical Areas (SMSAs) reporting to the DAWN system (Newmeyer, 1988). Implicit in the method is an estimator for the number of IVDUs nationally. Newmeyer's method is essentially as follows. Let

Y_i = total number of IVDUs in SMSA i (to be estimated),

U_i = total reported emergency room mentions of heroin/morphine for SMSA i,

V_i = total medical examiner mentions of opiates for SMSA i, except for Newark and Chicago (whose data were deemed problematic),

U^* = sum of U_i over all SMSAs except Newark and Chicago,

V^* = sum of V_i over all SMSAs except Newark and Chicago,

V_i = $\frac{U_i V^*}{U^*}$ for Newark and Chicago SMSAs,

U^{**} = sum of U_i over all SMSAs,

V^{**} = sum of V_i over all SMSAs, and

X_i = $.5(\frac{U_i}{U^{**}} + \frac{V_i}{V^{**}})$.

Newmeyer defines X_i as $\frac{U_i}{U^{**}}$ for Newark and Chicago and as $.5(\frac{U_i}{U^{**}} + \frac{V_i}{V^*})$ for the other SMSAs, which is theoretically slightly inferior but probably of no practical importance. Newmeyer then derives an external estimate of the number of IVDUs in New York City, A_{NY}, which he refers to as an anchor. The ratio $R = A_{NY}/X_{NY}$ is then computed. The estimated number of IVDUs for SMSA i is simply $\hat{Y}_i = RX_i$, and the estimated number for all 17 SMSAs is simply R. The method could be used with SMSAs other than New York as the anchor.

Suppose that $Y_i = \beta X_i + \varepsilon_i$, with ε_i having zero mean. The accuracy of the method depends critically on (1) the accuracy of the anchor A_{NY} and (2) the stability of the assumed relationship (i.e., the variance of ε_i). Both factors are important. Even if A_{NY} were known accurately (Newmeyer uses 160,000 for A_{NY}), if ε_{NY} is very large (small) then the overall estimate will be too large (small). One could attempt to improve the method by using principal components of several indicators or a multivariate ratio estimator, but the critical dependence on items (1) and (2) would remain.

Newmeyer's estimated anchor for New York is critical and may be controversial. As he notes (Newmeyer, 1988),

> There seems to be a consensus among experts in New York that there are about 200,000 IVDUs in that metropolis. I disagree. I have worked hard at modelling the AIDS epidemic among IVDUs in New York, and find that a base population of 120,000 users is as large a figure as can adequately account for the observed small size of their AIDS caseload. Even to make that base number work, I have to assume (1) that the 1982–83 estimates of their HIV seropositivity were too high, (2) that their rate of progression from infection to AIDS diagnosis is no faster than for the gay men in the San Francisco hepatitis study, and (3) that fully 35% of all New York IVDUs who die of HIV-related causes are not enumerated in the AIDS caseload. In this paper, I have used a midpoint between my 120,000 and the 200,000 figure of New York experts. Since the whole analysis depends on the New York "anchor," my estimate of the nation's infected IVDU population would be 25% higher if the New York experts are right—but it would be 25% lower if my New York model is the correct one.

Lange's estimate of the number of IVDUs in the 16 SMSAs with the largest X_i is 910,000 compared to Newmeyer's national figure of 625,000. Newmeyer estimated a total of 140,000 seropositive IVDUs in the 16 SMSAs. Using New York City's estimate of 240,000 for the number of IVDUs there would increase Newmeyer's figures by 50 percent.

CONCLUSIONS

The accuracy of the estimates of the number of IVDUs is not objectively ascertainable, but the estimates (of about 1 million) could well be off by a factor of 2; that is, the true number could conceivably be smaller than 500,000 or greater than 2 million. The closeness of several of the estimates is not persuasive because they cannot be regarded as independent estimates. *The question that persists is who counts as an IVDU; what definition is being used?* The judgment made here about the accuracy is based on a review of the estimation methods. Other reasonable people could read the review presented here and come to different conclusions.

REFERENCES

Brookmeyer, R., and Gail, M. H. (1986) Minimum size of the acquired immunodeficiency syndrome (AIDS) epidemic in the United States. *Lancet* 2:1320–1322.

Brookmeyer, R., and Gail, M. H. (1988) A method for obtaining short-term projections and lower bounds on the size of the AIDS epidemic. *Journal of the American Statistical Association* 83:301–308.

Butynski, W., Record, N., Bruhn, P., and Canova, D. (1987) *State Resources and Services Related to Alcohol and Drug Abuse Problems, Fiscal Year 1986.* Washington D.C.: NASADAD.

Centers for Disease Control (CDC). (1987) Human immunodeficiency virus infection in the United States: A review of current knowledge. *Morbidity and Mortality Weekly Report* 36(Suppl. S-6):1–48.

Dougherty, J. (1987) Estimates of Numbers of IV Drug Users Infected with HIV: Preliminary Data. Unpublished manuscript, December 5.

Gerstein, D. R. (1976) The structure of heroin communities in relation to methadone maintenance. *American Journal of Drug and Alcohol Abuse* 3:571–587.

Medley, G. F., Anderson, R. M., Cox, D. R., and Billard, L. (1987) Incubation period of AIDS in patients infected via blood transfusion. *Nature* 328:719–721.

Mosteller, F. (1977) Assessing unknown numbers: Order of magnitude estimation. In W. Fairley and F. Mosteller (eds.), *Statistics and Public Policy.* Reading, Mass.: Addison-Wesley.

Newmeyer, J. (1988) Estimating the Total of Seropositive IVDUs from SMSA Data. Unpublished manuscript, May 1988.

Schmeidler, J., and Frank, B. (n.d.) Estimating the Number of Narcotic Abusers. New York State Division of Substance Abuse Services, undated.

Schmeidler, J., Frank, B., Johnson, B., and Lipton, D. S. (1978) Seeking truth in heroin indicators: The case of New York City. *Drug and Alcohol Dependence* 3:345–358.

Shreckengost, R. C. (1983) *Heroin: A New View.* Washington, D.C.: U. S. Central Intelligence Agency.

Woodward, J. A., Retka, R. L., and Ng, L. (1984) Construct validity of heroin abuse indicators. *The International Journal of the Addictions* 19:93–117.

Wolter, K. M. (1986) Some coverage error models for census data. *Journal of the American Statistical Association* 81:338–346.

Monitoring the Spread of HIV Infection

Charles F. Turner and Robert E. Fay

The current picture of the AIDS epidemic is clouded. In 1986, the U.S. Public Health Service (PHS, 1986) estimated that approximately 1.0 to 1.5 million Americans are infected by the HIV virus. These infected persons, often unaware of their illness, can transmit the disease to others. (Indeed, high rates of transmission have been observed [Fischl et al., 1987] even when one partner had been diagnosed with AIDS and both partners had been counseled about the dangers of unprotected sexual intercourse.) Current studies suggest that a large proportion of this infected population may eventually develop AIDS. Thus, in terms of both the spread of the epidemic and its ultimate cost, the estimate that there are 1.0 to 1.5 million infected persons presents an even grimmer picture than the actual number who have developed AIDS (72,645 reported cases in the

---

This paper was prepared during the spring of 1987 in reaction to proposals for routine (or mandatory) testing of all hospital patients, marriage license applicants, and others, in order to obtain "better" epidemiological data on the spread of HIV. The paper was widely circulated in manuscript form during the summer and fall of 1987. This background paper is the same manuscript that was originally circulated (save for updating of numbers and copyediting); thus it does not review recent experiences of the National Center for Health Statistics and the Research Triangle Institute in their efforts to implement a survey program of the type described in this manuscript. This manuscript is included as a background paper to the committee's report because it describes the design problems that must be solved in order to use sample surveys to monitor HIV prevalence (see Chapter 1). Where appropriate, editorial notes have been appended to describe significant events that have occurred since the paper was prepared in 1987.—*ED.*

At the time the original manuscript was prepared, Charles Turner was a Scholar in Residence and Robert Fay a consultant at the National Research Council.

United States as of September 5, 1988, according to the Centers for Disease Control [CDC, 1988]).

Regrettably, there appears to be far less certainty about national estimates of the number of infected individuals than about estimates of the number of AIDS cases. At present there exists no comprehensive system for monitoring the prevalence of human immunodeficiency virus (HIV) in the United States or any other nation.

In this paper, we briefly review the uncertainties inherent in current estimates of the prevalence of HIV infection in the United States. Subsequently, we identify some of the statistical requirements of a reliable system for monitoring the spread of HIV infection in the U.S. population and the pitfalls involved in reliance upon data derived from mandatory (or routine) screening of convenient populations such as applicants for marriage licenses, hospital patients, and so on. We will then outline some considerations involved in mounting a practical survey program to provide the raw data required for such a monitoring system.

While this discussion draws upon the situation that prevailed in the United States in early 1987, the issues and methods we discuss continue to be of relevance in this country (see Chapter 1), and may have applications in other nations.

CURRENT ESTIMATES

Various attempts have been made to estimate the total number of persons infected with HIV. Table 1 presents three such estimates for the United States, in addition to the PHS estimates. It will be noted that these estimates vary widely; the largest estimate (2.49 million) is more than three times larger than the smallest (0.75 million).

We will briefly review some of the sources of uncertainty in these estimates. We commence by observing that the estimates are highly discrepant, and, therefore, insufficient to provide reliable monitoring of the spread of HIV infection in the population. Furthermore, it appears that the uncertainties in these estimates follow from the procedures (and data) that have been used to generate the estimates.

Proportional Model

A key element in the calculations of Curran et al. (1985) and Sivak and Wormser (1985), for example, was the fraction

$$\frac{N_{AIDS}}{N_{HIV}},$$

TABLE 1 Estimates of Number of Persons Infected with HIV in the United States

Source	Population	As of	Estimate
Curran et al. (1985)	Total population	May 1985	750 thousand[a]
PHS (1986)	IV drug users and homosexual men	June 1986	1.25 million[b]
PHS (1987)	IV drug users and homosexual men	Nov. 1987	1.17 million[c]
Sivak and Wormser (1985)	Total population	July 1985	1.76 million
Rees (1987)	Total population	Dec. 1984	2.49 million

[a]Estimated as the interval from 0.5 million to 1.0 million. The midpoint of the interval is listed in the table.
[b]Estimated as the interval from 1.0 million to 1.5 million. The midpoint of the interval is listed in the table.
[c]Estimated as the interval from 945,000 to 1.41 million. The midpoint of the interval is listed in the table.

where N_{AIDS} is the total number of reported AIDS cases and N_{HIV} is the total number of persons infected with the AIDS virus (HIV). This fraction can change substantially as an epidemic progresses. For infectious diseases with long latency periods such as AIDS, the fraction will be zero for a long time after the infection enters a new population. This occurs because the denominator (number of infections) can increase rapidly while the numerator (number of diagnosed cases) remains zero. Similarly, in a static population that has been saturated with infection, the denominator of the fraction may remain constant since all vulnerable members of the population have been infected, however, the numerator (diagnosed cases) will continue to grow. The instability of this fraction makes its use problematic, particularly when estimates from one subpopulation are applied to another subpopulation in which the infection may have been established for a different length of time.

Multiplicative Model

A different procedure was used to derive the most widely quoted estimate of HIV prevalence in the United States (presented in the Public Health Service's [1986] Coolfont report). That report concluded that "by extrapolating all available data, we estimate that there are between 1 and 1.5 million infected persons in those groups [IV drug users and homosexual men] at present." Although explicit calculations are not shown, the Coolfont report indicates that its authors estimated that 2.5 million American men between the ages of 16 and 55 are exclusively homosexual throughout their lives and 5 to 10 million more have some homosexual contact. Similarly, they estimated (without explicit reference to a source) that 750,000 Americans inject heroin or other intravenous (IV) drugs at least once a week and that similar numbers inject drugs less frequently. These estimates of population size were then multiplied by estimates of the prevalence of HIV infections among these groups in order to generate the widely quoted estimate that there are 1.0 to 1.5 million infected persons in these two groups. (The prevalence rates used in these calculations were not published but the report states that HIV prevalence estimates range from 20 to 50 percent for homosexual men and from 10 to 50 percent for users of IV drugs.)

This procedure (and a hybrid employed in the calculations of Sivak and Wormser) is vulnerable to errors of unknown magnitude in both multiplicands. Note, for example, that the Coolfont estimate used data collected by Kinsey and coworkers (1948) in the 1940s in order to estimate the *current* number of male homosexuals in the United States. Even 30 years ago, Kinsey's data were widely regarded as unreliable for use in making such estimates because the research did not employ probability sampling and because the respondents were disproportionately drawn from the Midwest and from the college-educated segment of the population (see Terman, 1948; Wallis, 1948; Cochran et al., 1953). Today, a further leap of faith is required since the relative size of the (self-reported) homosexual population must be assumed to have remained unchanged since the 1940s. Furthermore, we note that estimates of the prevalence of HIV infection among homosexual men were not derived from representative samples.

These factors introduce substantial uncertainty into the resultant estimates of HIV prevalence. Indeed, the multiplication used in this estimation introduces some unique problems in that errors in the two multiplicands are related, although the form of the relationship is not known with any precision. Consider, for example, the definition of what has loosely been termed the "homosexual population." If the definition of this population is restricted to persons whose sexual contacts have been exclusively (or predominantly) homosexual, the population will be smaller than if men who have had any homosexual contacts since the onset of the epidemic are included. Clearly, however, the estimates of HIV prevalence will also change (by unknown amounts) depending upon which definition is used. (May and Anderson [1987] provide useful models representing the underlying processes.) Parallel uncertainties afflict estimates of the number of persons who use IV drugs and the rates of infection in this subpopulation.

Temporal Distribution Model

The most recent estimate (as of June 1987) of the number of persons infected with HIV in the United States was produced by Rees (1987) using a different approach. Rees fit a normal distribution to the frequency of AIDS cases as a function of time elapsed between the initial HIV infection and the diagnosis of AIDS. The parameters of this distribution ($\mu = 15$, $\sigma = 5$) were selected on the basis of a relatively small sample ($n = 144$) of persons who developed AIDS from blood transfusions.

The resultant estimate that 2.49 million Americans are infected with HIV is the largest of the four estimates in Table 1. Indeed, this estimate is actually more extreme than it appears since it refers to an earlier date than the other estimates (December 1984) and it includes only "HIV infections that will result in AIDS over the next 30 years or so" (Rees, 1987:345).

Although the procedures proposed by Rees open another avenue for modeling, his estimates must be treated with caution. Note that Rees's selection of the normal distribution and its parameters ($\mu = 15$, $\sigma = 5$) was based upon the relative timing of AIDS onset for those who have developed AIDS from transfusions. The usual appropriate denominators (i.e., the number of persons infected via transfusions *or* the total number of persons infected via transfusion who will *eventually* develop AIDS) were not available.

An important implication of Rees's choice of parameters is that only 5.3 percent of those eventually developing AIDS (under his model) would be expected to do so in the first seven years after infection. This rate appears quite low. Such a low presumed rate of AIDS onset in the early years after infection implies large multipliers for each AIDS case observed during this period. It will be several years before the validity of Rees's assumptions can be fully tested;[1] however, the fit of Rees's model is particularly poor in the first year. Rees's fitted values for the first year of infection add up to 20.98 AIDS cases through 1983, compared to 8.5 observed cases. (Fractional observed cases result from Rees's splitting of ambiguous cases between adjacent years.)

---

[1]For present purposes, the committee concluded that a mean of 8 may be more appropriate (see Chapter 2, and Lui et al., 1988).—*ED.*

Because of such uncertainties in estimation procedures, it is, perhaps, not surprising that the estimates shown in Table 1 vary by a factor of 3. Nor is it surprising that similar uncertainties exist in other nations. (Rees's model, for example, estimates that 109,000 U.K. residents were infected by mid-1985. Rees observes, however, that "there seems to be a general opinion that there were about 30,000 infections in the middle of 1986, between a quarter and a third of my estimate for a year earlier" (Rees, 1987:345).

PROPOSAL

Inaccurate estimates of the size of the population infected with HIV are potentially dangerous because (among other reasons) such estimates may generate a false sense of security—or a false sense of alarm—among those charged with formulating policies to cope with the epidemic. The 1986 report of the Institute of Medicine/National Academy of Sciences (IOM/NAS, 1986) concluded that better information is needed to quantify the number of persons infected with HIV. This report recommended undertaking "extensive and repeated surveys of seropositivity to determine the incidence and prevalence of infection by age, race/ethnicity, geographic area, and sex" (p. 200). Epidemiological precedence for this approach is somewhat limited, but several factors specific to the AIDS epidemic argue for the use of *national sample surveys* to obtain these data. Specifically,

- For many infectious diseases there is only a short period between infection and manifestation of symptoms. For HIV infection, however, the latency period is several years; thus, the size of the currently infected population will remain unknown if one relies solely upon systems that monitor the number of AIDS cases.
- Sample surveys are typically ineffective at measuring very rare characteristics unless the specific subpopulation can be identified in advance. Regrettably, it appears that HIV infection is no longer extremely rare. Sample survey methods can now give effective estimates of the size of this population, without the need to explicitly identify high-risk individuals, such as homosexual males or intravenous drug users.
- Controlling the spread of the AIDS epidemic will depend critically upon public education programs and other social interventions. Periodic sample surveys of the prevalence of HIV infection in the population will provide

one important indicator of the overall impact of these programs.

A clearer picture of the magnitude of the epidemic in terms of the prevalence and incidence of infection and its distribution by age, sex, geographic area, ethnic group, and other distinguishing characteristics is a prerequisite for designing and targeting intervention efforts in a rational and cost-effective manner. Without such information, risk reduction efforts will always be targeted less than optimally. Additionally, there will be no way of monitoring on a broad scale how effective our interventions are in combatting the spread of the epidemic. Information on trends in HIV prevalence will also be essential in planning for the provision of health care.

REQUIREMENTS

Given the range of estimates shown in Table 1, few thoughtful observers would question the need for *more reliable* evidence on the current prevalence of HIV infection in the American population. With a minimal amount of reflection, most observers would also conclude that our need for up-to-date information on HIV prevalence will continue into the future—at least until such time as AIDS ceases to be a medical threat. Thus, reliable estimates of HIV prevalence must be *obtained at regular intervals* in order to track the spread of the epidemic.

In addition to the requirement that HIV prevalence estimates be generalizable to the population and regularly updated, it is also desirable that the estimates permit disaggregation sufficient for prevalence (and changes in prevalence over time) to be monitored in particular demographic (and other) subgroups of the population. Thus, prevalence estimates that allow us to *separately* track the spread of the infection among unmarried youth, for example, may be as critical as estimates of prevalence in the entire population.

Even this minimal set of *desiderata* constrains our data-gathering activity in several important ways. It requires that our estimates be

- representative of the entire population that is at risk,
- based on data collected at regular intervals, and
- capable of providing estimates for subpopulations of interest.

LIMITATIONS OF SAMPLES OF CONVENIENCE

The requirement that prevalence for the American population be characterized demands that *probability samples* be drawn from that population. Samples of convenience—even when they are extremely large—are not sufficient to satisfy the preceding list of statistical needs. Prevalence data derived from blood donors, armed forces recruits, persons voluntarily seeking testing, and other special populations are constitutionally incapable of providing reliable information on the key question: What is the prevalence of HIV infection in the general population?

The assumption that prevalence *per se* or trends in prevalence in these special populations will be mirrored in the general population requires a leap of faith. Given the seriousness of the AIDS epidemic, such leaps should be discouraged to the extent scientifically possible. What is needed are better data. With better data such assumptions can be avoided.[2]

It follows from such considerations that proposals to initiate mandatory or routine HIV-antibody testing of hospital patients, applicants for marriage licenses, and so forth will not provide reliable evidence on the prevalence of HIV infection in the population.[3]

These convenient populations provide pieces of information from a larger puzzle, but they provide this information in a manner that does not readily permit us to reassemble that puzzle. We know, for example, that hospital patients are a population that is both substantially older and sicker than the general population. We also know that some patients may be admitted to hospitals several times during a brief period and thus may be double- or triple-counted with such an approach. Healthy adults, on the other hand, are unlikely to be hospitalized.

---

[2]This is not to say that HIV prevalence data should no longer be collected from these convenient sources. However, careful studies are needed that document the nature of the interrelationships (if any) between trends in HIV prevalence in the general population (estimated from probability samples) and trends in HIV prevalence in convenient (but self-selected) samples such as blood donors and military recruits. Over time, such studies might provide an empirical basis for broadening the interpretation of trend data derived from such special populations.

[3]Mandatory (or routine) testing of hospital patients has been proposed for monitoring the course of the epidemic as well as for other purposes, such as "protecting health care workers." The deficiency of such proposals for epidemiological purposes does not, of course, imply that such testing might not serve these other purposes. It should be noted, however, that the recent report of the Institute of Medicine/National Academy of Sciences (1986:124) recommended that "the question of whether to undergo [HIV] testing should be a personal health care decision to be made by an individual, ideally following counselling by health care professionals."

The fact that the hospital population is considerably older than the general population will doubtlessly introduce a downward bias in prevalence estimates for any sexually transmitted disease that has been introduced recently into the population. On the other hand, persons with AIDS are more likely to be hospitalized than members of the general population. Furthermore, persons with HIV infection (but not diagnosed as having AIDS) may also be more likely to be hospitalized.[4] Such factors would introduce an upward bias in prevalence estimates derived from hospital populations (versus estimates derived from the general population). Finally, one cannot rule out the possibility that a program of routine screening as a condition of hospital admission would discourage persons from seeking hospital care if they believe they may be infected. Besides the terrible impact this would have on the individuals involved, it would introduce another source of bias into hospital-based prevalence measures.

Adjustments of hospital prevalence data might be attempted. For example, projections to the national population might adjust the hospital data to match the age distribution of the national population. Even the most ingenious adjustments, however, could not escape the essential uncertainties of using HIV prevalence rates for persons who pass through hospitals to estimate rates for persons who are not hospitalized. Age (or other) adjustments merely restrict the domain of our assumptions. Thus an age-adjustment procedure might have us assume that the prevalence of HIV infection among hospitalized 20- to 29-year-olds, for example, is equivalent to that for 20- to 29-year-olds in general. The validity of such assumptions would remain unknown.

Doubtlessly, other restrictions could be introduced. For example, diagnosed AIDS patients might be excluded from the hospital estimates (relying on the CDC case-reporting system for an estimate of the number of persons who are both HIV-antibody positive and diagnosed with AIDS). We might also derive estimates of HIV prevalence using only patients admitted for reasons that appear medically unrelated to HIV infection (e.g., accidental injuries).

Even such seemingly attractive strategies have the potential for introducing bias. We know, for example, that the propensity of individuals to seek medical care (given similar symptoms) is correlated with a number of factors including socioeconomic status. The

---

[4] Subsequent to the preparation of this draft (in early 1987) Des Jarlais and coworkers (1988) reported a sharp rise in non-AIDS deaths from pneumonia (not *pneumocystis carinii*), tuberculosis, and endocarditis among HIV-infected IV drug users.—*ED.*

prevalence of HIV infection is unlikely to be the same in all social classes, and prevalence estimates derived from hospital samples necessarily reflect the joint operation of socioeconomic variations in hospital admission rates and differences across social classes in the rates of HIV infection. Furthermore, although using "accidental" injury cases may *seem* to introduce an element of randomness into the sampling, the probability of accidental injury may not be independent of HIV antibody status. For example, IV drug users may be at greater risk of accidental injury due to impaired cognitive functioning (and, therefore, more likely to appear in a sample of hospitalized accident victims). Since IV drug users are at risk of HIV infection due to needle-sharing practices, prevalence rates could be biased by the joint operation of these two factors.

Inventive readers will be able to imagine a myriad of other potential biases, methods that might reduce them, further biases that remain or are newly introduced, and so forth *ad infinitum*. Such exercises are limited only by the fertility of one's imagination. The lesson taught by such exercises is that data from hospital and other seemingly "convenient" populations can never provide completely trustworthy evidence of the prevalence of HIV infection in the general population.

A concrete example of the limitations of convenience samples is provided by recent reports in the popular media that the prevalence of infection detected among military recruits in the United States did not increase during the first 15 months of the military's testing program (see, for example, *Washington Post*, May 15, 1987).[5] Although this result may appear encouraging, it is actually quite difficult to interpret. We cannot, for example, rule out the possibility that potential military recruits who had engaged in high-risk behaviors were discouraged from volunteering for military service by publicity about the mandatory testing of recruits.

Rather than expanding the quixotic enterprise of mandatory testing to include other "convenient" populations, we believe a program of regularly conducted surveys that obtain blood for testing from probability samples of the national population *should be considered*. Such a research program might, if properly designed and executed, provide a simpler, more reliable, less controversial, and less costly way of monitoring the spread of HIV infection in the population. In the following pages we outline some of the factors that should be considered and tested in planning such an endeavor.

---

[5] "AIDS Rate Remains Stable Among U.S. Military Recruits Since Testing Started in 1985; Statistics Puzzle Experts," *Washington Post*, May 15, 1987:A1.

DESIGN CONSIDERATIONS

Overview

An (*oversimplified*) summary of such a survey program might involve the following steps. The population to be surveyed would be identified. An appropriate probability sampling procedure would be designed, and survey procedures would be pretested. During this preliminary stage, a decision might be made to exclude certain segments of the total population from the survey (e.g., the elderly and young children). If the survey used a household sampling frame as one component of its sample design, sampled households would subsequently receive a letter which would (1) advise them that an interviewer would be calling at their household and (2) inform them of the purpose of the survey and the safeguards ensuring their anonymity. Subsequently, a survey interviewer (together with a phlebotomist) would visit the household. The interviewer would ascertain how many eligible respondents lived in the household (excluding persons outside the target population), and a respondent would be selected at random from among the eligible respondents (if any). The survey interviewer would ask the designated respondent a short series of demographic questions and subsequently request that the respondent provide a blood sample.

Results of HIV testing of these blood samples would provide a basis for estimating HIV prevalence in the total population and selected demographic subgroups.[6] Repeated annually (or at another suitable interval), such surveys might provide a reliable way of monitoring the spread of HIV infections in the population.

With this oversimplified summary of the procedure in mind, let us review in greater detail some of the important considerations in the design and execution of such a survey.

Sample Size and Efficiency

For purposes of initial discussion, a sample of approximately 10,000 persons might be considered for HIV screening. We might, in addition, restrict the sample to persons age 18 to 54. This restriction would avoid problems of consent below age 18 and reflect the practical judgment that those 55 and over are likely to contribute little

[6]In addition to providing statistical data on prevalence, the stored sera from this program could provide a valuable resource for future biomedical and epidemiological researchers. It is important, therefore, that plans be made for long-term storage of the sera collected in these surveys.

to the overall total of seropositive individuals. (As discussed below, samples that are substantially larger than 10,000 may be desirable in order to provide reliable estimates of prevalence in important subpopulations.)

Because the survey estimate will be based on a sample, some random error due to the selection of the sample will be present. If approximately 1.5 million Americans are infected at the time the first survey is done, the reliability of a survey estimate based on a sample of 10,000 could be stated as a relative standard deviation of about 10 percent. In other words, if the expected sample estimate (averaged over all possible samples) were 1.5 million persons, then two times out of three the sample estimate should be within 150,000 persons of this value, that is, within the interval from 1.35 to 1.65 million persons. Furthermore, 95 percent of the time, the sample estimate should fall within the wider interval from 1.2 to 1.8 million persons.

This random variation is an inevitable consequence of survey work. A survey estimate with this degree of reliability would be tremendously more informative, however, than currently available estimates. As Table 1 indicates, current estimates vary over a much wider range.

Such a survey could also provide separate estimates for demographic subgroups (e.g., for different age groups, marital statuses, minority groups, and genders). The relative reliability of these estimates, however, would be less than that for estimates based on the whole sample. To provide more reliable estimates for such subpopulations, larger samples (and oversampling of certain subpopulations) are required. Consider, for example, estimates of HIV prevalence for females. If 90 percent of HIV infections are assumed to be found in males, then only 150,000 of the presumed 1.5 million infected persons would be female. If half of our survey sample of 10,000 were female, estimates might have a coefficient of variation of about 30 percent. This variation is too large for most purposes (although, arguably, it might be an improvement over present estimates).[7] If, however, the sample included 20,000 women, the coefficient of variation should be in the range of 15 percent, yielding a 95 percent confidence interval of $105,000 \leq n \leq 195,000$ (if 150,000 is the expected value averaged over all possible samples).

[7] The launching in 1989 of a large-scale neonatal HIV screening program (see Chapter 1) will allow the HIV serostatus of childbearing women to be estimated directly. (Newborns carry the maternal antibodies to HIV, whether or not the newborn itself is infected.) This new development may reduce the need for such information from a sample survey. Although it should be noted that the newborn screening can provide no information on the HIV status of women who have not borne children.—*ED.*

Sample sizes of 10,000 (or even 50,000), it should be noted, are not large in comparison to other surveys conducted by federal statistical agencies. The Bureau of the Census, for example, interviews a sample of over 60,000 respondents *each month* to provide data for the monthly unemployment estimates. Similarly, approximately 40,000 households are interviewed each year in the Health Interview Survey program of the National Center for Health Statistics (NCHS).

Design

The proposed survey might profitably employ a complex sampling design. Oversampling of groups with high risk, followed by appropriate weighting of these groups in forming the survey estimates can improve the overall reliability. So, for example, oversampling younger, unmarried persons relative to older married couples could produce substantial gains in overall sampling efficiency (on the assumption that the former will yield a higher proportion of HIV-positive cases than the latter). Oversampling could also improve the reliability of estimates for specific demographic groups (e.g., blacks and Hispanics).

To take one simple example of the nature of such a sample design, let us suppose that the geographic distribution of HIV infections mirrored the distribution of AIDS cases (as of April 6, 1987). A complex sample design considering only this one factor might divide the United States into three geographic strata:

1. the New York and San Francisco Standard Metropolitan Statistical Areas (SMSAs), which had a population of 12.37 million in the 1980 census and 12,680 AIDS cases as of April 6, 1987;
2. the SMSAs ranked third to seventeenth in number of diagnosed AIDS cases, which had a total population of 44.27 million and 11,663 AIDS cases; and
3. the rest of the United States, which had a population of 173.47 million in the 1980 census and 9,377 AIDS cases diagnosed as of April 6, 1987.

If only this geographic distribution is considered, an optimum sample allocation would assign approximately 15 percent of the survey sample to the first stratum, 30 percent to the second, and 55 percent to the third. This allocation would reduce sampling variation in estimates of the prevalence rate by disproportionately drawing samples from geographical areas where there is presumptive evidence that the prevalence rate is high. Thus stratum 3, which has a lower (presumed) prevalence rate, would be allocated 55 percent of the sample even though it represents 75 percent of the total population. (The final survey estimates, of course, would employ an appropriate reweighting to derive national estimates that take account of the disproportional allocation of the sample to these geographic strata.) A complex sample design employing only these three geographical strata could reduce the sampling variance by as much as 24 percent (compared to a design that allocated the sample in proportion to the total population of these areas). Further refinements of the sample design (e.g., taking into account variations in AIDS prevalence by age, marital status, or race and ethnicity) might reduce the sampling error even further, perhaps by as much as 40 to 50 percent in total.[8]

Interview Data

Such a survey should collect, at a minimum, information on age, race and ethnicity, gender, and marital status from the respondents. Respondents are almost always willing to supply such information, so these questions should not threaten respondent cooperation. The resulting information about the spread of HIV infection in different geographic areas and among various demographic subgroups could be of great practical and scientific value. Questions on sexual practices and IV drug use, on the other hand, would also be highly informative but could reduce the level of cooperation. Hence, we suggest that such sensitive questions should be omitted from the national probability sample proposed here, *unless pretesting indicated that these data could be obtained without decreasing the response rate for the blood test.*

Cost

An HIV survey of the sort outlined is likely to cost *less than* $400 per sample case (this includes development and processing costs). Thus, the cost of an annual survey of 10,000 respondents should not

[8]Care must be exercised to ensure that decisions to decrease the sampling error of the overall estimate do not compromise the ability to obtain adequately reliable estimates of HIV prevalence in important subpopulations. So, for example, the design should not allocate sample disproportionately to male respondents, even though men make up the preponderance of current AIDS cases. (Changes over time in HIV prevalence among women can provide an important indicator of the extent of heterosexual transmission in the population. Thus, estimates must be reliable enough to track changes in the prevalence rate for women.)

exceed $4 million. (Because some of the costs of the survey are fixed, increasing the sample size by a factor of four should not produce a fourfold increase in survey costs.)

With the annual federal budget for AIDS projected to exceed $1 billion in the near future and with even larger costs being borne by individual AIDS victims, state and local governments, insurers, and the health care system), the proposed expenditure does not seem prohibitively expensive. When compared to the costs of mandatory testing programs that have recently been discussed, the costs of even a vastly expanded survey program would be small. The cost of HIV testing performed at alternative sites with appropriate pre- and posttest counseling averages approximately $40 per individual (IOM/NAS, 1986:17). Even if the cost of blood tests and counseling for persons applying for marriage licenses were only one quarter of this amount (i.e., $10 per individual), the total annual cost would be only approximately $50 million in the United States. Mandatory screening of all patients admitted to hospitals would be much more expensive (in 1982 there were 39 million such admissions).

Auspices

In most cases, government statistical agencies obtain higher levels of cooperation from the public than other survey organizations (see, for example, National Research Council, 1978:42, Table 1). We think therefore that an effort by one or more federal statistical agencies might be a reasonable approach. The possibility of using a private survey research firm, with a well-established record for quality, to carry out this work should not be excluded. Indeed, there are circumstances (see below) in which such a strategy would be mandatory.

The possibility of adding HIV testing to an ongoing survey should also not be excluded. Survey designers, however, would need to be sensitive to possible adverse reaction to such "piggybacking." Surveys are frequently perceived as involving an implicit social contract between the survey taker and the respondent. Respondents contacted to take part in an immunological health survey may more readily appreciate the importance of blood testing than respondents in another survey who might view an added request for a blood sample as irrelevant to their original commitment. Furthermore, researchers gathering survey data for other purposes might justifiably worry about the effects that such piggybacking might have on their own data collection.

Pretesting

Most surveys require a period of "pretesting" to evaluate the effect of the questionnaire and other survey procedures on the quality of the data to be collected. Such testing would be especially critical in developing an effective strategy for this survey, given the emotionally charged atmosphere surrounding public discussions of AIDS. Thus, greeting respondents at the door with "Good afternoon. May I please have a sample of your blood?" is unlikely to yield the desired results. A carefully structured interview, conducted by a well-trained interviewer and followed by blood sampling by a qualified health professional, *may* succeed. A letter stating the purposes and importance of the survey and detailing privacy and confidentiality provisions may help to set the stage for the interview, if mailed to the respondents in advance of the initial contact. Supplemental reading material (or a videotaped presentation) on the importance of the survey may also help to inform respondents of their expected roles. We would anticipate that many details of the survey strategy would be refined and tested in a pilot phase (prior to the formal data-gathering phase of the survey). We will not attempt to anticipate all of those details here. However, three issues are sufficiently important to merit further discussion: (1) assuring the completeness of survey coverage, (2) guaranteeing the confidentiality of survey data, and (3) providing blood test results to interested respondents. We briefly discuss each of these issues below.

Adequacy of Survey Coverage

Some readers may wonder whether it is feasible to achieve high levels of respondent cooperation in surveys that ask randomly selected respondents to provide blood samples. Although it may seem unusual to request that survey respondents provide blood samples, precedent suggests that such surveys are possible and do produce relatively high levels of cooperation. The National Health and Nutrition Examination Survey (NHANES), for example, performs physical examinations and administers a range of tests (including blood tests) to large probability samples of the U.S. population (approximately 21,000 examinations were performed in the most recent surveys). The recent experience of the NHANES program has been that approximately 91 percent of the public consent to a lengthy household health interview, and approximately 73 percent subsequently report to the survey's medical facility for examinations. (It should be noted that although NHANES could provide HIV prevalence estimates, its sampling schedule would not yield timely estimates. According to NCHS personnel, national estimates from the next NHANES survey will not be available until 1991.)

Nonresponse to the NHANES medical examination occurs for various reasons. Empirical studies suggest that nonresponse rates do not vary substantially by sex or race. Examination rates were 71.8 percent for females, 74.4 percent for males, 72.7 percent for whites, 75.6 percent for blacks, and 74.3 percent for other racial groups. There is, however, a monotonic decrease in examination rates with increasing age. Medical examinations were completed with 81 percent of designated respondents aged 6 months to 17 years, 74 percent of 18- to 34-year-olds, 69 percent of 35- to 54-year-olds, and 64 percent of persons aged 55 or older. The NCHS (1982:Appendix 1) reports, nonetheless, that various comparative studies indicate that respondents who do not undergo medical examinations in the NHANES program have self-reported health characteristics similar to respondents who do undergo those examinations. Similarly, Forthofer (1983:507) finds that after standard NCHS nonresponse and poststratification adjustments, "there is excellent agreement in the marginal distribution of variables between NHANES-II for examined persons and the 1976 National Health Interview Survey (NHIS)" (which achieved a 96 percent response rate).

The response rates from the NHANES demonstrate that most respondents are willing to provide blood samples in a national health survey. Three features of the proposed HIV survey might encourage even higher response rates than those obtained in the NHANES. First, the survey focuses on a health problem of pressing national importance. Second, restricting the survey interview to a few questions will minimize the burden on respondents. Finally, by drawing blood samples in the respondents' homes, the survey eliminates the need for respondents to travel to a central site for testing.

Although these factors encourage the belief that blood samples can be obtained from a substantial proportion of eligible respondents, it must be recognized that HIV blood testing is an emotionally and politically charged issue. As noted above, careful pretesting (and other measures) will be required to explore the feasibility and refine the details of any such measurement program. *It is vital that sufficient time and resources be devoted to these preliminary research activities* because they will have a major impact on the quality and usefulness of the resultant data.

Several potential impediments to adequate survey coverage can be identified at the outset. First, household-based sampling frames will not obtain data from persons who are not attached to a household. Such sampling frames will miss persons who are homeless or who live in prisons, hospitals, and other institutions. An HIV prevalence survey using a household sampling frame will, therefore, underrepresent some important subgroups (e.g., current or past IV drug users) if those subgroups are disproportionately homeless or institutionalized. In designing a survey, separate estimates must be obtained for important subpopulations that will be missed or underrepresented in household surveys (e.g., by drawing samples from prisoners or persons in drug treatment centers).

More troubling than the loss of identifiable segments of the population from the sampling frame is the loss of an *unidentifiable* fraction of the population because some respondents choose not to cooperate with the survey. As this fraction increases, the claim that the survey "represents" the general population is weakened. For our purposes, this threat is particularly serious because we are seeking to assess a relatively uncommon characteristic (HIV seropositivity) in a situation where one might expect noncooperation to be correlated with the respondent's known or suspected seropositivity. That is to say, persons who know or suspect that they are infected may be more likely to refuse to participate in the survey.[9]

Minimizing such refusals will be major challenge. Indeed, it must be recognized at the outset that it is both impossible to eliminate refusals entirely and likely, even under the best of circumstances, that these refusals will introduce some bias. As a consequence, estimation of HIV prevalence will require some imputation of missing data.[10]

Furthermore, it is important to recognize that *the survey effort could fail completely because of substantial noncooperation by members of the public.* Hopefully, this failure would be detected during pretesting, so that the cost of failing would be minimized.

Guaranteeing Anonymity

A first step in reducing noncooperation is to ensure that *both* in fact and in the perceptions of potential respondents, the survey poses no actual or potential threat. Given the level of public concern about

[9]Subsequent to the drafting of this paper, Hull and coworkers (1988) Reported results demonstrating this phenomenon in a situation in which *confidential* testing was offered to clients of an STD clinic—*ED.*

[10]To assist in this process, the suggestion has been made that a recent sample of respondents from another survey (e.g., the Health Interview Survey) might profitably be used. Data from the previous interview would assist in the analysis of the biases caused by nonresponse to the HIV survey.

AIDS and the particular vulnerabilities of the groups presently experiencing the bulk of AIDS cases, we believe it is essential that blood test data be collected in a way that ensures the *anonymity* (not merely the confidentiality) of these data. Even if persons familiar with the excellent record of the federal statistical system in preserving confidentiality are reassured by past history, it is unlikely that their trust will be shared by all members of the public. This may be particularly true for respondents who feel vulnerable to discriminatory actions as a result of being identified as carriers of the AIDS virus.

Obviously, as a practical matter one must know the addresses of respondents in order to draw a sample. Thus, total anonymity of the respondents is impossible. We would propose, however, that the blood test *results* be obtained in a manner that guarantees those results will be anonymous. Procedures to achieve this end might include the following:

- To the fullest extent possible, no linkage should be allowed *at any stage of the fieldwork or data processing* between addresses and the identification numbers assigned to respondents.
- As soon as practical after completion of the relevant portion of fieldwork, all materials that might allow the identification of addresses should be destroyed. If practicable, this should be done on a continual basis at the local sites.
- No information allowing linkages between addresses and identification numbers should be transmitted from the fieldwork sites to the central site.
- All blood samples should be identified only by encrypted identification numbers.
- All sampling records should be destroyed as soon as practical after completion of the relevant portion of the fieldwork.
- Blood samples should be tested by one central laboratory, and its testing procedures should be subject to strict security and quality control measures. Tests should not be performed until sampling, fieldwork, and other survey records have been destroyed. The results of the blood testing should be transmitted only to the central site (not to the fieldwork sites).
- *All* interview data obtained from respondents (e.g., age, sex, race) when entered into a data file and combined with all remaining geographic information, must conform to present standards for *public use* tapes released by the Bureau of the Census.

The foregoing are initial suggestions for the types of precautions that will be required to guarantee anonymity of the data records. The ultimate test will be whether or not the most knowledgeable members of the sampling, fieldwork, and statistical staffs of the survey agency can state with certainty that they would be unable to identify the data derived from any individual respondent (using all records that remained available from the survey, together with the data file). This litmus test should be satisfied prior to the merging of the encrypted HIV test results with the information obtained in the survey interview.

Perception of Anonymity

In addition to guaranteeing the anonymity of the survey data records, it is crucial that the public at large, all respondents to the survey, and key social groups (especially those presently bearing the brunt of the AIDS epidemic) be *convinced* that the design of the survey precludes any threat to the respondents in the survey. Moreover, each of these audiences must be convinced that the resultant data will play an important role in the U.S. attempt to cope with the AIDS epidemic.

We suggest that representatives of these different audiences should be appointed to review the design and execution of the survey. This group should be provided with access to survey sites and appropriate staff to allow them to undertake an independent review to ensure that the anonymity of survey respondents has been fully protected. Their certification of this fact should be made a prerequisite for the merging of the encrypted blood test results with the other survey data.

To further ensure that the anonymity of the data gathering would not be compromised (and to further reassure the respondents on this point), it may be desirable for the survey to be performed in cooperation with the Bureau of the Census so that the protections of Title 13 of the U.S. Code would apply (Title 13 provides criminal penalties under federal law for violations of the confidentiality of census data). Careful pretesting should be undertaken, however, to ascertain whether the "reassurance" provided to respondents by such legal protections will outweigh any reluctance of respondents to provide sensitive information directly to employees of a federal statistical agency. If a substantial fraction of the population (particularly groups with atypical HIV prevalence rates) feels threatened by the request to provide blood samples to interviewers from a federal statistical agency, it may be advisable for data gathering to be done by a nongovernmental survey research organization.

Informing Respondents of Test Results

There is an inevitable tension between the desire to provide fail-safe protection of a respondent's anonymity and the desire to provide test results to individuals who want this information. The design we have outlined precludes direct notification of individual survey respondents (because names are never obtained and address records would be destroyed). Nonetheless, there are ways in which test results might be provided without directly recontacting respondents. We believe, however, that it would be inadvisable to provide such information without appropriate counseling and support services. Counseling, of course, requires personal contacts that would jeopardize anonymity.

Alternative procedures should be considered that would protect the anonymity of the survey data while permitting respondents to use the blood samples drawn in the survey to obtain information about their HIV status (together with appropriate counseling). Any proposed procedure should have the following characteristics:

- It should eliminate the need to ask respondents for their names.
- It should eliminate the need to retain survey records that might permit the personal identification of blood samples for any respondent. It thereby ensures that all such records can be destroyed prior to testing of the blood samples.
- It should ensure that respondents who wish to know their HIV status can use the sample drawn during the survey to find that out, and it should do so without requiring that respondents reveal to the interviewer their interest in learning the test results.
- It should not force blood test results upon respondents who may not wish to know their status.
- It should guarantee that appropriate counseling will be provided along with blood test results.

This list of requirements might be used as a preliminary screening device for vetting proposed procedures. Survey development and pretesting are likely to reveal other requirements that should be met. One approach that satisfies these preliminary requirements would provide respondents with an encrypted identification number to be presented at a local medical facility if they wished to learn their blood test results. (They would, of course, be counseled at that time.) The encrypted number could be given to respondents in a sealed envelope so that it would not be seen by the interviewer. Obviously, this number should be different from the serial number on the survey interview form or the encrypted identification number placed on the blood sample. This number might also be printed on a distinctive form so that it could not be copied, and the respondent might be instructed to place some personal information (e.g., height, eye color, sex) on the form so that it could not be used by anyone else to obtain the respondent's blood test results.

An alternative strategy might involve dividing blood samples in half. One half of the sample would be taken for testing by the survey organization. The other half of the blood sample would be left with respondents, who would be given the address of a local medical facility that would provide free testing of the blood sample together with appropriate counseling. Respondents could then choose for themselves whether they wished to know their HIV test results. (HIV tests presently under development may make this alternative quite practical because future tests may require only droplets of blood lanced from a finger and blotted on filter paper.)

The foregoing suggestions are only two of a large number of possible strategies. There is no need to commit to any particular strategy prior to beginning the design and pretesting of the survey. However, the five attributes listed above are a reasonable starting point for vetting any strategies proposed for informing respondents of their test results. Further consideration might also be given to the option of not providing test result data in order to provide more assured protection of the anonymity of the blood test results.

CONCLUSION

Public and scientific awareness of the impending magnitude of the AIDS epidemic has increased substantially in recent years. Yet an aspect of unreality remains. Thus, many individuals and whole nations must face critical decisions without trustworthy information on the prevalence of the AIDS infection in the population. If the infection is as pervasive as the present fragmentary evidence suggests, a series of annual estimates based upon representative national samples can serve to remind us all of how real and threatening the AIDS epidemic will become in the near future. Such estimates will permit more reliable tracking of the spread of the infection, and they will facilitate evaluation of the overall impact of educational and other interventions designed to retard the spread of the AIDS epidemic.

REFERENCES

Centers for Disease Control (CDC). (1987a) Human immunodeficiency virus infection in the United States: A review of current knowledge. *Morbidity and Mortality Weekly Report* 36(Suppl. S-6):1–48.

Centers for Disease Control (CDC). (1987b) Human Immunodeficiency Virus Infections in the United States: Review of Current Knowledge and Plans for Expansion of HIV Surveillance Activities. Report to the Domestic Policy Council. Atlanta, Ga., November 30, 1987.

Centers for Disease Control (CDC). (1988) *AIDS Weekly Surveillance Report—United States.* Atlanta: AIDS Program, Center for Infectious Diseases, September 5.

Cochran, W. G., Mosteller, F., and Tukey, J. W. (1953) Statistical problems of the Kinsey Report. *Journal of the American Statistical Association* 48:673–716.

Curran, J. W., Morgan, W. M., Hardy, A. M., Jafte, H. W., Darrow, W. W., and Dowdle, W. R. (1985) The epidemiology of AIDS: Current status and future prospects. *Science* 229:1352–1357.

Des Jarlais, D. C., Friedman, S. R., and Stoneburner, R. L. (1988) HIV infection and intravenous drug use: Critical issues in transmission dynamics, infection outcomes, and prevention. *Reviews of Infectious Diseases* 10:155.

Fischl, M. A., Dickinson, G. M., Scott, G. D., Kitmas, N., Fletcher, M. A., and Perk, W. (1987) Evaluation of heterosexual partners, children, and household contacts of adults with AIDS. *Journal of the American Medical Association* 257:640–644.

Forthofer, R. N. (1983) Investigation of non-response bias in NHANES-II. *American Journal of Epidemiology* 117:507–515.

Hull, H. F., Bettinger, C. J., Gallaher, M. M., Keller, N. M., Wilson, J., and Mertz, G. J. (1988) Comparison of HIV-antibody prevalence in patients consenting to and declining HIV-antibody testing in an STD clinic. *Journal of the American Medical Association* 260:935–938.

Institute of Medicine/National Academy of Sciences (IOM/NAS). (1986) *Confronting AIDS: Directions for Public Health, Health Care, and Research.* Washington, D.C.: National Academy Press.

Kinsey, A. C., Pomeroy, W. B., and Martin, C. E. (1948) *Sexual Behavior in the Human Male.* Philadelphia: Saunders.

Lui, K., Darrow, W. W., and Rutherford, G. W. (1988) A model based estimate of the mean incubation period for AIDS in homosexual men. *Science* 240:1333–1335.

May, R. M., and Anderson, R. M. (1987) Transmission dynamics of HIV infection. *Nature* 326:137–142.

National Center for Health Statistics. (1982) Hematological and nutritional biochemistry reference data for persons 6 months–74 years of age: United States, 1976–80. *Vital and Health Statistics,* Series 11, No. 22, DHHS Pub. No. 83-1682. Washington, D.C.: U.S. Government Printing Office.

National Research Council. (1978) *Privacy and Confidentiality as Factors in Survey Response.* Washington, D.C.: National Academy Press.

Public Health Service. (1986) Coolfont Report: A PHS plan for the prevention and control of AIDS and AIDS virus. *Public Health Reports* 101:341–348.

Rees, M. (1987) The sombre view of AIDS. *Nature* 326:343–345.

Sivak, S. L., and Wormser, G. P. (1985) How common is HTLV-III infection in the United States? *New England Journal of Medicine,* 313:1352.

Terman, L. M. (1948) Kinsey's "Sexual Behavior in the Human Male": Some comments and criticisms. *Psychological Bulletin* 45:443–459.

Wallis, W. A. (1948) Statistics of the Kinsey Report. *Journal of the American Statistical Association* 44:463–484.

Cost-Effectiveness Analysis of AIDS Prevention Programs: Concepts, Complications, and Illustrations

Milton C. Weinstein, John D. Graham, Joanna E. Siegel, and Harvey V. Fineberg

The enormity of the AIDS problem and the limited resources available to finance a potentially large number of intervention programs, each likely to have some degree of effectiveness in preventing future cases of AIDS, have led policymakers at national, state, and local levels to seek a rational basis for setting priorities for prevention. Cost-effectiveness analysis is a quantitative approach to resource allocation under constrained resources (Weinstein and Stason, 1977; Warner and Luce, 1982; Drummond et al., 1987). The premise of this paper is that cost-effectiveness analysis can be a useful tool in guiding resource allocation for AIDS prevention.

Most AIDS prevention measures share the characteristic of promoting desirable behavioral changes that reduce the risk of HIV transmission. Prevention measures may be applied in a variety of population groups, in a variety of ways. *HIV antibody screening* may be regarded as a preventive measure, to the degree that knowledge of one's HIV status results in desirable behavioral change. Screening of high-risk groups, such as homosexual men, intravenous (IV) drug users, and visitors to sexually transmitted disease clinics, as well as screening of more heterogeneous population segments at a time at which transmission would be especially likely—for example, couples entering marriage and blood donors—have all been advocated. Pro-

The authors are from the Harvard School of Public Health.

motion of *safer sex practices* is exemplified by programs of condom distribution and safer sex education in schools, as well as community education through media such as television or the pamphlet recently mailed to all households by the U.S. Public Health Service. Programs to limit HIV spread among needle-sharing drug users, such as *bleach distribution* by outreach workers or *needle exchange*, are also very much under consideration. Another type of prevention program is *contact tracing,* which has been used with some success in dealing with other sexually transmitted diseases.

In this paper, the concepts, complications, and potential use of cost-effectiveness analysis in three of these areas are illustrated: premarital screening, condom promotion in secondary schools, and bleach distribution among IV drug users. Appendix A gives an illustrative cost-effectiveness analysis for premarital screening, and Appendix B illustrates an approach to modeling the benefits of condom promotion in schools. The authors' research on all three examples is used throughout the paper to illustrate key points.

The paper is structured as follows: the first section is a brief exposition of the general model for cost-effectiveness, and the next section is a discussion of problems involved in assessing program effectiveness. One key issue in measuring effectiveness is the choice of outcome measure: What measures of final health outcome exist? Can intermediate outcome measures be used as proxies? Another set of issues in estimating effectiveness concerns modeling the spread of infection in populations: What data are needed? Are long-term effects different from short-term effects? Must secondary spread of infection be modeled? What types of heterogeneity in the target population influence program effectiveness? Still another set of issues in estimating effectiveness relates to the scientific uncertainty that surrounds the biological, epidemiological, and behavioral variables which determine the number of AIDS cases that will occur under different program scenarios: How can this uncertainty be reflected responsibly in cost-effectiveness analyses of prevention programs? Does this uncertainty vitiate the entire cost-effectiveness modeling approach?

The third section introduces and illustrates the possibility of important "collateral" program effects—health or social consequences that relate to diseases or problems other than HIV (e.g., other sexually transmitted diseases or drug use) and that follow from interventions aimed at HIV. These collateral effects may significantly affect the relative desirability of a program option. In the fourth section, the emphasis changes from issues of program effects to issues of estimating program costs. Special problems of valuation, such as weighting effects on the quality of life, interpersonal comparisons across population groups including some (e.g., IV drug users) that impose substantial externalities on the rest of society, and valuation of avoiding births of infected or uninfected infants, are described in the last section.

A COST-EFFECTIVENESS MODEL FOR AIDS PREVENTION

The purpose of applying cost-effectiveness analysis to AIDS prevention programs is to guide the setting of priorities for the use of finite resources, with the objective of achieving the maximum reduction in AIDS-related mortality and morbidity. The cost-effectiveness model used herein assumes the societal perspective, according to which all program costs and consequences are recognized, irrespective of the beneficiary or payor. This is a broader perspective than that, for example, of a municipal health department (which does not realize all of the savings in AIDS treatment resources and which may not have to pay full program costs because of federal grants). However, the model is easily adapted to other perspectives by excluding costs and consequences that are extraneous to a given decision maker and by including costs and savings realized by one decision-making entity at the expense of another.

Cost-effectiveness analysis applies when four key ingredients are present: (1) an identifiable decision-making entity; (2) a measure of program effectiveness, such as number of cases prevented, number of years of life saved, or number of quality-adjusted years of life (QALYs) gained; (3) a constrained resource that limits the number of programs that can be implemented (e.g., cost); and (4) a set of independent programs from which to choose, each of which produces some degree of net expected effectiveness (e.g., lives saved or QALYs gained) and each of which consumes some of the constrained resource (e.g., dollars). When these conditions are met, the optimal allocation rule (i.e., the allocation rule that achieves maximum effectiveness subject to the resource constraint) is to select programs in ascending order of their cost-effectiveness ratio (net program cost/net program effectiveness) until the resource budget is exhausted. In other words, highest priority would go to the programs for which the net cost per unit of desired effect is lowest.

When the societal perspective is adopted and QALYs are the measure of effect, the following formulation of a cost-effectiveness ratio for AIDS prevention may be used:

$$\frac{\binom{Net}{Cost}}{\binom{Program}{Effectiveness}} = \frac{\binom{Program}{Cost} - \binom{Cases}{Prevented}\binom{Costs}{per\ Case}}{\binom{Cases}{Prevented}\binom{QALYs}{per\ Case} \pm \binom{Change\ in\ Quality}{of\ Life\ to\ Others}}. \quad (1)$$

Each term in the ratio should be interpreted as a present value, at a suitable time discount rate, of a stream of future benefits or costs. This interpretation enables comparison of programs that may have different lags in the appearance of benefits and different patterns over time in the investments required to make them work. Issues that arise in estimating each term in this ratio, as well as refinements of the ratio to account for considerations such as population dynamics and collateral costs and consequences, are discussed in the following sections.

ASSESSING PROGRAM EFFECTIVENESS

Measures of Health Outcome

Various measures of outcome can be used to assess the effectiveness of prevention programs directed at AIDS. These include both measures of final outcome and intermediate outcome measures. Possible final outcome measures include number of lives saved, number and discounted number of life-years saved, and discounted QALYs saved. Intermediate outcome measures include reductions in risk-taking behaviors and incidence of HIV infection. The virtues and limitations of these outcome measures, as they apply to AIDS prevention programs, are discussed below.

Final Outcome Measures

The number of lives saved is a simple and intuitively appealing measure because it corresponds with a basic and important purpose of public health intervention. Because lives are visibly lost as a result of AIDS, the number of lives saved offers a concrete representation of the success of a program. However, the number of lives saved has several drawbacks as an outcome measure. First, it does not reflect the timing of life saving. Cost-effectiveness analyses generally incorporate the assumption that it is preferable to use available resources to save a life now rather than in the future. This is both because improvements in technology will likely enable the savings of future lives at a lower cost and because lives saved now can contribute to the pool of resources that will be available in the future. Authors such as Keeler and Cretin (1983) describe the logical impossibility of recognizing the greater present value of money, reflecting its potential for investment, without concurrently recognizing the greater value of saving present as opposed to future lives. These authors recommend what has become a generally accepted practice, namely, discounting health effects to reflect the point at which they occur.

As a measure of outcome, the number of lives saved also falls short in failing to reflect the proportion of a person's life that is saved or, more precisely, the amount of life expectancy saved. This quantity can be represented as the number of discounted life-years saved, rather than discounted lives saved. Using the number of life-years saved to evaluate program effectiveness is often controversial, because it seems to discriminate against groups with lower remaining life expectancy, notably the elderly. When comparing interventions against AIDS, this issue assumes secondary importance because a large proportion of AIDS cases fall within a narrow age range. The distinction becomes more important, however, when programs to prevent AIDS are compared with other programs such as those against heart disease or cancer. Using the number of discounted life-years saved is preferable to using the number of discounted lives saved because, in the opinion of the authors, the former more accurately reflects society's disproportionate concern about causes of untimely or premature death.

One further complication of using discounted life-years saved as an outcome measure is that life expectancy may vary for groups of the same age, depending upon how groups are defined. This is an important concern in evaluating the effectiveness of AIDS prevention programs. For example, apart from any value judgments regarding the comparative worth of individuals to society, the life expectancy of a male 35-year-old IV drug user is lower than that of a 35-year-old gay man. The difference is due to the violence prevalent in the hazardous life-styles associated with drug abuse. Use of this lower life expectancy in calculating the effectiveness of AIDS programs, however, implies that preventing a case of AIDS among IV drug users is a less effective use of societal resources (i.e., results in fewer life-years saved) than preventing a case among the gay male population.

Such an analysis might be perceived as biased against lifesaving programs targeted at drug users. Perhaps a greater dilemma arises when one considers the life expectancy of a drug user with AIDS, which is only about one-third that of a non-drug user with AIDS. To incorporate this differential into an analysis is to accept the current disadvantages faced by drug users in recognizing AIDS and seeking care. The value judgments involved are discussed further in the section "Problems in Valuing Program Consequences."

One additional characteristic that should arguably be included in an outcome measure is the quality of life-years saved. Using QALYs saved implies favoring preventive programs, which save healthy life-years, over treatment programs that allow increased survival with AIDS. Because both AIDS and AIDS-related complex (ARC) can be extremely debilitating, it would be difficult to justify an equal preference for saving life-years with AIDS and saving the same number of life-years through prevention. Yet people with AIDS are identifiable individuals with visible needs, and our society may find it difficult to assign a lower priority to programs that benefit them. This dilemma can be mediated to some extent by adjusting the actual QALY value assigned to life with AIDS.

A final use of QALYs that deserves mention is in assigning a societal valuation to life-years saved, apart from the relative valuation of life years with and without AIDS. The clearest example of this use is in evaluating programs for IV drug users. Some would argue that the value of a saved life-year for a drug user is lower than that of a non-drug user because drug users impose substantial costs upon society (e.g., crime, fear). Alternatively, drug use can be seen as a disease that lowers the quality of life just as other illnesses do. One may, therefore, not believe it is appropriate to "penalize" drug users for suffering from a disease over which they may have limited control.

Intermediate Outcome Measures

Whereas final outcome measures reflect ultimate program goals, the effect of a given program on discounted life-years or QALYs saved is often difficult to assess. Programs are directed toward accomplishing intermediate objectives, which in turn are believed to achieve or contribute to the larger societal objectives. Intermediate outcome measures frequently have the advantage of being more immediate and potentially more measurable. Their disadvantage is that their relationship either to the larger goal or to the program itself is often indirect or elusive. This disadvantage will be described in greater detail as related to specific examples of two types of intermediate outcome, frequency of risk-taking behavior and incidence of HIV infection.

Many programs designed to prevent AIDS are directed at eliminating or reducing the frequency of behaviors that place individuals at risk of exposure to HIV infection. To prevent infection by means of sexual transmission, for example, programs may promote condom use, encourage safer sex practices, or encourage having fewer partners. Intermediate outcome measures of the effectiveness of these programs may describe the frequency of condom use before and after an educational campaign or the numbers of partners before and after the circulation of a "safer sex" pamphlet. The importance of these and other behavioral changes, however, depends on how these results actually translate into prevention of AIDS cases. Although condom use is theoretically effective in preventing HIV infection, for example, effectiveness may actually depend on the number of partners, the stage of infection of an infected partner, and the number of exposures per partner. Measures of risk-taking behavior thus indicate the success of a program in achieving the intermediate objective, but do not necessarily predict the program's effectiveness in achieving the larger societal goal. The value of this type of intermediate outcome measure for assessing program effectiveness depends on the relationship between the intermediate and the ultimate goals.

The incidence of HIV infection is a type of intermediate outcome closely related to the incidence of AIDS. The problem with this measure is its distance from more immediate programmatic objectives. There is no doubt that if a condom distribution program results in decreased incidence of HIV infection, it is a successful program. However, a causal link between such a program and HIV incidence is often difficult to establish. Many intervening factors may be involved, including other environmental influences (e.g., media coverage, concurrent prevention activities), the timing of HIV testing and seroconversion, the prevalence of HIV positivity, and factors related to the sample selected. This type of measure thus provides information on the spread of the virus but is difficult to relate to a particular program.

Modeling Program Effects on HIV Transmission

A major task in measuring the effectiveness of AIDS prevention is to estimate the number of incident cases of HIV infection expected to occur, over time, in both the presence and the absence of the program being assessed. This task is complicated by gaps in our basic knowledge of the biology of HIV transmission, the epidemiology of the infection in populations, and especially, the determinants of high-risk behaviors and the use of protective measures.

Data Requirements

As illustrated in Appendix A, key variables for which estimates are required in order to calculate the number of cases prevented by a premarital screening program include the following:

- current prevalence of HIV infection in the male and female partner at the time of marriage (including possible transmission prior to marriage;
- probability of HIV transmission during marriage, in the absence of preventive or protective action, from male to female or from female to male;
- probability of adopting preventive (e.g., abstention) or protective (e.g., condom use) action upon knowledge of a positive antibody test and appropriate counseling;
- efficacy of protective action against sexual transmission during marriage;
- sensitivity and specificity of HIV antibody test systems; and
- probability of conception and ultimate infection of a child of the marriage.

Some of these variables (e.g., test sensitivity and specificity, HIV prevalence) can be estimated from available data with reasonable precision and accuracy, although not entirely without uncertainty. (For example, HIV prevalence could vary considerably between populations of marriage candidates and populations of blood donors, although preliminary data from the premarital testing program in Illinois are consistent with prevalence estimates based on blood donors.) Other variables (e.g., probability of transmission by sexual contact with and without protection) have been studied to a limited degree, but wide variation in reported data exists. Still other variables (e.g., probability of adopting preventive or protective behavior) have hardly been studied at all. One value of performing cost-effectiveness analysis would be to identify those variables to which program cost-effectiveness is most sensitive, and thereby to identify areas in which field evaluations and further research would be most informative. Behavioral response variables almost surely fall into the high-priority category for further research. Formal approaches to assessing cost-effectiveness in the face of uncertainty, and their implications for targeting areas of research, are described in the following subsection.

Dynamic Modeling

The cost-effectiveness formula (Equation 1) suggests a naive and potentially misleading approach to modeling benefits, namely, that the health benefit associated with the prevention of a case of HIV infection at any point in time is the difference between the number of (quality-adjusted) years that would be lived without infection and the number of (quality-adjusted) years that would be lived with infection. The number of QALYs with infection can be estimated from models both of HIV latency prior to AIDS onset and of AIDS survival, but can the number of QALYs without infection be estimated from the usual method of life-table analysis in the general population? As a first-order approximation in low-risk populations (e.g., heterosexual partners of transfusion recipients), perhaps general life tables can be used to estimate the number of life-years potentially saved by preventing an instance of HIV infection. However, in populations in which the risk of HIV infection is an ongoing process, preventing infection at time t does not guarantee a normal life expectancy if the risk at time $t+1$ remains high. Dynamic, rather than static, models of the benefits of disease prevention are, therefore, needed.

In general, more complex modeling techniques may be useful in generating the estimates of cost and effectiveness that enter the cost-effectiveness ratio. State-transition models (in which disease status is modeled probabilistically in a population), epidemic models based on differential equations, and other computer-based approaches are available to assist in the projection of cost and effectiveness through time.

Assessment of the cost-effectiveness of prevention programs in IV drug user communities has revealed the importance of these considerations. The aggregate gain in life expectancy attributable to preventing a case of HIV infection in a relatively low-prevalence population of drug users (as in Houston, where HIV prevalence among IV drug users is estimated at 3 percent) is greater than that attributable to preventing a case in New York City (where HIV prevalence among IV drug users exceeds 50 percent). The reason is that IV drug users in Houston have a higher probability of avoiding (or delaying) infection than their New York City counterparts and, therefore, have more years of life to gain if they are spared infection at a point in time. Analogous considerations apply when comparing the life expectancy gained per infection avoided among homosexuals in San Francisco versus that in communities with lower HIV prevalence among homosexuals.

An important insight from this reasoning is that the most cost-effective communities in which to implement AIDS prevention programs may be those with intermediate levels of HIV prevalence. If prevalence is too low, resources are squandered in preventing very low probability events. However, if prevalence is too high, the gain (in terms of life expectancy) from preventing single-hit transmission today is attenuated by the high risk of eventual infection and premature death. Even if programs continue at a high relative efficacy, residual infection rates with the program in place may be high enough to diminish considerably the benefit per infection prevented. Further modeling of this phenomenon will yield other specific guidelines for targeting prevention efforts according to preexisting spread in the community.

Epidemic Control

First-order estimates of program effectiveness may be based on the assumption that preventing the spread of infection to an individual has the effect of averting the consequences of that single case of HIV infection. This assumption is correct only if that individual has a negligible probability of infecting others, either because anyone with whom the individual has intimate contact is already infected or because the individual engages in protective or preventive behavior immediately after becoming infected. In reality, the process of secondary spread has the effect of producing a "multiplier effect"; that is, each primary case prevented would otherwise multiply into some larger number of cases over time. To estimate the effects of AIDS prevention accurately, models are required that can yield estimates of these multipliers under various assumptions about number of contacts, frequency of contact, and probability of transmission per contact. As long as these multipliers are approximately constant across AIDS prevention programs, however, their relative cost-effectiveness will not be distorted by omitting the multiplier from the calculation. To the degree that multipliers do vary across programs, failure to consider them will tend to result in underestimating the relative cost-effectiveness of programs with large multiplier effects.

Heterogeneity

The models the authors have used to estimate the effectiveness of protective measures such as condom use and needle sterilization are based on a number of parameters that govern the probability of HIV transmission in a population of interest. With regard to condom use (Appendix B), for example, such parameters include the probability of transmission during unprotected intercourse, the probability of condom use during a given sexual act, and the probability of prevalent infection in a given sexual partner. The simplest model assumes that these parameters are constant across all members of a target population, such as a high school population. This homogeneity assumption, although simplifying the calculations and requiring only data on population means rather than frequency distributions, may distort the true effects of an intervention. It would be better to assume, for example, that the probability of transmission varies from individual to individual and that this probability is, in itself, distributed in the population according to some frequency distribution.

Although data do not permit estimation of these frequency distributions, it is important to model the possibility of heterogeneity in order to obtain reasonable bounds on the likely effects of intervention. In general, heterogeneity in the probability of transmission tends to diminish the effectiveness of preventive interventions, if it is not possible to identify the "superinfectors" and to target the interventions at them. Heterogeneity of compliance (e.g., condom use, needle sterilization) and heterogeneity of prevalence (e.g., nonrandom mixing within subpopulations with higher than average or lower than average prevalence) cause smaller deviations from estimates of program effectiveness (Appendix B).

Limited study populations make it extremely difficult to estimate underlying frequency distributions of such population characteristics as the infectivity rate. Therefore, in the absence of empirical data, modeling remains the only viable approach to exploring the implications of heterogeneity.

COLLATERAL PROGRAM EFFECTS

An important issue in applying cost-effectiveness analysis to AIDS prevention programs is the appropriate treatment of collateral program effects. In particular, many programs designed to prevent AIDS have other benefits or costs unrelated to AIDS itself. The behaviors that place individuals at risk for AIDS are frequently a source of risk for other illnesses and undesirable outcomes. To the extent that such programs intervene by reducing or eliminating these behaviors, they confer additional (side) benefits.

One program in which collateral benefits are particularly important is condom distribution among heterosexual teenagers. The effectiveness of such a program in preventing the spread of AIDS among this low-prevalence group may be modest compared to the effect condom use would have in preventing teenage pregnancy. Although averting even unwanted births is a consequence of debatable value, the reduction of teenage abortions is clearly desirable. In addition, reduction in teenage pregnancy would be beneficial in terms of reducing the societal costs of teen births and the excess in infant mortality resulting from pregnancy during teen years versus at an older age. Maternal mortality associated with abortion would also be reduced.

Another program in which collateral benefits are important is drug treatment for IV drug users. The goal of drug treatment—abstinence from IV drug use—is unquestionably the most effective means of eliminating the possibility of contracting AIDS by sharing needles. However, transmission of HIV among drug users can also be reduced or prevented by much less expensive means. These include provision of sterile needles and bleach distribution. Comparing programs on the basis of their ability to prevent AIDS would most probably lead to the conclusion that drug treatment is the least cost-effective program. However, bleach distribution and needle exchange have little effect on underlying drug use, which has many adverse consequences besides serving as a vehicle for HIV transmission. Some would even argue that such programs promote drug use—which would be a collateral disadvantage—although there is no evidence supporting this claim. Thus it would be necessary to consider the collateral benefits and costs of drug treatment in assessing the full benefit to be gained by society from an investment in drug treatment programs.

ESTIMATING NET PROGRAM COSTS

In estimating program costs, an important issue is the separation of fixed and variable costs. This distinction is important when the prevention program is part of an existing program. For example, a condom promotion program might be linked to existing sex education programs. In this case, it would not be correct to ascribe the full costs of the existing program to the new program. A similar circumstance arises with bleach distribution, which often makes use of existing community outreach programs. Because the outreach worker is an integral part of the bleach program, the costs of implementing bleach distribution where an outreach program exists and where it does not will be different.

The distinction between fixed and variable costs is also important in estimating the eventual costs of programs of various sizes. If a program has relatively large fixed costs, as is often the case when substantial design, research, or administrative costs are incurred, the incremental cost of the program will be considerably less than its average cost. As a result, the average cost of the program will decrease as it is expanded, and it will become more cost-effective. In this instance, however, it is also important to note at what point additional fixed (or semifixed) costs are incurred.

The other component of net program costs concerns the resources saved by preventing a case of AIDS. Issues of fixed and incremental costs are also important in this calculation. In New York City and San Francisco, for example, the large numbers of AIDS patients will likely necessitate expansion of medical facilities: the opening of hospital AIDS wards, the establishment of hospices, and the initiation of new home care programs. In cities where the impact of AIDS is lower, incremental costs will constitute a larger proportion of costs resulting from AIDS cases. Even in communities with relatively small numbers of AIDS patients, the AIDS epidemic imposes fixed costs on hospitals in such forms as personnel training, universal precautions, and protective clothing.

Whereas the large burden of AIDS in some cities will result in more fixed costs, greater experience and specialization of care in these cities are likely to have the opposite effect. Greater use of hospice and home care, less frequent and earlier hospitalization, and decreased reliance on diagnostic tests will help to lower average costs. These variations are important in estimating net programs in different geographical areas.

PROBLEMS IN VALUING PROGRAM CONSEQUENCES

Several thorny problems in outcome valuation raise difficult ethical questions. The cost-effectiveness framework does not prescribe a "correct" way to value these consequences, but it can accommodate a wide range of value judgments. Depending on the values selected, the analysis can reveal the benefits attainable by alternative investments.

Consider first the question of how to value the prolongation of life of an IV drug user. The years of life gained could (but need not) be weighted according to society's valuation of the "quality" of these years compared to the years of a non-drug user's life. Alternatively, by using the actual life expectancy of IV drug users in calculating the number of years of life saved, instead of national averages by age and sex, the value of these lives could be reduced. Then too, instead of adjusting the denominator of the cost-effectiveness ratio (health effectiveness), the numerator (net societal cost) could be adjusted by subtracting the economic costs imposed on the rest of society—in terms of crime—during those added years of life. Also, just as the incremental benefit of preventing secondary spread of HIV could be modeled, so might the cost of keeping an IV drug user alive who may spread drug use in the community. The model does not determine which, if any, of these adjustments to make, but it does accommodate all of them.

Another difficult valuation concerns newborns. If a program averts the birth of an HIV-infected child, what is the measure of benefit? If the mother was infected so that the birth of an uninfected child is unlikely in any case, then the change caused by the program is from an infected child with a brief and horrible life span to no child. Whether this is regarded as a gain or loss of quality-adjusted life years may depend on whether life with AIDS is judged worse than death, especially when considering the effect on parents and others. On the other hand, if the program results in preventing an infected man from impregnating a susceptible woman, and the woman later gives birth to a child with a different father, should this transaction be viewed as a "substitute" birth, so that the gain in QALYs is the difference between the normal life span of the "substitute" child and the impaired life span of the averted diseased child? The ethical aspects of this discussion ought to dominate the policy debate, and alternative value judgments can be reflected in the measures of program consequences and costs within the framework of cost-effectiveness analysis.

APPENDIX A

Illustrative Cost-Effectiveness Analysis: Premarital Screening

Several states have adopted mandatory premarital HIV screening laws with the presumed objective of detecting and interrupting the spread of HIV at a point in life at which the probability of heterosexual transmission increases. To the extent that sexual activity is not significantly different during the postmarital years from other stages of adult life, the cost-effectiveness of premarital screening would approximate the cost-effectiveness of universal screening of young adults.

The constrained resource, for purposes of this illustrative analysis, is health care cost, including the costs of screening and counseling, and the net savings in AIDS treatment. Reductions in indirect costs of AIDS (i.e., avoidance of lost productivity due to premature death or disability) are not considered pertinent to the constrained resource but are reflected in the measure of the program's health consequences.

The health outcome measure employed here is the gain in quality-adjusted life-years, including gain in life expectancy and quality of life due to prevention of AIDS cases, as well as loss in quality of life due to anxiety among false positives. Prevention of the birth of HIV-infected children is not assigned either a positive or a negative value, although the direct cost savings associated with their treatment are incorporated into the calculation of net resource cost.

This simple model limits the potential benefit of screening to prevention of transmission to the spouse or child of an infected person. Effects on spread by extramarital intercourse or needle-sharing are not considered. (It is possible, paradoxically, that knowledge of infection could lead to increased sexual promiscuity and resultant increased spread of infection, but positive or negative effects on HIV spread outside marriage are not considered.) Also excluded are the costs of repeated testing and counseling for false positives, although the effects on their quality of life are included.

Assumptions

The crucial assumption upon which there are virtually no data to draw is the effect of a positive screening result on behavior. Some fraction of test-positives will abstain from sexual intercourse; another fraction may employ protective sexual practices (i.e., condoms); the rest will make no change. Studies of screened homosexual males have found up to 75 percent reductions in high-risk behaviors compared to 33 percent in unscreened controls. For purposes of this illustrative analysis, it is assumed that 25 percent of test-positives will abstain and that 50 percent will use condoms regularly. Other assumptions and data used in the analysis are as follows:

(1a) Prevalence of HIV infection in male partners:[1] 0.0007
(1b) Prevalence of HIV infection in female partners: 0.00007
(2a) Enzyme immunoassay (EIA) test sensitivity:[2] 0.983
(2b) Western blot test sensitivity among EIA positives: 0.92
(2c) EIA false-positive rate: 0.002
(2d) WB false-positive rate among EIA positives: 0.05
(3a) Probability of premarital intercourse:[3] 0.6
(3b) Probability of HIV transmission during premarital intercourse: 0.1 (M to F) and 0.04 (F to M)
(4a) Probability of transmission during marriage:[4] 0.5 (M to F) and 0.2 (F to M)
(4b) Probability of transmission during marriage, with condom use:[5] 0.06 (M to F) and 0.025 (F to M)
(5a) Probability of abstention given positive test:[6] 0.25
(5b) Probability of condom use given positive test: 0.50
(6a) Probability of childbirth during marriage without screening:[7] 0.75
(6b) Probability of transmission (M to F) before first child: 0.20
(6c) Probability of maternal–fetal transmission: 0.50
(7) Latency distribution of AIDS onset from time of HIV infection, based on San Francisco Hepatitis B Cohort Study, with extrapolation according to a Weibull probability distribution; data consistent with median latency of approximately 8 years[8]

[1](1a) and (1b) are based on Centers for Disease Control reports of prevalence in first-time blood donors.

[2](2a)–(2d) are based on a review by Ward et al. (1986).

[3](3a) and (3b) are required in order to adjust downward the potential number of cases prevented because transmission has already occurred at the time of marriage. The estimates are consistent with data on the frequency of extramarital intercourse prior to age 20, a mean probability of transmission of 1 per 800 unprotected contacts (M to F) and 1 per 2,000 (F to M), and an estimated 100 premarital contacts. Risks of transmission per sexual contact are derived from data in Peterman et al. (1988).

[4](4a) is based on the transmission probabilities per contact cited above and a mean of 500 contacts per marriage.

[5](4b) is based on 90 percent efficacy of condom use and 100 percent adherence.

[6](5a) and (5b) are guesses, based on behavioral changes observed in homosexual screenees in various studies reviewed by the Office of Technology Assessment. They are probably optimistic.

[7](6a)–(6c) are consistent with data reviewed by Cleary et al. (1987).

[8]Both the Weibull and exponential distributions fit the data rather well. The Weibull, which assumes increasing incidence with time, yields a greater cumulative incidence of

(8) Mortality probability with AIDS:[9] 50 percent per year
(9) Mortality from other causes: based on U.S. life tables
(10) Quality-of-life weight for years with AIDS:[10] 0.5
(11) Quality-of-life loss for false positives:[11] 0.25 for 15 years
(12) Cost per case of AIDS: $60,000
(13a) Cost of EIA test: $6
(13b) Cost of counseling: $25
(13c) Cost of Western blot test (for EIA positives): $50
(14) Costs and life-years discounted to present value at 5 percent per year.

Results

Calculations are for a population of 1 million 25-year-old couples. The expected numbers of HIV cases are 700 males and 70 females. Of these, 633 males and 63 females will test positive on the EIA and Western blot.

Of the 633 female partners of infected males, 38 will already have been infected by their spouses prior to marriage, leaving 595 females at risk. Of the 63 male partners of the infected females, 2 will already have been infected by their spouses prior to marriage, leaving 61 males at risk.

The expected numbers of spouses infected, without preventive or protective action, are 298 females and 13 males. With 25 percent abstention and 50 percent protection, these numbers are reduced to 92 females and 4 males.

The at-risk females will bear 44 infected children without preventive or protective action; with protection, this number is reduced to 14.

Health benefits are 2,144 life-years, with a quality-of-life adjustment of 125 QALYs, minus a loss of 520 QALYs in false positives, for a net gain of 1,749 QALYs.

Costs are $62.2 million for screening and counseling, less $7.4 million savings for treatment of adults with AIDS, less $1.8 million savings for treatment of newborns with AIDS, for a net cost of $53 million.

AIDS in the long run. Parameters of both distributions were estimated by ordinary least squares fit to the San Francisco Cohort data.

[9](8) is probably lower with availability of zidovudine (AZT).

[10](10) is selected arbitrarily.

[11](11) is selected arbitrarily.

The cost per quality-adjusted life-year saved is $30,000. This is comparable to the treatment of mild hypertension or screening for breast cancer by mammography; higher than screening for cervical cancer in 40-year-old women (Pap smear) or screening for phenylketonuria (PKU) in newborns; and lower than pharmacologic serum cholesterol reduction in asymptomatic patients or screening for pheochromocytoma in hypertensives. The meaning of this level of cost-effectiveness in the context of AIDS prevention must await analogous evaluations of other programs that compete for society's limited resources.

Moreover, sensitivity analyses are required to test the stability of this ratio compared to analogous ratios for other AIDS prevention programs, with resulting implications for field research. Clearly, this analysis is highly sensitive to the assumed behavioral change based on a positive HIV antibody screen. As an approximation, half of the behavioral response would double the cost-effectiveness ratio.

APPENDIX B

Effectiveness of Condoms Against HIV Infection Among Adolescents

Before oral contraceptives became widely available, condoms were the preferred method of birth control among millions of U.S. teenagers. With the advent of the pill and the feminization of adolescent sexuality in the 1970s, condom use declined substantially. Despite a modest resurgence in condom use in the late 1970s (perhaps in response to publicity about the health dangers of the pill), the rate of condom use among teenagers leveled off in the 1980s. One recent estimate is that one-fifth of sexually active teenage girls who practiced contraception had partners who used condoms at last intercourse.

The conventional wisdom is that condoms are not a very promising contraceptive method for most adolescents. Drawbacks of the condom include the following:

- condoms are perceived as difficult to use, and many teenagers believe that condoms must interfere with sexual pleasure;
- use of the condom requires both premeditation about sex and conscious protective action at the time of intercourse; and

- condoms are not 100 percent effective in preventing pregnancy, and misuse of the condom can result in a substantial risk of pregnancy.

Despite these drawbacks, it is well recognized that condoms have considerable virtues as a contraceptive method among teenagers. They are cheap, can be made readily available to adolescents, and can be used by teenagers without informing "establishment" figures such as physicians and parents. If used properly, condoms are quite effective at preventing both pregnancy and venereal disease. Condoms are perhaps the most effective contraceptive method during a couple's initial several encounters, before the girl elects a prescription method of contraception. In many adolescent relationships, women remain sexually active for more than a year before pursuing a prescription method.

The emergence of the AIDS epidemic is causing a serious reappraisal of the benefits and costs of increasing condom use among adolescents. Although the AIDS virus has so far penetrated only modestly beyond the traditional "high-risk" groups, there are reasons to target U.S. teenagers in the development of prevention activities. Adolescent life-style in the United States is characterized by sexual experimentation, multiple partners, frequent sexual intercourse, exposure to sexually transmitted diseases, and significant amounts of intravenous drug use. In light of all of the above, the potential role of condom use as an AIDS prevention strategy among teenagers needs to be analyzed.

A complete cost–benefit analysis of condom promotion and distribution programs is not attempted in this paper. Instead, some mathematical models are presented that are useful in simulating the potential HIV prevention benefits of increased condom use to the adolescent. The purpose is not to produce precise estimates of an adolescent's absolute risk of HIV infection, but rather to determine how much condom use might reduce an adolescent's risk of infection. These analyses also highlight what the data requirements of a comprehensive benefit analysis of condom use might be. Because the economic facets of AIDS prevention have already been examined in the previous example (premarital screening), the focus here is on the interrelationships among patterns of sexual behavior, extent of condom use, and rates of HIV infection.

Personal Risk of HIV Infection: A Simple Model of the Adolescent

Let us take the perspective of an uninfected teenager at the start of ninth grade, for example, and simulate the cumulative probability that he or she will become infected with the HIV virus prior to graduation (or four years later). In the equations that follow, let r be the risk of transmitting the virus (from an infected to an uninfected person) during a single act of vaginal intercourse, e the efficacy of condoms in preventing transmission of the virus, and f the fraction of sexual encounters protected (properly) by a condom.

Given the above, the probability of becoming infected by an infected partner during a single act of intercourse is

$$P = r(1 - fe). \tag{1}$$

If there are n exposures with the same infected partner, the risk of infection becomes

$$P = 1 - [1 - r(1 - fe)]^n. \tag{2}$$

If the uninfected teenager draws his or her partner randomly from the pool of U.S. adolescents and p is the prevalence of HIV infection among adolescents, the cumulative risk of infection then becomes

$$P = p\{1 - [1 - r(1 - fe)]^n\}. \tag{3}$$

Of course, many adolescents will have more than one partner. If the uninfected teenager has n exposures with each of m random partners, the cumulative risk of infection becomes

$$P = 1 - \{p[1 - r(1 - fe)]^n + (1 - p)\}^m. \tag{4}$$

Before computing some probabilities with Equation 4, the key simplifications made in this model will be summarized. They are

- no intravenous drug use;
- randomness in partner selection;
- no anal intercourse;
- partners drawn only from the adolescent population;
- a constant value of r, which applies to both males and females; and
- a constant value of p during the period of sexual activity.

To compute the cumulative probability of becoming infected during four years of adolescence, the following hypothetical values of the inputs are used:

TABLE 1 Cumulative Probability of HIV Infection During Adolescence (Ages 15–18) as a Fraction of the Number of Sexual Partners, the Number of Sexual Exposures per Partner, and the Frequency of Condom Use

Number of Sexual Partners	Number of Exposures per Partner	Frequency of Condom Use[a]		
		0	0.5	1.0
2	10	3.0×10^{-4}	1.6×10^{-4} (−45%)	3.0×10^{-5} (−90%)
	100	2.9×10^{-3}	1.6×10^{-3} (−44%)	3.0×10^{-4} (−90%)
	750	1.6×10^{-2}	1.0×10^{-2} (−36%)	2.2×10^{-3} (−86%)
5	10	7.5×10^{-4}	4.1×10^{-4} (−45%)	7.5×10^{-5} (−90%)
	100	7.1×10^{-3}	4.0×10^{-3} (−44%)	7.5×10^{-4} (−90%)
10	10	1.5×10^{-3}	8.2×10^{-4} (−45%)	1.5×10^{-4} (−90%)

[a]Values in parentheses are percent reductions from the cumulative probability of HIV infection under the baseline assumption of zero condom use.

$$
\begin{aligned}
p &= 0.015 \text{ (a constant rate)} \\
r &= 0.001 \\
e &= 0.90 \\
f &= [0, 0.5, 1.0] \\
n &= [10, 100, 750] \\
m &= [2, 5, 10]
\end{aligned}
$$

The corresponding hypothetical values of P are reported in Table 1. Note that hypothetical values have been used for the inputs because none of the true values for the U.S. teenage population is currently known with precision. The assumptions about teenage sexual behavior are roughly compatible with data reported in the 1987 National Academy of Sciences' report on adolescent sexuality and childbearing (Hayes, 1987; Hofferth and Hayes, 1987).

Given the hypothetical values for the inputs, condom use appears to be a highly effective AIDS prevention strategy. Among teenagers who are not very sexually active (e.g., $m = 2$, $n = 10$), half-time and full-time condom use cuts the cumulative risk of HIV infection by 45 and 90 percent, respectively. Among teenagers with a relatively large number of partners (e.g., $m = 10, n = 10$), half-time and full-time condom use cuts the cumulative risk of infection by 45 and 90 percent, respectively. Among those with high frequency of intercourse (e.g., $m = 2, n = 750$), half-time and full-time condom use cuts the cumulative risk of infection by 36 and 86 percent, respectively. Whereas the absolute probabilities of HIV infection in Table 1 may be off the mark, there is nonetheless a strong suggestion that even half-time condom use produces significant reductions in the risk of HIV infection.

In a recent analysis of 1,000 acts of anal intercourse with and without condoms, Fineberg (1988) showed that condom use is not always a highly effective prevention strategy. Where the prevalence of HIV infection is high among potential partners (e.g., 0.50), he found that half-time condom use produces virtually no benefit and full-time condom use cuts the cumulative risk of infection by 36 percent. He also found that the effectiveness of condoms against HIV infection diminishes rapidly among homosexuals who practice anal intercourse with large numbers of partners.

It is reasonable to expect the relative effectiveness of condoms against HIV infection to be greater among heterosexual adolescents than among homosexuals. Heterosexual adolescents draw partners from a population with relatively low rates of HIV prevalence compared to homosexuals. Moreover, homosexuals tend to practice sex more often and with more partners than heterosexual adolescents do. There is also reason to believe that anal intercourse is a more potent way to transmit the virus than vaginal intercourse. All of these factors help explain why the relative effectiveness of condom use (if not the absolute effectiveness) is larger among heterosexual adolescents than among homosexuals.

Sensitivity Analysis of HIV Prevalence and Condom Efficacy

To determine how confident one should be about condom effectiveness, sensitivity analysis was performed by increasing the value of p (HIV prevalence) from 0.015 to 0.2 and reducing the value of e (condom efficacy) from 0.9 to 0.5. The cumulative probabilities of HIV infection were then recalculated by using the same assumptions and Equation 4.

Results of the sensitivity analysis are reported in Table 2. As expected, the absolute risk of infection is influenced significantly by the new values of p and e. However, the relative effectiveness of the

TABLE 2 Sensitivity Analysis of P Under Alternative Assumptions About HIV Prevalence, Condom Efficacy, and Pattern of Sexual Activity

Sexual Activity	Condom Efficacy	Frequency of Condom Use[a] $f = 0$	$f = 0.5$	$f = 1.0$
	Assume HIV Prevalence = 0.015			
$m = 10, n = 10$	0.9	1.5×10^{-3}	8.2×10^{-4} (−45%)	1.5×10^{-4} (−90%)
	0.5	1.5×10^{-3}	1.1×10^{-3} (−25%)	7.5×10^{-4} (−50%)
$m = 5, n = 100$	0.9	7.1×10^{-3}	4.0×10^{-3} (−44%)	7.5×10^{-4} (−90%)
	0.5	7.1×10^{-3}	5.4×10^{-3} (−24%)	3.7×10^{-3} (−49%)
$m = 2, n = 750$	0.9	1.6×10^{-2}	1.0×10^{-2} (−36%)	2.2×10^{-3} (−86%)
	0.5	1.6×10^{-2}	1.3×10^{-2} (−18%)	9.4×10^{-3} (−41%)
	Assume HIV Prevalence = 0.200			
$m = 10, n = 10$	0.9	2.0×10^{-2}	1.1×10^{-2} (−45%)	2.0×10^{-3} (−90%)
	0.5	2.0×10^{-2}	1.5×10^{-2} (−25%)	9.9×10^{-3} (−50%)
$m = 5, n = 100$	0.9	9.2×10^{-2}	5.2×10^{-2} (−43%)	9.9×10^{-3} (−89%)
	0.5	9.2×10^{-2}	7.0×10^{-2} (−23%)	4.8×10^{-2} (−48%)
$m = 2, n = 750$	0.9	0.20	0.13 (−35%)	2.9×10^{-2} (−86%)
	0.5	0.20	0.16 (−18%)	0.12 (−39%)

NOTE: p = cumulative probability of HIV infection, m = number of partners, n = number of exposures.

[a]Values in parentheses are percent reductions from the cumulative probability of HIV infection under the baseline assumption of zero condom use.

condom remains quite significant. At $p = 0.015$ and $e = 0.5$, half-time and full-time condom use cut the cumulative risk of infection by 18–25 and 40–50 percent, respectively, depending on the sexual activity assumptions. If $e = 0.9$ and $p = 0.2$, half-time and full-time condom use cut the risk by 40–50 and 86–90 percent, respectively, again depending upon the sexual activity assumptions. Because it is unlikely that any adolescent population is currently at $p = 0.2$ and it is likely that $e \geq 0.5$, condom use appears to be a promising strategy for reducing the risk of HIV infection among adolescents.

Accounting for Variations in Condom Use Among Adolescents

Up to this point it has been assumed that condom use is uniform throughout the adolescent population (0, 50, or 100 percent). Suppose instead that condom use behavior in the population mirrors a probability distribution. To simplify, assume a discrete distribution, with three types of condom users—full-time users (f_1), half-time users (f_2), and nonusers (f_3). Each adolescent is assumed to be in one of these three groups, $Prob\{F = f_k\} = x_k$. Given the constraint that $\Sigma_{k=1}^{3} x_k f_k = f$, one must determine how different distributions of condom users influence the cumulative probability of HIV infection.

Suppose, for example, that 50 percent of adolescent sexual exposures are protected by condoms ($f = 0.5$). Although this could occur if all teens used condoms half the time, it could also result from half the teens using condoms all the time and the other half never using condoms.

Under these circumstances, the probability of infection can be modeled in two ways: (1) the frequency of condom use is linked to the person at risk of infection, or (2) the frequency of condom use is linked to the partners of those at risk. Both perspectives are modeled below.

Taking the first perspective (the person at risk) and recalling Equation 4 lead to:

$$P = 1 - \{p[1 - r(1 - f_k e)]^n + (1 - p)\}^m. \tag{5}$$

Here the value of f is conditional on being in condom use group k; hence, the value of P is computed by assuming that the person at risk is in condom group k. If the person at risk exhibits all three types of condom use at different times, the cumulative risk of infection is obtained by:

$$P = 1 - \sum_{k=1}^{3} x_k \{p[1 - r(1 - f_k e)]^n + (1 - p)\}^m. \tag{6}$$

This approach is somewhat awkward because it seems unnatural to assign the same person at risk to more than one condom-use group.

The second approach defines condom-using groups in terms of the behavior of partners. The probability of *no* infection after n exposures with partners in group k is then:

$$\overline{P} = p[1 - r(1 - f_k e)]^n + (1 - p). \tag{7}$$

If the partner is drawn randomly, the probability of infection is

$$P = p \sum_{k=1}^{3} x_k [1 - r(1 - f_k e)]^n + (1 - p). \tag{8}$$

Again, if m random partners are assumed,

$$P = 1 - \{p \sum_{k=1}^{3} x_k [1 - r(1 - f_k e)]^n + (1 - p)\}^m. \tag{9}$$

The quantitative implications of this complication have been explored for the case in which 50 percent of adolescent exposures are protected by condoms ($f = 0.5$). It was assumed that either half of teens were full-time condom users and half nonusers or, alternatively, that all teens were half-time users. An attempt was made to determine which pattern of condom use would be most effective in preventing HIV infection.

The hypothetical input values used to construct the probabilities in Table 1 were used again ($p = 0.015$, $r = 0.001$, $e = 0.90$), except that three groups of sexually active teens were examined ($m = 10$, $n = 10$; $m = 5$, $n = 100$; $m = 2$, $n = 750$). The results, reported in Table 3, indicate that this refinement in the model does not make much difference. Given a particular value of f, it is only slightly better to see the average rate of condom use generated by full-time condom users.

Accounting for Heterogeneity of HIV Prevalence

So far all members of the population at risk have been assumed to select partners from the same HIV "prevalence pool." Suppose instead

TABLE 3 Cumulative Probability of HIV Infection Under Alternative Assumptions About the Fraction of Adolescents in Various Condom-Using Groups, Given That Half of Exposures Are Protected by Condoms

	Sexual Behavior Assumptions		
Condom-Use Distribution	$m = 10$, $n = 10$	$m = 5$, $n = 100$	$m = 2$, $n = 750$
1. ($x_1 = 0, x_2 = 1.0, x_3 = 0$)	8.2×10^{-4}	4.0×10^{-3}	1.0×10^{-2}
2. ($x_1 = 0.5, x_2 = 0, x_3 = 0.5$)	8.2×10^{-4}	3.9×10^{-3}	9.0×10^{-3}

NOTE: m = number of partners, n = number of exposures, x_k = proportion of population in condom-use group k (1 = full-time user, 2 = half-time user, 3 = nonuser).

[a]Values in parentheses are percent reductions from the cumulative probability of HIV infection under the baseline assumption of zero condom use.

that each member selects partners from one of several prevalence pools, in which the prevalence of HIV is p_j. To simplify, let there be three pools with prevalence rates p_1, p_2, and p_3. The probability that an at-risk adolescent draws from pool j is v_j. Let the constraint be that:

$$\sum_{j=1}^{3} v_j p_j = p. \tag{10}$$

In previous calculations, it was assumed in effect that $p_1 = p_2 = p_3 = p = 0.015$. Suppose instead that there is a small population of adolescents ($v_1 = 0.02$) with high HIV prevalence ($p_1 = 0.5$), a large population ($v_2 = 0.48$) with low prevalence ($p_2 = 0.01$), and another large population ($v_3 = 0.50$) with zero prevalence ($p_3 = 0$). The relative effectiveness of condom use under these circumstances must then be determined.

To determine the cumulative probability of infection with three pools of HIV prevalence,

$$P = 1 - \sum_{j=1}^{3} v_j \{p_j[1 - r(1 - fe)]^n + (1 - p_j)\}^m. \tag{11}$$

To estimate P, the hypothetical input values in Table 1 were used, and a sexually active group was the focus ($m = 5$, $n = 100$).

Condoms were still found to be quite effective. The figures in Table 4 for the $m = 5$, $n = 100$ group illustrate this point. If $p_1 = 0.5$, $p_2 = 0.01$, $p_3 = 0$, and if $v_1 = 0.02$, $v_2 = 0.48$, and $v_3 = 0.50$, half-time and full-time condom use cut the risk of HIV infection by 42 and 89 percent, respectively. This rate of relative effectiveness is only slightly inferior to the relative effectiveness rates calculated in the case of a homogeneous HIV prevalence pool.

Accounting for the Possibility of "Superinfectors"

Suppose that all people infected with HIV are not equally infectious. In particular, assume that transmissibility (r) in the population of HIV positives exhibits a probability distribution. To simplify, assume a discrete distribution with three levels of transmissibility (r_1 = highly infectious, r_2 = somewhat infectious, r_3 = not infectious) and $Prob\{R = r_i\} = w_i$. Given that $\Sigma_{i=1}^{3} w_i r_i = r$, let us determine how the existence of "superinfectors" might influence the effectiveness of condoms against HIV.

The probability of no infection given n exposures with partner in group r_i is

$$\overline{P} = p[1 - r_i(1 - fe)]^n + (1 - p). \qquad (12)$$

If the partner is drawn randomly,

$$\overline{P} = p\sum_{i=1}^{3} w_i[1 - r_i(1 - fe)]^n + (1 - p). \qquad (13)$$

With m random partners, the probability of infection becomes

TABLE 4 Cumulative Probability of HIV Infection if Three "Prevalence Pools" Are Assumed, Given Mean Prevalence of 0.015, Alternative Rates of Condom Use, and Specified Sexual Behavior Pattern (n = 100, m = 5)

Frequency of Condom Use	One HIV Prevalence Pool	Three HIV Prevalence Pools
0	7.1×10^{-3}	6.6×10^{-3}
0.5	4.0×10^{-3}	3.8×10^{-3}
	(−44%)	(−42%)
1.0	7.5×10^{-4}	7.3×10^{-4}
	(−89%)	(−89%)

NOTE: m = number of partners, n = number of exposures.

[a]Values in parentheses are percent reductions from the cumulative probability of HIV infection under the baseline assumption of zero condom use.

$$P = 1 - \{p \sum_{i=1}^{3} w_i [1 - r_i(1 - fe)]^n + (1 - p)\}^m. \quad (14)$$

The quantitative implications of this complication were explored for the case in which $r = 0.001$. In one scenario (Table 1), it was assumed that all HIV positives were infectious at the same rate, $r_1 = r_2 = r_3 = r = 0.001$. The alternative scenario presumes a small group ($w_1 = 0.001$) of "superinfectors" who are certain to infect their partners with a single unprotected sexual exposure ($r_1 = 1.0$). Everyone else who is infected is assumed not to be infectious ($w_2 = 0, w_3 = 0.999, r_3 = 0$). Such an extreme case of heterogeneity in transmissibility substantially reduces the effectiveness of even full-time condom use, as long as n is fairly large (Table 5).

It is easy to visualize this phenomenon by considering the case in which the adolescent at risk has a "superinfectious" partner. Even if the person at risk is protected by full-time condom use, the cumulative probability of infection increases rapidly as the number of exposures increases. Although the condom may be 90 percent effective per exposure, repeated exposures will ultimately infect the person at risk due to condom failure. The cumulative risk of infection is 0.65 from 10 "protected" exposures, 0.93 from 25 exposures, 0.995 from 50 exposures, and 0.99997 from 100 exposures. In a potential population of partners that is known to include such superinfectors,

TABLE 5 Cumulative Probability of HIV Infection Under Alternative Assumptions About the Fraction of Partners in Various Transmissibility Groups ("superinfector" case)

	Sexual Behavior Assumptions		
Frequency of Condom Use	$m = 10$, $n = 10$	$m = 5$, $n = 100$	$m = 2$, $n = 750$
0	1.5×10^{-4}	7.5×10^{-5}	3.0×10^{-5}
0.5	1.5×10^{-4} (~0%)	7.5×10^{-5} (~0%)	3.0×10^{-5} (~0%)
1	9.8×10^{-5} (35%)	7.5×10^{-5} (~0%)	3.0×10^{-5} (~0%)

NOTE: $w_1 = 0.001$, $w_2 = 0$, $w_3 = 0.999$ and $r_1 = 1$, $r_2 = 0.5$, $r_3 = 0$, where w_k = proportion in population of transmissibility group k and r_k = the risk of transmitting the virus. m = number of partners, n = number of exposures.

the choice of partner is far more critical to risk reduction than is condom use.

Even if superinfectors are in the pool of potential partners, condom use is somewhat effective if the number of exposures per partner is small. Because many adolescent sexual relationships involve only several (or even one or two) exposures, condom use is still an effective protection strategy. Hence, even an extreme case of heterogeneity in transmissibility ("superinfectors") does not eliminate the promise of condom use as a method to prevent HIV infection.

REFERENCES

Cleary, P. D., Barry, M. J., Mayer, K. H., Brandt, A. M., Gostin, L., and Fineberg, H. V. (1987) Compulsory premarital screening for the human immunodeficiency virus. *Journal of the American Medical Association* 258:1757–1762.

Drummond, M. F., Stoddart, G. L., and Torrance, G. W. (1987) *Methods for the Economic Evaluation of Health Care Programs.* Oxford, England: Oxford University Press.

Fineberg, H. V. (1988) Education to prevent AIDS: Prospects and obstacles. *Science* 239:592–596.

Hayes, C. D. (ed.) (1987) *Risking the Future: Adolescent Sexuality, Pregnancy, and Childbearing,* Volume I. Washington, D.C.: National Academy Press.

Hofferth, S. L., and Hayes, C. D. (eds.) (1987) *Risking the Future: Adolescent Sexuality, Pregnancy, and Childbearing,* Volume II. Washington, D.C.: National Academy Press.

Keeler, E. B., and Cretin, S. (1983) Discounting of lifesaving and other nonmonetary effects. *Management Science* 29:300–306.

Peterman, T. A., Stoneburner, R. L., Allen, J. R., Jaffe, H. W., and Curran, J. W. (1988) Risk of human immunodeficiency virus transmission from heterosexual adults with transfusion-associated infections. *Journal of the American Medical Association* 259:55–58.

Ward, J. W, Grindon, A. J., Ferrino, P. M., et al. (1986) Laboratory and epidemiologic evaluation of an enzyme immunoassay for antibodies to HTLV-III. *Journal of the American Medical Association* 256:357–361.

Warner, K. E., and Luce, B. R. (1982) *Cost Benefit and Cost Effectiveness Analysis in Health Care: Principles, Practice, and Potential.* Ann Arbor, Mich.: Health Administration Press.

Weinstein, M. C., and Stason, W. B. (1977) Foundations of cost-effectiveness analysis for health and medical practices. *New England Journal of Medicine* 296:716–721.

Sexuality Across the Life Course in the United States

John H. Gagnon

In all societies one of the major axes on which sexual life is ordered is the age of individuals as organized into a socially constructed life course (Clausen, 1972; Reigel and Meachum, 1976). However, the timing in the life course in which various forms of sexual conduct will be learned, expressed, and disappear, and the relationship of sexual conduct to other aspects of social and psychological life vary from one society to another and from one period to another in the history of any specific society (Ford and Beach, 1951; Marshall and Suggs, 1971; Dover, 1978; Katz, 1983; Herdt, 1984; Duberman, 1986; D'Emilio and Freedman, 1988). Thus not only does the patterning of sexuality even across such a relatively narrow life stage as adolescence differ in an advanced industrial society with a predominantly Judeo-Christian religious tradition like the United States and in developing societies with differing religious traditions, but also important differences can be found in the sexual lives of adolescents in the United States and those in other Western industrial societies (Jones et al., 1986). Similarly, differences in the sexual life of adolescents can be found across relatively short time spans in the history of the United States; one need only contrast the 1920s with the 1950s or either of these decades with the 1980s.

As a result of this grounding in social and cultural processes, chronological age and the biological events associated with it rarely

John H. Gagnon is in the Department of Sociology, State University of New York at Stony Brook.

directly explain sexual conduct. For example, the biological changes associated with puberty interact with the social and cultural contexts that provide the framework for interpreting one's changing bodily characteristics and reproductive capacities (Gagnon and Simon, 1973). In the same fashion, the social and cultural expectations about the appropriate levels of sexual activity for the elderly often shape the sexual declines associated with aging (Verwoerdt et al., 1969; Brecher et al., 1984)

Understanding that variations in sexual conduct are stratified by culturally defined life stage groupings does not entail the acceptance of culturally universal sequences of human psychosocial development (Baltes and Brim, 1979). The staging of the life course in any culture, and the sexual activities that are linked to it, depend on social constructions within cultures rather than on the automatic biological unfolding of the organism (Nardi, 1973; Neugartan and Datan, 1973; Uhlenberg, 1978). Thus, in the United States, although the scripts for sexual conduct (the who, what, when, where, and why of conduct) and the interpersonal sexual networks through which they are expressed change across life course stages, both the sexual scripts and the networks can be matched only *partially* with age/stage periods in the life course (Gagnon, 1973; Simon and Gagnon, 1987).

The matching of life events to age/stage periods is most precise in strongly age-graded traditional societies with a relatively limited set of irreversible role transitions across the life course (Kagan, 1980). In industrial and postindustrial societies, such matchings of life events to age/stage periods seem most satisfactory early in life, which accounts for much of the success of age/stage variables in human development theory and research related to infancy and childhood. However, there is cross-cultural and historical evidence that even these early moments of the life course are not immune to change (for an instructive example, see Kett, 1978).

The complexity of life course stages has increased in the more advanced industrial societies. Both increases in discontinuities early in the life course (as a function of participation of sharply age-graded family and schooling practices) and a greater diffuseness of stage boundaries later in life (e.g., when relatively age-independent patterns of affectional and sexual coupling and recoupling) can be observed. With increases in societal complexity and social mobility, individuals turn out less often to be exactly what they might have been expected to be, given their life chances at birth (Brim and Wheeler, 1966). In contrast to more traditional societies with limited adult role sets, limited rates of individual mobility, and slow rates of sociocultural change, rapidly changing advanced industrial societies are characterized by individuals with wider role networks and less predictable life courses. In such cultures, personality structures themselves might be expected to be more fluid.

These differences in societies make it important to examine those social strata and experiences that crosscut age/stage periods and increase the variability of conduct within age and stage groupings. Some of these stratification systems begin early in life to allocate individuals into relatively fixed streams of individual development, isolating them from conventional life courses. For instance, some birth defects, when responded to by the society, often create specially segregated clusters of differentially abled individuals with quite different age/stage patterns. Other strata rest on characteristics such as race, religion, or the socioeconomic status of parents; sometimes this status is relatively easy to change, other times, it is not, depending on the social context (Featherman, 1980). Other stratifications that differentiate age groups appear later in life. College attendance by some young persons and going to work after high school by others often affirm prior, but less stringent, boundaries between young persons of different social classes in high school. Going to college or going to work creates new social and sexual networks that exclude former potential sexual partners and open slots for new ones.

One important division in the society that is particularly relevant to sexuality and crosscuts all other strata, including age, is gender (Rossi, 1985). The gendering of social life has seemed so natural that it appeared to most to be part of the biological background. It is only through the efforts of feminist scholars, both women and men, to denaturalize the gender order and point out its social origins, that one has been able to observe the importance of gender in structuring the conceptions of sexuality. Over the last 15 years there have been important changes in research and theorizing about gender and sexuality in most social science disciplines. In general, these reconsiderations have followed in a social constructionist tradition (Ortner and Whitehead, 1981; Tiefer, 1987), but important contributions have been made by those who have focused on what they consider to be "essential" differences between the genders and their sexuality (Rich, 1983).

Although much of this work has been theoretical or critical, important original empirical work has been published, particularly in social history. While it is not possible to review here in detail this extensive and theoretically rich literature, a number of points need to be made in light of it (some important recent works are by Rubin,

1975, 1984; English et al., 1981; Snitow et al., 1984; Vance, 1984; and Califia, whose works are cited in Rubin, 1984). Such work points out the necessary considerations that must be given to gender differences in sexuality as they are "found" to exist across the life course. In some cases these differences will be illusory; in others they will be real, but culturally transient; in still others they will be functions of the interests, both scientific and otherwise, of the observers. Such cautions should be kept in mind when considering the life course constructed below.

Linked to the issue of gender is the problem of violence and its sequelae in the lives of women. Some of this violence involves sexual acts, but large amounts of violence against women may not be specifically sexual and still be consequential for their sexual lives. Making too sharp a distinction between sexual and nonsexual violence may conceal rather than illuminate both the origins and the consequences of gender-related violence (Straus et al., 1980; Finkelhor et al., 1983). While some men are the victims of specifically sexual violence (perpetrated almost exclusively by other men), this is not a routine aspect of men's lives. Relatively unexamined, however, is the nonsexual violence between men (including games involving physical aggression), which is often traceable to the direct or indirect competition among men for the attention of, or access to, women. However, women of all ages, but more often the young, are relatively frequent targets of sexual coercion and violence (Groth, 1979; Russell, 1984). From being forced by lovers and spouses to perform sexual acts they do not wish to perform to acts of sexual violence by strangers, the specter or the experience of violence related to sexuality is part of the background of female sexuality. The climate of potential violence (heavily reinforced by, and represented in, the mass media), as well as the experience of actual violence by women, must have effects on their sexual lives. How to factor this climate and these individual events into a life course perspective on the sexual relations between women and men is not entirely obvious, but such experiences, on average, may be as important as other major life events (e.g., divorce) or life conditions (e.g., low income) in structuring women's sexuality.

The most important stratification of individuals on specifically sexual grounds is the result of an erotic preference for persons of either the other or the same gender. This cleavage begins to be sharply felt by many in adolescence but often only becomes fully articulated in young adulthood. The social cleavage between those who prefer sex with the same gender and those who prefer sex with persons of the other gender is extremely complex and has undergone considerable historical change since the end of World War II (D'Emilio, 1983). It should be noted that many persons having ongoing sexual experiences with persons of the same gender do not think of themselves as gay, lesbian, or homosexual. Some of these persons have such sexual relations out of a variety of motives and in a variety of contexts, some of them subcultural. Thus, young men who have regular sex with women may intermittently sell themselves (usually their penis) to persons of the same gender for sex, never thinking of themselves as homosexual (Reiss, 1961). Delinquents, young men in the military, young men down on their luck, and working-class men in need of sexual outlet in absence of women may engage in such "homosexual" activity. Some men from some Latin cultures and some aggressive men in prisons do not discriminate between the gender of their sexual partners as long as they are in the active/insertive sexual role (Carrier, 1976). Such persons, and others that could be identified, are often described as bisexual, but this is much too simple, except as a purely behavioral identifier (Schwartz and Blumstein, 1977). There are men who identify themselves as gay who have sex with women and women in lesbian relationships who may have sex with men on an intermittent basis (Gagnon, 1977; Califia, 1983).

Most people who have sex with partners of the same gender solely on a situational or contextual basis have only a limited portion of their social relationships with those having same-gender erotic preferences and often have most of their sexual activity with persons of the other gender. Prior to the early 1970s, this pattern of living a life hidden among the heterosexual majority was probably true of large numbers of persons who would have identified themselves as homosexual or at least predominantly interested in sex with persons of the same gender. Life entirely in the closet or at least concealing their predominant sexual preference to important persons in their lives (parents, spouses, children, other relatives, coworkers, good friends, members of the religious community) was the common condition of persons with same-gender sexual desires (Humphrey, 1978). Homosexuality was thought to be sinful, criminal, pathological, or deviant, and research was usually conducted by scientists holding these presumptions on persons living under these conditions of social repression (Bieber, 1962, Socarides, 1978). Many individuals participated clandestinely and fearfully in the limited institutions of the "homosexual community," whereas others lived in sexual relationships open to limited friendship circles and social groups (Warren, 1974). Fear of blackmail, robbery, police harassment or brutality, loss of jobs, and discovery by unknowing loved ones was endemic

(Kinsey et al., 1948; Gebhard et al., 1965; Simon and Gagnon, 1967; Weinberg and Williams, 1974).

The social transformations of the 1960s and 1970s created from the earlier homosexual community a new social collectivity that has come to be called the gay male and lesbian communities in which new sexual identities have been created (Plummer, 1981; Escoffier, 1985). Part of this social solidarity was the emergence of a more complex community in metropolitan centers based on a wide variety of needs and interests (Humphreys, 1972; D'Emilio, 1983). Gay and lesbian political groups, newspapers and book publishers, community service agencies, restaurants, employment and other agencies, and medical and legal professionals have flourished in these communities. As a tradition of greater openness emerged, it was possible for some gay men and lesbians to be "open" to all the important persons in their lives as well as to the general public, whereas others remained either selective or constrained in their openness. Despite these changes, however, there does not seem to have been a reduction in homophobia among the general population, at least as measured by attitude questions about homosexuality on national surveys (see Figure 7-2 in Chapter 7).

The relation of the gay male and lesbian communities to the larger society has come to look more like that of other minority communities based on ethnicity, religion, and race, which prized both their cultural singularity and their relation to the larger culture, polity, and economy (Paul et al., 1982; D'Emilio, 1983). Some gay men and lesbians live their entire lives within their own communities, spending the majority of their lives working and living with persons having the same sexual preference. Others work and live partially in the social world populated by a majority of heterosexuals, sometimes open, and sometimes not, but have most of their important affectional ties and interpersonal connections in the gay and lesbian communities. Still others retain strong ties to members of the heterosexual majority (including parents and children)—sometimes open about their sexual preference and sometimes not—and sustain connections of the widest variety with members of the larger society. Although an imperfect analogy, one might think of the relations of Jews to the non-Jewish majority in the United States at an earlier stage in history—a relationship that ranged (and still ranges, though with less anti-Semitism) from the insularity of the Hasidic communities to the invisibility of secular Jews in the larger society.

Given these restrictions on the universality of life course models or even the lack of a dominant model in the United States, it is still useful to attempt to characterize the sexual life course in the United States in order to identify modal sexual processes and experiences as well as those that vary substantially from them. It is important to point out that the presentation of the age/stage periods in a time order from early to late does not mean that earlier experience is always strongly determinative of later experience (Brim and Wheeler, 1966). The demands of current social circumstances are often more determinative of current sexual conduct than are early experiences that are *post hoc* thought to connect earlier to later behavior. Sexual conduct at later moments in the life course should not be thought of as a simple reenactment of, or as preformed by, earlier patterns of nonsexual or sexual conduct (Gagnon and Simon, 1973).

What follows then is a heuristic framework for the life course of those with other-gender and same-gender preferences in erotic relations in the United States for the last two decades and perhaps extending into the future until the turn of the century. There are many variations from this framework. It is not meant to be prescriptive or normative, although it may be treated by some as such, but rather descriptive and indicative of sexual patterns in one culture and at one point in time. In addition it should be emphasized that both the life course and the patterns of sexual conduct are changing in relatively unpredictable directions as a result of the influence of much larger social forces.

CHILDHOOD

Infancy

Infancy stretches in time from birth to the middle of the third year of life when independent locomotion and language skills have been developed. The center of the child's life moves from the mother (and less often a father or other caretaker) to a more extended group of individuals in and out of the family. Although, historically, the psychoanalytic tradition viewed these years as critical for mature psychosexual development, more contemporary research suggests that the importance of these early experiences (e.g., weaning, toilet training, parental attachment) to adolescent and adult sexual patterns is quite limited. This is in accordance with other work in human development which suggests that early experience may be less critical for later development than previously assumed, although this remains a serious point of controversy among developmental psychologists (Kagan, 1971). Perhaps of most importance in the United States is the successful acquisition of some elements of a conventionalized gender identity, and perhaps the most important of these is the preliminary sense of being a boy or a girl. Although it has been argued that this acquisition of gender identity is an all or none process somewhat like imprinting, a more cautious formulation would be that the components of the conventional gender identity package are probably learned in a more cumulative fashion over the entire period of childhood (Luria, 1979).

The intensity and consistency of environmental demands for conforming gender conduct among the young may make the acquisition of gender identity appear to be a form of natural development, but there is evidence that various elements of gender identity seem to be accessible to change later in life (Maccoby and Jacklin, 1974). Thus gender-linked differences in the behavior of small children, such as assertiveness, often wash out in the context of the demands of adult work lives (Epstein, 1981). In most Western societies and particularly in the United States, this earliest portion of the life course is linked to sexuality as expressed by most postpubertal individuals primarily through cumulative gender role and nonsexual learning, which serve as a frame for the future acquisition and practice of both heterosexual and homosexual conduct in adolescence (Money and Ehrhardt, 1972; Kessler and McKenna, 1974; Gagnon, 1979).

Preschool

In the preschool period, say from ages 3 to 6, children enter an expanding world of interpersonal and media experiences. Mothers, fathers, siblings, grandparents, same-age peers, the mass media through television, and preschool and day-care experiences rapidly complicate and enrich the world of children. Here, the differences among various cultures and points in the history of any given culture become more sharply focused. The presence or absence of the mass media, churchgoing, full-time care by mothers, and urban or village living shape not only the daily life of the child but also the ways in which knowledge about sexuality is acquired and the systems of meaning to which it is linked. (The historical study of sexual life is rapidly expanding; for examples, see Foucault, 1978; Boswell, 1980; Weeks, 1981; Gay, 1984; and Crompton, 1985.) Few children in the world are as bombarded with gender role models linked to the consumption of toys and other products, or to explicit models of personal attractiveness that become the basis of sexual attractiveness later in life, as are children in the United States (for a review, see Brown et al., 1988).

The aspects of the conventional gender identity package acquired in infancy are systematically reinforced and policed by the widest variety of audiences. Children first learn about modesty and shame, and systematic restrictions are placed on their access to various bodily pleasures. Their earliest inquiries about sexuality are commonly unanswered, their bodily parts and reproductive processes are either mislabeled or nonlabeled (Sears et al., 1957; Gagnon, 1965). It is characteristic of the majority of families to avoid references to sexual matters and protect children from sexual information. Nearly all retrospective studies of adolescents and adults on sources and timing of sexual learning indicate the limited role that parents play in these matters.

Later Childhood

The transition of children from the home to elementary school has clearly changed with the increase of working mothers and day-care or preschool programs. Many of the experiences that once characterized the first day of school are now spread out over a much longer period. The significance of the first six years of school has probably not changed a great deal, however. The elementary school in its normal practices extends and further reinforces the conventional gender role package in still another set of environments. School opportunities and peer relationships sharpen the gender divisions between boys and girls in both formal and informal school programs. Failure in schools for either academic or other reasons begins to set the stage for nonconformist and risk-taking behaviors that characterize young people who are reached inadequately by the schools themselves. Pressures toward general conformity to rules and regulations offer other opportunities for deviance among children.

There are still strong tendencies for children to spend the majority of their time and emotions in same-gender peer groups. Whereas the strength of gender divisions has been growing weaker among urban, upper middle class groups, the support for same-gender friendships remains strong among most social groups in the society (Hess, 1981). Schools tend to reinforce these patterns through both the cultural preferences of teachers and the institutionalized gender practices of the school itself.

Television maintains its continuing pressure on gender role conformity through Saturday morning programming for children, particularly the advertisements, as well as through programming directed toward adults that is seen by children. Of particular importance to sexuality are the effects of these materials on what children expect to happen in adolescence and adulthood. Indeed, perhaps the most important training that children receive about the social context of their sexual futures comes from the mass media, largely television, but also from the cinema shown on television. Thus, the importance of physical attractiveness, success with the opposite gender, falling in love, being a member of a couple, and high consumption standards are the staples of adult television that children watch (Brown et al., 1988).

Although there is evidence of an increase in more explicit sexual or sexuality-related mass media materials, the effect of these materials on prepubertal children is unknown. This new explicitness exists at two levels. The first is the one that attracts attempts at social control: programs or magazines that contain nudity, open references to sexuality, or language that may offend. Although this material often evokes attempts at censorship, the majority of prepubertal children may not understand much of it. The second aspect of the new explicitness is the relatively constant public debate conducted in the mass media about such topics as pornography, contraception, abortion, and adolescent sexuality, as well as public education programs about AIDS prevention. This openness of debate and public discussion about sexuality, without any explicitly sexual depictions, may offer more informal sexual information to older children than pornography. For example, the access of girls to mass market magazines intended for women, which heavily emphasize issues of sexual adjustment, orgasm, extramarital sex, and sexual dysfunction, may be more critical than the availability of more sexually open materials in movies or on television. The recency of this increased sexual openness means that we do not yet have a generation that has grown up under this informational regime. These mass media forces in sexual education of the prepubertal young are also relevant to the adolescent and young adult periods as well, but equally little is known about their consumption or influence. It may well be that exposure to these materials actually has no consequence for the current or future lives of children or young people; the dilemma is that there is no acceptable scientific evidence one way or the other.

This is also the period in life when sex play among children begins to take place. In the early years, most sex play among younger children has motives specific to their developmental stage (Gagnon, 1965). In these cases, adult interpretation of the conduct as sexually motivated (i.e., motivated by sexual desires possessed by adults) is probably in error. Among most children, even when they are close to puberty, the motivation for such exploration is probably not the full complement of adult sexual desires or preferences. However, there is evidence that some older children, who live in environments in which the sexual conduct of adults is more observable and acceptable or who are targets for the sexual interest of postpubertal youth, may be involved in sexual experimentation which in techniques and motives is more like that of adults. Much of this evidence comes from studies of child sexual abuse (Finkelhor, 1984).

Despite the growth of sexual knowledge from media sources, there is little evidence that either parents or schools have engaged in vigorous attempts to reduce the general sexual ignorance of children during these years, although this may be changing as a consequence of the dangers associated with AIDS. For example, the recent National Health Interview Survey found that approximately 60 percent of parents with children and adolescents from ages 10 to 17 reported that they had talked to these youngsters about AIDS (Dawson and Thornberry, 1988). It is not clear what their children would report about the same matter. Most pre-AIDS research reports that teaching about sex and reproduction remains limited in the schools (Jones et al., 1986:57–58). Even AIDS risk prevention programs for children tend to be less informative than they might be. Studies in the last decade suggest that even youthful parents rarely tell their children much about sexuality (Kline et al., 1978). What seem to be most strongly reinforced publicly are conventional marriage, family, and reproductive roles, whereas sexual knowledge remains part of a covert underground fed indirectly by the media and peers.

Both the physical assault of children and the sexual contacts of children with adults are important experiences that have only recently become the focus of intense public debate, criminal proceedings, and social movements (Finkelhor, 1984; Russell, 1984). Both of these experiences, in combination or separately, may have important consequences on adult social and sexual adjustment. There is estimated to be a substantial amount of sexual contact between adults (usually male) and young children of both genders which varies in duration, level of sexual intimacy, and degree of consanguinity (Finkelhor, 1979). However, the actual amount of such contacts and their impact are often obscured by research methods and classificatory decisions that have the possibility of inflating rates and conflating serious with less serious events (Cook and Howells, 1980).

YOUTH

The transition from childhood to adolescence, roughly the years from 12 to 15, is most clearly marked by the physical changes associated with puberty. These changes signal somewhat diffusely to most children and more precisely to most older persons that the child is now potentially a sexual being and might/can/should be treated as such. Such treatment can vary from an increasing protectiveness by parents in terms of association with the opposite sex (more likely for girls than boys) to an increased frequency of being the object of the expression of sexual interest by older peers. The interaction between biological changes and social context in the shaping of sexual conduct during this period is now beginning to be studied carefully, and there is discussion of the significance of biological potentiation in the context of newly available social roles and opportunities for sexual expression (Udry, 1985; for a general discussion of this period, see Kagan and Coles, 1973).

The timing of specific physical changes (breast development, axillary and genital hair, voice changes, changes in the genitalia) are spread out over the period from 11 to 14 years, with many changes occurring at ages 12 and 13 (Tanner, 1973). The first menstruation, increases in the frequency of erection, and the first ejaculation tend to be concentrated in this period, with the first orgasm somewhat less common in this early period for girls than boys due to lower rates of masturbation (Kinsey et al., 1953; Atwood and Gagnon, 1987; Gagnon, 1987).

The practice of social skills needed for heterosexuality begins during early adolescence through the *heterosocial* pattern of association with the opposite gender, pairing off from other young people, developing a strong emotional bond (falling in love), and sexual experimentation (for a summary of the pattern, see Gagnon and Greenblat, 1978:167–169). Conventionally, young people have a series of such relationships across the adolescent period, with each relationship increasing in its emotional–sexual intimacy. This pattern anticipates in some ways the pattern of serial monogamy found in adults. These levels of sexual activity at various ages differ substantially according to ethnicity and socioeconomic status. In some inner-city populations, sexual intercourse may begin at ages 13 and

14 for some boys and girls, whereas for others, from more affluent-groups interested in attending college, intercourse will not begin until the late teens or early 20s (Furstenberg et al., 1987; Udry and Billy, 1987; Weinberg and Williams, 1988).

It is unclear how much of the overt sexual activity of adolescence is motivated by sexual desire and how much results from the desire for peer acceptance and other nonsexual motives. This is particularly true among younger adolescents whose motivations for sexual activity still differ between girls and boys (Newcomer and Udry, 1985). Sexuality remains strongly colored by affection and caring among the former and by desires for sexual conquest and male peer approval among the latter (Jessor and Jessor, 1978; Jessor et al., 1983; Carroll et al., 1985). However, it is in the relationships young people have during this period that a somewhat greater commonality of sexual motives between girls and boys tends to emerge (Miller and Simon, 1974). At the same time, one should not underestimate the extraordinary power of gender differentiation in shaping the sexual relations even between women and men who have been married for many years. For example, Leiblum and Rosen (1988) report that many sexual difficulties among couples may be attributed to rigid gender role expectations about sexuality (see also Rubin, 1976).

These emergent sexual relations between male and female adolescents are generally not attended to by adults unless something untoward occurs that forces an adult to notice. Young people are often left on their own to work out their intrapsychic and interpersonal sexual adjustments (Fox, 1981). Evidence from clinical and other descriptive sources suggests that this period is often one of psychological and social confusion for many young people. This is probably even more true of those young people who find themselves, for one reason or another, attracted either sexually or emotionally to persons of the same gender or who find, for one reason or another, that other-gender relations are unattractive or implausible (Coleman, 1982). Young people who have unconventional desires often must adopt or modify the minimal social guideposts set up by the media and youth culture for the conventional heterosocial/heterosexual pattern to guide their early practice of sexuality. The "coming-out process" for those with same-gender preferences has always been a complex one (Dank, 1971) with many dimensions. One can recognize the preference privately, have overt sexual activity with a person of the same sex, be open with various other persons (from parents to strangers), and engage in political activity—in any combination and in any time order. The parallel process of coming out sexually is less marked among young people who have sex with persons of the opposite gender, appearing to be part of the natural order of things. Indeed many adolescents, simply by not disobeying the rules, can drift into conventional heterosexuality and find elements of this pattern acceptable without any strong sexual desires of their own.

In contrast, a great deal of unsystematic clinical and literary evidence produced even into the 1970s suggested that self-identification as "homosexual" and the expression of emotional and sexual desires for the same gender were often guilt producing and conflict laden (White, 1983). The sexual developmental pattern was often one in which adolescent sexual experience with persons of the same gender was intermittent and a fuller participation in a homosexual life-style occurred only in the very late teens or early 20s after some years of emotional difficulties. "Coming out" was often linked to participation in the institutions of the "homosexual community" (Hooker, 1966). It should be noted that the methods of gathering evidence used to select young persons in many clinical studies often overlooked untroubled and eager acceptance of same-gender desire and sexuality among some young people.

What has happened to young people with the feelings identified above since the emergence of the gay male and lesbian communities (there is overlap, but these communities are not identical) is relatively unknown. The visibility of gay and lesbian life-styles in the mass media (television, the cinema, and the press) may often provide young people a more concrete version of a possible sexual future and allow both intrapsychic and interpersonal experimentation with the emotional and sexual possibilities of being gay or being lesbian. This is particularly true in large cities where gay male and lesbian communities exist. The contemporary process of "coming out" should be more complex among young people, with some following the more traditional secretive path, whereas others find their way to a gay or lesbian identity both more openly and much earlier in life. Even in current circumstances, development of same-gender desires is often repressed by the overwhelmingly heterosocial and heterosexual character of the institutions of adolescent life and by adults who view same-gender sexual experience and desire as pathological. The reception that these desires receive is usually dependent on family and community factors that are well outside the control of the young person. Only recently has this period in the lives of young people been studied, and most of this research has been undertaken after the beginning of the AIDS crisis (see the work of Herdt, n.d.).

Such sexual experiences with persons of the same gender are, however, not uncommon even among those who ultimately become exclusively heterosexual as adults (Kinsey et al., 1948, 1953; Fay et al., in press). It should also be pointed out that many adolescent and adult males who have sexual experience with other men on some regular basis as adults do not view themselves as gay or homosexual (Schwartz and Blumstein, 1977). At the same time, many—though surely not all—men who, as adults, have substantial sexual experiences with other men usually have had some such sexual experience in their youth (Bell and Weinberg, 1978; Bell et al., 1980). The patterning of adolescent or adult female experiences with the same gender appears to be more diffuse; the acquisition of a strong commitment to sexual experiences with other women is spread out over adolescence and young adulthood (Wolf, 1979; Peplau and Gordon, 1983).

Equally concealed by the code of silence about sexuality in early adolescence is masturbation. Masturbation, in adolescence and adulthood, is usually defined, following Kinsey, as primarily genitally focused self-stimulation that results in orgasm. The infrequent inquiries about this form of sexual conduct until the middle 1970s found that the incidence of such conduct was far more common among males and that the frequency of masturbation (so defined) was also far higher among males than females (Kinsey et al., 1948, 1953; Atwood and Gagnon, 1987; Gagnon, 1987). These gender differences in the incidence and frequency of masturbation seemed to remain throughout the entire life course. Cross-sectional data on students in West Germany gathered in 1966 and 1981 suggest that there may have been a greater convergence in the masturbatory patterns of young people in the last two decades, but comparable recent data for the United States do not appear to be available (Clement et al., 1984). In the past, male masturbatory patterns were more often associated with explicit fantasies of unconventional sexual behavior than were those of women, but again few data on this matter exist for more recent periods.

This emphasis on genitality, erotic fantasy, and orgasm as the criteria for identifying masturbation may have effectively excluded from the sexual arena the more romantically focused fantasies of many adolescent women and their bodily activities that are more diffusely satisfying, but nonorgasmic. This difference points up the critical role of gender prescriptions in setting the normative boundaries of what is or is not a sexual experience for both sexual actors and sexual scientists. Many women scholars have pointed out that most research on sexuality has taken male sexual interests and models of desire as normative (Tiefer, 1987). Both Freud and Kinsey viewed women as somehow "less sexual" than men because they did not have the same repertoire of sexual activities and gratifications. Kinsey's concern with male sexual urgency and search for variety led him to pose differences in the central nervous systems of men and women to account for what were largely the results of social and historical differences in culture and social organization (Kinsey et al., 1953).

Although sexual conduct is shaped by gender and there are obvious gender patterns for all conduct in the society, gender differences are not monolithic, either psychologically or socially (Gagnon, 1979; Stoller, 1985). There is a great variety in the sexual lives of women, a variety which tends not to be noticed because of the usual focus on the tension that exists for women between passionate and reproductive sexuality. There is a tendency to see both women who are reproductively "out of control" (unplanned pregnancy) and women who are reproductively "in control" (successful contraception outside marriage) as sexually "out of control" (Snitow et al., 1984; Vance, 1984). This confusion between contraceptive and sexual readiness is only one of the double binds in which girls and women find themselves as they take greater control of their sexual lives.

Adolescence is the first period in the life course when variation from the conventional expectations of adults becomes explicitly supported, particularly by peers and the mass media. In some cases, adults find themselves nearly entirely separated from the important aspects of young people's lives by the grounding of the latter in youth culture, although more often, there continue to be important, although more attenuated, points of contact between parents or other adults and young people. This transitional character of contemporary adolescence makes it, unlike other periods in the life course, more devoted to various forms of risk taking, including the sexual. This is in contrast to other, more stable, stages in the life course when either status transitions or untoward events initiate changes in relationships that thrust persons into new forms of conduct which may involve risks of various sorts. During adolescence, overt sexual experimentation by relatively untutored young people is as common as experimentation with drugs, alcohol, and driving. Overt sexual activity is usually insulated from adult notice so that only the negative consequences of such conduct are identified—pregnancy, sexually transmitted disease (STD), and socioemotional crisis are the events that mobilize adult concern.

The mass media play an ambivalent role in facilitating adolescent sexuality and risk taking. Whereas the media often reinforce conventional adult roles and point up the dangers of deviating from sexual/gender norms, they usually do so in the course of portraying "attractive nuisances." In films such as *Fatal Attraction*, after displaying a good deal of exciting and provocative extramarital sex between very attractive people, one of the two persons (usually the woman) is somehow punished for the transgressions. In this way the audience may be sexually excited and still have the opportunity to see the deviants punished (Brown et al., 1988). Although reinforcing conventional outcomes, the media offer more explicit sexual models for conduct and, perhaps more important, attach sexual and gender success to particular norms of attractiveness, consumer values, and practices. The linkage of sex and gender to consumption probably permeates all adolescent subcultures.

As young people move closer to the end of high school, more and more of them are involved in the cycle of finding opposite-gender partners, pairing off with them in emotional–sexual relationships, and then breaking off these relationships (for changes since the 1940s, see Reiss, 1960, 1967; Cannon and Long, 1971; Simon et al., 1972; Udry et al., 1975; Chilman, 1978; Clayton and Bokemeier, 1980; Hofferth et al., 1987). There are both an increase in experimentation with novel sexual techniques (particularly oral sex, DeLamater and MacCorquodale, 1979:59; Newcomer and Udry, 1985; Gagnon and Simon, 1987) and increasing frequencies of sexual intercourse. Involvement in this cycle of coupling and recoupling also increases the numbers of both primary (relations of significant duration and emotional commitment) and secondary sexual partners that young persons have before the end of their teens (see Chapter 2 of this volume, and Zelnik et al., 1981). Perhaps the greatest change from the past is that much of the heterosexual activity that occurs can no longer be described simply as "premarital" intercourse. Although it does occur before marriage, only some of it is actually in service of the marriage institution. If, for instance, a young person's first intercourse occurs at 15 or 16 and first marriage in the mid-20s, with a number of affectional–sexual relationships (including intercourse) in between, the first experience and many of the later ones will have been undertaken for their own sakes, not in a search for marriage partners (Furstenberg, 1982). Even early cohabitations may not be directed toward finding a one and only partner. This sexual experimentation is in important ways no longer premarital in the sense that similar conduct might have been three decades ago.

Even though there has been a general change in the experience of the young with intercourse (in terms of both increasing incidence and numbers of partners), it does not appear that young persons are any better prepared by adults in the society for such relationships than they were in the 1950s. High rates of risk taking in terms of both pregnancy and STD are common, as are relatively weak sources of support when relationships are in emotional or sexual difficulty (Ooms, 1981; McClusky et al., 1983; O'Reilly and Aral, 1985). Although sex among adolescents is understood to be widespread, it remains covert and largely supported by peer groups and the youth culture of the school or of the mass media.

Although prior discussion describes the modal pattern, it should be understood that there is considerable heterogeneity in adolescent sexual patterns, depending on ethnicity, religion, income, education, and class. Some of these differences may be substantial enough to create quite different patterns of sexual life. Indeed, there are increasing numbers of young people who, by the end of adolescence, have moved into parental roles with and without marriage. In minority communities, this has resulted in an increase in young women and children in poverty and a serious decline in the life chances of these young people (Rainwater, 1964; Hofferth and Hayes, 1987; Wilson, 1988). The role of early pregnancy and its contribution to the cycle of poverty are now well understood.

The impact of the schools (both middle and high schools) is extraordinarily complex because they are the primary institutional context in which the sexual development of young people takes place. The school has two important stratifying effects, one systematic and the other adventitious, on the general lives of young people and on their sexuality. The former is the effect of academic tracking in schools, which directs young people into college or into the labor force after high school, or forces young people out of high school before graduation; this can occur either within a school or between different schools that serve different race/ethnic/class strata of young people. The delay of marriage, the improved social placement, and the "liberalizing" sociosexual attitudes offered college attenders will systematically change their future sexual lives in a number of ways. The more adventitious effects of the high school on sexuality depend on the level of sex-related educational, social, and health services that the school offers young people, particularly disadvantaged young people. Limiting these services makes sexual development more problematic during this period, even though the provision of services does not provoke additional sexual activity (Jones et al., 1986; Marsiglio and Mott, 1986).

YOUNG ADULTHOOD AND FAMILY FORMATION

Young Adulthood

At the end of high school, that is, from ages 17 to 19, young people have begun to be stratified along socioeconomic lines independent of the socioeconomic status of their family, and this early stratification will be associated with important differences in their sexual present and future. Many young people will not have completed high school, and some portion of these will have been sexually very active and may even have children. Of the far larger number who have finished high school and will enter the job market, many will cohabit or marry in the five years after completing high school. Those going on to various levels of higher education (two-year, four-year, and professional or graduate education) will differentially delay marriage to fit with their educational and occupational goals. The pattern of social life during this period between the end of high school and about age 23 is increasingly heterogeneous socially as young people disperse in terms of their life-styles. Some go to work in the labor force; some start work in the household; some enter the military; some live at home and work toward a two-year college degree; others enter Ivy League colleges and plan careers in law, medicine, or business—each life-style carries with it different patterns of sexual opportunities.

The sexual lives of nearly all young people who are sexually and emotionally interested in the other gender will continue in the cycle of finding new sexual partners with relationships of differential durability (Hofferth and Upchurch, 1988; Tanfer and Schoorl, n.d.). Some young people will already have completed this cycle, married, and started families; others will continue the pattern begun in high school of having a mix of transient and more permanent sexual relationships, a pattern that often concludes in cohabitation or marriage; still others may have sexual lives that involve many transient sexual relationships; others remain virgins until marriage. The duration of the period prior to marriage and the social contexts within which this period is spent often determine the numbers of these sexual partners and the characteristics of these relationships. The sexual careers of young people who marry their high school sweethearts in June after graduating from the twelfth grade look very different from the sexual career of a young person who enters the military, serves overseas, returns to the United States to attend college, and marries in the late 20s.

This period is one in which there is increased legitimation of sexual activity by peers, media, and, in some cases, parents. Parental values and wishes may be more attended to as young people come closer to marriage; however, usually the longer marriage is delayed, the lower is the influence of parents over the characteristics of the person their child marries. Parents often find themselves dealing with their children's cohabitational and sexual–emotional partners while understanding that these relationships may not turn into marriages. There is a sharp tension in this period between the freedoms offered to the young and the responsibilities attached to growing up (Simon et al., 1972). Young people are often torn between the attractions of youth and those of adulthood, and this is expressed in their sexual patterns during this period. The mass media, particularly films and music directed toward the young, emphasize these themes of male freedom (the rowdy sexuality of *Animal House*), party life (beer advertisements on television), and passionate sexual attachments (cosmetic advertisements), as opposed to the values of settling down with one true love, finding a place to live, and having children. These opposed attractions are expressed in practice by patterns of sexual risk taking by young adults, usually between, but sometimes during, coupled affectional relationships.

Persons with strong same-gender erotic desires and experience often separate some parts of their lives from the heterosexual world during this period. The end of high school and the ability to move away from home are often used as an opportunity to explore the social, emotional, and sexual possibilities of the gay and lesbian communities that can be found in larger cities. There is also the possibility of migration from small towns and cities to environments that are more tolerant of gay and lesbian life-styles. Prior to the AIDS epidemic, this period often involved high levels of sexual activity and large numbers of sexual partners as young men entered the gay male community in which their own sexual interests could be expressed (Bell and Weinberg, 1978; Goode and Troiden, 1980). This burst of sexual activity associated with entry into community membership seems less common at the present time, but rigorous data do not exist. Current studies of the lives of gay men focus almost entirely on the cohorts of men over 30 in the epicenters of AIDS, who are most at risk for infection (Hessol et al., 1987; Joseph, 1987); younger cohorts and minority men are relatively unstudied. Even in the recent past when large numbers of sexual partners were common among gay men, many gay men (and the majority of lesbians) engaged in patterns of sexual–affectional coupling that were quite like those of heterosexuals (Gagnon and Simon, 1967; Bell and Weinberg, 1978; Peplau and Amaro, 1982; McWhirter and Mattison, 1984; Kurdek and Schmitt, 1985–1986). Gay men and lesbians have shared most of the socialization experiences of heterosexuals and, as a consequence, believe in and may search for (whereas others reject) durable sexual–affectional relationships with other persons.

Cohabitation, Marriage, and Family Formation

Although the average age at first marriage is no longer such a precise measure of a change in sexual life-style, it remains at least a rough marker of when most heterosexuals have settled down into a relatively durable and (what is expected to be) permanent relationship. By their late 20s nearly all persons in the society who will marry have already been married for the first time. This involves the legitimization, regularization, and, often, routinization of sexual activity for the couple. Rates of intercourse often start fairly high during these years and decline over time, influenced by the presence of children and the escalation of work and other obligations (James, 1981; Greenblat, 1983). In such relationships a relatively conventional repertoire of sexual techniques evolves and stabilizes as part of the usual sexual practices of the couple. Experiences of modest sexual disappointment may begin in this period, as do the beginnings of sexual dysfunction in some relationships (Masters and Johnson, 1970; Leiblum and Rosen, 1988). Most individuals are "settling down" sexually in this period. The move into a coupled relationship occurs most often with a married partner, but also through cohabitation (about one-third of men now in their 30s have reported cohabiting at least once: Michael and Willis, 1988). This is a continuation of the dominant national heterosexual pattern of having one stable partner at a time and appears to be becoming part of the coupling process among a substantial portion of the youthful population (Bumpuss and Sweet, 1988).

As children are born and the marriage/cohabitation turns into a family, family values are reinforced both by the presence of children and by the attitudes of the families of origin. In many such relationships there is a decline in the erotic character of the relationship which is replaced by the increasing importance of paternal and maternal roles (Byrne, 1977). This is reinforced by changes in friendship patterns in which there is a decrease in social contact with unmarried persons of the other gender unless they are in couples (Bell, 1981; Hess, 1981). There is a general escalation of interaction with same-gender friends (men with men, women with women) and with persons who also are married and have children.

Cohabitation is more likely to be less permanent than marriage during this period, and in most cases the differences between cohabitation and marriage are probably qualitative; it has been argued (Blumstein and Schwartz, 1983) that as long as marriage retains its economic and legal advantages, cohabitation among heterosexuals will remain unequal to it (see also Risman et al., 1981). Some marriages terminate within the first year as do many cohabitations; however, other cohabitations turn into marriages (about three-quarters, Michael and Willis, 1988; Thornton, 1988). What both cohabitation and marriage imply is sexual fidelity, and such quasipermanent couplings offer the opportunity to have sexual relationships outside of the couple.

These extracouple relationships vary enormously in duration, emotional commitment, and impact on the primary relationship (Thompson, 1983; Richardson, 1985). Most are with persons of the other gender, although some are with same-gender partners. Some of these same-gender contacts are signals of a change in the gender of the preferred sexual partner for both women and men. This pattern of extramarital or extracouple sexual relationships seems to be relatively common throughout the life course, at least until the early 50s for both men and women (for earlier data, see Kinsey et al., 1948, 1953; later data are more anecdotal and sparse: Atwater, 1982, Reiss, 1983; for data from a convenience sample of older persons, see Brecher et al., 1984). Recent increases in the rate of nonmarital contacts on the part of women are thought to be associated with increased participation in the labor force.

For some couples this sexual activity will be a signal of the impending termination of the relationship, whereas for others the sexual relations outside the couple will have little effect on the duration of the relationship; this, however, varies by culture (Reiss, 1986). Existing evidence about the interaction between sexual activity outside a coupled relationship and the stability of the couple over time suggests that extramarital relationships often lead to the breakup of couples, but many of these studies depend on samples of divorced or separated persons (Spanier and Margolis, 1983). Whatever the impact of such relationships on marriages, it is clear that they are disapproved by a large majority of the population (Singh et al., 1976; Reiss et al., 1980).

There are similarities between some marriages and cohabitations of equivalent duration during these years, especially among those who do not have children, particularly in the ways in which couples break up and return to single status. In both cases there is considerable emotional and social disruption (although cohabitants cannot divorce, they can have emotional and material experiences similar to a married couple when dissolving a relationship); however, both parties reenter the world of the child-free unmarried. This means that their social and sexual relations will look quite similar to those who have been continuously single and who are the same age. Among those who have children, and this is more common among the married, couple disruption has quite different consequences. In this case, both partners may be burdened with the expenses of child care and the woman in particular becomes a single mother rather than a single woman. This will affect her economic status as well as her value in the sexual marketplace in contrast to women without children (Weitzman, 1985).

First breakups of cohabiting and married couples are followed by a period of looking for new partners and, in most cases, by new sexual relationships, some of which eventuate in new cohabitations or marriages (Michael and Willis, 1988). In these periods between coupled status, there is an increased likelihood of additional sexual partners for both men and women (Tanfer and Schoorl, n.d.).

Some of the extracouple sexual relationships by men in this period, as well as in later life, are with partners whom they pay (Winick, 1962; Gagnon, 1968; James, 1977). This is more characteristic of men who do not marry or who are between coupled relationships. The patterns of contact with women for pay differ substantially by class and ethnic groupings, as well as by more adventitious factors. Participation in military service early in this period and membership in all male groups also increase the frequency of sexual contacts of men with women for pay. These all male groups can be college fraternities, men's organizations, or conventioneers, as well as occupational groups such as sailors, migrant workers, and others separated for periods of time from "appropriate" sexual partners.

The period from the late teens to the late 20s is one in which there is some reshuffling of an individual's sexual preference as well as patterns of social and sexual relations within gay and lesbian groups. Historically many persons who adopted an other-gender sexual preference early in life found it less satisfactory after unsuccessful marriages or after participating more fully in heterosexual life. In some cases a heterosexual life-style was adopted to satisfy the wishes of others or because it was thought that heterosexual participation would limit homosexual desires. These factors account for some of the numbers of married persons, many of whom have children, who leave their spouses to live as lesbians and gay men both in their 20s and in their 30s (it is estimated from convenience samples of gay men and lesbians that up to one in five have been married in the past: Bell and Weinberg, 1978). In the past, during this period many lesbians lived in quite stable relationships with relatively low rates of turnover, whereas gay men participated in a wider variety of couples (some only sexual, others sexual–affectional, others purely affectional). There is some evidence that, more recently, lesbians have more sexual partners and less stable relationships, whereas because of the AIDS epidemic many gay men have fewer sexual partners and are concentrating somewhat more on coupled relationships (Wolf, 1979; Levine, 1988). How extensive these practices are outside the metropolitan areas where research is being conducted is not known.

ADULTHOOD

Middle Adulthood

The period from the late 20s and early 30s into the late 40s and early 50s is rather poorly understood. In part, this may be more a measure of limited data and a limited perspective on life course changes than of the actual potential for complex changes in the status of individuals that affect their sexual lives. Adulthood is a curiously unmapped terrain even though the lives of adults are transformed in a variety of ways by an extraordinary number of life events (Albrecht and Gift, 1975; Einhorn et al., 1981). Perhaps this is because the microdramas of childbearing, divorce, work change, or love affairs reverberate through small networks rather than being reflected in larger scale collective effects such as the more synchronized cohort changes that characterize more youthful groups.

Life course markers and collective transitions become increasingly difficult to identify between ages 30 and 50 because persons are moving in and out of stable relationships based on individualized contingencies often dependent on short-run historical or biographical processes (Elder, 1979; Furstenberg, 1982). Even transitions relevant to larger collectivities (e.g., divorce and remarriage) are not keyed to ages or institutional settings in the same way as transitions in the preadult years (for general reviews of this period, see Neugarten, 1968; Smelser and Erikson, 1980). Other events (changes in health, death of parents, accidents) signaling life course transitions are entirely independent of age cohorts and occur probabilistically at many different points in time (Hultsch and Plemons, 1979; Brim and Ryff, 1982; Reese and Smyer, 1983).

Further, the multiplicity of roles that people play in these years complicates our understanding of their lives. Persons in this period of life may have both primary and secondary sexual and affectional partners (with some turnover through divorce and remarriage); they often have children (and stepchildren) of various ages whose demands are quite different; they have a set of relations with other couples and work peers (often both the husband and the wife), leisure time pursuits, and obligations to their families of origin. Such high densities of role demands are probably more characteristic of this period in the life course. This does not mean that there are no developmental changes to be faced during this period (Smelser and Erikson, 1980); however, the issues to be dealt with are increasingly unlinked with chronological age. The crisis of midlife does not occur exactly on a person's 40th birthday, but can range from the late 30s to the early 50s.

This is the period when there are often declining levels of sexual activity in continuous relationships and the emergence of identifiable sexual dissatisfactions that may be ignored or dealt with in a variety of ways (Trussel and Westoff, 1980; Udry, 1980; Jasso, 1985, 1986; Kahn and Udry, 1986). Sexuality in the couple is experienced less and less as erotic and more and more as a routine sexual experience, signaling reassurance and affection rather than passion (Leiblum and Rosen, 1988). There are increases in nonmarital or noncoupled sexual experiences by both men and women, although not necessarily as a response to the technical qualities of coupled sexuality. The erotic and romantic desires in nearly all coupled relationships conflict with increases in occupational commitments, a child-centered family life, and the demands of maturing children (Atwater, 1982).

For most people, their first experiences with visible declines in physical attractiveness and aging occur in the 40s, along with their first anxieties about aging. These are sharpened by the emphasis on youth and beauty in the mass media, which contrast with their own aging.

During this period there is a relatively constant rate of couple dissolution and formation of new couples, with many men finding younger female partners. Women with children are increasingly left out of the market for heterosexual partners and in some cases fall into poverty during this period.

Later Adulthood

For the majority of persons in coupled heterosexual relationships the patterns of social life during their early 50s do not differ dramatically from the mid-40s. Intergenerational relationships grow more complex as children enter adulthood and as older parents often grow dependent both psychologically and economically. There is an intensification of leisure, work, and family commitments as primary sources of life satisfaction move away from children.

Sexuality seems to have a declining salience after the midlife crises of the 40s. Although a variety of more "exciting" patterns do appear, particularly among the more affluent, the picture one gets from the limited data is a "settling in" by the coupled and a somewhat more sexualized life among the divorced and remarried (Luria and Meade, 1984). The important point is that little new is happening socially as the same pattern of coupling, uncoupling, and recoupling is repeated. Something new is happening in individual networks, but less so in social structure.

There is a continuing decline in the rate and significance of sexual activity in marriages and in other stable coupled relations. This is often a period of difficult sexual adjustment as some men and women experience increases in anxiety about their failed sexual aspirations, which are often accentuated by invidious comparisons with the youthfulness constantly emphasized by the media. These difficulties are expressed in complicated and often contradictory ways; some men and women experience the decline in marital sexuality with considerable relief, glad to be relieved of sexual responsibilities, whereas others increase their desire for affectional–sexual relations both in and out of marriage. The midlife crisis is often expressed by attempts at sexual rejuvenation to compensate for the increased evidence of physical aging and decline in attractiveness.

This crisis is often reflected in the desire for, and enactment of, sexual relationships outside the couple. There seems to be considerable potential in these relationships for emotional commitment and, in some cases, disruption of ongoing marriages. In other cases, men who do not wish to disrupt a marriage will engage in paid relationships with women which do not involve emotional complications and may offer the eroticism that is absent in the long-term relations.

The marital dissolutions that occur during this period continue to result in remarriage, particularly for men. As in earlier periods, such remarriages may occur with younger women, whereas the women in these divorces are often left with the full care of adolescent children. Women who divorce in this period are often much less marriageable than their former spouses.

The importance of the mass media as a source of fantasy or reassurance may increase in these years. Soap operas and sporting events may serve similar functions for gender-segregated audiences.

The crisis of aging may be particularly acute for gay men among whom youth, at least in the recent past, was an important aspect of sexual relations. This may not be as acute among lesbians, particularly of the same generation, who may be involved in quite stable long-term relationships. What impact the AIDS epidemic will have on the traditional focus on youth in the gay community is unclear. Sharp declines in the number of partners of older gay men may well have impact on the youthful orientation of gay life, at least in practice if not in fantasy. In this period, both gay men and lesbians with children will experience the transition of these children into young adults. Depending on the relationships to their families of origin, they will share the same problems as male–female couples in dealing with aging parents. The problem of aging particularly among gay men has been addressed by McWhirter and Mattison (1984) and Kimmel (1978).

THE LATER AGES

Middle Age

As most individuals move into their middle 50s and early 60s, they move out of the parenting role and their lives increasingly rotate around their primary affectional–sexual partners, friends, and work peers. Grandchildren may be reminders of family life, but for most this is far more attenuated than their own experiences of child rearing. Their adult children and their grandchildren are independent markers of a transition in the life course.

This is a period of continuing reduction in sexual relations in marriage, and some marriages may be almost entirely asexual. It is also a period when sexual relationships outside the couple decline in number and intensity, regardless of gender preference. There is a steady increase of nonsexual commitments between the individuals in the couple as the erotic core of their relationship disappears. At least some individuals in this period have ceased to conceive of themselves as sexual actors. This may be connected to declines in health and physical attractiveness. Nonmarital or noncoupled sex may be affected by this process because the psychological plausibility of an individual being a potential sexual partner does rest upon attractiveness and health.

The Young Old

As individuals move out of the labor force in their middle 60s, there is often a reduction in their interaction with persons younger than they are. This accentuates the importance of their spouse or long-term partner, friends, and adult children. This is true of those with same- or other-gender sexual preferences. Traditionally, during this period in the life course, there is often the substitution of nonsexual commitments, leisure, hobbies, memories, and sometimes grandchildren, as the basis for the couple.

There is some evidence that in the past there was a substantial reduction in sexual relations among most older couples and that the majority of couples may have been entirely asexual by age 70 (Kinsey et al., 1948, 1953; Christensen and Gagnon, 1965). There is, however, some more recent longitudinal data suggesting that stable, low rates of sexual activity do occur among some couples and that asexuality is not a necessary accompaniment of aging (George and Weiler, 1981).

Health status is absolutely critical to sexual life in these years (as it is in earlier portions of the life course), because life-threatening illnesses are psychological as well as physical threats to sexuality (Martin, 1981; Weizman and Hart, 1987). However, it is important to note that changes in the general health of the population are also changing the life course itself. Thus the phenomena of "youth creep" (i.e., healthy 70-year olds in 1980 are more like 60-year olds were in 1960; healthy 60-year olds in 1980 are more like 50-year olds were in 1960; and so forth, to some upper limit, in both the physical health and the social desires of older persons) will have unknown consequences for sexuality. This process may well reduce the "desexualization" of older persons commonly noted in earlier generations (Brecher et al., 1984).

The business sector of the society has been taking notice of this more affluent and active older population by providing new leisure, housing, travel, and mass media products for them. Each of these products focuses on the greater youthfulness and continued sexual potential of this group.

Women are being widowed at a relatively high rate during this period, and some recoupling that involves sexuality does occur.

There is often some intergenerational conflict with children about these recouplings because they provoke both sexual and property anxieties.

Among the elderly after age 70, the forces that affected sexuality in the years after 60 should retain their impact. What consequences the very large number of persons of this age in the early years of the twenty-first century will have on their sexuality is unknown.

AFTERWORD

The density of references in the latter half of this preliminary attempt to suggest some links of sexuality to the life course decreases steadily as the focus of discussion moves from childhood and youth to later life. This decline follows the national cultural prejudice that finds sexual learning and sexual conduct among the young far more interesting than the changes in the sexual life of their elders. This may be due to the fact that the sexual activities of the young seem to generate more passion as well as more social problems. Whatever the reasons, the research literature on sexuality (which is not very abundant in any case) nearly evaporates as our attention moves from the first 25 years of life. Perhaps the graying of the population will redress this imbalance, but given the dominant cultural representations of sexuality in which sexual desire after 40 appears slightly comic, one cannot be entirely sure. However just because the sexual pleasures and problems in the last two-thirds of the life course are private and socially invisible does not mean that they are not important parts of the lives of most women and men.

REFERENCES

Albrecht, G., and Gift, H. (1975) Adult socialization: Ambiguity and adult life crises. In N. Datan and L. Ginsberg (eds.), *Life Span Developmental Psychology: Normative Life Crises.* New York: Academic Press.

Atwater, L. (1982) *The Extramarital Connection: Sex, Intimacy and Identity.* New York: Irvington.

Atwood, J., and Gagnon, J. H. (1987) Masturbatory behavior in college youth. *Journal of Sex Education and Therapy* 3:35–42.

Baltes, P., and Brim, O. G. (eds.) (1979) *Life Span Development and Behavior,* Vol. 2. New York: Academic Press.

Bell, A. P., and Weinberg, M. (1978) *Homosexualities: A Study of Diversity Among Men and Women.* New York: Simon and Schuster.

Bell, A. P., Weinberg, M., and Kiefer-Hammersmith, S. (1980) *Sexual Preference,* 2 vols. New York: Simon and Schuster.

Bell, R. R. (1981) *Worlds of Friendship.* Beverly Hills, Calif.: Sage.

Bell, R. R., Turner, S., and Rosen, L. A. (1975) A multivariate analysis of female extramarital coitus. *Journal of Marriage and the Family* 37:375–384.

Bieber, I. (1962) *Homosexuality: A Psychoanalytic Study.* New York: Basic Books.
Blumstein, P. W., and Schwartz, P. (1983) *American Couples.* New York: William Morrow.
Boswell, J. (1980) *Christianity, Social Tolerance, and Homosexuality: Gay People in Western Europe from the Beginning of the Christian Era to the Fourteenth Century.* Chicago: University of Chicago Press.
Brecher, E., and the Editors of Consumer Reports Books (1984) *Love, Sex and Aging.* Boston: Little Brown.
Brim, O. G., and Ryff, C. D. (1982) On the properties of life events. In P. Baltes and O. C. Brim (eds), *Life Span Development and Behavior,* Vol. 3. New York: Academic Press.
Brim, O. G., and Wheeler, S. (1966) *Socialization After Childhood: Two Essays.* New York: John Wiley & Sons.
Brown, J., Childers, K. W., and Waszak, C. S. (1988) Television and Adolescent Sexuality. Preliminary Findings on Cohabitation from the 1987 National Survey of Families and Households. Presented at the Conference on Television and Teens, Manhattan Beach, Calif. June 22–24.
Bumpuss, L., and Sweet, J. (1988) Presented at the Annual Meeting of the Population Association of America, New Orleans.
Byrne, D. (1977) Social psychology and the study of sexual behavior. *Journal of Abnormal and Social Psychology* 62:158–160.
Califia, P. (1983) Gay men, lesbians and sex: Doing it together. *The Advocate* July 7:24–27.
Cannon, K. L., and Long, R. (1971) Premarital sexual behavior in the sixties. *Journal of Marriage and the Family* 33:36–49.
Carrier, J. (1976) Family attitudes and Mexican male homosexuality. *Urban Life* 5:359–375.
Carroll, J. L., Volk, K., and Hyde, J. S. (1985) Differences in males and females in motives for engaging in sexual intercourse. *Archives of Sexual Behavior* 6:53–65.
Chilman, C. S. (1978) *Adolescent Sexuality in a Changing American Society.* Washington, D.C.: National Institutes of Health.
Christensen, C. V., and Gagnon, J. H. (1965) Sexual behavior in a group of older women. *Journal of Gerontology* 20:251–256.
Clausen, J. (1972) The life course of individuals. In M. W. Riley, M. Johnson, and A. Foner (eds.), *Aging and Society,* Vol. III. New York: Russell Sage.
Clayton, R. R., and Bokemeier, J. L. (1980) Premarital sexual behavior in the seventies. *Journal of Marriage and the Family* 42:759–775.
Clement, U., Schmidt, G., and Kruse, M. (1984) Changes in sex differences in sexual behavior: A replication of a study on West German students (1966–1981). *Archives of Sexual Behavior* 13:99–120.
Coleman, E. (1982) Developmental stages of the coming out process. In W. Paul et al. (eds.), *Homosexuality: Social, Psychological and Biological Issues.* Beverly Hills, Calif.: Sage.
Cook, M. and Howells, K. (eds.) (1980) *Adult Sexual Interest in Children.* New York: Academic Press.
Coxon, A. P. M. (1986) *Report of a Pilot Study: Project on Sexual Lifestyles of Non-Heterosexual Males.* Social Research Unit, University College, Cardiff.
Crompton, L. (1985) *Byron and Greek Love: Homophobia in 19th Century England.* Berkeley: University of California Press.
Dank, B. (1971) Coming out in the gay world. *Psychiatry* 34:180–197.

Dawson, D., and Thornberry, O. T. (1988) AIDS knowledge and attitudes for December 1987, Provisional data from the National Health Interview Survey. *NCHS Advance Data* 153(May 16).

Delamater, J., and MacCorquodale, P. (1979) *Premarital Sexuality: Attitudes, Relationships, Behavior.* Madison: University of Wisconsin Press.

D'Emilio, J. (1983) *Sexual Politics, Sexual Communities: The Making of a Homosexual Minority in the United States, 1940–1970.* Chicago: University of Chicago Press.

D'Emilio, J., and Freedman, E. (1988) *Intimate Matters: A History of Sexuality in America.* New York: Harper & Row.

Dover, K. J. (1978) *Greek Homosexuality.* Cambridge: Harvard University Press.

Duberman, M. B. (1974) The bisexual debate. *New Times* (June 28):34–41.

Duberman, M. B. (1986) *About Time: Exploring the Gay Past.* New York: Gay Presses of New York.

Einhorn, D. H., Clausen, J., Hann, N., Honik, N., and Mussen, P. (eds.) (1981) *Past and Present in Middle Life.* New York: Academic Press.

Elder, G. H. (1979) Historical changes in life patterns and personality. In P. Baltes and O. G. Brim (eds.), *Life Span Development and Behavior,* Vol. 2. New York: Academic Press.

Elder, G. H. (1984) Family history and the life course. In R. Parke et al. (eds.), *The Family.* Chicago: University of Chicago.

English, D., Hollibaugh, A., and Rubin, G. (1981) Talking sex. *Socialist Review* (July–August).

Epstein, C. F. (1981) *Women in Law.* New York: Basic Books.

Escoffier, J. (1985) Sexual revolution and the politics of gay identity. *The Socialist Review* 82:119–153.

Fay, R., Turner, C. F., Klassen, A., and Gagnon, J. H. (in press) Prevalence and patterns of homosexual contact among men. *Science.*

Featherman, D. (1980) Schooling and occupational careers: Constancy and change in worldly success. In O. G. Brim and J. Kagan (eds.), *Constancy and Change in Human Development.* Cambridge, Mass.: Harvard University Press.

Finkelhor, D. (1979) *Sexually Victimized Children.* New York: Free Press.

Finkelhor, D. (1984) *Child Sexual Abuse, New Theory and Research.* New York: Free Press.

Finkelhor, D., Gelles, R. J. Hotaling, G. T., and Straus, M. A. (1983) *The Dark Side of Families: Current Family Violence Research.* Beverly Hills, Calif.: Sage.

Ford, C. S., and Beach, F. A. (1951) *Patterns of Sexual Behavior.* New York: Harper & Row.

Foucault, M. (1978) *The History of Sexuality, Vol. 1, An Introduction.* New York: Pantheon.

Fox, G. L. (1981) The family's role in adolescent sexual behavior. In T. Ooms (ed.), *Teenage Pregnancy in a Family Context.* Philadelphia: Temple.

Furstenberg, F. F., Jr. (1982) *Conjugal Succession: Reentering Marriage After Divorce, Life Span Development and Behavior,* Vol. 4. New York: Academic Press.

Furstenberg, F. F., Jr., Morgan, S. P., Moore, K. A., and Peterson, J. L. (1987) Race differences in the timing of adolescent intercourse. *American Sociological Review* 52:511–518.

Gagnon, J. H. (1965) Sexuality and sexual learning in the child. *Psychiatry* 28:212–228.

Gagnon, J. H. (1968) Prostitution. In *The International Encyclopedia of the Social Sciences,* Vol. 14. New York: Crowell-Collier.

Gagnon, J. H. (1973) Scripts and the coordination of sexual conduct. In J. K. Cole and R. Dienstbier (eds.), *Nebraska Symposium on Motivation.* Lincoln: University of Nebraska Press.

Gagnon, J. H. (1977) *Human Sexualities.* Glenview, Ill.: Scott Foresman.

Gagnon, J. H. (1979) The interaction of gender roles and sexual conduct. In H. Katchadourian (ed.), *Human Sexuality: A Comparative and Developmental Approach.* Berkeley: University of California Press.

Gagnon, J. H. (1987) Masturbation in Two College Cohorts. Presented at the meeting of the International Academy of Sex Research, Tutzing, G.D.R.

Gagnon, J. H., and Greenblat, C. S. (1978) *Life Designs.* Glenview: Scott Foresman.

Gagnon, J. H., and Simon, W. (1967) Femininity in the lesbian community. *Social Problems* 15:212–221.

Gagnon, J. H., and Simon, W. (1973) *Sexual Conduct: The Social Sources of Human Sexuality.* Chicago: Aldine.

Gagnon, J. H., and Simon, W. (1987) The scripting of oral genital sexual conduct. *Archives of Sexual Behavior* 16:1–25.

Gay, P. (1984) Education of the Senses, Vol. 1 in *The Bourgeois Experience, Victoria to Freud.* New York: Oxford University Press.

Gebhard, P. H., Gagnon, J. H., Pomeroy, W. B., and Christensen, C. (1965) *Sex Offenders: An Analysis of Types.* New York: Harper.

George, L. K., and Weiler, S. J. (1981) Sexuality in middle and late life. The effects of age, cohort and gender. *Archives of General Psychiatry* 38:919–923.

Goode, E., and Troiden, R. (1980) Correlates and accompaniments of promiscuous sex among male homosexuals. *Psychiatry* 43:51–59.

Greenblat, C. S. (1983) The salience of sexuality in early marriage. *Journal of Marriage and the Family* 43:121–132.

Groth, A. N. (1979) *Men Who Rape: The Psychology of the Offender.* New York: Plenum.

Herdt, G. (1984) *Ritualized Homosexuality in Melanesia.* Berkeley: University of Calfornia Press.

Herdt, G. (n.d.) Gay and Lesbian Teenagers. Committee on Human Development, University of Chicago.

Hess, B. B. (1981) Friendship and gender roles over the life course. In P. Stein (ed.), *Single Life: Unmarried Adults in Social Context.* New York: St. Martin's Press.

Hessol, N., et al. (1987) The natural history of human immunodeficiency virus in a cohort of homosexual and bisexual men: A 7-year prospective study. Presented at the Third International Conference on AIDS, Washington, D.C., June.

Hofferth, S. L., and Hayes, C. D. (1987) *Risking the Future: Adolescent Sexuality, Pregnancy, and Childbearing,* Vol. II. Washington, D.C.: National Academy Press.

Hofferth, S. L., Kahn, J. R., and Baldwin, W. (1987) Premarital sexual activity among U.S. teenage women over the past three decades. *Family Planning Perspectives* 19:46–52.

Hofferth, S. L., and Upchurch, D. M. (1988) Breaking Up: Dissolving Non-Marital Unions. Presented at the Annual Meeting of the Population Association of America, New Orleans, April.

Hooker, E. (1966) The homosexual community. In J. C. Palmer and M. J. Goldstein (eds.), *Perspectives in Pathology.* Oxford, England: Oxford University Press.

Hultsch, D., and Plemons, J. (1979) Life events and life span development. In P. Baltes and O. G. Brim (eds.), *Life Span Development and Behavior,* Vol. 2. New York: Academic Press.

Humphrey, L. (1978) *Tea Room Trade: Impersonal Sex in Public Places.* Chicago: Aldine.

Humphreys, R. A. L. (1972) *Out of the Closets: The Sociology of Homosexual Liberation.* Englewood Cliffs, N.J.: Prentice-Hall.

James, J. (1977) Prostitutes and prostitution. In E. Sagarin and F. Montanino (eds.), *Deviants: Voluntary Actors in a Hostile World.* Glenview, Ill.: Scott Foresman.

James, W. (1981) The honeymoon effect on marital coitus. *The Journal of Sex Research* 17:114–123.

Jasso, G. (1985) Marital coital frequency and the passage of time: Estimating the separate effects of spouses' ages and marital duration, birth and marriage cohorts and period influences. *American Sociological Review* 50:224–241.

Jasso, G. (1986) Is it outlier deletion or is it sample truncation? Notes on science and sexuality (reply to Kahn and Udry). *American Sociological Review* 51:738–742.

Jessor, R., and Jessor, S. L. (1978) *Problem Behavior and Psychological Development: A Longitudinal Study of Youth.* New York: Academic Press.

Jessor, R., et al. (1983) Time of first intercourse: A prospective study. *Journal of Personality and Social Psychology* 44:608–626.

Jones, E. F., et al. (eds.) (1986) *Teenage Pregnancy in Industrialized Countries.* New Haven, Conn.: Yale University Press.

Joseph, J. G. (1987) Two-Year Long Longitudinal Study of Behavioral Risk Reduction in a Cohort of Homosexual Men. Presented at the Third International Conference on AIDS, Washington, D.C., June.

Kagan, J. (1971) *Change and Continuity in Infancy.* New York: John Wiley & Sons.

Kagan, J. (1980) Perspectives on continuity. In O. G. Brim and J. Kagan (eds.), *Constancy and Change in Human Development.* Cambridge, Mass.: Harvard University Press.

Kagan, J. (1981) *Infancy.*

Kagan, J., and Coles, R. (eds.) (1973) *Twelve to Sixteen: Early Adolescence.* New York: Norton.

Katz, J. (1983) *Gay/Lesbian Almanac: A New Documentary.* New York: Harper & Row.

Kahn, J. R., and Udry, J. R. (1986) Marital coital frequency: Unnoticed outlier and unspecified interactions lead to erroneous conclusions (Comment). *American Sociological Review* 51:734–737.

Kessler, S. J., and McKenna, W. (eds.) (1974) *Gender.* New York: John Wiley & Sons.

Kett, J. (1978) Curing the disease of precocity. In J. Demos and S. Boocock (eds.), In *Turning Points: Historical and Sociological Essays on the Family.* Vol. 84, Supplement. Chicago: American Journal of Sociology.

Kimmel, D. (1978) Adult development and aging: A gay perspective. *Journal of Social Issues* 34:113–130.

Kinsey, A. C., Pomeroy, W. B., and Martin, C. E. (1948) *Sexual Behavior in the Human Male.* Philadelphia: Saunders.

Kinsey, A. C., Pomeroy, W. B., Martin, C. E., and Gebhard, P. H. (1953) *Sexual Behavior in the Human Female.* Philadelphia: Saunders.

Kline, D., Roberts, E., and Gagnon, J. (1978) *Family Life and Sexual Learning, a Report of the Project on Human Sexual Development,* 3 vols. Cambridge, Mass.: Project on Human Sexual Development.

Kurdek, L. A., and Schmitt, J. P. (1985–1986) Relationship quality of gay men in closed or open relationships. *Journal of Homosexuality* 12:85–99.

Leiblum, S. R., and Rosen, R. C. (1988) *Sexual Desire Disorders.* New York: Guilford.

Levine, M. (1988) The Heterosexualization of Gay Desire. Presented at the Annual Meeting of the American Sociological Association, Atlanta.

Luria, Z. (1979) Psychosocial determinants of gender identity, role and orientation. In H. Katchadourian (ed.) *Human Sexuality: A Comparative and Developmental Perspective.* Berkeley: University of California Press.

Luria, Z., and Meade, R. G. (1984) Sexuality and the middle aged woman. In G. Baruch and J. Brooks-Gunn (eds.), *Women in Midlife.* New York: Plenum.

Maccoby, E. E., and Jacklin, C. (1974) *The Psychology of Sex Differences.* Stanford, Calif.: Stanford University Press.

Macklin, E. D. (1978) Review of research on non-marital cohabitation in the United States. In B. J. Murstein (ed.) *Exploring Intimate Lifestyles.* New York: Springer.

Marshall, D., and Suggs, R. (eds.) (1971) *Human Sexual Behavior, Variations in the Ethnographic Spectrum.* Englewood Cliffs, N.J.: Prentice-Hall.

Marsiglio, W., and Mott, F. L. (1986) The impact of sex education on sexual activity, contraceptive use and premarital pregnancy among American teenagers. *Family Planning Perspectives* 18:151–161.

Martin, C. E. (1981) Factors affecting the sexual functioning in 60–79 year old married males. *Archives of Sexual Behavior* 10:399–400.

Masters, W., and Johnson, V. (1970) *Human Sexual Dysfunction.* Boston: Little, Brown.

McCluskey, K., Killarney, J., and Papini, D. (1983) Adolescent pregnancy and parenthood: Implications for development. In E. J. Callahan and K. McCluskey (eds.), *Life Span Developmental Psychology, Nonnormative Life Events.* New York: Academic Press.

McWhirter, D., and Mattison, D. (1984) *The Male Couple.* Englewood Cliffs, N.J.: Prentice-Hall.

Michael, R., and Willis, R. (1988) Presented at the Annual Meeting of the Population Association of America, New Orleans.

Miller, P. Y., and Simon, W. (1974) Adolescent sexual behavior: Context and change. *Social Problems* 22:52–76.

Modell, J., Furstenberg, F. F., and Strong, D. (1978) The timing of marriage in the transitions to adulthood: Continuity and change, 1860–1975. In J. Demos and S. Boocock (eds.), *Turning Points: Historical and Sociological Essays on the Family,* Vol. 84, Supplement. Chicago: American Journal of Sociology.

Money, J., and Ehrhardt, A. A. (1972) *Man and Woman/Boy and Girl.* Baltimore, Md.: Johns Hopkins University Press.

Nardi, A. (1973) Person perception research and the perception of the life span. In P. Baltes and K. Schaie (eds.), *Life Span Developmental Psychology: Personality and Socialization.* New York: Academic Press.

Neugarten, B. (ed.) (1968) *Middle Age and Aging.* Chicago: University of Chicago Press.

Neugarten, B., and Datan, N. (1973) Sociological perspectives on the life course. In P. Baltes and K. Schaie (eds.), *Life Span Developmental Psychology: Personality and Socialization.* New York: Academic Press.

Newcomer, S. F., and Udry, J. R. (1985) Oral sex in an adolescent population. *Archives of Sexual Behavior* 14:41–46.

Ooms, T. (ed.) (1981) *Teenage Pregnancy in a Family Context.* Philadelphia: Temple.

O'Reilly, K., and Aral, S. (1985) Adolescence and sexual behavior, trends and implications for STD. *Journal of Adolescent Health Care* 6:262–270.

Ortner, S. B., and Whitehead, H. (eds.) (1981) *Sexual Meanings: The Cultural Construction of Gender and Sexuality.* Cambridge, England: Cambridge University Press.

Paul, W., Weinrich, J. D., Gonsiorek, J. C., and Hotvedt, M. E. (eds.) (1982) *Homosexuality: Social, Psychological and Biological Issues.* Beverly Hills, Calif.: Sage.

Peplau, L. A., and Amaro, H. (1982) Understanding lesbian relationships. In W. Paul, et al. (eds.), *Homosexuality: Social, Psychological and Biological Issues.* Beverly Hills, Calif.: Sage.

Peplau, L. A., and Gordon, S. L. (1983) The intimate relationships of lesbians and gay men. In E. R. Allgeier and N. B. McCormick (eds.), *Changing Boundaries: Gender Roles and Sexual Behavior.* Palo Alto, Calif.: Mayfield.

Plummer, K. (1981) *The Making of the Modern Homosexual.* Totowa, N.J.: Barnes and Noble Books.

Plummer, K. (1984) Sexual diversity: A sociological perspective. In K. Howells (ed.), *Sexual Diversity.* London: Basil Blackwell.

Rainwater, L. (1964) Marital sexuality in four "cultures of poverty." *Journal of Marriage and the Family* 26:457–466.

Reese, H., and Smyer, M. (1983) The dimensionalisation of life events. In E. J. Callahan and K. McCluskey (eds.), *Life Span Developmental Psychology, Nonnormative Life Events.* New York: Academic Press.

Reigel, K. F., and Meachum, J. A. (eds.) (1976) *The Developing Individual in a Changing World, Vol. I: Historical and Cultural Issues; Vol. II: Social and Environmental Issues.* Chicago: Aldine.

Reiss, A. (1961) The social organization of queers and peers. *Social Problems* 9:102–120.

Reiss, I. L. (1960) *Premarital Sexual Standards in America.* New York: Free Press.

Reiss, I. L. (1967) *The Social Context of Premarital Permissiveness.* New York: Holt, Rinehart & Winston.

Reiss, I. L. (1983) Heterosexual Relationships Inside and Outside of Marriage. Morristown, N.J.: General Learning Press.

Reiss, I. L. (1986) *Journey into Sexuality.* New York: Prentice-Hall.

Reiss, I. L., Anderson, R. E., and Sponaugle, G. C. (1980) A multivariate model of the determinants of extramarital sexual permissiveness. *Journal of Marriage and the Family* 45:395–411.

Rich, A. (1983) *Compulsory Heterosexuality and Lesbian Existence.* San Francisco: Antelope.

Richardson, L. (1985) *The New Other Woman.* New York: The Free Press.

Risman, B. J., Hill, C., Rubin, Z., and Peplau, L. A. (1981) Living together in college: Implications for courtship. *Journal of Marriage and the Family* 43:77–83.

Roebuck, J., and McGee, M. G. (1977) Attitudes toward premarital sex and sexual behavior among black high school girls. *Journal of Sex Research* 13:104–114.

Rossi, A. S. (ed.) (1985) *Gender and the Life Course.* Hawthorne, N.Y.: Aldine.

Rubin, G. (1975) The traffic in women. In R. R. Reiter (ed.), *Toward an Anthropology of Women.* New York: Monthly Review.

Rubin, G. (1984) Thinking Sex. In C. Vance (ed.), *Pleasure and Danger.* London: Routledge & Kegan Paul.

Rubin, L. (1976) *Worlds of Pain: Life in the Working Class Family.* New York: Basic Books.

Russell, D. E. H. (1984) *Sexual Exploitation: Rape, Child Abuse and Workplace Harrassment.* Beverly Hills, Calif.: Sage.

Schwartz, P., and Blumstein, P. (1977) Bisexuality. *Journal of Social Issues* 33:132–145.

Sears, R. R., Maccoby E., and Levin, H. (1957) *Patterns of Childrearing.* Evanston, Ill.: Row, Peterson.

Simon, W., Berger, A., and Gagnon, J. H. (1972) Beyond fantasy and anxiety: The coital experiences of college youth. *Journal of Youth and Adolescence* 1:203–222.

Simon, W., Buff, S., and Gagnon, J. H. (1972) Son of Joe: Continuity and change among working class adolescents. *Journal of Youth and Adolescence* 1:13–34.

Simon, W., and Gagnon, J. H. (1967) Homosexuality: The formulation of a sociological perspective. *Journal of Health and Social Behavior* 8:177–185.

Simon, W., and Gagnon, J. H. (1987) Sexual scripts, permanence and change. *Archives of Sexual Behavior* 15:97–120.

Singh, K. B., Walton, B. L., and Williams, J. S. (1976) Extramarital sexual permissiveness: Conditions and contingencies. *Journal of Marriage and the Family* 38:701–712.

Smelser, N. J., and Erikson, E. H. (1980) *Themes of Love and Work in Adulthood.* Cambridge, Mass.: Harvard University Press.

Snitow, A., Stansell, C., and Thompson, S. (eds.) (1984) *Desire: The Politics of Sexuality.* London: Virago.

Socarides, C. W. (1978) *Homosexuality.* New York: Aronson.

Spanier, G. B., and Margolis, R. L. (1983) Marital separation and extra-marital sex. *Journal of Sex Research* 19:28–48.

Stoller, R. (1985) *Presentations of Gender.* New Haven, Conn.: Yale University Press.

Straus, M., Gelles, R., and Steinmetz, S. (1980) *Behind Closed Doors: Violence in the American Family.* New York: Anchor/Doubleday.

Tanfer, K., and Schoorl, K. (n.d.) The Extent and Context of Sexual Promiscuity. Unpublished manuscript.

Tanner, J. M. (1973) Sequence, tempo and individual variation in growth and development in boys and girls between twelve and sixteen. In J. Kagan and R. Coles (eds.), *Twelve to Sixteen: Early Adolescence.* New York: Norton.

Thompson, A. B. (1983) Extramarital sex: A review of the scientific literature. *Journal of Sex Research* 19:1–22.

Thornton, A. (1988) Dynamics of Cohabitation and Marriage in the 1980s. Presented at the annual meeting of the Population Association of America, New Orleans.

Tiefer, L. (1987) Social constructionism and the study of human sexuality. In P. Shaver and R. Kendrick (eds.), *Sex and Gender.* Beverly Hills, Calif.: Sage.

Trussel, J., and Westoff, C. (1980) Contraceptive practice and trends in coital frequency. *Family Planning Perspectives* 12:246–249.

Udry, J. R. (1980) Changes in the frequency of marital intercourse from panel data. *Archives of Sexual Behavior* 9:319–325.

Udry, J. R. (1985) Serum androgenic hormones motivate sexual behavior in adolescent boys. *Fertility and Sterility* 43:90–94.

Udry, J. R., Bauman, K. E., and Morris, N. M. (1975) Changes in premarital coital experience of recent decade-of-birth cohorts of urban American women. *Journal of Marriage and the Family* 37:783–787.

Udry, J. R., and Billy, J. O. G. (1987) Initiation of coitus in early adolescence. *American Sociological Review* 52:841–855.

Uhlenberg, P. (1978) Changing configurations of the life course. In T. Haraven (ed.), *Transitions.* New York: Academic Press.

Vance, C. (1984) *Pleasure and Danger.* London: Routledge & Kegan Paul.

Verwoerdt, A., Pfeiffer, E., and Wang, H. S. (1969) Sexual behavior in senescence: Patterns of sexual activity and interest. *Geriatrics* 24:137–144.

Warren, C. A. B. (1974) *Identity and Community in the Gay World.* New York: John Wiley & Sons.

Weeks, J. (1981) *Sex, Politics and Society: The Regulation of Sexuality Since 1800.* London: Longmans, Green.

Weinberg, M. S., and Williams, C. J. (1974) *Male Homosexuals: Problems and Adaptations.* New York: Oxford University Press.

Weinberg, M. S., and Williams, C. J. (1988) Black sexuality: A test of two theories. *Journal of Sex Research* 25:197–218.

Weitzman, L. (1985) *The Divorce Revolution.* New York: Free Press.

Weizman, R., and Hart, J. (1987) Sexual behavior in healthy married elderly men. *Archives of Sexual Behavior* 16:39–44.

Westoff, C. F. (1974) Coital frequency and contraception. *Family Planning Perspectives* 6:136–141.

White, E. (1983) *A Boy's Own Story.* New York: E. P. Dutton.

White, E. (1980) *States of Desire.* New York: E. P. Dutton.

Willis, R., and Michael, R. (1988) Innovation in Family Formation: Cohabitational Unions from the 1986 Follow-Up of the NLS/72 Sample. Presented at the annual meeting of the Population Association of America, New Orleans.

Wilson, W. J. (1988) *The Truly Disadvantaged: The Inner City, The Underclass and Public Policy.* Chicago: University of Chicago Press.

Winick, C. (1962) Prostitutes clients' perception of the prostitutes and themselves. *International Journal of Social Psychiatry* 8:289–297.

Wolf, D.G. (1979) *The Lesbian Community.* Berkeley: University of California Press.

Zelnik, M., Kantner, J. F., and Ford, K. (1981) *Sex and Pregnancy in Adolescence.* Beverly Hills, Calif.: Sage.

Sex Counts: A Methodological Critique of Hite's *Women and Love*

Tom W. Smith

In the fall of 1987, with a media campaign more sagely planned and successfully executed than those of most of the 1988 presidential candidates, Shere Hite (1987) launched the final book of her Hite Report trilogy, *Women and Love: A Cultural Revolution in Progress.* The overall conclusion of the book is that women are deeply dissatisfied with their relationships with their husbands and male lovers. Hite reports that 84 percent were not emotionally satisfied with their relationships, that 84 percent of their husbands/lovers frequently responded to what they said with ridicule or condescension, and that 95 percent had faced "emotional and psychological harassment." In contrast Hite found that relations between women and their female friends were warm and emotionally supportive. Hite reports that 87 percent said these friendships were emotionally closer than those with husbands/lovers. In addition, in perhaps her most widely cited statistics, Hite asserts that 70 percent of women married five years or more "are having sex outside of their marriages" (pp. 395–396, 856).

To evaluate how much credence to give this finding of infidelity, as well as her other figures and conclusions, the methodology employed must be considered and a determination made of whether it was scientifically sound and likely to yield reliable, valid estimates and whether appropriate conclusions were drawn from the data.

Tom W. Smith is with the National Opinion Research Center, University of Chicago. This is a revised and extended version of a paper initially prepared for the American Association for Public Opinion Research, annual meeting, Toronto, May 1988.

METHODOLOGY: GENERAL OBSERVATIONS

Hite's methodology is described and defended in a 18-page appendix, "Essay on the Methodology of the Hite Report," as well as in an essay by Gladys Engel Lang, "Quantifying the Emotions: Methodological Observations on the Hite Trilogy." Unfortunately Hite's methodological essay consists largely of a defense of her general hermeneutical and feminist approach and a criticism of other approaches. She presents only the barest glimmer of documentation about how her study was conducted and analyzed.

Sampling

Hite asserts that her research could not have been carried out if she had tried to employ random probability sampling. She charges that with such a sampling approach it would have been impossible (1) to guarantee anonymity (pp. 774, 778) and (2) to have an essay or open-ended questionnaire (p. 777). She also contends (1) that true random probability samples do not exist (pp. xxx and 778) and (2) that the social sciences are swinging behind her type of research methodology (pp. xxx, 769–773). These criticisms are, at best, extreme. Ensuring respondents of confidentiality and gaining their cooperation for surveys on sensitive topics are challenging tasks, but national probability samples have been carried out on such difficult topics as drug addiction (including urine tests), homosexual behavior, and alcoholism, to mention only a few. Similarly, although closed-ended questions are more common than open-ended ones, in contemporary survey research open-ended questions are used. For example, over the years about one-sixth of the attitude questions on American National Election Studies have been open-ended (Converse and Schuman, 1984:305).

Instead Hite used a combination of haphazard sampling and volunteer respondents to collect her cases. First, she sent questionnaires to a variety of organizations and asked them to circulate the questionnaires to their members. She does not list all organizations solicited but mentions that they included "church groups in thirty-four states, women's voting and political groups in nine states, women's rights organizations in thirty-nine states, professional women's groups in twenty-two states, counseling and walk-in centers for women or families in forty-three states, and a wide range of other organizations, such as senior citizens' homes and disabled people's organizations, in various states" (p. 777). There is no information on the comparative representation of these groups either among the initial distribution of questionnaires or among the completed cases (on response rates, see below), but these groups would not seem to be representative of women in general, with an overrepresentation of feminist groups and of women in troubled circumstances. In addition, the use of groups to distribute the questionnaires apparently meant that gatekeepers (and perhaps a single person) had the power of assuring a zero response rate (by deciding not to distribute the questionnaires) or, conversely, of perhaps greatly stimulating returns by endorsing the study in some fashion. However, since no information is presented on such matters, the actual role of gatekeepers cannot be ascertained.

Second, Hite also relied on volunteer respondents who wrote in for copies of the questionnaire. These volunteers seem to have been recruited from readers of her past books and from those who saw her interviews on television and in the press. This type of volunteer respondent is the exact opposite of the randomly selected respondent utilized in standard survey research and even more potentially unrepresentative than the group samples cited above.

Response Rates

Hite reports that she distributed 100,000 questionnaires and obtained 4,500 responses for a final response rate of 4.5 percent. While admitting that this response rate is lower than that obtained on full-probability surveys (which she states would not have been possible to use, given her research methodology; see above), she claims that "this is almost twice as high as the standard rate of return for this kind of questionnaire distribution, which is estimated at 2.5 to 3 percent" (p. 777). Given the highly unusual nature of her questionnaire and the unusual nature of her "sample," it is doubtful that there is any standard rate of return. While the source of the 2.5–3 percent return figure is not certain, it probably represents the percentage of people placing orders or making contributions in response to direct mail solicitations.

In general a response rate as low as 4.5 percent is extremely unlikely to yield a representative sample since nonresponse bias is a function of how different the respondents are from nonrespondents and the size of the nonresponse group. Hite supplies no direct information about the differences between her respondents and nonrespondents and, given her sample design, any such comparison would be virtually impossible (although one of her statistical information questions—Where did you obtain this questionnaire?—might have shed some light on the comparative response rates from the groups she selected). Standard survey experience suggests, however, that respondents are typically different from nonrespondents and that the degree of difference is probably inversely associated with the response rate (Smith, 1983, 1984). In particular, responses usually come disproportionately from those who are agitated by, or concerned about, an issue. It is thus likely that the small minority of women who responded would be heavily drawn from those who were dissatisfied with their personal relationships with men.

Representativeness and Census/Demographic Comparisons

Hite argues that "sufficient effort was put into the various forms of distribution that the final statistical breakdown of those participating according to age, occupation, religion, and other variables known for the U.S. population at large in most cases quite closely mirrors that of the U.S. female population" (p. 777, see also p. 801). She gives two pages (pp. 802–803) of tabular comparisons of the attributes of her respondents to the U.S. census and other sources. At first glance, one is impressed by how well her figures match the census, but closer inspection raises serious questions about this favorable impression.

The first question that arises is whether Hite's data are weighted to match those of the census. In her introductory statement, Lang indicates that the data were weighted (p. xxx: "Most survey research today tries to match its samples demographically to the general population in other ways by, for example, weighting responses to conform to the population profile, as Hite does"). Hite herself comes close to admitting this directly when she closely echoes Lang's statement: "Most survey research now tries to match its sample demographically to the general population in other ways; for example, by weighting responses to conform to the population profile, somewhat similarly to the methods used here" (p. 778). If the demographics were merely weighted to match the census, then of course nothing is known about the representativeness of the raw data. However, since the evidence is not conclusive (on this point as elsewhere because of a lack of documentation), one must proceed to examine the statistical comparisons on pp. 802–803 under the assumption that these comparisons are not weighted and, therefore, are of some interest.

Once again, the continual problem of inadequate documentation arises. One is often unsure of how terms are defined or where the census comparisons come from and what they represent exactly. Some problems start when the first comparison of age is made. Hite's respondents are generally adults, but since she includes a few cases (4 percent) under 18 she apparently compares her respondents to the age distribution of the entire female population from infants on up. This naturally indicates that her sample "underrepresents" females under 18. Of course, she did not really intend to cover this segment of the population, so the mismatch is not important. In attempting to see how the age distribution among adults compared, it was found that the percentages for her study added up to only 97 percent and those for the census to only 96.5 percent. Since the rest of her percentages total 100 percent (within what might be attributed to rounding error), it is not clear why both of these figures are off by so much.

Her second comparison on education shows the only major deviation from census results reported in her tables. Those with a high school degree or less are underrepresented by 11.7 percent. This result is to be expected given her sample design and the fact that even full-probability surveys tend to underrepresent the less educated, although not typically to this degree. It is more surprising, however, that variables such as income and race, which are highly associated with education, do not show a similar pattern of underrepresentation.

The third comparison, with income, raises the most serious questions. Hite shows a virtually perfect match to the census. However, what the census income figures measure and what Hite's figures cover are not the same and not comparable. The census figures represent the total money income (i.e., both earned and unearned) of women 15 years and older in 1985 (U.S. Bureau of the Census, 1987:105). Hite, on the other hand, asked her respondents to report what the approximate total income of their household was, before taxes, in the previous year. Household income is dramatically higher than individual income and would not come close to matching the census figures for women with money income. For example, from the same Census Bureau publication that Hite used, the percentage of households with incomes over $25,000 was 47.6 percent in 1985, compared to the 8.5 percent she reported. (Of course, Hite does state that she used four different versions of the questionnaire, and since she presents only one version in the book the possibility cannot be ruled out that respondent income was collected in other versions. This seems unlikely, however; see p. 775.)

In the next comparison on race, the lack of definitions and of specification of the Census Bureau publications utilized makes any evaluation difficult. By many definitions of the Hispanic population, the 1.5 percent census figure and the 1.8 percent in her study are both low. The census typically uses a Spanish-origin question to determine the Hispanic share of the population, and this measure shows Hispanic women making up a little over 6 percent of adult women (U.S. Bureau of the Census, 1985).

With respect to geographic area, it is very unclear how Hite was able to match the census figures. She did not ask information on geographical location and apparently coded both type of area and region from postmarks on the letters (p. 777). To have coded postmarks into categories that matched the census would have been a major (and needlessly inefficient) task involving the correct geographic coding of many, if not most, of the ZIP codes in the country and would have produced much error from questionnaires mailed from a nonresidential address and from the many letters that do not have readable or codable postmarks. (On geographic region, see the comments immediately above.)

With regard to marital status, the most peculiar thing is the strange note that makes inappropriate references to such things as "life expectancy tables" and "projected divorce rate." It appears that these comments are directed toward the issue of calculating the proportion of marriages that will end in divorce, or some similar matter, and have nothing to do with the simple marital distributions that she is presenting.

The next comparison is the percentage of women in the labor force under various marital and child-caring circumstances. Although her vague census references have not been checked, on the face of it there appear to be no problems with the numbers presented.

Finally, the comparison of party identification is problematic on two counts. First, it is unclear where in her questionnaire she collected this information. It is not one of her demographics, and the only other questions that would yield any political identification information are the global ones "Who are you? What is your description of yourself?" It seems dubious that these would have yielded any extensive and readily codable partisan information. Second, it is hard to figure where she obtained the comparison figures. She cites "CBS News poll, May, 1987, distributed by the Eagleton Foundation [sic], New Jersey." This apparently refers to a fact sheet on the gender gap prepared by the Center for the American Woman and Politics (1987) of the Eagleton Institute. This document presents figures from a May 1987 CBS poll that match the percentages for women who are Republicans and Democrats, which Hite includes in her table. The fact sheet does not, however, give the percentages for independents, conservatives, or radicals that she reports; also, CBS does not even code political identifications such as conservative and radical (Kathleen Frankovic, personal communication, 1988).

In brief, the statistical comparisons are riddled with peculiarities: in a number of cases, Hite does not appear to have collected the information that she matched with the census; in other cases, the matches, although possible, would have been extremely difficult; and in still other instances, either numbers fail to add up or definitions do not fit the data.

ESSAY QUESTIONNAIRE AND ANALYSIS

Hite's questionnaire consists of 127 open-ended questions, many with numerous subquestions and follow-ups. (At one point she refers to 180 questions [p. 779], and her questionnaire has over 400 queries and follow-ups.) It would have been a gargantuan task for anyone to complete. By Hite's own estimate her respondents spent over 20,000 hours completing the questionnaire, an average of at least 4.4 hours per person. Hite instructed respondents that "it is not necessary to answer every question! There are seven headings; feel free to skip around and answer only those sections or questions you choose." Hite provides no information about how frequently the respondents skipped over questions; thus, we do not know if a particular question was answered by all 4,500 or only a small fraction of the total. Given the extreme burden of completing the entire questionnaire, it is probable that many respondents did skip over questions. This item nonresponse would probably introduce more bias into the study.

As difficult as the completion of the questionnaire was for respondents, it was even more challenging to code and analyze. Hite indicates that 40,000 person-hours were spent analyzing the answers. Much of this would have been needed just to code the open-ended answers. Hite indicates that individual answers were copied onto a "large chart" for each question. Once so compiled the responses were examined for "patterns and 'categories'." She indicates that usually the "categories more or less formed themselves" (p. 779). This coding of the complex, open-ended material might be the most problematic part of the entire study. Taking the voluminous and variegated essay material, it is not only possible but likely that one could find whatever results one wanted within the responses. Given the strong ideological positions of the author, it would have taken the greatest care and the most exacting coding criteria to have avoided subjective and biased coding of the data. (On the difficulties of handling open-ended questions and coding, see Duncan et al., 1973; Schuman and Presser, 1981.)

Wording of Essay Questions

Hite's questions have a distinctive style, a kind of brisk, rapid-fire type of probing and following-up that throws out queries, follow-ups with possible answers, and digs for more details. This style is much more leading and less studiously neutral than open-ended questions usually are, but although atypical, this general style probably does not in itself seriously mold and shape responses. Individual questions pose more serious problems, however. Often there is a lack of balance in questions. For example, consider the following two questions about mothers and fathers:

> 9. Was your mother affectionate with you? Did she speak sweetly to you? Sing to you? Bathe you and do your hair? Were there any clashes between you? When was she angriest? What do you think of her today? Do you like to spend time with her?
> 10. Was your father affectionate? Did you talk? Go places together? Did you like him? Fear him? Respect him? What did you argue about? What do you think of him today?

The questions cover substantially different ground and have a very traditionalist perspective. Mothers talk sweetly and groom you. Fathers are to be feared and/or respected. What can be learned about mothers and fathers is not equivalent and is severely limited by the traditionalist cast of the questions. In another example (question 40), Hite asks who performs several traditional female household tasks (doing dishes, beds, cooking, etc.) but fails to inquire about any traditional male tasks (yard work, repairs, automobile upkeep, etc.). Again, only one-sided analysis is possible from these questions. Many other questions suffer from a host of nagging technical problems such as unclear referents, being double-barreled, and vagueness.

Analysis of Essay Questions

Many of the statistical tables describe topics and categories that are vague and confusing. For example, at one point we learn that "87 percent of women say they feel they are not really 'seen' by the men they are with" (p. 812). What does that mean and how was it coded from which questions? We also learn that 95 percent have faced "emotional and psychological harassment" but that only 56 percent are being "undermined or sabotaged psychologically" (pp. 810, 811). What do these terms mean and what is the difference between the two that leads to quite different percentages? Also, on the basis (apparently) of question 50 ("Do you believe in monogamy? Have you/are you having sex outside the relationship? Known to your partner? How do you feel about it? What is it/was it giving you?"), how did Hite decide that for 60 percent of men their reaction to finding out about their wife's infidelity was "low-keyed" or "very low-keyed" (pp. 417–418), while 40 percent reacted "stormily" (p. 865). Then too, what is the difference between the statements "only about one-fourth of women having affairs had ever had their husbands find out about them. In fact, most affairs (74 percent) are never discovered or openly recognized . . ." (p. 417, note) and "89 percent of married women keep their affairs secret and/or are never 'found out' (or at least never confronted) by their husbands" (p. 861)?

Other than the statements that 4,500 women answered the questionnaire, that respondents were told they did not have to answer all questions, and that some questions were added only after much data had been collected, nothing is known about how many people answered particular questions. Often the number left in a particular table had to be but a small percentage of the entire 4,500. For example, all questions about married women were asked of a maximum of about 2,200 (if no item nonresponse is assumed). If 70 percent of all married women cheat and if only 11 percent of husbands find out, the "how-did-he-react" table cited above covered a maximum of about 170 husbands ($2,200 \times .7 \times .11 = 169$). This again, of course, is only approximate since it assumes no item nonresponse and strings together statistics from several of Hite's tables. Similarly, the table on p. 892 was probably based on a few hundred cases, depending on the definition of "gay women" and other undocumented issues. The problem is not that some questions refer only to small subsets, but that Hite's report does not mention the large shifts in case bases and makes it difficult to determine even the approximate number of cases involved in virtually any of the tables.

Cross Tabulations of Essay Questions

Hite presents nearly 100 pages of cross tabulations of her essay questions, typically showing how responses varied by age, income, race/ethnicity, education, occupation/employment, and marital status/duration of marriage. Responses to the essay questions show remarkably little variation by these demographics. A random sample of 93 cross tabulations showed that the average percentage difference between the extreme response categories was only 3.25. One might well expect to find greater variation than that by chance alone.

In addition, differences repeatedly fail to appear when well-established theories and previous empirical research have demonstrated subgroup differences. For example, whites report greater happiness than blacks (Davis, 1984; Freudiger, 1979; Singh et al., 1981), but this pattern fails to emerge in Hite's tabulations. Similarly, Hite finds no racial or class variations in spousal violence (p. 821), again contrary to well-established patterns (Gelles and Cornell, 1985:73, 109; Strauss, 1980).

CONCLUSION

Hite's substantive findings about the current state of "women and love" and about such specific matters as the infidelity rate and level of female homosexuality or bisexuality must be considered problematic and questionable because of the methodology employed. The extreme lack of documentation, the use of nonrandom or volunteer respondents and other suspect methodologies, the vague and contradictory reporting of findings, and the inconsistencies in the statistical comparisons to the U.S. census and other sources, all seriously undermine her figures and conclusions. In the marketplace of scientific ideas, Hite's work would be found in the curio shop of the bazaar of pop and pseudoscience.

REFERENCES

Center for the American Woman and Politics, Eagleton Institute (1987) *The Gender Gap, Fact Sheet.* New Brunswick, N.J.: Eagleton Institute.

Converse, J. M., and Schuman, H. (1984) The manner of inquiry: An analysis of survey question form across organizations and over time. In C. F. Turner and E. Martin (eds.), *Surveying Subjective Phenomena,* Vol. 2. New York: Russell Sage and Basic Books.

Davis, J. A. (1984) New money, an old man/lady, and "Two's Company": Subjective welfare in the NORC general social surveys, 1972–1982. *Social Indicators Research* 15:319–350.

Duncan, O. D., Schuman, H., and Duncan, B. (1973) *Social Change in a Metropolitan Community.* New York: Russell Sage and Basic Books.

Freudiger, P. T. (1979) Life Satisfaction Among American Women. Unpublished Ph.D. dissertation, North Texas State University.

Gelles, R. J., and Cornell, C. P. (1985) *Intimate Violence in Families.* Beverly Hills, Calif.: Sage Publications.

Hite, S. (1987) *Women and Love: A Cultural Revolution in Progress.* New York: Knopf.

Schuman, H., and Presser, S. (1981) *Questions and Answers in Attitude Surveys: Experiments on Question Form, Wording, and Context.* New York: Academic Press.

Singh, B. K., Adams, L. D., and Jorgenson, D. E. (1981) Epidemiology of marital unhappiness. *International Journal of Sociology of the Family* 8:207–218.

Smith, T. W. (1983) The hidden 25%: An analysis of nonresponse on the 1980 general social survey. *Public Opinion Quarterly* 47:386–404.

Smith, T. W. (1984) Estimating nonresponse bias with temporary refusals. *Sociological Perspectives* 27:473–489.

Smith, T. W. (1988) Speaking out: Hite vs. Abby in methodological messes. *AAPOR News* 15:3–4.

Strauss, M. (1980) *Behind Closed Doors: Violence in the American Family.* Garden City, N.Y.: Anchor Press.

U.S. Bureau of the Census (1985) *Statistical Abstract of the United States: 1986.* Washington, D.C.: U.S. Government Printing Office.

U.S. Bureau of the Census (1987) Money income of households, families, and persons in the United States: 1985. *Current Population Reports, Series P-60,* No. 156. Washington, D.C.: U.S. Government Printing Office.

Trends in Premarital Sexual Behavior

Albert D. Klassen, Colin J. Williams, Eugene E. Levitt, Laura Rudkin-Miniot, Heather G. Miller, and Sushama Gunjal

Information on the patterns of premarital sexual activity over the past century has been derived from data sources of varying pedigree (see the review in Chapter 2). Although it is difficult to make definitive statements about the magnitude of change in premarital sexual behavior in the U.S. population, it appears that both the prevalence of premarital sex and the number of premarital sexual partners have increased over time, while the age at which the first premarital sexual activity occurs has decreased. Variations in these patterns and trends between the sexes and across other subgroups have also been described. For example, data presented by Kinsey and colleagues (1948, 1953), while not generalizable to the national population or to more recent periods, show gender-differentiated patterns of sexual behavior.

It has been difficult enough to map patterns of behavior over time and across subgroups—understanding the forces that shape

Albert Klassen is from the Department of Sociology, University of North Dakota at Grand Forks; Colin Williams is from the Department of Sociology, Indiana University–Purdue University at Indianapolis; Eugene Levitt is from the Department of Psychiatry, School of Medicine, Indiana University (Indianapolis). The development and original analyses of the 1970 Kinsey survey were carried out by these authors and are reported fully in a book by Klassen, Williams, and Levitt currently in press. Laura Rudkin-Miniot is from the Department of Sociology, Princeton University. Heather Miller and Sushama Gunjal are from the National Research Council.

these behaviors is an even more formidable task. Many sexual behaviors, including heterosexual activity before marriage, reflect complex interactions among religious and cultural standards, patterns of courtship and marriage, gender roles, legal sanctions associated with sexual behavior, and sex-related cultural values related to self-respect and the moral reputation of society's members. Some historical–cultural analyses of U.S. national survey data have posited a male-dominant pattern of suppression of female sexuality (e.g., Klassen, 1982; Klassen and Wilsnack, 1986). In this brief paper, we describe some trends in premarital heterosexual behavior based on survey data collected in 1970 for the Kinsey Institute (Indiana University) by the National Opinion Research Center (University of Chicago). These data permit us to derive an overview of changes in premarital sexual behavior in America during this century by comparing the reported behaviors of different birth cohorts. Some findings regarding trends in premarital sexual activity and numbers of premarital heterosexual partners are reported. A full report of the results of this survey is forthcoming (Klassen, Williams, and Levitt, in press.)

METHODS

Survey data were collected in 1970 from 3,018 adults in the United States. The sampling frame included noninstitutionalized adults (age 21 or older) residing in the continental United States. A multistage sampling strategy provided a probability sample to the block or segment level. At the block (or segment) level, interview quotas were used for men over and under age 30, and for employed and unemployed women. For more detailed information on the sample design and execution, see the forthcoming book by Klassen, Williams, and Levitt (in press).

Although no data are available on the potential respondents who refused to participate in this survey, Fay and colleagues (in press) have assessed the adequacy of sample design and execution by comparing the distributions for age, race, education, and marital status for men in this sample to the distributions obtained in the 1970 census. They found considerable agreement between the survey and the census, except for an overrepresentation of blacks, persons with one to three years of college education, and men 65 years of age or older.

Respondents in this survey were interviewed privately in their homes with only the interviewer and respondent in attendance. Initial questions requested demographic information about the respondents, their households, and their parents. The respondent's opinions on a variety of topics were also obtained. Approximately 70 questions concerning participation in different sexual behaviors were included in a self-administered booklet. Interviewers introduced the booklet at the end of the interview with the following instructions:

> In order to make a true evaluation of this entire survey, it is important to know something about people's experience. We would greatly appreciate your filling out this booklet, which is, of course, completely confidential. I will give you an envelope in which you, yourself, will seal the completed booklet. The answers from all sorts of people are really needed for statistical purposes.

Questions in the booklet addressed the respondent's experiences with sex play as a child, masturbation, premarital heterosexual activity, heterosexual experiences with the spouse, homosexual experiences, sexual orientation, and general enjoyment of sexual experiences.

This paper makes use of data from the questions on premarital heterosexual activity. Specifically, the booklet asked respondents:

- How old were you the first time you had sexual activity with someone of the opposite sex, when either you or your partner came to a sexual climax? If the first time was when you got married, please give your age at that time. This includes other sexual activity, as well as intercourse, if one of you had a climax (orgasm).
- If you *never* had this experience before you were married, check (box) and skip (next questions).
- Was there a period of time, before marriage, when you had this experience fairly often, occasionally, or rarely—maybe once or twice?
- With about how many *persons* altogether did you have this sexual experience before you were married? If it happened with your husband or wife before you were first married, this counts as one person, too.
- If this happened *only* with a person you later married, check (box).

Respondents were also asked about their feelings regarding their premarital sexual experiences or lack of experiences.

Several possible sources of error that may affect the data used in this paper merit discussion. These problems concern sampling biases and both intentional and unintentional reporting errors.

First, it should be noted that the survey provides information on sexual behaviors for a wide range of birth cohorts (from before 1900 to 1949), but that the information was gathered in 1970. Thus, different proportions of each birth cohort would have survived until 1970 to be included in the survey sample. Interpretation of the survey results requires the assumption that the sexual behaviors of those who did and did not survive were the same.

Second, different proportions of the birth cohorts may be living in noninstitutional situations. Specifically, more individuals in the older cohorts may be institutionalized. Thus, an assumption must be made that the sexual behaviors of the now-institutionalized population did not differ significantly from the behaviors of those available for the sample.

Third, the cross-sectional structure of the survey means that older individuals are being asked about events that happened further back in their past than are younger individuals. Errors in recall (particularly by the older individuals) may mean the data do not accurately reflect what happened.

Fourth, the highly personal nature of the material covered in the survey may have caused some respondents to inaccurately report their experiences. In attempting to conform to self-perceived norms for their gender and cohort, some individuals may have either under- or overreported their sexual experiences.

Fifth, the phrase "sexual activity . . . when either you or your partner came to a sexual climax," though seemingly specific, could be interpreted in different ways by respondents. The most problematic situation would be one in which interpretations differed systematically by birth cohort or gender. For example, an individual may equate sexual climax with intercourse and exclude other types of sexual activity, despite specific instructions not to do so. Alternately, an individual may not have recognized or remembered a partner's sexual climax or, not having experienced orgasm him- or herself, may fail to report the experience.

FINDINGS

Abstinence from Premarital Sexual Activity

Judeo-Christian religious traditions prohibit sexual activity outside marriage. In practice, however, Western societies have traditionally imposed a double standard, anticipating that men would more often seek heterosexual experience before marriage and insisting that women avoid such experience. Data from the 1970 survey indicate that women were indeed more likely than men to report abstaining from premarital sexual activity, although the proportions of *both* men and women reporting abstinence before marriage have decreased throughout this century (Table 1).[1] Premarital sexual abstinence was reported by 45.6 percent of ever-married men and 92.4 percent of ever-married women born before the turn of the century. These figures are markedly lower for ever-married respondents born in the 1940s, with 10.5 percent of men and 37.1 percent of women reporting premarital abstinence.[2]

The pace and timing of the change in the proportions abstaining from premarital sexual activity may be considered using the decade decrement figures found in Table 1. The decade decrements are the percentage point declines between cohorts in the proportions abstaining from sexual activity before marriage. For example, the proportion of men premaritally abstinent declined 9.3 percentage points between the cohort born before 1900 and the cohort born between 1900 and 1909. The pace of the change slowed over time for men, with the largest changes occurring between the older cohorts. The picture is much different for women, however, with the most dramatic change coming between the youngest cohorts. The proportion premaritally abstinent fell 24 percentage points between the 1930–1939 and 1940–1949 birth cohorts. Decrements between other female cohorts ranged from 3.3 to 11.6 percentage points.

[1]To provide a crude statistical test of gender and cohort differences in premarital sexual behavior, log-linear models were fitted (using the procedures of Goodman [1978] and Goodman and Fay [1973]) to the 3-way tabulation of Abstinence (A: 2 categories, abstained–did not abstain) by Gender (G: 2 categories, male–female) by Cohort (C: 6 cohorts, see Table 1). As a crude adjustment for design effects of the clustered sample, cell counts in the analysis were reduced by one third: that is, we have assumed that this clustered sample is equivalent to a simple random sample with two thirds as many cases. Fitting a full set of models (with abstinence as the dependent variable), we found significant effects of cohort on abstinence and of gender on abstinence, as indicated in the above discussion. The observed data thus did not require a model that posited that patterns of change in abstinence over time varied by gender (although there was an overall gender difference in abstinence for each cohort). Thus a model constrained to fit the three 2-way marginals $\{AC\}\{AG\}\{GC\}$ fit the observed data (likelihood-ratio chi-square: $L^2 = 4.69$, $d.f. = 5$, $p > .4$).

[2]The tabulations in Table 1 exclude the premarital experiences of those respondents who failed to report the number of premarital partners. All of those excluded indicated that they were sexually active before marriage. Including these respondents in a retabulation of proportions abstaining from sexual activity before marriage yields proportions 1 to 7 percentage points below those reported in Table 1.

The trends described are unlikely to be explained by changes across cohorts in age at first marriage. If the cohort members were marrying successively later over time, the younger cohorts would have more premarital years in which to engage in sexual activity. In short, they would spend more time "at risk" of premarital sex. However, the median, 1st, and 3rd quartiles for ages at first marriage for the cohorts are generally stable or declining over time (Table 2). This suggests that with age at marriage held constant, the changes over time may be even greater. (It should be noted, however, that age at first marriage may explain a portion of the male–female differences in proportions premaritally abstinent. Men typically have married at a later age and therefore spend more time "at risk" of premarital sexual activity.)

A modified form of premarital abstinence (perhaps an alternative that is more consistent with post-World War II norms) is sexual experience with only the spouse-to-be. Of women and men who were sexually active before marriage, women were more likely to limit their premarital experience to only their future spouse (see Table 1). Approximately half of the premaritally active women in each cohort reported that their future husbands were their only premarital partners. In contrast, roughly 10 percent of premaritally active men in each cohort reported that their wives were their sole partners. It is interesting to note that these ratios were stable over time.

If reports of "spouse-only" premarital sexual experience are combined with reports of abstinence (representing a modified form of premarital abstinence), then male–female differences in premarital sexual abstinence are even more pronounced. Almost all of the ever-married women (97.5 percent) but only half of the ever-married men (51.7 percent) born before the turn of the century "abstained" from sexual activity before marriage.[3] For the 1940–1949 cohort, the proportions of respondents who could be similarly categorized were much smaller, but women were still more likely to "abstain" from premarital sex. Two thirds (67.6 percent) of ever-married women and less than one quarter (22.5 percent) of ever-married men "abstained."

As mentioned previously, traditional Judeo-Christian norms discourage premarital sexual activity. Therefore, one might assume that people who consider themselves strongly religious would be less

[3]Figures reported for the cohort born before 1900 (aged 70 and older at the 1970 survey date) refer only to those individuals who survived to be included in the survey sample and who were not living in institutions (i.e., nursing homes, hospitals, etc.). Generalizing these figures to the entire cohort requires the assumption that the sexual behaviors of those excluded from the sample did not differ from those in the sample.

TABLE 1 Tradition Compliance and Number of Heterosexual Partners Before First Marriage Reported in 1970 Kinsey Survey by Decade of Birth, Gender, and Marital History

	Part A						
	Birth Cohorts of Ever-Married Women						Never-Married Women
	Before 1900	1900–1909	1910–1919	1920–1929	1930–1939	1940–1949	1940–1949
Tradition Compliance (%)							
Strict: No partners	92.4	85.5	73.9	70.6	61.1	37.1	30.0
Decade decrement		**6.9**	**11.6**	**3.3**	**9.5**	**24.0**	N.A.
Spouse only	5.1	7.6	12.4	14.7	19.5	30.5	N.A.
Modified (0 or spouse)	97.5	93.1	86.3	85.3	80.6	67.6	N.A.
Decade decrement		**4.4**	**6.8**	**1.0**	**4.7**	**13.0**	N.A.
No. of partners (accumulated %s)							
1 (not spouse) or more	2.5	6.9	13.7	14.8[a]	19.5[a]	32.6[a]	69.9[a]
2 or more	2.5	2.3	8.7	11.0	15.1	25.8	56.6
3 or more	—	0.8	5.5	5.3	7.0	15.7	49.9
4 or more	—	0.8	4.1	3.8	4.7	7.8	39.9
5 or more	—	—	3.2	2.3	3.0	5.3	26.6
6 or more	—	—	2.3	0.8	1.0	4.2	26.6
10 or more	—	—	1.4	0.4	1.0	1.7	26.6
15 or more	—	—	0.9	0.4	0.3	0.6	6.6
20 or more	—	—	0.9	—	0.3	0.3	6.6
30 or more	—	—	—	—	—	—	3.3
40 or more	—	—	—	—	—	—	3.3
50 or more	—	—	—	—	—	—	—
60 or more	—	—	—	—	—	—	—
Base of percentage (*N*)	79	131	218	265	298	367	30
Partner data missing (*N*)	2	6	17	14	17	13	5

Part B

	Birth Cohorts of Ever-Married Men						Never-Married Men
	Before 1900	1900–1909	1910–1919	1920–1929	1930–1939	1940–1949	1940–1949
Tradition Compliance (%)							
Strict: No partners	45.6	36.3	28.2	19.5	14.6	10.5	11.8
Decade decrement		**9.3**	**8.1**	**8.7**	**4.9**	**4.1**	N.A.
Spouse only	6.1	5.6	7.2	7.4	9.4	12.0	N.A.
Modified (0 or spouse)	51.7	41.9	35.4	26.9	24.0	22.5	N.A.
Decade decrement		**9.8**	**6.5**	**8.5**	**2.9**	**1.5**	N.A.
No. of partners (accumulated %s)							
1 (not spouse) or more	48.3	58.1	64.5[a]	73.0[a]	76.1[a]	77.9[a]	88.3[a]
2 or more	43.9	51.8	58.4	70.7	71.6	72.6	82.4
3 or more	36.0	42.4	51.8	61.9	62.6	64.9	76.5
4 or more	29.0	35.5	44.1	53.5	54.7	57.2	70.6
5 or more	25.5	32.4	37.5	47.5	46.8	50.5	66.2
6 or more	20.2	26.8	29.8	40.5	38.9	43.3	58.8
10 or more	14.9	21.2	19.9	31.2	28.0	31.3	45.6
15 or more	5.3	10.6	9.4	19.6	16.4	19.3	26.5
20 or more	5.3	6.2	7.7	14.5	11.9	12.6	20.6
30 or more	—	0.6	1.1	4.7	2.9	4.9	5.9
40 or more	—	0.6	1.1	2.8	1.8	2.5	5.9
50 or more	—	0.6	1.1	2.3	1.1	1.5	5.9
60 or more	—	—	—	—	—	0.5	4.4
Base of percentage (*N*)	114	160	181	215	267	209	68
Partner data missing (*N*)	23	37	29	41	25	14	22

NOTE: Total female *N*, age 21 + = 1,490; total male *N*, age 21 + = 1,450. N.A. = not applicable.

[a]Accumulated sums are discrepant due to rounding error.

TABLE 2 Median, First, and Third Quartiles for Age at First Marriage by Gender and Birth Cohort

	Birth Cohort					
	Before 1900	1900–1909	1910–1919	1920–1929	1930–1939	1940–1949
Women						
First quartile	18	18	18	18	18	18
Median	20	20	21	21	20	19
Third quartile	25	24	24	23	22	22
Men						
First quartile	22	22	21	21	20	21
Median	25	25	25	24	22	22
Third quartile	28	30	29	27	25	[a]

[a]Of men born in the 1940s, more than 25 percent had not yet married as of the survey date.

likely to be sexually active before marriage than would less religious individuals. However, data from the 1970 survey do not show a clear relationship between strength of self-reported religiosity and levels of premarital sexual activity for either men or women (Table 3). Men and women who describe themselves as strongly religious are not consistently more likely to report abstaining from sexual activity before marriage than those who describe themselves as being less religious. Furthermore, no simple relationship between religiosity and age at first premarital sexual activity is evident.

Age at First Premarital Sexual Activity

Data from the 1970 survey also indicate that across the cohorts both men and women[4] became sexually active at increasingly younger ages (see Table 3). However, at every age and for every cohort a smaller proportion of women than men reported premarital sexual activity.[5]

Nearly one quarter (24 percent) of the men born before 1900 reported engaging in premarital sexual activity at or before age 16

[4]Table 3 has been restricted to persons who married at age 21 or later or who were never married.

[5]Using the procedure described previously (see footnote 1), a series of log-linear models were fitted to the 3-way tabulation of Gender (G) by Cohort (C) by Abstinence *to age 21* (A). Again, we found significant effects of gender and cohort on the likelihood that respondents would report sexual abstinence to age 21. However, we also found that a model constrained to fit the three 2-way marginals $\{AC\}\{AG\}\{CG\}$ provided an acceptable fit to the observed data ($L^2 = 2.21$, $d.f. = 5$, $p > .5$).

TABLE 3 Percentage of Men and Women Reporting Having Heterosexual Experience to Climax by Ages 16, 18, and 20 by Strength of Religious Belief in Childhood Household and Birth Cohort

Gender, and Religious Belief in Childhood Home	Birth Cohort	Age at First Premarital Sexual Experience					
		16 or Before	(*N*)	18 or Before	(*N*)	20 or Before	(*N*)
Males							
Total	Pre-1900	24.0%	(129)	36.8%	(125)	44.8%	(116)
	1900–1909	23.9	(184)	40.2	(174)	49.4	(156)
	1910–1919	28.7	(209)	51.3	(197)	61.4	(176)
	1920–1929	45.0	(258)	66.1	(251)	73.0	(207)
	1930–1939	47.4	(285)	69.1	(265)	74.4	(207)
	1940–1949	50.2	(295)	76.6	(273)	83.9	(224)
Not strongly religious	Pre-1900	[a]	(12)	[a]	(12)	[a]	(12)
	1900–1909	[a]	(20)	[a]	(20)	[a]	(19)
	1910–1919	[a]	(18)	[a]	(18)	[a]	(16)
	1920–1929	53.3	(30)	64.3	(28)	[a]	(23)
	1930–1939	38.6	(44)	69.1	(42)	84.6	(26)
	1940–1949	56.8	(44)	88.4	(43)	97.8	(33)
Moderately religious	Pre-1900	22.5	(40)	41.0	(39)	55.9	(34)
	1900–1909	16.7	(42)	45.0	(40)	48.7	(37)
	1910–1919	26.2	(61)	50.9	(57)	65.4	(52)
	1920–1929	48.4	(64)	76.2	(63)	82.7	(52)
	1930–1939	48.7	(78)	72.2	(72)	73.6	(53)
	1940–1949	49.0	(98)	77.2	(92)	85.7	(77)

Continued

TABLE 3 *Continued*

Gender, and Religious Belief in Childhood Home	Birth Cohort	Age at First Premarital Sexual Experience: 16 or Before	(*N*)	18 or Before	(*N*)	20 or Before	(*N*)
Males							
Strongly religious	Pre-1900	24.7	(77)	35.1	(74)	41.4	(70)
	1900–1909	24.6	(122)	36.8	(114)	49.0	(100)
	1910–1919	29.2	(130)	48.4	(122)	56.5	(108)
	1920–1929	42.1	(164)	62.5	(160)	69.7	(132)
	1930–1939	49.1	(163)	67.6	(151)	72.7	(128)
	1940–1949	49.0	(153)	72.5	(138)	81.6	(114)
Females							
Total	Pre-1900	2.7%	(75)	3.3%	(60)	5.1%	(39)
	1900–1909	4.8	(124)	6.5	(92)	8.8	(68)
	1910–1919	6.3	(205)	9.6	(167)	14.1	(121)
	1920–1929	4.9	(243)	12.4	(193)	22.1	(140)
	1930–1939	10.0	(281)	21.0	(210)	22.7	(132)
	1940–1949	19.1	(362)	37.2	(261)	46.2	(143)
Not strongly religious	Pre-1900	[a]	(5)	[a]	(5)	[a]	(3)
	1900–1909	[a]	(6)	[a]	(4)	[a]	(2)
	1910–1919	[a]	(24)	[a]	(20)	[a]	(12)
	1920–1929	6.3	(16)	[a]	(14)	[a]	(10)
	1930–1939	17.7	(34)	21.4	(28)	[a]	(17)
	1940–1949	20.0	(45)	34.5	(29)	[a]	(18)

Moderately religious	Pre-1900	[a]	(12)	[a]	(8)	[a]	(6)
	1900–1909	[a]	(18)	[a]	(14)	[a]	(12)
	1910–1919	2.0	(49)	10.0	(40)	24.1	(29)
	1920–1929	1.3	(76)	12.7	(55)	20.9	(43)
	1930–1939	7.9	(76)	19.2	(52)	18.5	(27)
	1940–1949	26.6	(113)	41.6	(77)	50.0	(36)
Strongly religious	Pre-1900	1.7	(58)	2.1	(47)	3.3	(30)
	1900–1909	6.0	(100)	6.8	(74)	9.3	(54)
	1910–1919	7.6	(132)	10.3	(107)	10.0	(80)
	1920–1929	6.6	(151)	11.3	(124)	18.4	(87)
	1930–1939	9.4	(171)	21.5	(130)	20.5	(88)
	1940–1949	14.7	(204)	35.5	(155)	46.1	(89)

NOTE: The table includes males and females age 21 and over at the time they were interviewed.

TECHNICAL NOTE: The religion variable (04/23) was recoded into three categories as to whether the religious beliefs were *not strong* (which includes respondents "against or rejecting religion" [0], those who did *not* feel the belief strongly at all [1], and those who did not feel the beliefs "so strongly" [2]), moderate (3), and strong (which includes respondents with strong [4] and very strong [5] beliefs). A new variable (PAGE) was created to define whether the respondent had any sexual experience before a certain age using Question 5 (09/27). If the question about sexual experience (09/31) was answered "no," the new variable PAGE was given a high value, 70. Three ages for first premarital sex (sex before marriage or never married) were selected: 16, 18, and 20. Respondents who did not answer the questions on religion (04/23), sexual experience frequency (09/32), age at first sexual experience (09/27), or current age (01/13) were excluded from the analysis.

[a]Percentages are not shown because $N < 25$.

and 44.8 percent reported such experience at or before age 20. Men born in the 1940s were roughly twice as likely to have had a premarital sexual experience by these specific ages: half (50.2 percent) of them reported premarital sexual activity at age 16 or earlier and 83.9 percent reported it at or before age 20.

The increases across cohorts in the proportions of people engaging in premarital sexual activity by specific ages are even more dramatic for women than for men. Only 2.7 percent of women in the oldest birth cohort reported premarital sexual activity at age 16 or earlier and just 5.1 percent had engaged in such activity at or before age 20. In marked contrast, 19.1 percent of the women born in the 1940s reported premarital sexual experience at or before age 16, and 46.2 percent reported it at or before age 20. Male premarital sexual activity by specific ages had increased by a factor of 2 across the cohorts, while female activity had risen approximately by a factor of 8.

Data from the 1970 survey indicate an association between age at first premarital sexual activity and age at marriage (Table 4): those who become sexually active at young ages are more likely to marry at young ages. For example, 22.8 percent of women who married at age 16 reported sexual experience before age 16, compared to only 1.5 percent of women who married at age 24. More than half (53.9 percent) of the men who married at age 18 reported sexual experience before age 16, while only 26.1 percent of men who married at age 24 were sexually active before age 16.

The direction of this relationship is not clear. Does sexual activity at an early age lead to marriage at an early age, perhaps through unplanned pregnancies or by intensifying the couple's relationship? Do plans for or the anticipation of marriage at an early age prompt young people to become sexually active before marriage? Or do other unspecified factors contribute to both a young age at first sexual experience and a young age at marriage?

Number of Premarital Sexual Partners

Having multiple sexual partners before marriage is another type of noncompliance to traditional sexual norms, especially for women. It is unlikely that an expectation of marriage was associated with each premarital sexual relationship, especially for those individuals who reported five or more premarital partners. Therefore, involvement with multiple partners before marriage is a departure from both the strict and modified standards of premarital abstinence. This aspect of sexual behavior (particularly if intercourse is unprotected by condoms and spermicide) is potentially important in understanding the spread of sexually transmitted diseases, including HIV infection.

The 1970 survey data on numbers of premarital sexual partners reveal marked differences over time and between the sexes. As Table 1 shows, the proportions of both male and female respondents reporting multiple premarital sexual partners increase steadily over time. In addition, men report more premarital sexual partners than women in each cohort.

In the oldest cohorts, the number of sexual partners reported by women reflect that a small but growing proportion allowed themselves one partner before marriage, generally their future husband. The proportion of women reporting premarital partners other than their spouse-to-be increased over the decades. The percentage of women who reported at least one premarital partner other than their spouse rose from 6.9 percent for women born between 1900 and 1909 to 32.6 percent for women born in the 1940s. However, the younger women still did not report a large number of partners. The percentage of women reporting five or more premarital sexual partners increased only slightly, rising from 3.2 percent for women born between 1910 and 1919 to 5.3 percent for women born in the 1940s.[6]

Male patterns of premarital partnering are markedly different. Among men born before 1900, 25.5 percent reported having had 5 or more premarital sexual partners and 5.3 percent reported 20 or more partners. Those figures were roughly doubled for the cohort of men born in the 1940s, with 50.5 percent reporting 5 or more partners and 12.6 percent reporting 20 or more.[7]

[6]As a crude test of the time trend in the number of premarital partners reported by ever-married women, we fitted the simple linear regression equation $P = b_1 A + c$, where P was the number of premarital partners reported, and A is age (in years) in 1970. As previously, we assume that the effective sample size is 0.66 of the actual sample size to allow for effects of the complex sample design. This analysis indicated a significant linear trend in number of partners by age—with older respondents reporting fewer partners ($\hat{b} = -.0232$, *s.e.* = 0.0039; $\hat{c} = 1.779$, *s.e.* = 0.1796). When dummy variables for the birth cohorts were introduced into the equation, it was found that women born between 1940 and 1949 had more partners than predicted by a simple linear model. The equation estimated was $P = b_1 A + b_2 C_{1940} + c$, with C_{1940} being coded 1 if the respondent was born between 1940 and 1949, and coded zero otherwise; $\hat{b}_1$ was estimated at $-.01476$ (*s.e.* = .0054), $\hat{b}_2$ was estimated at +.4266 (*s.e.* = .1886), and $\hat{c}$ was estimated as 1.2966 (*s.e.* = .2787).

[7]As for women (see footnote 6), we carried out a crude test for linear trends and deviations from the linear trend for particular birth cohorts of men. We again estimated the equation, $P = b_1 A + c$, and obtained estimates of $\hat{b}_1 = -.0858$ (*s.e.* = .0190); $\hat{c} = 10.3512$ (*s.e.* = .9472). (The variable A is age in 1970.) No birth cohort of men evidenced significant deviations from the linear trend.

TABLE 4 Age at First Premarital Heterosexual Experience to Climax by Age at Marriage for Men and Women Who Married Between the Ages of 16 and 24

Gender, Age at First Premarital Sexual Experience	Age at Marriage								
	16	17	18	19	20	21	22	23	24
Males									
Never	[a]	[a]	11.5%	12.8%	17.8%	19.7%	19.4%	20.6%	19.8%
Pre-13	[a]	[a]	9.6	4.6	6.7	6.0	7.8	4.9	5.2
13	[a]	[a]	5.8	5.5	4.4	5.5	6.2	7.8	3.1
14	[a]	[a]	15.4	11.0	4.4	7.1	3.9	6.9	6.3
15	[a]	[a]	23.1	14.7	12.2	10.9	9.3	5.9	11.5
16	[a]	[a]	15.4	21.1	20.0	10.9	15.5	12.7	9.4
17	—	[a]	13.5	10.1	16.7	13.1	12.4	10.8	11.5
18	—	—	5.8	13.8	8.9	11.5	12.4	12.7	12.5
19	—	—	—	6.4	3.3	4.9	3.1	6.9	5.2
20	—	—	—	—	5.6	6.0	3.9	3.9	2.1
21	—	—	—	—	—	4.4	3.9	2.9	5.2
22	—	—	—	—	—	—	2.3	1.0	2.1
23	—	—	—	—	—	—	—	2.9	1.0
24	—	—	—	—	—	—	—	—	5.2
Total	100%	100%	100%	100%	100%	100%	100%	100%	100%
N	9	24	52	109	90	183	129	102	96

Females									
Never	59.5%	63.0%	60.0%	57.9%	59.1%	59.6%	66.4%	65.5%	65.2%
Pre-13	2.5	2.4	1.1	0.5	0.0	1.3	0.0	0.0	0.0
13	0.0	0.0	1.1	0.5	0.6	0.0	0.0	0.0	0.0
14	11.4	2.4	0.0	0.5	2.5	1.3	0.0	0.0	1.5
15	8.9	3.9	3.9	3.3	1.3	0.7	0.8	1.1	0.0
16	17.7	15.0	6.1	7.1	4.4	2.0	1.7	2.3	4.5
17	—	12.6	14.4	9.8	7.5	3.3	0.8	3.4	4.5
18	—	—	13.3	9.3	9.4	4.6	5.9	3.4	1.5
19	—	—	—	10.9	8.8	7.9	3.4	8.0	4.5
20	—	—	—	—	6.3	7.3	7.6	3.4	1.5
21	—	—	—	—	—	11.9	5.0	4.6	3.0
22	—	—	—	—	—	—	8.4	4.6	1.5
23	—	—	—	—	—	—	—	3.4	4.5
24	—	—	—	—	—	—	—	—	7.6
Total	100%	100%	100%	100%	100%	100%	100%	100%	100%
N	79	127	180	183	159	151	119	87	66

NOTE: The table includes only persons age 21 and over at the time of the interview who reported being married between the ages of 16 and 24.

TECHNICAL NOTE: Analysis includes cases if age (card/col = 1/13) greater than or equal to 21; marital status (1/19) was coded as "currently married" (0), "widowed" (1), "divorced" (2), or "separated" (3) (ever married); and respondents indicated in response to Question 6.a (9/32) that they had rarely, occasionally, or often had premarital sex to the point of climax. Two hundred and twenty persons did not answer Question 6.a (9/32) about the frequency of premarital sex (even though they had not checked a box indicating they never had premarital sex); 1,173 persons (including 886 currently married, 169 widowed, 53 divorced, 26 separated, and 39 single, never married) reported not having premarital sex. Persons who did not answer Question 5 (9/27), which asked about age at first sexual experience, or who did not give their current age or age at marriage were also excluded.

[a]Percentages are not shown because $N < 25$.

For every cohort, men reported having many more premarital partners than did women. This raises a question: With whom were these men partnering? The possible explanations, some more plausible than others, include

- men overreported and/or women underreported their number of partners;
- the women who provided the excess "partnering" in the male reports of sexual activity might not be represented in the sample (i.e., they refused to be interviewed; they did not survive to be included in the 1970 survey due to risks associated with childbirth, abortion, hardships associated with brothel life or "a bad reputation"; or they were in institutions, which excluded them from the sampling frame);
- the women who provided the excess "partnering" never married and thus were excluded from the tabulations presented in Table 1 (see the discussion in the following section);
- men found female partners from birth cohorts other than their own;[8] and
- men were having their premarital relationships with married women.

There is reason to believe that a substantial portion of the premarital partners reported by the older cohorts were prostitutes.[9] However, from the 1970 survey data, it is not possible to determine the extent to which "one-night stands," cohabitation, or other forms of coupling replaced sexual activity with prostitutes.

---

[8]While this might conceivably account for cases in any one cohort, it is an inadequate explanation for the total pattern because the number of men reporting large numbers of partners from all cohorts vastly exceed the number of women reporting similar numbers of partners.

[9]In Kinsey and coworkers' (1948) analyses of the sexual behavior of men, accumulative incidence rates for lifetime experience with prostitutes were calculated. While the level of education and "generation" were taken into account, marital status, unfortunately, was not. However, if one assumes that most men have not yet married at age 20, the Kinsey data suggest a high incidence of premarital experience with prostitutes. Approximately 20 percent of both generations with some college education and 50 percent of men who did not enter high school reported having sex with prostitutes by age 20 (see Kinsey et al., 1948:402, Table 100). Unfortunately, neither the 1953 Kinsey publication on female sexual behavior nor the 1970 NORC survey provide data on women's experience as prostitutes.

Sexual Activity of Never-Married Respondents

While there are relatively few never-married respondents, twice as many men as women (135 versus 63) in the sample had never married. The never-married could not respond to the question about premarital sex with the spouse-to-be and were therefore excluded from the main tabulations presented in Table 1. The never-married respondents obviously also were excluded from Table 4, which relates age at first sexual experience to age at marriage. Data on the never-married, however, are presented in the last column of Table 1. Other than in the youngest cohort, there are not enough never-married respondents to allow analysis. Even in the youngest cohort, their numbers are extremely small (30 women and 68 men) and these data should be treated as suggestive, at best.

In general, never-married men born in the 1940s reported more sexual partners than did ever-married men in the same cohort who reported on premarital partners. Among never-married men, 82.4 percent reported having 2 or more partners and 20.6 percent reported 20 or more partners. In contrast, 72.6 percent of the ever-married men listed 2 or more premarital partners and 12.6 reported 20 or more such partners.

Never-married women from this cohort had fewer partners than the men, but reported more partners than their ever-married female counterparts. Among the never-married women, 56.6 percent reported 2 or more partners and 26.6 percent reported 10 or more. Of ever-married women in the 1940s cohort, 25.8 percent reported 2 or more premarital partners and only 1.7 percent reported 10 or more premarital partners.

It is not surprising that the never-married respondents reported larger numbers of sexual partners than the number of premarital partners reported by the ever-married respondents. Those individuals who were not yet married had spent more time "at risk" of engaging in sexual activity outside marriage. However, a certain portion of the differences between the two groups also may be due to different patterns of sexual behavior independent of the amount of time spent unmarried.

CONCLUSIONS

There are two primary inferences to be drawn from the data we have presented. The first is that as of 1970, this century had already seen significant increases over time in the proportion of adults reporting premarital heterosexual experiences (to climax). The second is that, despite the trend, the proportion of ever-married women who reported experience with several partners did not rise dramatically. Thus the proportion of ever-married women reporting 5 or more partners increased from 0 percent in the cohorts born prior to 1910 to 5.3 percent among the cohorts born in 1940–1949; nonetheless, this proportion remained considerably lower than that found among men (50.5 percent in the 1940–1949 cohort).

There are many factors that might have contributed to the observed increases in premarital sexual experience. During World War I and the decades that followed, many men and women left rural communities and traditional life-styles for more urban environments. National radio networks and the growing movie industry brought with them increased exposure to new, nontraditional ideas for nearly all Americans. During World War II and the postwar period, the diffusion of new ideas continued with additional rural-to-urban migration, the advent of television, and the greater inclusion of women in the labor force. Young people exposed to various nontraditional ideas may have begun to question, and possibly reject, the norms that had previously regulated their sexual behavior.

The writings of Freud and the research of Kinsey and coworkers (1948, 1953), augmented by that of later sex researchers, may have contributed to a questioning and modification of traditional values by describing sexuality as healthy human behavior. Indeed, Freud and others raised questions about whether repressed sexuality and sexual inactivity were normal or healthy for either men or women (Yerkes and Corner, 1953). The sex research of Masters and Johnson (1966) and Sherfey (1966), along with the earlier work of Kinsey and colleagues, raised the possibility that the sexual response potential of women might exceed that of men. While acknowledging the male tendency to focus on sexuality and women's interest in intimacy, more recent work has speculated on the possible convergence of male and female views (Gagnon and Simon, 1973; Klassen, 1977; Reiss, 1967, 1973, 1976).

While the precise causes of the trends identified in this paper remain unclear, the trends themselves provide important historical information on changing patterns of sexual behavior in the United States. Just as social trends and historical events have seemingly contributed to past changes in sexual behavior, so, too, AIDS may affect future sexual behavior. Further research is needed to refine and update our understanding of how complex social forces shape human sexual behavior.

REFERENCES

Fay, R., Turner, C. F., Klassen, A. D., and Gagnon, J. H. (In press) Prevalence and patterns of male homosexual contact. *Science.*

Gagnon, J. H., and Simon, W. (1973) *Sexual Conduct: The Social Sources of Human Sexuality.* Chicago: Aldine.

Goodman, L. A. (1978) *Analysing Qualitative/Categorical Data.* Cambridge, Mass.: Abt Books.

Goodman, L. A., and Fay, R. (1973) ECTA program: Description for users. Unpublished manuscript, Department of Statistics, University of Chicago.

Kinsey, A. C., Pomeroy, W. B., and Martin, C. E. (1948) *Sexual Behavior in the Human Male.* Philadelphia: Saunders.

Kinsey, A. C., Pomeroy, W. B., Martin, C. E., and Gebhard, P. H. (1953) *Sexual Behavior in the Human Female.* Philadelphia: Saunders.

Klassen, A. D. (1977) Intimacy, Loving, and Sexuality. Presented in Distinguished Lecturers in Psychology series. University of Windsor, Windsor, Ontario, Canada, March.

Klassen, A. D. (1982) The Undersocialized Conception of Woman. Presented at the annual meeting of the Midwest Sociological Society, Des Moines, Iowa, April.

Klassen, A. D., and Wilsnack, S. C. (1986) Sexual experience and drinking among women in a U.S. national survey. *Archives of Sexual Behavior* 15:363–392.

Klassen, A. D., Williams, C. J., and Levitt, E. E. (In press) *Sex and Morality in the United States: A Study Conducted at the Kinsey Institute,* edited by H. J. O'Gorman. Middletown, Conn.: Wesleyan University Press.

Masters, W. H., and Johnson, V. E. (1966) *Human Sexual Response.* Boston: Little, Brown.

Reiss, I. L. (1967) *The Social Context of Premarital Sexual Permissiveness.* New York: Holt, Rinehart & Winston.

Reiss, I. L. (1973) *Heterosexual Relationships: Inside and Outside Marriage.* Morristown, N.J.: General Learning Press.

Reiss, I. L. (1976) *Family Systems in America,* 2d ed. Hinsdale, Ill.: Dryden Press.

Sherfey, M. J. (1966) The evolution and nature of female sexuality in relation to psychoanalytic theory. *Journal of the American Psychoanalytic Association* 14:28–128.

Yerkes, R. M., and Corner, G. W. (1953) Foreword. Pp. vii–viii in A. C. Kinsey, W. B. Pomeroy, C. E. Martin, and P. H. Gebhard, *Sexual Behavior in the Human Female.* Philadelphia: Saunders.

Index

D

E

F

G

H

I

J

K

L

N

Q

R

S

T

U

W